ENCYCLOPEDIA OF

BIOETHICS

3RD EDITION

EDITORIAL BOARD

ENCYCLOPEDIA OF
BIOETHICS

3RD EDITION

EDITED BY

STEPHEN G. POST

VOLUME

5

T - X
APPENDICES
INDEX

MACMILLAN REFERENCE USA™

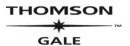
THOMSON
GALE

New York • Detroit • San Diego • San Francisco • Cleveland • New Haven, Conn. • Waterville, Maine • London • Munich

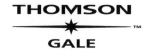

THOMSON
™
GALE

Encyclopedia of Bioethics, 3rd edition

Stephen G. Post

Editor in Chief

Library of Congress Cataloging-in-Publication Data

Encyclopedia of bioethics / Stephen G. Post, editor in chief.— 3rd ed.
    p. cm.
Includes bibliographical references and index.
    ISBN 0-02-865774-8 (set : hardcover : alk. paper) — ISBN
0-02-865775-6 (vol. 1) — ISBN 0-02-865776-4 (vol. 2) — ISBN
0-02-865777-2 (vol. 3) — ISBN 0-02-865778-0 (vol. 4) — ISBN
0-02-865779-9 (vol. 5)
    1. Bioethics—Encyclopedias. 2. Medical ethics—Encyclopedias. I.
Post, Stephen Garrard, 1951-
QH332.E52 2003
174′.957′03—dc22

                                                            2003015694

This title is also available as an e-book.
ISBN 0-02-865916-3 (set)
Contact your Gale sales representative for ordering information.

Printed in the United States of America
10 9 8 7 6 5 4 3 2

Front cover photos (from left to right): Custom Medical Stock;
Photo Researchers; Photodisc; Photodisc; AP/Worldwide Photos.

T

TEAMS, HEALTHCARE

• • •

A healthcare team is two or more health professionals (and, when appropriate, other lay or professional people) who apply their complementary professional skills to accomplish an agreed-upon goal. Coordinated, comprehensive patient care is the primary goal of most teams. Other goals may include education of health professionals, patients, or families; community outreach; advocacy; abuse prevention; family support; institutional planning; networking; and utilization review in hospitals. The team approach to patient care has been viewed as a means of building and maintaining staff morale, improving the status of a given profession (for example, nurses and allied health professionals may become team collaborators with the physician rather than working under the physician), or improving institutional efficiency.

Some teams are ongoing, such as a psychiatric care team, home visit team, ventilator patient care team, child development team, or rehabilitation team. Such teams may be responsible for following the person throughout the entire process of healthcare interventions, including diagnosis, goal setting and planning, implementation, evaluation, follow-up, and modification of goals for the patient. Other teams form around an event (for example, a disaster plan team or organ transplant team), or focus on a single function, such as discharge planning or the initiation of renal dialysis. Some teams are undisciplinary; others are multidisciplinary, and may include lay people.

Though taken for granted today, a team approach to healthcare has appeared only recently in many places where Western medicine is practiced. The development of team approaches in the United States reflects the history of that development in North America and Europe as well. In the first period, between World War I and World War II, a multiprofessional approach appeared that later developed into the team model. Major sources of impetus included the proliferation of medical specialties, an increase in expensive, complex technological interventions, and the ensuing challenge of providing a coordinated and comprehensive approach to patient care management. A second period of development occurred between the 1950s and the 1980s, when teamwork became the norm: healthcare became increasingly hospital-based, enabling a large corps of health professionals in one place to minister to the patient. In addition, new professional groups were generated in the belief that healthcare should be attentive to patients' social as well as physical well-being. The third period, which continues to the present, has focused on the appropriate goals and functions of the healthcare team and evaluation of the team's effectiveness (Brown).

Ethical issues regarding teams arise in four major areas: challenges arising from the team metaphor itself; the locus of authority for team decisions; the role of the patient as team member; and mechanisms for fostering morally supportable team decisions.

The Team Metaphor

It is generally agreed that the healthcare team idea and rhetoric arose from assumptions about sports teams and military teams (Nagi; Erde). This metaphor is not completely fitting because the healthcare team is not in competition with another team. However, it is fitting insofar as members experience their affiliation as entailing *team loyalty,* a moral obligation to other members and to the team itself. They may believe that they have voluntarily committed themselves to a type of social contract requiring a member not only to perform maximally but also to protect team secrets, thereby promoting a tendency for cover-ups or protection of weaker members. In the military team, obedience to and trust in the leader is an absolute.

A troubling ethical conflict arises when the member's moral obligation of faithfulness to other team members or "captain" does battle with moral obligations to the patient. This may manifest itself in questions of whether to cover up negligence or a serious mistake by some or all of the team. Overall, holding peers morally accountable for incompetence or unethical behavior may be made more difficult by the team ideal. Therefore, teams must foster rules that require and reward faithfulness to patient well-being, and balance and value of team membership with that of maintaining high ethical standards.

Feminist analyses of bureaucratic structures and bioethical issues highlight a related ethical challenge. The team metaphor entails assumptions about relationships, rules, and "plays" that often exclude women from full participation because their childhood and later socialization did not prepare them for this "game" and its insiders' rhetoric. Noteworthy is the sports or military team ethos of ignoring the personal characteristics of fellow team members (within limits), provided each person is technically well suited to carry out assigned functions. Many women find it almost impossible to function effectively with team members whom they judge as morally deplorable, no matter the latter's technical skills; for such women, the relationships among and integrity of team members is as important as the external goal (Harragan).

Sometimes a further breakdown of communication and effectiveness accrues because of the team leader's allegiance to scientific rigor and specificity at the expense of subjective attentiveness to caring. Since many team leaders are physicians, on multidisciplinary teams the problems may become interpreted as pointing to serious differences in orientation between physicians and other healthcare professionals (addressed in the next section). Whatever its cause, marginalization of some team members results in team dysfunction.

Locus of Authority for Decision Making

Roles involve ongoing features and conduct appropriate to a situation, and create expectations in the self and others regarding that conduct. Each role has an identity and boundaries, giving rise to the question of whose role carries the authority for team decision making (Rothberg). The challenge applies to both unidisciplinary and multidisciplinary

teams but is highlighted in multidisciplinary ones, particularly those involving physicians and other health professionals. Traditionally the physician was the person in authority by virtue of his or her office. The team metaphor reinforces the nonmovable locus of authority vested in one who holds such office (for example, *captain*).

At the same time, the team metaphor created expectations of more equality among members based on competence to provide input. Each member becomes an authority on the basis of professional expertise instead of office, and should be in a position to provide leadership at such time as expertise indicates it. In ethical decisions regarding patient care, the question of authority must be viewed in terms of who should have the morally authoritative voice. Technical expertise does not automatically entail ethical expertise. In both types of decision-making situations, the locus of authority is movable.

Clarification of role identity and boundaries helps to create reasonable expectations and mitigate this type of conflict regarding locus of authority (and concomitant locus of accountability) regarding team decisions (Green). A further complication arises, however, because teams usually have several members. A critical question regarding such collective decision making is whether team decisions are the sum of individual members, with accountability allocated only to the individuals, or whether a team itself can be regarded as a moral agent (Pellegrino). Lively debate continues regarding this topic (Abramson; Newton; Green).

Sometimes teams have difficulty coming to consensus about the appropriate course of action. The moral responsibility of the team members is to assure that further role clarification, further attempts at consensus building, and other collective decision-making mechanisms are instrumental only to maximizing patient well-being (or any other appropriate goal of teamwork). Negotiation strategies must be built into the team process so that the authority of any one or several members, or even the team as a whole, does not govern at the cost of the competent, compassionate decision geared to the appropriate ends of that team's activities.

The Patient as Team Member

There is much discussion about whether and in what respect patients/clients and their families are members of healthcare teams. The doctrine of informed consent and its underlying legal and ethical underpinnings dictate that patients and families should have input into decisions affecting themselves and their loved ones. At the same time, much of the team's work proceeds without direct involvement of patients and families. Some have argued that a primary care orientation places the patient as focus and arbiter of the care, and that present team practices fall short of that essential condition (Smith and Churchill). Others argue that conceptually a primary care approach is consistent with the goals of good teamwork (Barnard).

Moral Education for Teams

The team ideal provides a widely used model for effective and efficient patient care. Ethical issues are an inherent part of clinical decision making. In preparation for facing ethical issues the team can (1) develop a common moral language for discussion of the issues; (2) engage in cognitive and practical training in how to articulate feelings about pertinent ethical issues; (3) clarify values to uncover key interests among team members; (4) participate in common experiences upon which to base workable policies; and (5) refine a decision-making method for the team to use (Thomasma).

It appears that team approaches to a wide variety of healthcare issues and events will continue to develop and grow. The emergence of ethics committees as a type of team approach focusing explicitly on ethical decisions should help further in these deliberations.

RUTH B. PURTILO (1995)
BIBLIOGRAPHY REVISED

SEE ALSO: *Consensus, Role and Authority of; Long-Term Care; Medicine, Profession of; Nursing, Profession of; Palliative Care and Hospice; Trust; Women as Health Professionals*

BIBLIOGRAPHY

Abramson, Marcia. 1984. "Collective Responsibility in Interdisciplinary Collaboration: An Ethical Perspective for Social Workers." *Social Work in Health Care* 10(11): 35–43.

Barnard, David. 1987. "The Viability of the Concept of a Primary Health Care Team: A View from the Medical Humanities." *Social Science and Medicine* 25(6): 741–746.

Becker-Reems, Elizabeth D., and Garrett, Daniel G. 1998. *Testing the Limits of Teams: How to Implement Self-Management in Health Care.* Chicago: American Hospital Association.

Brown, Theodore. 1982. "An Historical View of Health Care Teams." In *Responsibility in Health Care,* ed. George J. Agich. *Philosophy and Medicine,* vol. 12. Boston: D. Reidel.

Doucet, Hubert; Larouche, Jean-Marc; Melchin, Kenneth R.; Larouche, Jean-Claude. 2000. *Ethical Deliberation in Multiprofessional Health Care Teams.* Ottawa, Ontario: University of Ottawa Press.

Erde, Edmund. 1982. "Logical Confusions and Moral Dilemmas in Health Care Teams and Team Talk." In *Responsibility in*

Health Care, ed. George J. Agich. *Philosophy and Medicine,* vol. 12. Boston: D. Reidel.

Gilligan, Carol. 1982. *In a Different Voice: Psychological Theory and Women's Development.* Cambridge, MA: Harvard University Press.

Green, Willard. 1988. "Accountability and Team Care." *Theoretical Medicine* 9:33–44.

Harragan, Betty L. 1977. *Games Mother Never Taught You: Corporate Gamesmanship for Women.* New York: Warner.

Heinemann, Gloria D., and Zeiss, Antonette M., eds. 2002. *Team Performance in Health Care: Assessment and Development (Issues in the Practice of Psychology).* New York: Plenum Publishers.

Nagi, Saad Z. 1975. "Teamwork in Health Care in the United States: A Sociological Perspective." *Milbank Memorial Fund Quarterly* 53:75–81.

Newton, Lisa H. 1982. "Collective Responsibility in Health Care." *Journal of Medicine and Philosophy* 7(1): 11–21.

Pellegrino, Edmund D. 1982. "The Ethics of Collective Judgments in Medicine and Health Care." *Journal of Medicine and Philosophy* 7(1): 3–10.

Purtilo, Ruth B. 1988. "Ethical Issues and Teamwork: The Context of Rehabilitation." *Archives of Physical Medicine and Rehabilitation* 69(5): 318–326.

Purtilo, Ruth B. 1998. "Rethinking the Ethics of Confidentiality and Health Care Teams." *Bioethics Forum* 14(3–4): 23–27.

Rothberg, June. 1985. "Rehabilitation Team Practice." In *Interdisciplinary Team Practice: Issues and Trends,* ed. Pedro J. Lecca and John S. McNeil. New York: Praeger.

Siegler, Eugenia L.; Myer, Kathryn; Fulmer, Terry., eds. 1998. *Geriatric Interdisciplinary Team Training.* New York: Springer.

Smith, Harmon L., and Churchill, Larry R. 1986. *Professional Ethics and Primary Care Medicine: Beyond Dilemmas and Decorum.* Durham, NC: Duke University Press.

Thomasma, David. 1981. "Moral Education in Interdisciplinary Teams." *Prospectus for Change* 6(5): 1–4.

Wagner, Joan; Rafter, Roseanne Hanlon; and Saveriano, Juliana. 1999. *Interdisciplinary Team in the Long Term Continuum: A Collaborative Approach.* New York: Springer.

TECHNOLOGY

• • •

I. History of Medical Technology

II. Philosophy of Medical Technology

I. HISTORY OF MEDICAL TECHNOLOGY

Medical technologies are objects, directed by procedures, that are applied against the hazards of illness. The object is the tangible dimension of technology. The procedure is the focused and standardized plan that guides the use of the object according to defined purposes.

Some medical technologies are more object-embedded. In them the tangible portion is the principal functional component. The X ray, artificial kidney, and penicillin are examples. Others technologies are more procedure-embedded. Their main function is to organize facts, individuals, and/or other technologies. Examples are the medical record, hospital, and surgical procedures. Indeed, the common synonym for the surgical procedure, the operation, connotes actions that are related as parts in a series.

It is important to distinguish technologies from another medium through which actions are taken in medicine—techniques. Medical techniques are procedures mediated through the human senses rather than through objects. Examples are percussion, pulse-feeling, and psychoanalysis. This perspective on medical technology will be used in this entry.

Technology, Nature, and Ethics

The works of the Hippocratic corpus, a group of essays on medical theory and therapy written between the fifth and third centuries B.C.E., analyze the relation between nature and the agents of the medical art, from the viewpoints of effectiveness and ethics.

The ancient Greek concepts of health and illness were based on a theory postulating four humors or basic elements of the body: blood, phlegm, yellow bile, and black bile. In health, these were in a stable equilibrium. Illness occurred when one or more of these humors increased or decreased and thus changed their proportional relation. This change caused an instability of the equilibrium state synonymous with health, and the breakdown produced illness. Nature—the force that inclined the humors toward remaining in or returning to the proportional relations of the healthful state—was viewed as the most powerful agent of healing. The purpose of the medical art was to assist nature to reestablish the proportional relationship of health among the humors.

Works in the Hippocratic corpus cautioned physicians against misapplying medical means. Such behavior constituted an offense that could harm both the patient and the reputation of medicine. In the essay "The Art," the following observation is made:

> For in cases where we may have the mastery through the means afforded by a natural constitution or by an art, there we may be craftsmen, but nowhere else. Whenever therefore a man suffers from an ill which is too strong for the means at the disposal of medicine, he surely must not even expect that it can be overcome by medicine. (Hippocrates, 1923a, p. 203)

To exceed the rational limits of the means of medicine was to commit the sin of hubris.

The technology of Greek doctors was relatively simple. They used ointments, compresses, bandages, surgical instruments, simple and compound drugs, and bloodletting in moderation. They used the techniques of history taking, visual observation, and palpation to learn the circumstances of illness, and prescribed diets, bathing, and exercise to maintain health and combat illness.

The Greeks also recognized that the manner in which physicians dressed, approached the bedside, and discussed illness with a patient could influence their success at healing by producing help and avoiding harm, and thus had an ethical meaning. Accordingly, attention to the effects of the physician as a person on the patient as a person became a significant aspect of Greek medical practice. The physician is told "to have at his command a certain ready wit, as dourness is repulsive both to the healthy and the sick." When coming into the sickroom, doctors should consider their "manner of sitting, reserve, arrangement of dress, decisive utterance, brevity of speech." The doctor was to perform all duties "calmly and adroitly, concealing most things from the patient while you are attending him," lest such revelations cause the patient to take "a turn for the worse" (Hippocrates, 1923b, pp. 291–299).

The Hippocratic Greek physicians recognized that appropriate applications of technology required a searching analysis of its capabilities, of the ethical canons that should guide its use, and of the relation between technology and nature in treating patients. Consideration of these three factors was the significant contribution of Greek civilization to the use of medical technology.

Anatomy and Specialization

The content of the technologies used in medical practice did not change appreciably for two thousand years. Indeed, the Hippocratic works and other Greek texts, in Latin translations, formed the core of medical learning in Europe through the Middle Ages.

As the sixteenth century began, however, a growing interest in firsthand exploration of nature, and learning and questioning the authority of tradition, created what we call the Renaissance, generating a perspective that would eventually exert a profound influence on the development and use of technology in medicine. Although the study of the structural composition of the body through anatomic dissection was thwarted by cultural, social, and religious constraints against dismemberment, Renaissance scientific and artistic interest in the body's physical makeup overcame these restrictions and encouraged its exploration.

The leading figure in this movement was Andreas Vesalius, a physician and professor at Padua, who in 1543 published *De humani corporis fabrica.* In it the structure of the body was analyzed in detail and portrayed through illustrations that were far in advance of any previous work. Its illustrations, the work of a still unknown Renaissance artist, were startling in their beauty and detail. In contrast, the typical anatomical illustrations of the day were inaccurate and crude outlines, with organs drawn in more as symbols than as representations. Vesalius corrected over two hundred errors in the work that had been the standard, authoritative text in use for almost fifteen hundred years. Written by the Greek doctor Galen in the second century, it reflected typical restrictions on human dissection, for its content was based on animal dissection (mainly pigs and apes) extrapolated to human structure.

Vesalius' book, devoted to the normal anatomy of the body, fostered within medicine an interest in bodily structure, particularly in the changes it underwent when attacked by illness. During the next two hundred years, physicians examined bodies and wrote texts commenting on the pathological transformation of anatomic structure. These efforts were brought together in a 1761 text by the Italian physician Giovanni Battista Morgagni, *The Seats and Causes of Diseases Investigated by Anatomy.* The work's principal objective was to demonstrate that the symptoms of illness in the living were determined by the structural changes produced within the body by disease. Morgagni demonstrated this relation through a tripartite analysis of cases. Typically, he began by reporting on the clinical course of an illness experienced by a patient who eventually died. This was followed by the autopsy findings. Then came a synthetic commentary in which he connected clinical and autopsy results.

Morgagni asserted that through anatomic examination, particular diseases could be recognized by their telltale footprints on the landscape of the body. As the title of Morgagni's work suggests, the author believed that diseases had "seats" in the body, and that they were expressed through characteristic disruptions of the body's fabric in discernible sites. This perspective ran directly counter to that prevailing under the humoral theory of illness, dominant since Hippocratic times.

Anatomy, beginning in the sixteenth century, when it departed from this whole-body perspective, focused the doctor's vision on the search for sites in the body where a change in structure had occurred. The leading question for anatomists and the physicians who adopted their outlook was *Where is the disease?* This question and viewpoint paved the way for the modern specialization of medicine, beginning in the nineteenth century and undergirded by a new technology. It justified a retreat by the doctor from patients as individuals to aspects of their anatomy, giving rise to the practice of having different physicians for the eyes, heart, kidneys, and other organs and organ systems.

Technology and the Nineteenth Century

With the anatomic ideology firmly established, the nineteenth century became one of the great centuries for medicine, a time of significant advance and change fueled largely by technologic innovation.

The transformation of diagnosis by technology was one of the century's most important features. The symbol and initiator of this change was a simple instrument used to enhance the conduction of sound, the stethoscope. Its transforming effect was as much caused by the new relationship it generated between physicians and patients as by the new information it provided. Before the stethoscope, the evidence that physicians acquired about illness came mostly from two sources: the visual inspection of the motions and surface of the body, and the story told by the patient of the events, sensations, and feelings that accompanied the illness. It was this encounter with the life of the patient that was at once enlightening, troubling, and engaging for physicians.

The patient's story provided significant diagnostic evidence that often determined the doctor's judgment. But physicians expressed concern about the authenticity of this evidence, which usually could not be confirmed. Who could know if a patient really heard a buzzing in the ears? Diagnosis was prone to the distortions of memory and whim. For all of its evidentiary faults, however, the narrative of the patient's journey through illness connected the doctor with the life of the patient.

The stethoscope challenged the place of the narrative of illness. It was introduced into practice through 1819 treatise (*De l'auscultation médiate*), written by the inventor of the stethoscope, the French physician René Laennec. Laennec claimed that physicians who placed their ear to one end of the foot-long wooden tube that was the first stethoscope and the other end to the chest of a patient, would hear sounds generated by the heart and lungs indicative of health or disease within them. He demonstrated through autopsy evidence that a particular sound perceived in the chest corresponded to a particular lesion within its anatomic structure. He asserted that his technology enabled physicians to diagnose illness not only precisely but often without the help of other symptoms. Doctors need depend on no one else. They could be scientifically self-reliant. The findings of their own senses, extended by a simple instrument, were adequate to reach diagnostic judgments.

This technological advance reduced the significance of the patient's narrative. Why should physicians painstakingly acquire this story and its subjective and unverifiable verbal evidence, if they could use more objective sonic evidence they gathered themselves? With the stethoscope, physicians stepped back from the lives of patients. They began to engage patients through the anatomic and physiologic signs detected by their instruments.

Other simple technologies to extend the doctor's senses into the body, such as the ophthalmoscope (1850), the clinical thermometer (1867), and the sphygmomanometer (1896), were introduced during the nineteenth century. By the century's end physicians had become skillful diagnosticians, seekers of physical clues they used to deduce the source of their patients' troubles. The doctor's black bag contained the technologies to explore the body physically and to obtain evidence that greatly improved diagnostic accuracy. It was, in fact, through witnessing great skill in the analysis of physical evidence by one of his instructors, Joseph Bell, that a physician-in-training, Arthur Conan Doyle, was led to create the fictional character Sherlock Holmes.

Still, therapy remained limited. In the 1860 address to the Massachusetts Medical Society, Oliver Wendell Holmes, Harvard professor of anatomy, proclaimed: "I firmly believe that if the whole materia medica, *as now used,* could be sunk to the bottom of the sea, it would be all the better for mankind,—and all the worse for the fishes" (Holmes, p. 203).

The only major bright spot to emerge in the nineteenth century on the therapeutic side of medicine was in surgery. Radical change in the ability of surgeons to perform the dangerous and delicate work of cutting into the body occurred through two separate innovations, one introduced in 1846 and the other in 1867. At the beginning of the nineteenth century, pain had become so inseparably linked with surgical incision that several reports of an anesthetic effect produced by nitrous oxide and ether were disregarded by practitioners. Surgical pain was dealt with by efforts to shorten its presence. Techniques of rapid surgery were developed, with some surgeons capable of detaching a limb in minutes. The conclusive demonstration (in a surgical procedure for a tumor of the neck) at the Massachusetts General Hospital in 1846 of the ability to control operative pain through use of ether, was made by the American Dentist William Morton, who administered the ether. It ameliorated the trauma of surgery for patient and surgeon alike, but cutting into the cavity of the body still was limited by infection.

To control infection, insight was needed into the causal role of bacteria. Joseph Lister, a British surgeon, wrote a paper in 1867 in which he described eleven operations on compound fractures of the limbs in which nine patients recovered without amputation, one required it, and one died. These startling results were made possible by treating the operating space—wound, instruments, surgeon's hands, and air—with the antiseptic carbolic acid. In 1882, the German scientist Robert Koch published a paper that proved through rigorous experiments the causal link between the tubercle bacillus and tuberculosis—a disease that at the time was responsible for about one out of seven deaths in Europe. This essay established the pivotal role played by bacteria in infection. It not only gave further impetus to the practice of antiseptic surgery and liberated surgeons, no longer thwarted by pain or infection, to perform extensive operations within the body cavity. It also produced a new workshop for surgery and all of medicine—the hospital.

The Technologies of Twentieth-Century Medicine

The origins of the hospital reside in military hospitals put up by Roman soldiers on their routes of march, and hospices established early in the history of Christianity to care for the homeless, travelers, orphans, the hungry, and the sick. These multiple activities gradually became divided among separate institutions, one of which was the hospital. It flourished greatly through the medieval period but began a decline afterward, due to diminished church support of its activities.

By the nineteenth century the hospital's medical role was restricted. It was a place for those who could not afford either to call a physician or surgeon to the house for treatment or to employ servants to administer needed bedside care at home. There were two kinds of medicine: home care for the well-to-do and hospital care for the indigent. Hospitals were dangerous places. Infections could rage through them, killing large numbers of patients and making work there dangerous for staff. Hospitals were also feared for the moral dangers said to be posed to women and children by the rough patients they housed.

New technologies transformed the hospital medically and socially. Surgery could no longer be done on kitchen tables at home: it required an antiseptic environment, sterilized instruments, and a staff of skilled nurses for the aftercare of patients undergoing more extensive procedures than were possible in the past.

As the twentieth century dawned, diagnosis and therapy of nonsurgical disease could not be readily done in the home with technology carried in a doctor's bag. diagnostic technology now entered a new phase of development. The simple instruments to extend the senses of the physicians were being replaced by sensing machines too large and expensive to be housed anywhere but in hospitals.

This new technology automatically recorded the data of illness, leaving the reading of its results to the doctor. The X ray, discovered in 1895; the ward laboratory, with its microscopes and chemical tests of the body fluids, which came together as a hospital space in the early 1900s; and the electrocardiograph, introduced in 1906, all converted medical diagnosis from a personal act to a scientific event. The physician leaning over the bedside, at least physically connected to the patient through the stethoscope and similar technologies, became an increasingly anachronistic image as the twentieth century wore on. The physician holding an X ray up to light, studying it, was more in keeping with physicians' growing self-image as scientists. Where was the patient? There was less need for personal medical encounters; the best evidence available to medicine was increasingly not what the patient said, nor what the physician sensed, but what the pictorial or graphic image reported.

As it entered this new technologic phase, medicine required a location within which patients, the increasingly specialized medical staff, and technology could be brought together. The hospital became that place. Its success was dramatic. While there were about four hundred hospitals in the United States in 1875, by 1909 the number grew to over four thousand, and by 1929 surpassed six thousand. No longer shunned but sought by communities, the hospital became the workshop of medicine. By the mid-twentieth century not only patients and technology but also doctors' offices were placed in hospitals. Home care and the house call, no longer adequate as means to apply new medical knowledge, were disappearing as the hospital, perhaps the quintessential technology of the twentieth century to organize medical care, enfolded medicine.

Several other innovations critical to the functions of hospitals and medicine were in place by the mid-twentieth century. One—having integrative influence like the hospital—was the technology of organizing the data of medicine—the medical record. It was fundamentally reformed in the 1920s by the work of the American College of Surgeons (Reiser, 1991). In an era of growing specialization, not only among

physicians but also among nurses and the technical experts needed to run the hospital and its machines (there were over two hundred separate healthcare specializations by the mid 1970s), communication was of great importance. How to learn what each had done? Through the record, which was the main agent of synthesis in medicine. In its pages the thoughts and actions of a diverse staff were recorded.

But for all its integrative significance, the medical record remains a problem. It shows the results of the information explosion. These data literally burst the confines of the chart. Hundred-page records abound. They contain the details of medical care, but their order often makes following the course of an illness, or locating a particular bit of information, difficult and frustrating. Innovations such as the unit record (having all hospital encounters of a patient recorded in a single place rather than dispersed through separate charts in each clinic); the problem-oriented record (ordering medical data problems—physical, psychologic, or social—rather than by data source, such as putting laboratory data in one place, X-ray data in another); and the computerized record have yet to solve the problem of what to do with the avalanche of technologic evidence.

Another critical innovation available by mid-century was antibiotics. The mass production of penicillin in 1944 (it had been discovered by Alexander Fleming in 1928) inaugurated the antibiotic era in medicine. Antibiotic drugs flowed from the laboratories of the pharmaceutical industry, finally breaking the hold of bacterial illness. Penicillin was called a wonder drug when it was introduced. Given the drug, a patient gravely ill with meningitis or pneumonia would be up and about and home in a week. Not only was it fast-acting and fully curative, but it was safe and cheap. It was commonly thought that penicillin would be the first innovation of a pharmaceutical revolution to produce not only antibacterial drugs but also drugs to deal as effectively with other human ailments. However, the symbol of medicine in the second half of the twentieth century would not be penicillin but a machine that made its debut in the mid-1950s.

The artificial respirator had a long history, dating back to the mid-nineteenth century, when rudimentary forerunners were fashioned to deal mainly with the respiratory crisis of drowning. A tank respirator introduced by Philip Drinker and Charles McKhann in 1929, which used negative-pressure techniques to secure respiration, became the "iron lung" that sustained victims of poliomyelitis. Its effectiveness was variable, and its use was complicated. But by the mid-1950s, using new machines based on positive-pressure technology, clinicians had a far better means of dealing with diseases and accidents that threatened lives through respiratory failure.

Initially, this machine was intended to assist critically ill persons by temporarily sustaining a vital physiologic function and giving them time to recover. For the first time in medical history, physicians acquired a technology that, allied to other advances in nursing, monitoring, and drug therapy, and all brought together by an integrative technique of care embodied in the intensive care unit (ICU), permitted the long-term sustenance of desperately ill people who had no chance of recovery. Now families and medical staff waited by ICU beds, where the main signs of life were not manifest in the expressions or movements of the patient but in the mechanical sounds, motions, and readouts of the new machinery of rescue.

Ethical Issues in Applying Medical Technologies

As families and medical staff assimilated the consequences of the life-support technology represented by the artificial respirator that could prolong dying or life without cognition, they reached out to the ethical traditions of religion, medicine, and society for help (Pius XII, pp. 501–504). Physicians particularly began to see that the ethical problems to be solved in these crises were as great as or greater than the technical problems of treatment. How to decide whether in a hopeless case to remove the technology that maintained the person's life? On what values should this judgment be based, and who should decide?

Other machines developed in this period posed a similar mix of ethical and technical issues. The artificial kidney was created as a device for acute, intermittent dialysis by Willem Kolff in The Netherlands in 1944. However, it was introduced as a clinically usable machine in the early 1960s in Seattle, Washington, by Belding Schribner. He added an arteriovenous shunt that allowed long-term access to it and made continuing hemodialysis possible. The limited number of machines and personnel to run them led to moral agonizing over developing criteria for selection. Someone had to choose which of the thousands of individuals in the United States having chronic renal failure and able to benefit from dialysis would gain access to a technology that could save their lives. Thirteen years after the machine's introduction, American society decided how to resolve this crisis. In 1973, U.S. congressional legislation provided funds to provide dialysis to all who required it.

Technologies such as the artificial kidney and the respirator have been criticized as offering expensive but partial solutions to fundamental problems of biologic breakdown. The American physician Lewis Thomas calls them "halfway technologies," because they represent only a partial (halfway) understanding of a biologic puzzle that, once solved, will do away with the expense and the disadvantages of such therapies (Thomas, p. 37).

The extraordinary and growing expense of the healthcare system that followed the development of such technologies may be reduced when biomedical research produces comprehensive biologic answers to problems such as organ failure. But in the twentieth century, we have acquired few such complete technologies. One group, already mentioned, is penicillin and other antibiotics, which offer total solutions, that also are inexpensive and rapidly acting, to the problems of bacterial infection. A second generic complete technology is the vaccine. Those invented to prevent smallpox (first introduced in the eighteenth century) and poliomyelitis (developed in the mid-1950s) have in the twentieth century eradicated the first disease and almost wholly contained the second.

The emerging field of genetic research promises fundamental solutions to a host of disorders, with the prospect of their early detection and correction. Finally, the growing ability to visualize the basic structures of the body through endoscopes and computer-driven imaging machines such as the MRI and PET scans provides diagnostic knowledge facilitating the use of therapeutic technologies that promise complete cures. Indeed, genetic and imaging technologies have taken the anatomic concept of illness to its ultimate terminus. To the question "Where is the disease?" the answer now can be "In this particular gene!"

Conclusion

Technologies, history shows, can be imperative: We may be impelled to use the capacities they provide us without adequate reflection on whether they will lead to the humane goals of medical care. The ancient Greeks understood this issue. They recognized that technologic means must be used in consonance with articulated, ethically informed ends. Their example remains worth following.

STANLEY JOEL REISER (1995)
BIBLIOGRAPHY REVISED

SEE ALSO: *Artificial Hearts and Cardiac Assist Devices; Artificial Nutrition and Hydration; Cybernetics; Dialysis, Kidney; Deep Brain Stimulation; DNR; Electroconvulsive Therapy; Enhancement Uses of Medical Technology; Fertility Control: Medical Aspects; Genetic Testing and Screening; Life Sustaining Treatment and Euthanasia; Organ Transplants, Medical Overview; Pediatrics, Intensive Care in;*

Psychosurgery, Medical and Historical Aspects of; Reproductive Technologies; Tissue Banking and Transplantation, Ethical Issues in; Transhumanism and Posthumanism; Virtue and Character; and other *Technology* subentries

BIBLIOGRAPHY

Grace, P A. 1997. "Men, Medicine and Machines." *Irish Journal of Medical Sciences* 166(3): 152–156.

Hippocrates. 1923a. "The Art." In Vol. 2 of *Hippocrates,* 4 vols., tr. William H. S. Jones. Cambridge, MA: Harvard University Press.

Hippocrates. 1923b. "Decorum." In Vol. 2 of *Hippocrates,* 4 vols., tr. William H. S. Jones. Cambridge, MA: Harvard University Press.

Holmes, Oliver Wendell. 1883. "Currents and Counter Currents in Medical Science." In his *Medical Essays,* 2nd edition. Boston: Houghton Mifflin.

Jeffrey, Kirk. 2001. *Machines in Our Hearts: The Cardiac Pacemaker, the Implantable Defibrillator, and American Health Care.* Baltimore: John Hopkins University Press.

Koch, Robert. 1886. "The Etiology of Tuberculosis." In *Recent Essays by Various Authors on Bacteria in Relation to Disease,* ed. W. Watson Cheyne. London: New Sydenham Society.

Laennec, René. 1821. *A Treatise on Diseases of the Chest,* tr. John Forbes. London: T. & G. Underwood.

Lister, Joseph. 1867. "On the Antiseptic Principle in the Practice of Surgery." Lancet 2: 353–356.

Morgagni, Giovanni Battista. 1960. *The Seats and Causes of Diseases Investigated by Anatomy,* tr. Benjamin Alexander. New York: Hafner.

Nightingale, Florence. 1863. *Notes on Hospitals,* 3rd edition, rev. London: Longman, Green, Longman, Roberts, & Green.

Pius XII. 1977 (1958). "The Prolongation of Life." In *Ethics in Medicine: Historical Perspectives and Contemporary Concerns,* eds. Stanley Joel Reiser, Arthur J. Dyck, and William J. Curran. Cambridge, MA: MIT Press.

Reiser, Stanley Joel. 1978. Medicine and the Reign of Technology. New York: Cambridge University Press.

Reiser, Stanley Joel. 1991a. "The Clinical Record in Medicine. Part I: Learning from Cases." *Annals of Internal Medicine* 114(10): 902–907.

Reiser, Stanley Joel. 1991b. "The Clinical Record in Medicine: Part II: Reforming Content and Purpose." *Annals of Internal Medicine* 114(11): 980–985.

Sandelowski, Margarete. 2000. *Devices & Desires: Gender, Technology, and American Nursing (Studies in Social Medicine).* Raleigh: University of North Carolina Press.

Stanton, Jennifer, ed. 2002. *Innovations in Medicine and Health: Diffusion and Resistance in the Twentieth Century (Studies in the Social History of Medicine).* London: Routledge.

Thomas, Lewis. 1977. "On the Science and Technology of Medicine." In *Doing Better and Feeling Worse: Health in the United States,* ed. John H. Knowles. New York: Norton.

Vesalius, Andreas. 1980 (1543). *De humani corporis fabrica.* Stuttgart: Medicina Rara.

II. PHILOSOPHY OF MEDICAL TECHNOLOGY

Philosophy of technology aspires to comprehensive reflection on the making and using of artifacts. Medicine is increasingly defined not just by the character of its human interactions (physician—patient relationships) or professional expertise (knowledge of illness and related therapies) or its end (health), but also by the type and character of its instruments (from stethoscope to high-tech imaging devices) and the construction of special human-artifact interactions (synthetic drugs, prosthetic devices). Indeed, the physician-patient relationship, medical knowledge, and the concept of health are all affected by technological change. There is even debate about whether the term *artifact* should include nonmaterial as well as material human constructions, in which case all of the above might well be interpreted as technologies. From either perspective, medicine and the issues of bioethics fall within the purview of the philosophy of technology.

Historical Development

Philosophy of technology as a distinct discipline originated with the publication of Ernst Kapp's *Grundlinien einer Philosophie der Technik* (1877), the first book to be entitled a "philosophy of technology." A left-wing Hegelian contemporary of Karl Marx, whose thought includes important analyses of human-machine systems, Kapp left Germany in the mid-1800s to become a pioneer and "hydrotherapist" on the central Texas frontier. Returning to Europe two decades later, he elaborated a general theory of technology as "organ projection"—from the hammer as extension of the fist to railway and telegraph as extensions of the circulatory and nervous systems—thereby promoting analysis of the philosophical-anthropological foundations of technology.

Another major formative figure was Friedrich Dessauer, whose *Philosophie der Technik* (1927) and *Streit um die Technik* (1956) reflect his experience as the inventor of deep penetration X-ray therapy. For Dessauer the philosophical core of technology is the act of invention, for which he sought to provide a Kantian analysis of transcendental preconditions. Dessauer's argument that the fact inventions work shows how inventors depend on insight into a supernatural realm of "pre-established solutions" to technical problems raises basic epistemological and metaphysical issues.

José Ortega y Gasset and Martin Heidegger, two major philosophers of the twentieth century, also contributed texts dedicated to the theme of technology. Ortega's "Meditación de la técnica" (1939) presents technical activity as a means for realizing some supernatural human self-conception, and modern technology as generalized knowledge of how to create such means. Ortega thus pushes anthropological reflection to new depths. Heidegger's "Die Frage nach der Technik" (1954) argues that both traditional technics or craft and modern technology are forms of truth, revealing different aspects of Being. Modern technology in particular is a "challenging" and "setting-upon" that reveals Being as "resource"—that is, the world as a reservoir of materials subject to indefinite human manipulations. In this argument Heidegger likewise carries epistemological and metaphysical reflection well beyond Kantian terms.

Lewis Mumford, Jacques Ellul, Herbert Marcuse, Jürgen Habermas, and Michel Foucault have made further contributions to the development of philosophy of technology from the perspective of social theory. Mumford (1934) focuses attention on technological materials and processes as major elements in the historical development of modern civilization. Ellul (1954) argues that the pursuit of technical efficiency is the defining characteristic of the contemporary world, which constitutes a milieu distinct from the natural and social milieus that preceded it. For Ellul, just as the Hebrew-Christian tradition once demythologized the two earlier milieus, now it called upon to demythologize technology.

Marcuse (1964) and Habermas (1968) have debated the character of technology as ideology. Foucault (1988) views all technologies and sciences as masking power manipulations, and develops a special analysis of technologies as historical transformations and determinations of the self. Such ideas exercise continuing influence in debates over the extent to which technology is properly conceived as an autonomous determinant of human affairs (see Winner, 1986) or as a social construction (see Feenberg). Such debates in turn influence fundamental orientations with regard to practical questions about the assessment and control of technology that find expression in such applied fields as medical ethics, environmental ethics, engineering ethics, and computer ethics.

Ortega and Heidegger are leading figures in the Continental or phenomenological tradition in the philosophy of technology. Further analyses of phenomenological inspiration can be found in the work of Don Ihde (1979) on human-technics interactions and of Albert Borgmann (1984) on the political-cultural implications of contemporary technological formations.

A different, equally strong tradition in the philosophy of technology is constituted by Anglo-American analytic reflection on artificial intelligence (AI). Here questions center on the extent to which brains are computers and thinking processes can be modeled (see, e.g., Simon; Dreyfus). In contrast to the phenomenological tradition, the Anglo-American analysis of AI exhibits considerable interactions with biomedical theory of neurological processes and, to a lesser extent, with biomedical practice.

Theoretical Perspectives

Throughout its diverse strands, philosophy of technology, like philosophy generally, includes theoretical and practical issues, from epistemology and metaphysics to ethics and politics, all of which can helpfully inform bioethics. Comprehensive understanding nevertheless grows out of partial understandings. The making and using of artifacts involve not only the artifacts themselves but also technological knowledge, technological activity, and technological volition. Theoretical analyses can thus conveniently be described by referencing tendencies to interpret technology in one of four primary forms.

TECHNOLOGY AS OBJECT. The theory that identifies technology with particular artifacts, such as tools, machines, electronic devices, or consumer products, is the commonsense view. Initially it involves a classification of artifacts into different types, according to their own internal structures, different kinds of human engagement, impacts on the environment, or other factors. Mumford, for instance, distinguishes utilities (roads, electric power networks), tools (artifacts under immediate human power and guidance), machines (nonhuman power with immediate human guidance), and automatons (nonhuman power and no immediate human guidance).

Taking a different tack, Borgmann argues a distinction between things and devices. An example of a thing, in Borgmann's special sense, is a traditional fireplace, which engages a variety of human activities ranging from cutting wood to cooking food, functions in a clearly understandable manner, and is an explicit center of daily life. By contrast, a device, such as a heat pump, simply makes available some commodity (hot and cold air) by nonobvious processes and disappears into a background of quotidian activities. The device is a special instance of what Heidegger called a "resource."

Ihde, in a different but equally provocative manner, distinguishes embodiment and hermeneutic relations between humans and their instruments. Embodiment relations experience the world through instruments, as exemplified by eyeglasses, which disappear into and become an unconscious part of the experience of seeing. In hermeneutic relations, by contrast, the instrument itself—for instance, a camera—becomes part of the world with which one engages; a user consciously focuses on the operation and interpretation of this instrument. Both Borgmann's and Ihde's distinctions obviously provide frameworks within which to interpret the myriad tools and instruments of high-technology medicine.

TECHNOLOGY AS KNOWLEDGE. Etymologically, however, the word *technology* implies not objects but "knowledge of techne," or craft skill. Epistemological analyses of such knowledge distinguish between knowing how (intuitive skill) and knowing that (propositional knowledge). The transition from premodern technics to modern technology can thus be argued as defined by the development of propositional knowledge about techne through the unification of technics and science.

This theory of modern technology as applied science is particularly influential among scientists and engineers, and has been given detailed philosophical exposition by Mario Bunge (1967). For Bunge, modern technology develops when the rules of prescientific crafts, originally discovered by trial-and-error methods, are replaced by the "grounded rules" or technological theories. Technological theories can be formulated by applying either the content or the method of science to technical practices. The former application takes preexisting scientific knowledge (e.g., fluid dynamics) and adapts it under certain boundary conditions to formulate an engineering science (aerodynamics). The latter uses the methods of science to formulate distinctive engineering analyses of human-machine interactions, such as operations research and decision theory.

Medicine can readily be incorporated within such an epistemological analysis. Prior to the nineteenth century, most medical practice relied on rule-of-thumb experience. But twentieth-century medicine has involved the progressive grounding of medical practice in the sciences of anatomy and physiology as well as the development of such distinctive fields as epidemiology and biomedical engineering. Indeed, José Sanmartín (1987), for instance, analyzes genetic engineering exactly as an embedding of techniques in scientific theory.

TECHNOLOGY AS ACTIVITY. The transformation of some technics (such as medicine) into an applied science is not, however, simply an epistemic event. As Foucault (1963) argues, for example, modern medicine "is made possible as a form of knowledge" by the reorganization of hospitals and new kinds of medical practices. This emphasis on technology as activity or a complex of activities is characteristic of social theory. Ellul's "characterology of technique" and analysis of the central role played by the rational pursuit of technical efficiency in the economy, the state, and what he terms "human techniques" (ranging from education to medicine) is another case in point, as are the Marxist and neo-Marxist analyses of Marcuse, Habermas, and Andrew Feenberg.

The emphasis on technology as activity has roots in Max Weber's observation that there are techniques of every conceivable human activity—from artistic production and performance to mass manufacturing and bureaucratic organization—even education, politics, and religion. One classic problem for social theorists is to explain the character and limits of *technicalization*—that is, the movement from traditional societies, in which techniques are situated within and delimited by nontechnical values, to modern societies, in which techniques are increasingly evaluated solely in technical terms. In traditional societies, for example, animals can be eaten only if butchered in a ritually prescribed manner; in modern societies animal slaughter is largely subject to calculations of efficiency.

Efficiency can also be conceived in economic terms and applied at micro or macro levels. The former is typical of analyses internal to business corporations (including hospitals and clinics); the latter, of social assessments of technology. In regard to technology assessments especially, there arise questions of the limits of technicalization and possible alternative forms of technical institutions (see Feenberg), as well as of responsible agency and risk.

TECHNOLOGY AS VOLITION. A fourth element in the interrelationship of knowledge, object, and activity is that of volition. The human activity of making and using artifacts depends not only on knowledge but also on volition. Indeed, it can be argued that volition is even more important in this respect than knowledge, that is, that human action can be ignorant but not unwilled.

The philosophical analysis of volition distinguishes between volition in the weaker senses of wishing, hoping, longing, and desiring, and the stronger or more decisive intending and affirming. Volition in the second or stronger senses is constituted by self-reflective identification with some particular wish, hope, or desire that takes on the character of a project. Ortega, Mumford, and Frederick Ferré (1988) argue that technology is essentially a matter of volition in one or more of these senses. According to Ferré, for instance, technology is grounded in "the urge to live and to thrive." For Ortega, technology is based in the willed attempt at a worldly realization of some specific self-image. For Mumford, technology in a distinctive sense emerges when human beings subordinate their traditional polytechnical activities of craft, religious ritual, and poetry to the monotechnical pursuit of physical power—something that first happened about five thousand years ago in Egypt, with the construction of the pyramids by means of large, rigid, hierarchical social organizations that he terms "megamachines."

Defining technology in terms of volition makes possible the perception of broad historical continuities more than does a focus on the elements of knowledge or object or even activity. It is inherently more believable that the *will* to fly was coeval with human existence than that technical knowledge of how to fly, flying machines, or the human performance of flying or flying-like actions have existed from time immemorial. Such an approach once again has immediate implications for the interpretation of medicine. If medicine is interpreted primarily as grounded in volition, then it is inherently more believable that there exists a fundamental continuity between premodern and modern medicines.

Nevertheless, one of the most sustained critiques of modern medicine is precisely that as volition, it is fundamentally different from all previous kinds of medicine. Ivan Illich's *Medical Nemesis* (1976) argues that modern medicine arises from a basic "social commitment to provide all citizens with almost unlimited outputs." Indeed, the nemesis of rising iatrogenic disease is a direct result of "our contemporary hygienic hubris," which can be reversed only "through a recovery of the will to self-care." In the 1990s, however, Illich becomes critical of the idea of self-care when it serves as an ideological support for what has been termed "health fascism."

Practical Perspectives

Not theoretical analysis, however, but ethical and political concerns predominate in philosophy of technology. Ethics has from its beginnings in the West involved at least marginal considerations of technology. Aristotle's *Nicomachean Ethics,* for instance, in passing identifies *techne* as an intellectual virtue. More than two thousand years later Immanuel Kant distinguished moral and technical imperatives. But in line with such marginal attention, from Plato and Aristotle to the Renaissance, technology was widely accepted as properly subject to ethical constraints. From the Renaissance to the Enlightenment, by contrast, traditional restraints were effectively replaced with an ethical commitment to the unfettered pursuit of technology for what Francis Bacon called "the relief of man's estate." It is precisely this modern commitment, along with its subsequent questioning in response to a series of increasingly prominent problems, that frames the contemporary prominence of ethical issues in the philosophy of technology.

ALIENATION. Historically, the first problem of modern technology involved the industrial revolution and alienation. At the basis of modern technological making lies a belief that the world as it is given does not provide a suitable home for human beings; humanity must construct a home for itself. The problem is that human beings do not immediately find themselves at home in the worlds they technologically create. The resulting alienation is especially problematic to the extent that it is grounded in attempts to overcome alienation.

The two most extensive critiques of technological alienation are Romanticism and socialism. The Romantic critique, an early version of which appears in Jean-Jacques Rousseau's *Discourse on the Sciences and the Arts* (1750), focuses on how technology alienates the individual from feelings and sentiments, as manifested in relationships with nature, the past, or other human beings. This is caused, according to the Romantic argument, by a one-sided development of rationality. Romanticism thus perceives technology as an extension of reason and proposes to enclose it within a larger affective life.

By contrast, in the socialist critique of alienation, Marx, like Kapp, explicitly conceives technology as a human organ projection. Marx thus focuses on the separation of human beings from control over the tools and products of their labor, as manifested in an economy based on money and the "fetishism of commodities." In response, socialism argues for a comprehensive restructuring of society to promote worker control of the means of production.

In biomedical practice the use of technological instruments and rationalized systems of diagnosis raises the issue of alienation in the form of questions about the depersonalization of healthcare techniques and organizations. Responses can exhibit characteristically Romantic or socialist features. Exemplifying Romanticism are proposals to situate diagnostic techniques within a more humanistic framework, perhaps one of beautiful buildings and a pleasant environment. Exemplifying a socialist response might be arguments for the promotion of patient autonomy by granting patients more direct control over their own healthcare institutions.

WARFARE. A second ethical problem has centered on technology and war. There are two basic theories about the relationship between war and technology: First, technological weapons make war so horrible that it becomes unthinkable; rational self-interest leads to deterrence of their use. Second, human beings will always tend to miscalculate their self-interests and go to war; weapons production must therefore be limited, and a higher ideal of global human unity promoted.

Prior to World War I, naive versions of the first theory largely supported the pursuit of technology. The trauma of the war contributed to pessimistic criticisms of technological civilization and led to emphasis on the second theory. This pessimistic critique, coupled with idealist attempts at world government, failed to avoid World War II and a technological practice of genocide, the invention and use of the atomic bomb, and a subsequent Cold War spread of nuclear weapons. As a result, much more sophisticated versions of deterrence policy were developed in alliance with management and decision theories. Advanced technological weapons development projects also stimulated science and technology policy and management studies, while the practice of nuclear deterrence was subject to extended moral criticism. One of the more idealistic criticisms argues that human unity and peace, which in the past could remain as moral exhortations, have now become necessities, lest human beings obliterate themselves from the face of the planet. In this argument the rational self-interest of the first theory appears to merge with the idealism of the second.

Prospects for social and genetic engineering call forth similar arguments between pragmatic deterrence management and idealistic delimination. The progressive refinements of conditioning techniques and sophisticated drug therapies create behavior-control technologies of immense potential power. Developments in recombinant DNA technology and the Human Genome Project offer opportunities to extend this power to the biological creation of human life. As Sanmartín has pointed out, this attack on the vagaries of human nature can be seen as developing new technologies for the prevention of "social diseases" such as war.

TECHNOLOGY AND SOCIAL CHANGE. Concerns about the relatively specific issues of alienation and warfare have been complemented by more general analyses of the causal relations and patterns of interaction that obtain between technology and social change. Such analyses include bottom-up case studies of changes related to bureaucracy, urbanization, work (from mass production to automation to customized production), leisure and mobility, secularization, communications (from telephone and radio to television and computer), and medical technologies, as well as top-down theoretical reflections on the same dimensions of social life and on the social order as a whole. Within both approaches it is common to find descriptions of disorder between technology and society brought about by technological change along with arguments for addressing such disorder by means of some intellectual and/or volitional adaptations.

In the period between the two world wars, for instance, William F. Ogburn's *Social Change* (1922) described a "cultural lag" between technological development and social adaptation across a variety of indicators, and argued for a more intelligent appropriation of technology. A decade later Henri Bergson's *Two Sources of Morality and Religion* (1932) argued that the vices of industrial civilization as a whole could be corrected only by what he termed a "supplement of soul" that is at once ascetic (against luxuries) and charitable (for eliminating inequalities).

To stress the need for intellectual or rational adaptations is no doubt more characteristic of advanced industrial society, with its concomitant large-scale educational institutions and activities. The kind of piecemeal social engineering advocated by John Dewey and Karl Popper, and the many theories of economic rationality from Pareto efficiency to risk-benefit analysis, and of postindustrial organization from Daniel Bell to Habermas, likewise advocate effective increases in the rational control of modern technology. By contrast, a follower of Bergson such as Ellul argues that technology has become a kind of totalitarian milieu that requires comprehensive demythologizing. Others suggest the need for expansions of affective sensibility. Some theories of postmodern culture exhibit certain affinities with this approach.

With regard to increasing rationality, Kristin Shrader-Frechette (1991) has drawn an explicit parallel between the requirements of informed consent in the practice of medically risky procedures and the general societal adaptation to technological change. With regard to affective responses to technological change, the work of Illich is illustrative.

POLLUTION AND THE ENVIRONMENTAL CRISIS. Perhaps even more demanding of attention than warfare, and adding a new dimension to analyses of technological change, are problems associated with environmental pollution and global climate transformation. The environmental crisis has obvious and fundamental impacts on human health and safety, and thereby on biomedicine. Indeed, outside medical ethics, perhaps the single most intensively explored area of applied philosophy is that of environmental ethics.

Beyond intensified self-interest, environmental change has engendered the new science of ecology and extended ethical concern both temporally (for future generations) and ontologically (for nonhuman entities). As analyzed by Hans Jonas (1979), this extension is grounded in "the altered nature of human action" brought about by the "novel powers" of modern technology. Although all human life requires some technical activity, not until the advent of modern scientific technology did the technical power to create become so explosive as to be capable of fundamentally transforming nature and the future of the human condition. On the basis of this power there arises what Jonas terms an "imperative of responsibility" to "ensure a future."

Jonas explicitly argues the application of this principle of responsibility in the field of bioethics. Applications might also be adumbrated for other discussions in environmental ethics, such as those that distinguish shallow versus deep ecology movements and argue the rights of nature understood as wilderness. Could one not, for instance, distinguish a shallow versus a deep bioethics? Would it not be possible to argue, against excessive medical intervention, a defense of wildness in biology?

ENGINEERING ETHICS. A second well-developed field of applied ethics with potential implications for the medical dimensions of bioethics is that of engineering ethics (see Martin and Schinzinger). Here a basic shift has taken place in the interpretation of the primary responsibility of the professional engineer—from loyalty to a company or client (patterned after the ethics of the medical and legal professions) to responsibility to public health, safety, and welfare. Could this shift, resting on a recognition of engineering as social experimentation, have implications for new understandings of professional medical obligation? Is it not the case that technological medicine is, as much as the treatment of individual patients, to some extent a social experiment? If so, then the engineering ethics defense of the rights and role of the whistle-blower might well have analogous applications in the biomedical field.

COMPUTERS AND INFORMATION TECHNOLOGY. A third well-developed area of applied ethics deals with computers. One defining book in this field was written by a computer scientist (see Weizenbaum) and based on Mumford's philosophical anthropology of the human as a polyvalent being for whom calculating is only a very small part of thinking and a limited dimension of technics. Key issues in the philosophical analysis of computers concern the degree to which human thinking can be modeled by computers and the extent to which human beings should properly rely on computer programs, especially in areas such as weapons. Subsequent development, as summarized by Deborah Johnson (1985), has emphasized issues of individual privacy and corporate security, the formulation of ethical codes for computer professionals, and liabilities for the malfunctioning of computer programs. The computerization of medical practice calls for the application of such reflection to many aspects of high-tech medical diagnosis and treatment.

DEVELOPMENT AND DIVERSITY. The ambiguities of technology in developing countries, together with reassessments of the impacts of advanced technological transformations in relation to women and ethnic minorities, especially in the United States and Europe, raise new issues regarding the abilities of scientific technology to accommodate true diversity. On the one side, there are questions of equity. In advanced technological countries, technological power and affluence are not equally shared between men and women and among different ethnic communities. Nor does there appear to be equality of opportunity among advanced and developing countries. On the other side, technological development tends to set up national and international economic orders that homogenize personal and world cultures. Distinctions among markets and ways of life are subsumed within the financial structures of transnational corporations and global communications systems. This paradox of inequity and homogenization poses a fundamental challenge to both reflection and action.

Attempts to address this challenge can be found in the alternative technology movement, arguments regarding the ethics and politics of development, and in diverse feminist contributions to the philosophy of technology (as collected, for instance, in Rothschild). Feminist critiques of technology, for instance, emphasize both the need for equity and the threats of homogenization. Technologies of the workplace are to a large extent sexually differentiated; those of the home are designed and used in ways that confirm masculine and feminine roles. But technological culture creates images of androgynous liberation while medical procedures diminish the experiences of gendered bodies. In the face of this paradox, what some feminists argue is the need for a new theory and practice of technology itself, a truly alternative technology, one that transforms both its masculine biases and its characteristically modern commitments. The ideals and pursuit of alternative medicines can be interpreted as concrete attempts to achieve such a goal.

Conclusion

Successive technological problems have provoked a series of ethical analyses and moral responses. Reflections on these problems and their emerging responses, because they have been focused on a particular technology, have tended to remain isolated from each other and untested by generalization. Philosophies of technology that have attempted to bridge such particularities, and that include a substantial role for bioethics, can be found in the work of Jonas, Sanmartín, Gilbert Hottois (1990), and Friedrich Rapp (1990).

Complementing such work, problems addressed by the varied discussions of practice have been approached from within a variety of ethical frameworks, among which are natural-law theory, deontologism, and consequentialism. With natural-law theory, one tends to assess technological change in terms of its harmony with some given lawful order perceived in nature. With deontological theory the emphasis is on evaluating the rightfulness and wrongfulness of technological change in accord with some inner criteria of the action. With consequentialism there is an effort to look to the goodness or badness of future results that flow from some particular technology. Each such ethical framework can exhibit selective affinities with different basic theoretical conceptions of technology.

Environmental ethics, for instance, tends to be distinguished by criticisms of technologies that do not harmonize with preexisting natural order. The emphasis here is easily placed on human activity, with nonhuman realities taking on special moral significance. Computer ethics, by contrast, tends to put forth deontological principles about the wrongness, for instance, of the invasion of privacy. Such an ethics emphasizes human intention or volition with respect to technology. Finally, technology policy studies are likely to stress the evaluation of technologies in terms of results, and thus to call attention to the physical consequences of technological decisions. Here the issue of risk becomes a special challenge to the accepted cost-benefit calculus typical of consequentialist analysis.

The suggestive character of such relationships points toward the need for a more systematic pursuit of the philosophy of technology in ways that integrate epistemological, metaphysical, ethical, and political analyses. They also indicate the opportunities for more extended interactions between general philosophies of technology and the issues of biomedical ethics, interactions that have the potential for deepening and increasing the fruitfulness of both.

CARL MITCHAM (1995)
BIBLIOGRAPHY REVISED

SEE ALSO: *Human Dignity; Human Nature; Medicine, Philosophy of; Natural Law; Posthumanism and Transhumanism; Virtue and Character;* and other *Technology* subentries

BIBLIOGRAPHY

For more extensive introductions to philosophy of technology, see Friedrich Rapp (1978), Carl Mitcham (1980), and Frederick Ferré (1988), which can be complemented with the collections of readings by Carl Mitcham and Robert Mackey (1972) and Friedrich Rapp (1974). The most important serials are *Research in Philosophy and Technology* (1978–present) and *Philosophy and Technology* (1981–present). There is also a "Philosophy of Technology" monograph series from Indiana

University Press (1990–present). For bibliography, consult Carl Mitcham and Robert Mackey, *Bibliography of the Philosophy of Technology* (Chicago: University of Chicago Press, 1973; paperback reprint with author index, Ann Arbor: Books on Demand, 1985), and supplements that have appeared in *Research in Philosophy and Technology.*

Achterhuis, Hans, ed. 2001. *American Philosophy of Technology: The Empirical Turn,* tr. Robert P. Crease. Bloomington: Indiana University Press.

Bergson, Henri. 1932. *Les deux sources de la morale et de la religion.* Paris: F. Alcan. Translated by Ruth Ashley Audra, Cloudesley S. H. Brenton, and William H. Carter under the title *The Two Sources of Morality and Religion.* London: Macmillan, 1935.

Bilsker, Richard. 2002. *On the Philosophy of Technology.* Belmont, CA: Wadsworth.

Borgmann, Albert. 1984. *Technology and the Character of Contemporary Life: A Philosophical Inquiry.* Chicago: University of Chicago Press.

Bunge, Mario. 1967. "Action." In *The Search for Truth,* vol. 2 of his *Scientific Research.* Berlin: Springer-Verlag.

Bunge, Mario. 1985. "Technology: From Engineering to Decision Theory." In *Life Science, Social Science, and Technology,* part 2 of *Philosophy of Science and Technology,* vol. 7 of his *Treatise on Basic Philosophy.* Boston: D. Reidel.

Edelbach, Ralph; Wainwright, Steve; Hawes, Worth; and Winston, Morton Emanuel, eds. 2002. *Society, Ethics, and Technology.* Belmont, CA: Wadsworth.

Dessauer, Friedrich. 1927. *Philosophie der Technik: Das Problem der Realisierung.* Bonn: Friedrich Cohen. 2nd enl. edition, *Streit um die Technik.* Frankfurt am Main: J. Knecht, 1956.

Dreyfus, Hubert L. 1972. *What Computers Can't Do: A Critique of Artificial Reason.* New York: Harper and Row. Rev. ed., *What Computers Can't Do: The Limits of Artificial Intelligence.* New York: Harper and Row, 1979. 2nd rev. edition. *What Computers Still Can't Do: A Critique of Artificial Reason.* Cambridge, MA: MIT Press, 1992.

Ellul, Jacques. 1954. *La technique; ou, l'enjeu du siècle.* Paris: Armand Colin. 2nd rev. edition. Paris: Economica, 1990. Translated by John Wilkinson under the title *The Technological Society.* New York: Alfred A. Knopf, 1964.

Ellul, Jacques. 1977. *Le système technicien.* Paris: Calmann-Lévy. Translated by Joachim Neugroschel under the title *The Technological System.* New York: Continuum, 1980.

Ellul, Jacques. 1988. *Le bluff technologique.* Paris: Hachette. Translated by Geoffrey W. Bromiley as *The Technological Bluff.* Grand Rapids, MI: W. B. Eerdmans, 1990.

Feenberg, Andrew. 1991. *Critical Theory of Technology.* New York: Oxford University Press. Carries forward the ideas of Marx, Marcuse, and Habermas.

Fellows, Roger, ed. 1995. *Philosophy and Technology.* New York: Cambridge University Press.

Ferré, Frederick. 1988. *Philosophy of Technology.* Englewood Cliffs, NJ: Prentice-Hall.

ENCYCLOPEDIA OF BIOETHICS 3rd Edition   2509

Foucault, Michel. 1963. *Naissance de la clinique: une archéologie du regard médical.* Paris: Presses Universitaires de France. Translated by A. M. Sheridan Smith under the title *The Birth of the Clinic: An Archeology of Medical Perception.* New York: Pantheon, 1973.

Foucalt, Michel. 1988. *Technologies of the Self: A Seminar with Michel Foucault,* eds. Luther H. Martin, Huck Gutman, and Patrick H. Hutton. Amherst: University of Massachusetts Press.

Habermas, Jürgen. 1968. *Technik und Wissenschaft als "Ideologie."* Frankfurt am Main: Suhrkamp. Translated by Jeremy J. Shapiro as the last three essays in *Toward a Rational Society: Student Protest, Science, and Politics.* Boston: Beacon Press, 1970.

Harding, Sandra and Figueroa, Robert, ed. 2003. *Science and Other Cultures: Diversity in the Philosophy of Science and Technology.* New York: Routledge.

Heidegger, Martin. 1954. "Die Frage nach der Technik." In his Vorträge und Aufsätze, pp. 13–44. Pfullingen: Günther Neske. Translated by William Lovitt under the title "The Question Concerning Technology." In The Question Concerning Technology and Other Essays. San Francisco: Harper & Row, 1977.

Hottois, Gilbert. 1984. Le signe et la technique: La philosophie à l'épreuve de la technique. Paris: Aubier.

Hottois, Gilbert. 1990. *Le paradigme bioéthique: Une éthique pour la technoscience.* Brussels: De Boeck.

Ihde, Don. 1979. *Technics and Praxis.* Boston: D. Reidel.

Ihde, Don. 1990. *Technology and the Lifeworld: From Garden to Earth.* Bloomington: Indiana University Press.

Illich, Ivan. 1973. *Tools for Conviviality.* New York: Harper and Row.

Illich, Ivan. 1976. *Medical Nemesis: The Expropriation of Health.* New York: Pantheon.

Johnson, Deborah G. 1985. *Computer Ethics.* Englewood Cliffs, NJ: Prentice-Hall.

Johnson, Deborah G., ed. 1991. *Ethical Issues in Engineering.* Englewood Cliffs, NJ: Prentice-Hall.

Johnson, Deborah G., and Snapper, John W., eds. 1985. *Ethical Issues in the Use of Computers.* Belmont, CA: Wadsworth.

Jonas, Hans. 1979. *Das Prinzip Verantwortung: Versuch einer Ethik für die technologische Zivilisation.* Frankfurt am Main: Suhrkamp. Translated by Hans Jonas and David Herr under the title *The Imperative of Responsibility: In Search of an Ethics for the Technological Age.* Chicago: University of Chicago Press, 1984.

Jonas, Hans. 1985. *Technik, Medizin und Ethik: Zur Praxis des Prinzips Verantwortung.* Frankfurt am Main: Insel.

Kapp, Ernst. 1877. *Grundlinien einer Philosophie der Technik: Zur Entstehungsgeschichte der Kultur aus neuen Gesichtspunkten.* Braunschweig: G. Westermann.

Marcuse, Herbert. 1964. *One-Dimensional Man: Studies in the Ideology of Advanced Industrial Society.* Boston: Beacon Press.

Martin, Mike W., and Schinzinger, Roland. 1989. *Ethics in Engineering.* 2nd edition. New York: McGraw-Hill.

Mitcham, Carl. 1980. "Philosophy of Technology." In *A Guide to the Culture of Science, Technology, and Medicine,* ed. Paul T. Durbin. New York: Free Press.

Mitcham, Carl. 1996. "The Philosophical Challenge of Technology." *American Catholic Quarterly* 70(Supp): 45–58.

Mitcham, Carl, and Mackey, Robert, eds. 1972. *Philosophy and Technology: Readings in the Philosophical Problems of Technology.* New York: Free Press. Paperback reprint, 1983.

Mumford, Lewis. 1934. *Technics and Civilization.* New York: Harcourt Brace.

Mumford, Lewis. 1967. *Technics and Human Development.* Vol. 1 of *The Myth of the Machine.* New York: Harcourt Brace Jovanovich.

Mumford, Lewis. 1970. *The Pentagon of Power.* Vol. 2 of *The Myth of the Machine.* New York: Harcourt Brace Jovanovich.

Ogburn, William F. 1922. *Social Change with Respect to Culture and Original Nature.* New York: Viking.

Ortega y Gasset, José. 1939. "Meditación de la técnica." In his *Ensimismamiento y alteración.* Buenos Aires: Espasa-Calpe. Collected in vol. 5 of *Obras completas.* Madrid: Alianza, 1946.

Rapp, Friedrich J. 1978. *Analytische Technikphilosophie.* Freiburg: Karl Alber. Translated as *Analytical Philosophy of Technology.* Boston Studies in the Philosophy of Science, vol. 63. Boston: D. Reidel, 1981.

Rapp, Friedrich J. 1982. "Philosophy of Technology." In vol. 2 of *Contemporary Philosophy: A New Survey,* ed. Guttorm Floistad. The Hague: Martinus Nijhoff.

Rapp, Friedrich J., ed. 1974. *Contributions to the Philosophy of Technology: Studies in the Structure of Thinking in the Technological Sciences.* Boston: D. Reidel.

Rapp, Friedrich J., ed. 1990. *Technik und Philosophie.* Düsseldorf: VDI Verlag. A cooperative overview with contributions by Rapp, Alois Huning, Ernst Oldemeyer, Hans Lenk, and Walther Ch. Zimmerli.

Rothschild, Joan, ed. 1983. Machina ex Dea: Feminist Perspectives on Technology. New York: Pergamon.

Sanmartín, José. 1987. Los nuevos redentores: Reflexiones sobre la ingeniería genética, la sociobiología y el mundo feliz que nos prometen. Barcelona: Anthropos.

Scharff, Robert C., and Duske, Val, eds. 2002. *Philosophy of Technology, the Technological Condition: The Technological Condition: An Anthology* (Blackwell Philosophy Anthologies). Malden, MA: Blackwell.

Shrader-Frechette, Kristin S. 1991. *Risk and Rationality: Philosophical Foundations for Populist Reforms.* Berkeley: University of California Press.

Simon, Herbert A. 1969. *The Sciences of the Artificial.* Cambridge, MA: MIT Press. 2nd enl. edition, Cambridge, MA: MIT Press, 1991.

Tiles, Mary, and Oberdiek, Hans. 1995. *Living in a Technological Culture: Human Tools and Human Values.* New York: Routledge.

Weizenbaum, Joseph. 1976. *Computer Power and Human Reason: From Judgment to Calculation.* New York: W. H. Freeman.

Winner, Langdon. 1977. *Autonomous Technology: Technics-out-of-Control as a Theme in Political Theory.* Cambridge, MA: MIT Press.

Winner, Langdon. 1986. *The Whale and the Reactor: A Search for Limits in an Age of High Technology.* Chicago: University of Chicago Press.

TISSUE BANKING AND TRANSPLANTATION, ETHICAL ISSUES IN

• • •

Although the transplantation of solid organs such as kidneys and hearts is familiar to the general public, knowledge about transplants of tissues such as bone, skin, veins, and heart valves is only beginning to be disseminated broadly. In the first decade of the twenty-first century the tissue transplant industry grew rapidly as tissue transplantation became a standard treatment option for thousands of patients. Spurred by technological developments and new clinical applications, the transplantation of human tissue grew from a $20 million industry in the early 1990s to one that was approaching $1 billion. In 1994 an estimated 6,000 persons were tissue donors upon death; by 1999 that number had grown to 20,000, more than tripling.

The great majority of cadaveric organs come from brain-dead, heart-beating donors who are maintained on ventilators, of whom there are an estimated 10,000 to 20,000 each year. The pool of potential tissue donors is in the hundreds of thousands because tissue can be retrieved up to 24 hours after death, assuming that the donor is medically suitable and meets generally applied age criteria. With tissue from one donor going to as many as 50 to 100 recipients, the number of tissue transplants dwarfs that of organ transplants. It is estimated that there were more than 850,000 tissue transplants in 2002. The immunological properties of most tissue are reduced greatly or eliminated in the processing of tissue. Therefore, unlike recipients of solid organs, tissue recipients are not required to take antirejection drugs for the rest of their lives.

With this growth in transplantation have come changes in organization, financing, and regulation, and those changes

have led to unique ethical concerns. Those concerns arise in great measure from the stark contrast between the selfless gift of human tissue by donor families and the commercial forces at play as tissue passes down a complex chain of distribution from donor to recipients.

This entry describes the history, organization, technological developments, clinical applications, and regulation of the tissue industry and then dicusses the ethical issues that have emerged. It is concerned solely with the transplantation of tissues that come as gifts from families whose members have died recently. Other human tissues also may be used for medical and research purposes, including gametes (sperm and eggs), tissue discarded during surgery, blood and blood products, and cell lines grown in laboratories. The collection, distribution, financial implications, regulation, and ethical issues raised by those tissues are different from those which apply to tissues transplanted from newly dead donors to recipients.

History

Although many human tissues can be transplanted, including corneas, heart valves, veins, and skin, the most common type of transplant by far involves musculoskeletal tissue. Legend has it that Saints Cosmos and Damian performed the first transplant (a leg) in 287 C.E., but the first documented successful transplantation of musculoskeletal tissue was performed by the Scottish surgeon William Macewan in 1881. In 1908 the U.S. surgeon Eric Lexer reported transplanting an entire knee joint. Although Inclan established a surgical bone bank (storing bone from living patients) in Cuba in 1942, the U.S. Navy Tissue Bank in Bethesda, Maryland, established in 1949, was the first modern tissue bank. The Navy Tissue Bank recovered and preserved tissues to treat injured servicemen and servicewomen and advanced the science of tissue banking through research programs.

Tissue banks have always attempted to provide tissues needed by surgeons in the form in which they can be used best. The organization and operation of tissue banks have changed in response to changes in practice and demand. In the 1960s and 1970s many hospitals maintained their own surgical discard bone banks, storing primarily femoral heads that were removed during hip replacement surgery. Advances in orthopedic surgery, especially the treatment of primary large bone (e.g., femur, humerus) cancers by replacing entire bones with those obtained from cadavers, increased the need for more sophisticated tissue banking. In the 1980s, local tissue banks began to proliferate and a few regional tissue banks were established. Over time banks began to distribute outside their traditional service areas. Currently, many U.S.

tissue banks have allocation systems that return high-demand tissue to the area that provided the donation and distribute other tissue throughout the country. Some tissue banks distribute tissue to other countries.

Clinical and Organizational Developments

As the proportion of older patients in the United States has grown, there has been a dramatic increase in the types of tissues used for joint replacement surgery, which often requires transplanted bone in combination with a metallic prosthesis. There also has been a major increase in spinal fusion surgery. Some reports estimate that more than 200,000 patients in the United States have received cadaveric bone for spinal surgery. Enhanced techniques for limb salvage surgery in cancer patients have increased the demand for large tissue grafts. Sports medicine uses increasing amounts of *soft tissues,* primarily patellar and Achilles tendons, to repair damaged knee ligaments.

The 1990s saw the development of proprietary processing technologies, patented tissue configurations, and advanced processing systems that result in tissue grafts with very specific dimensions and shapes designed by biomechanical engineers that are used primarily in spinal fusion surgery and sports medicine. These and other developments have resulted in the need to hire new and different kinds of personnel, the move by tissue banks to affiliate with traditional competitors to gain access to new technologies, the elimination of smaller tissue banks, and the consolidation of tissue banks. They also have facilitated the entry into the field of for-profit companies. In 1992 Grafton® demineralized bone matrix (DBM) was introduced by the for-profit company Osteotech. Grafton® and similar DBM products are made from demineralized cortical bone combined with various types of carriers that are designed to function as defect fillers or as adjuncts to traditional bone-grafting techniques to promote bone healing. This type of tissue originally was designed for use in dental and periodontic applications but now is being used broadly in orthopedics and neurosurgery. By 2000 at least five other DBM products were on the market, usually codeveloped and promoted by a nonprofit tissue bank and a for-profit device partner.

Another development that has spawned controversy has been the use of tissue for enhancement purposes. Deep layers of skin can be processed into an acellular form that can be used by plastic surgeons to reconstruct deep dermal defects and scars as well as to smooth out wrinkles and temporarily "puff up" lips. Despite the debate that this use of donated tissue has generated, the industry reports that this type of surgery accounts for only a minuscule proportion of tissue transplants.

By the 1990s larger tissue banks, most of which are nonprofit organizations, were moving toward a more traditional medical device–pharmaceutical sales and marketing system, using professionally trained sales representatives or agents to promote their tissue and services, developing advertisements and brochures, and implementing controversial market-driven practices such as consignment, discounting, and bundling. Nonprofit tissue banks also have entered into relationships with orthopedic and medical device companies, sometimes allowing a device company to process, package, market, and sell the tissue. These activities and relationships have blurred the line between an altruisitic gift and the distribution of a medical device and created ethical challenges relating to the handling of the gift. In 1996 the American Association of Tissue Banks (AATB) adopted a set of principles intended to provide guidance in the growing commercialization of tissue, Ethical Guidelines for Commercial Advertising and Activities.

Regulation and Safety

Although tissue safety is not the only medical and ethical issue in which regulation may come into play, it is a crucial one. The avoidance of potential infection has always been of paramount importance. This is not a simple task because transplant tissue is removed from a dead body that may have been exposed to bacteria, viruses, and other pathogens before death or during the decomposition process. Until the late 1980s processing techniques primarily entailed sterilization, which was felt by many to be mandatory despite concerns that sterilization techniques damage the biological and/or biomechanical properties of tissue.

In the late 1980s the construction of pharmaceutical-grade processing facilities allowed *aseptic processing,* which eliminated the need for sterilization of tissues while maintaining the biomechanical and biological properties of tissue. *Clean room* technology provides an environment with 10 to 100 microorganisms per cubic foot of air. In comparison, a standard operating room, normally the "cleanest" place any patient will enter, provides an environment with 1,000 to 10,000 microorganisms per cubic foot. As tissue transplantation becomes an increasingly integral part of modern medical treatment, processors must strike a balance between the goals of maximal tissue safety and viability.

Regulation of organ transplantation began in the mid-1980s with the passage of the National Organ Transplantation Act and other legislation that initiated federal influence on and regulation of organ procurement and transplantation policy and practice. A national Organ Procurement and Transplantation Network (OPTN) was created at government expense to set organ transplantation policy and gather data on organ transplantation events. The transplant community formed the United Network of Organ Sharing (UNOS), which obtained the OPTN contract. None of this authority, however, has been extended to tissue transplant practices. In addition, organ procurement organizations (OPOs) were given the authority to operate within a designated territory by the Health Care Financing Administration (HCFA, now the Centers for Medicare and Medicaid Services, or CMS), which also provided for financial reimbursement for the costs associated with kidney transplantation. Tissue banks, in contrast, were not and still are not compensated directly by the federal government for their operations, and there are no governmental regulations or guidelines that govern the organization of tissue banks.

Despite their safety risks, tissue banks were subject to very little federal regulation until the 1990s. In 1976 the AATB was founded as scientific nonprofit peer group organization to address issues of donor criteria and recovery and processing systems with an eye toward maintaining quality and safety. In the mid-1980s it established standards for acceptable norms of technical and ethical performance, including a program of inspection and accreditation. However, the AATB is strictly voluntary. In 2002 it listed 73 accredited banks among the estimated 100-plus banks in the United States. Among the unaccredited banks are some of the largest tissue processors. Only a handful of states have any type of tissue bank regulation.

A seminal event occurred in 1991 with the report of the transmission of human immunodeficiency virus (HIV) from an organ and tissue donor who had tested negatively for the antibody to HIV. This focused the public's attention on the potential for disease transmission, especially the need for more rigorous donor screening. In 2001 safety issues resurfaced. The Federal Drug Administration (FDA) and the Centers for Disease Control (CDC) reported several cases of infection, possibly caused by donor tissue in recipients, including one that resulted in the death of the patient. In 2002 the CDC issued a report documenting fifty-four tissue infections that had occurred over several years, noting, however, that out of an estimated 650,000 annual tissue transplants, bacterial infection was a rare complication. Later in 2002 there were reports involving six organ and tissue recipients who contracted hepatitis C from an organ and tissue donor, and several organ recipients who were infected with West Nile virus, including a number who died. Creutzfeldt-Jakob disease, the human variant of mad cow disease, looms as a potential hazard, and new testing regimens to screen out potential donors with these diseases are awaited by the tissue banking and surgical communities.

FDA regulation of tissue banking began in earnest in 1993 with the Interim Rule for Banked Human Tissue, which was intended to require infectious disease testing, donor screening, and record keeping. Among the things required were extensive interviews about a potential donor's sexual history, use of illegal drugs, and other exposure to infectious diseases. This rule was finalized in 1997 and resulted in in-depth training of tissue bank and hospital staff and a lengthy interview (between thirty and sixty minutes) with a grieving family member. During that time the FDA also began routinely inspecting tissue banks, suggesting changes, and conducting mandatory recalls at large tissue banks that remained out of compliance. It is anticipated that additional FDA regulations for good tissue banking practices will be issued in 2004.

In 1997 the Centers for Medicare and Medicaid Services (CMS) established regulations that changed the system of organ and tissue donation dramatically. The Conditions of Participation (CoP) required that all hospital deaths be reported to the OPO that serves the hospital and that all those deaths be evaluated as potential donors. The results of the CoPs were most notable among tissue banks, which often experienced an increase of over 50 percent in their tissue donors.

Ethical Issues

As tissue transplantation has gained visibility, it has attracted the attention of critics. In April 2000 the *Orange Country Register* ran a series of articles titled "The Body Brokers." With provocative headlines such as "Assembly Line" and "Skin Merchants," the newspaper raised concern that the tissue industry was commodifying the human body, making outrageous profits, and irresponsibly allocating skin for "cosmetic" purposes. According to those and other allegations, the industry was violating the trust of grieving families that altruistically had donated tissue. The tissue industry replied that those allegations were inflammatory and inaccurate. However, press coverage brought the the industry to public attention. Several senators approached the secretary of the U.S. Department of Health and Human Services (DHHS), Donna Shalala, who asked the DHHS's inspector general to investigate. Out of that investigation came two thorough 2001 reports, *Oversight of Tissue Banking* and *Informed Consent in Tissue Donation: Expectations and Realities.*

As was mentioned above, the ethical issues of tissue banking arise largely from the apparent contrast between the way society views the source of human tissue and the industrial and commercial aspects of tissue processing and distribution. Like organs, tissue comes as an altruistic gift from grieving families. The notion of altruistic donation has been the bedrock of the ways in which organs and tissues are obtained. The National Organ Transplant Act specifically prohibited the sale of human organs and tissues, allowing only reasonable charges for the costs of retrieval, processing, and the like. Whereas some would argue that financial incentives and even outright payment should be allowed to increase the supply of organs, the law continues to recognize only altruistic donation.

Commerce is not absent from organ transplantation, however. Surgeons, hospitals, OPOs, and pharmaceutical companies, among others, make money from their participation in the transplantation process. However, with tissue transplantation, commodification and commercialization are much more evident. Unlike organs, which remain identifiable as organs in their relatively brief journey from donor to recipient, many tissue forms are highly processed and machined into forms that no longer resemble the bones or skin from which they were derived. Tissue forms are packaged much like pharmaceutical products and medical devices and can be stored for distribution years later. As they pass down the chain of distribution from donor to recipients, for-profit companies enter into the process. Many of those companies have invested capital to develop new processes for which they hold patents.

Unlike organs, tissue is rarely lifesaving, with skin for severe burn victims being the major exception. Instead, tissues are used to treat medical and surgical illnesses that are debilitating but not necessarily life-threatening. Sometimes tissue products are employed for cosmetic or enhancement purposes.

In summary, the chain of distribution of tissue from donor to recipient involves multiple players, including organ procurement organizations, nonprofit and for-profit tissue banks, and publicly held companies that process and distribute tissue. Tissue often is changed from its original form into packaged grafts that may sit on shelves to be distributed months or years later. Value is thus added to tissue as it passes along the chain of distribution. Sometimes donated tissue can be used for enhancement rather than saving lives or the treatment of serious medical and surgical conditions.

These characteristics make the commodification and commercialization of tissue much more evident than those of solid organs and, most important, present a stark contrast to the altruistic gifts of grieving families that make the entire enterprise possible. This contrast forms the basis for much of the criticism of the tissue industry. For example, if the families that selflessly donate do not make money, why should others? Another criticism is that families would not want their gifts used for cosmetic purposes.

Two potential solutions to these problems are not acceptable in the current legal and cultural context. On the one hand, society could abandon altruism and allow families to sell tissue at its fair market value. On the other hand, financial incentives could be eliminated from the processing and distribution of tissue. The first solution would eliminate the traditional basis of organ and tissue procurement: the gift. The second would bring an increasingly successful and desired clinical intervention to a halt.

Informed Consent

As a more realistic alternative many have suggested a rigorous informed consent process. If families were informed about the commodification and commercial aspects of their gifts, they would have the freedom not to give them. This would avoid the abandonment of both altruism and the market forces that have allowed the tissue industry to flourish. Although this suggestion has great merit, it also has several limitations.

First, the informed consent model does not fit the situation perfectly. People think of informed consent as the principle governing the decision of patients to consent to treatment or that of research subjects to consent to research. With tissue donation, the patient is dead and no treatment or research is involved. The decision to donate generally is made by a family member. Second, the request is made under less than ideal conditions: The family is in the middle of a crisis, and the request most often is made by a stranger, frequently over the telephone. In these circumstances the ability and willingness of the family to receive and process large amounts of information are limited. Third, issues involving the financial aspects of donation are complicated and to some extent dependent on the political views of the requestor and the family member. Is it possible, for example, to give a robust description of the structure and function of the tissue transplant industry in the context in which the request is made? Even if one attempted to do that, what words and tone should be used? Should the difference between for-profit and not-for-profit organizations be explained? Should the realities of the market economy be presented? Should those realities be praised or criticized, and in what balance? Words such as *for profit* and *making money* used out of context can be provocative and even manipulative. However, avoiding a discussion of these issues might allow people to naïvely imagine that their gifts of tissue make their way to grateful recipients without money changing hands or acting as an incentive.

Some things are known about what families want to be told. In 2000 the University of Florida Tissue Bank released the results of two telephone surveys of 507 persons who had been offered the option of tissue donation at the death of a family member. Among those who donated, 86 percent said they had enough time to make a decision, whereas 73 percent of nondonors said they did not. Twenty-eight percent of donors and 36 percent of nondonors said they did not receive enough information. Thirty-five percent of donors and 43 percent of nondonors said it would have been helpful to know that recovered tissue is "sent to companies" and in that group10 percent of donors said that knowing would have made a difference in their decisions. Forty-one percent of donors and 49 percent of nondonors said they would have wanted to know costs are associated with recovery, preparation, distribution, and surgery, including salaries, materials, shipping, and administration. Nineteen percent of donors said that knowing those facts would have made a difference in their decisions. Forty-eight percent of donors and 24 percent of nondonors said that profits should be permitted.

Donor families that have written on the subject point out that not all donor families think alike and acknowledge their ambivalence about their right to information versus their ability to process information in the middle of a tragedy.

After interviewing 30 organizations involved in tissue recovery and receiving more than 50 responses to a questionnaire from donor families, the inspector general of the DHHS concluded that the expectations of altruistic motives among donor families are the foundation of tissue banking. The report, *Informed Consent in Tissue Banking: Expectations and Realities,* said that, among other things:

- Large-scale financial operations may overshadow the underlying altruistic nature of tissue donation.
- After processing, tissue and products containing tissue often are marketed and sold as a medical supply rather than as a donation.
- Some tissues, particularly skin, may be processed into products that are used for cosmetic puposes.

The inspector general concluded that the special nature of tissue and the way in which it is made available call for steps beyond those which apply to most other businesses and philanthropic enterprises. He called for the HHS Division of Transplantation to identify principles and guidelines that should underpin consent requests; make suggestions about the type, format, and content of written information that should be shared with families; make recommendations about training tissue bank staff and external requestors; and make recommendations about ways to evaluate the effectiveness of requestors. He also called on the tissue industry to give written materials to families at the time of a request or in the days immediately afterward, including a copy of the consent form, a full description of the uses to which donated

tissue may be put, and a list of other companies and entities with which the bank has relationships, and to indicate clearly on all tissue packaging and marketing materials that the contents are derived from donated human tissue. Finally, the report called for the tissue banking industry to explore a process for public disclosure of tissue banks' financing and research into what types and how much financial information would be useful for families and to consider the impact of that disclosure on the rate of donation.

The report also asked the tissue banking industry to work with groups representing the interests of donor families. The most prominent of those groups is the National Donor Family Council of the National Kidney Foundation. The council is an organization of over 8,000 donor families whose mission is to nurture and protect the interests of donor families as well as to promote donation. In 2000 the Donor Family Council issued a report titled *Informed Consent Policy for Tissue Donation* that called for full disclosure of the facts, including the ways in which tissue is recovered, processed, stored, and distributed. The report also said that families should have the right to restrict use of the tissue they donate. It did not mention financial issues.

In response to those suggestions the transplant community has begun to strengthen the process of informed consent. Many tissue banks now offer informational brochures to donor families that more clearly outline the specifics of donation, including the fact that tissue may be processed into many forms and sizes and may be stored for extended periods and the fact that for-profit companies may be involved in the processing. Education for tissue requestors also has been expanded. Tissue banks routinely offer donor families follow-up information, including copies of the consent form. The AATB, the Association of Organ Procurement Organizations (AOPO), and the Eye Bank Association of America (EBAA) established guidelines for obtaining informed consent on tissue donation that formed the basis of many recovery agencies' consent policies. In addition, the AOPO established suggested guidelines for its members to use in selecting a tissue processor or tissue banking partner.

Many commentators think that the inherent limitations of those recommendations call for other mechanisms to protect potential donors and the integrity of the industry. One of those mechanisms is public education. If the general public better understood the way tissue is altered and the financial realities of tissue processing and distribution, there would be less need to place the burden for sharing that information only at the moment of the actual request. The inspector general, for example, recommended that the tissue banking industry work with groups representing donor families to explore a process for disclosure of tissue banks' financing, including knowledge about the sources of tissue banks' funding and other entities with which tissue banks have financial arrangements. Proposed legislation in California would mandate that families be given information about the involvement of for-profit companies and the possibility of cosmetic uses of tissue and be given the option to "opt out" of those scenarios.

Many states have passed laws that may further change the landscape as it relates to obtaining consent. Known as designated donation or first person consent, those laws give individuals an opportunity to declare their intention (or consent) to donate upon death and do not allow the next of kin to override that declaration. These laws present an entirely new set of challenges for OPOs, tissue banks, and eye banks: If an individual has declared his or her desire to "be an organ donor," does that necessarily refer to any body part that can be transplanted? Did that person receive full information about tissue donation so that the decision to donate was fully informed? What if the family objects strongly? Should the recovery agency move forward without regard for their feelings?

Good Stewardship

In the essay "The Gift and the Market" Courtney Campbell argues against the industrial perception of tissue banking, emphasizing instead that the tissue industry should "act in accordance with a model of 'stewardship of the gift'" (Campbell, p. 207). The acceptance of the gift of tissue, he writes, involves harmony between donor and recipient in regard to the meaning of the gift, the intention for its use, and the relationship of giver and recipient. Others also have emphasized this point. For example, Helen Leslie and Scott Bottenfield from LifeNet, one of the United States' leading tissue banks, in the essay "Donation, Banking and Transplantation of Allograft Tissues" note that "it is only through the humanitarian actions of donors and donor families—people helping people, the noblest of principles—that tissue transplantation is made possible" (Leslie and Bottomfield, p. 281). Stewardship mediates the relationship of the donor to the recipient. It provides a moral connection between the gift and the use of the gift and establishes a framework for enhancing the value of the gift as long as the intent of the donor is respected and the benefits of the gift are directed toward the larger community, not claimed solely as proprietary interests by tissue bankers, processors, and distributors.

Good stewardship in the context of human tissue for transplantation means that the industry should take collective responsibility by doing the following:

- Minimizing commodification by insisting that all packaged tissue prominently reveal its origin as an altruistic gift;
- Adopting nationwide rules for the just allocation and distribution of tissues, for example, making sure that purely cosmetic uses of tissue occur only after more worthy needs are met;
- Working to make tissue as safe as possible;
- Making sure that all tissue recovery is done by nonprofit organizations whose finances are publicly known;
- Maintaining a publicly accessible national database against which potential problems can be assessed rationally; and
- Providing a public forum for discussion and debate of controversial issues.

Although the industry has begun to adopt some of these aspects of good stewardship, there is much room for improvement and it remains to be seen how active a role the federal government will assume in pushing for these important moral and social goals.

MARTHA ANDERSON
STUART J. YOUNGNER
SCOTT BOTTENFIELD
RENIE SHAPIRO

SEE ALSO: *Human Dignity; Organ and Tissue Procurement; Organ Transplants, Medical Overview of; Organ Transplants, Sociocultural Aspects of*

BIBLIOGRAPHY

American Association of Tissue Banks, Eye Bank Association of America, and Association of Organ Procurement Organizations. 2000. *Model Elements of Informed Consent for Organ and Tissue Donation: Joint Statement.*

Campbell, Courtney. 2003. "The Gift and the Market: Cultural Symbolic Perspectives." In *Tissue Transplantation, Ethical Issues,* ed. Stuart Youngner, Martha Anderson, and Renie Schapiro. Oxford: Oxford University Press.

Leslie, Helen W., and Bottenfield, Scott. 1989. "Donation, Banking and Transplantation of Allograft Tissues." *Nursing Clinics of North America* 24: 891–905.

National Donor Family Council, Executive Committee. 2000a. *Position Statement on Tissue Donation.* New York: National Kidney Foundation.

National Donor Family Council, Executive Committee. 2000b. *Informed Consent Policy for Tissue Donation.* New York: National Kidney Foundation.

National Organ Transplantation Act of 1984 (PL 98–507).

Scott, M.; Oppenheim, A.; and Rodrigue, J. 2000. *Adequacy of Informed Consent for Tissue Donation: A Survey of Donor Families.* Gainesville: University of Florida Tissue Bank, Inc.

Tomford, W. W. 1993. "A History of Musculoskeletal Tissue Banking in the United States." In *Musculoskeletal Tissue Banking,* ed. W. W. Tomford. New York: Raven Press.

U.S. Congress. 1984. *National Organ Transplantation Act* (PL 98–507).

U.S. Department of Health and Human Services, Office of the Inspector General. 2001. *Informed Consent in Tissue Donation: Expectations and Realities.* Washington, D.C.: Author.

U.S. Department of Health and Human Services, Office of the Inspector General. 2001. *Oversight of Tissue Banking.* Washington, D.C.: Author.

Youngner, Stuart; Anderson, Martha; and Schapiro, Renie. 2003. *Tissue Transplantation: Ethical Issues.* Oxford: Oxford University Press.

INTERNET RESOURCES

American Association of Tissue Banks, Eye Bank Association of America, and Association of Organ Procurement Organizations. 2000. *Model Elements of Informed Consent for Organ and Tissue Donation: Joint Statement.* Available from <http://www.aatb.org>.

Office of the Inspector General, Department of Health and Human Services. 2001a. *Informed Consent in Tissue Donation: Expectations and Realities.* Available from <http://www.fda.gov/cber/tissue/infrmcnsnt.pdf>.

Office of the Inspector General. 2001b. *Oversight of Tissue Banking.* Available from <http://www.fda.gov/cber/tissue/ovrst0101.pdf>.

TRANSHUMANISM AND POSTHUMANISM

• • •

At one time or another, most people have dreamed of having the ability to fly (without technological assistance), of never having to have to age or die, or of having bodies and minds that transcend human limitations. Yet in the end people move on with their lives, trying to learn to deal with the realities of finitude and mortality. This is necessary, given the lack of means to significantly alter biological constraints. Yet new technologies may soon begin to enable people to transcend such limitations. With such technologies, however, come questions about the appropriateness of actually pursuing and employing them to experience greatly extended longevity—perhaps even some form of physical immortality—and to re-engineer the human body to expand

its functional capacity. Transhumanism and posthumanism are worldviews, or philosophies, that strongly favor an affirmative reply to these questions and that look forward to the day when *homo sapiens* have been replaced by biologically and technologically superior beings.

Transhumanism has been defined as "the intellectual and cultural movement that affirms the possibility and desirability of fundamentally improving the human condition through applied reason, especially by using technology to eliminate aging and greatly enhance human intellectual, physical, and psychological capacities" (Bostrum, 1999). A posthuman would no longer be a human being, having been so significantly altered as to no longer represent the human species. Underlying this worldview is a core belief that the human species in its current form does not represent the end of our development, but rather its beginning (Bostrum, 1999).

The tools transhumanists would use to achieve their ends include genetic manipulation, nanotechnology, cybernetics, pharmacological enhancement, and computer simulation. The most ambitious—and controversial—transhumanist vision involves the concept of *mind uploading.* According to proponents, advances in computing and neurotechnologies will, within several decades, enable individuals to completely read the synaptic connections of the human brain, enabling an exact replica of the brain to exist and function inside a computer. This simulation could then "live" in whatever mechanical body-form it desired (Kurzweil). In his book *The Enchanted Loom* (1981), Richard Jastrow speculated about this future time: "At last, the human brain, ensconced in a computer, has been liberated from the weakness of the mortal flesh.... It is in control of its own destiny.... Housed in indestructible lattices of silicon, and no longer constrained in its span of years, ... such a life could live forever" (p.166–167).

Origins of Transhumanism

While the terms *transhumanism* and *posthumanism* are very recent in creation, the ideas they represent are anything but new. The underlying philosophical ideals are fully those of the Enlightenment, imbued with a healthy dose of postmodern relativism. From the Enlightenment comes a fully reductionistic view of human life characteristic of that movement's materialistic empiricism. In *L'Homme Machine (Man a Machine),* written in 1748, the French physician and philosopher Julien Offray de la Mettrie wrote that humans "are, at bottom only animals and machines," while the Marquis de Condorcet, another French Enlightenment philosopher, wrote in 1794 that "no bounds have been fixed to the improvement of faculties ... the perfectibility of man is unlimited." These eighteenth century ideas could be easily updated to recent transhumanist writings, such as Bart Kosko's *The Fuzzy Future* (1999), in which he proclaims: "Biology is not destiny. It was never more than tendency. It was just nature's first quick and dirty way to compute with meat. Chips are destiny" (p. 256). Consider also Kevin Warwick's declaration, written in 2000, "I was born human. But this was an accident of fate—a condition merely of time and place. I believe it's something we have the power to change" (p. 145). Derived from other Enlightenment ideals is a fierce libertarianism, supported by a postmodern moral skepticism, that proclaims that each individual is the final arbiter of what is right and appropriate for his or her life or body. One also sees a precedent for transhumanist thinking in Frederick Nietzche's thoughts on the will to power and the *ubermensche* (superman), particularly in *Thus Spake Zarathustra*, "man is something to be overcome"(p. 12).

As a named movement, transhumanism started in the 1980s with the writings of a futurist known as FM-2030, with the term *transhuman* being a shorthand for *transitional human* (Bostrom, 1999). Transhumans were "the earliest manifestation of new evolutionary beings, on their way to becoming posthumans" (FM-2030). Within the first years of the 1990s, a whole series of groups emerged embracing transhumanist ideology, including the Extropians, the Transtopians, and the Singularitarians, the latter group anticipating and working to bring about the technological "Singularity" predicted by Vernor Vinge. Writing in 1993, Vinge predicted that the exponential increase in scientific and technical knowledge, coupled with feedback loops from artificial intelligence systems, would soon lead to a massive destabilization and transformation of all social structures, technical devices, and human beings, who would be transformed into superior beings. While the Singularity is the most extreme of the transhumanist visions, the idea that humankind should engineer the next phase of its own evolution, and that human beings should be augmented and altered, even to the point of losing their humanity, has captured the thinking of numerous faculty and leaders in the engineering and scientific establishment. This can no better be illustrated than the National Science Foundation's (NSF) proposed plan for converging several technologies, including nanotechnology, biotechnologies, information technologies, and cognitive technologies (such as cybernetics and neurotechnologies) for the expressed purpose of improving human performance (Roco and Bainbridge).

Fundamentals of Transhumanism and Posthumanism

The first assertion of transhumanist thinking is a rejection of the assumption that human nature is a constant (Bostrom, 1999). There is nothing sacrosanct about *nature* in general, or about *human nature* in particular. Criticisms of attempts to modify nature as "playing God" or as the ultimate human hubris are therefore rejected as inappropriate.

Katherine Hayles, in her book *How We Became Posthuman* (1999), describes four characteristic posthuman, or transhuman, assumptions. First, information patterns are more important or essential to the nature of being than any "material instantiation, so that embodiment in a biological substrate is seen as an accident of history rather than an inevitability of life" (p. 2). Second, consciousness is an epiphenomenon. There is no immaterial soul. Third, the body is simply a prosthesis, albeit the first one we learn to use and manipulate. Consequently, replacing or enhancing human function with other prostheses is only a natural extension of our fundamental relationship with our begotten bodies. Lastly, the posthuman views the human being as capable of being "seamlessly articulated with intelligent machines. In the posthuman, there are no essential differences or absolute demarcations between bodily existence and computer simulation, cybernetic mechanism and biological organism, robot technology and human goals" (p. 3).

Ethical Issues

One of the first significant ethical issues relating to transhumanism and posthumanism is the question of enhancement or augmentation: should human beings augment or enhance themselves and future generations? This is not a simple question to answer, though humans have made a practice of augmenting and enhancing themselves throughout recorded history. This is the nature and explicit goal of all tool use and education. Yet there are some implicit boundaries that transhumanist modifications challenge.

As an example, consider correction of vision. The use of glasses or contact lenses to correct vision is an example of a commonly employed augmentation. Yet this intervention is only correcting a deficiency, returning the individuals function to species-normal levels. It is thus a healing intervention more than an enhancement. What becomes problematic for some is when the augmentation or enhancement in question potentially exceeds the function that could be achieved by the finest specimens of *homo sapiens* trained in the most rigorous fashion. People accept the use of some enhancing technologies, such as telescopy or microscopy, which may be used for a time, and for a specific purpose, but cannot become a permanent fixture of the human being. They remain tools, rather than becoming attributes. Thus it is acceptable to use a computer or personal digital assistant (PDA), which can be separated from the user, but permanently enhancing the brain with cybernetic connections or brain implants seems to many to cross a boundary that should not be violated. Why is this so?

Two criticisms of such permanent enhancements are that: (1) they are unnatural; and (2) they engage people in activities that should be the sole purview of the deity—"Playing God" is a frequent aspersion thrown at enhancement technologies. While these are both legitimate concerns, the rhetoric used in the critique typically misses the point, which is a concern about the appropriateness, personal and social consequences, and wisdom of pursuing the proposed modifications and are thus generally dismissed as irrelevant by transhumanists (without addressing the genuine issues).

Transhumanists dismiss the claim of *unnatural* because most of what human beings do with any technology is *unnatural*, yet these uses are accepted as benefits, not harms. As to the second argument, many, if not most, transhumanists are agnostic or atheists, and thus engaging in a supposed Promethean rebellion against the gods is not to them a legitimate concern. The issue is one of great concern to theists, however, though the way the argument is commonly expressed comes close to violating their own basic theological tenants. Can God be so easily dethroned? Can the creature really act outside the permissive will of the creator? Further, many theologians assert that part of the *Imago Dei,* the "image of God," that humankind is said to bear, is the creative impulse.

The real issue of concern to those who object to or are wary of transhumanist goals is that human beings are engaging in activities that may have a profound impact on the individuals involved, as well as on the surrounding environment, without balancing forces or divine wisdom that might minimize possible negative consequences of such activities. From the environmental, or naturalist, perspective, the changes are occurring too swiftly and too dramatically for ecosystems or individual creatures to evolve appropriate safeguards or counterbalances. From the more theistic perspective, these changes are occurring without proper understanding and respect for God's initial designs and plan, and certainly without God's foresight or wisdom. In the end, both arguments are expressing concern for the great harm that these interventions could potentially induce, calling into question activities that presuppose a significant degree of knowledge, foresight, and wisdom that may, and most likely will, be lacking. Hubris, therefore, not ingenuity or even a passion for change, is the fundamental problem.

For others, however, even if such enhancements would not be tried until there was careful prospective evaluation for, and protections against, undesirable consequences, any

intervention intended to move function beyond species-normal levels would be rejected. This leads to the next series of concerns: the social consequences of transhumanism. The pursuit of transhumanist goals could lead to individuals and communities possessing significant differences in the type and extent of biotechnological modifications. One consequence of these disparities will be the likelihood of discrimination—against both the enhanced and the unenhanced, as each community may feel threatened by the other. Claims of unfair competitive advantage are probable, potentially leading to attempts at restrictive legislation. Yet it is doubtful such restrictions would find sufficient consensus to be passed, let alone prevent the enhancements from taking place. According to Freeman Dyson, a British physicist and educator, "the artificial improvement of human beings will come, one way or another, whether we like it or not, as soon as the progress of biological understanding makes it possible. When people are offered technical means to improve themselves and their children, no matter what they conceive improvement to mean, the offer will be accepted.... The technology of improvement may be hindered or delayed by regulation, but it cannot be permanently suppressed.... It will be seen by millions of citizens as liberation from past constraints and injustices. Their freedom to choose cannot be permanently denied" (p. 205–206). Particularly powerful—especially in the United States, which is predicated upon the right to life, liberty, and the pursuit of happiness—is the argument posed by the transhumanist Anders Sandberg that freedom to pursue enhancing technologies is a fundamental matter of the right to life.

One likely consequence of this is that multiple communities will develop that adhere to certain values and agreed-upon levels of technological modification. But as some groups may choose lesser degrees of enhancement they may run the risk of becoming ghettoized or restricted from other goods of the larger society that they may still desire. While some transhumanists are quite clear that they do not wish to force their desires for enhancement onto others (Bostrom, 1999), as a group, or even as individual scholars, they have not satisfactorily resolved how tolerance will be maintained both within and outside their communities of choice. In fact, some transhumanists already display belligerent attitudes against skeptics and dissenters (Dvorsky; Smith; Shropshire).

This fact itself acknowledges one of the fundamental flaws of transhumanist, or any other, utopian thinking: the failure to understand the darkness, the fears, and the unpredictability of each human heart. The lesson of the twentieth century, such as the experience with eugenics, fascism, and communism, should have been to beware the power of utopian dreams to enslave, destroy, and demean, rather than provide the promised justice, freedom, and human flourishing. Now the transhumanists offer yet another form of human contrivance to provide salvation for all. This time the faustian bargain is with technology—what John McDermott, a professor emeritus in labor studies at the State University of New York at Old Westbury, has referred to as "the opiate of the intellectuals"—rather than with economic or political systems.

Technology is not inherently evil, and has in fact been the source of much good (as well as harm). It is but a tool, and as a tool must be carefully examined and carefully used. Transforming ourselves into our tools in the hopes of achieving immortality is an illusion. Decay cannot be forestalled indefinitely. If one must change the underlying substrate of the body to "live," then it is really something else that exists, not the original being, and death will still need to be confronted. Extended life may be achieved, but at what social cost? How will people deal with greatly enhanced life spans? What will be the impact on economic structures, the workforce, and reproduction? These questions are all, as yet, unanswered by the transhumanists and the Converging Technologies project of the NSF. While it is doubtful that consensus could ever be reached on enhancing or augmenting technologies, humankind must engage prospectively in a full and open dialogue concerning the coming technologies and their implications.

C. CHRISTOPHER HOOK

SEE ALSO: *Cybernetics; Enhancement Uses of Medical Technology; Nanotechnology*

BIBLIOGRAPHY

Broderick, Damien. 2001. *The Spike: How Our Lives Are Being Transformed by Rapidly Advancing Technology.* New York: Forge.

Dyson, Freeman J. 1997. *Imagined Worlds.* Cambridge, MA: Harvard University Press.

Hayles, N. Katherine. 1999. *How We Became Posthuman: Virtual Bodies in Cybernetics, Literature and Informatics.* Chicago: University of Chicago Press.

Jastrow, Richard. 1981. *The Enchanted Loom: Mind in the Universe.* New York: Simon & Schuster.

FM-2030. 1989. *Are You a Transhuman?* New York: Warner Books.

Kosko, Bart. 1999. *The Fuzzy Future: From Society and Science to Heaven in a Chip.* New York: Harmony Books.

Kurzweil, Ray. 1999. *The Age of Spiritual Machines: When Computers Exceed Human Intelligence.* New York: Viking.

McDermott, John. 1969. "Technology: The Opiate of the Intellectuals." *New York Review of Books.*

Nietzche, Frederick. 1995 (1883–1892). *Thus Spake Zarathustra,* trans. Walter Kaufmann. New York: Modern Library.

INTERNET RESOURCES

Bostrom, Nick. 1999. "The Transhumanist FAQ." Available from <http://www.transhumanism.org/resources/faq.html>.

Bostrom, Nick. 2001. "What Is Transhumanism?" Available from <http://www.nickbostrum.com>.

Condorcet, Marquis de (Marie Jean Antoine Nicholas Caritat). 1795. "The Future Progress of the Human Mind." Available from <http://www.fordham.edu/halsall/mod/condorcet-progress.html>.

de la Mettrie, Julien Offray. 1748. "L'Homme Machine (Man a Machine)." Available from <http://www.santafe.edu/˜shalizi/LaMettrie/Machine>.

Dvorsky, George. 2002. "Ending Biblical Brainwash." Available from <http://www.betterhumans.com>.

Foresight Institute. 2003. Available from <http://www.foresight.org>.

KurzweilAI.net. 2003. Available from <http://www.kurzweilai.net>.

Principia Cybernetic Project. 2003. Available from <http://www.pespmc.vub.ac.be>.

Roco, Mikail, and William Sims Bainbridge, eds. 2002. "Converging Technologies For Improving Human Performance." Available from <http://www.wtec.org/ConvergingTechnologies/Report/nbic-complete-screen.pdf>.

Sandberg, Anders. 2001. "Morphological Freedom—Why We Not Just Want It, but Need It." Available from <http://www.nada.kth.se/˜asa/Texts>.

Schropshire, Philip. 2002. "The Battle for Biotech." Available from <http://www.betterhumans.com>.

Smith, Simon. 2002. "Killing Immortality." Available from <http://www.betterhumans.com>.

Vinge, Vernor. 1993. "The Coming Technological Singularity." Available from <http://www.rohan.sdsu.edu/faculty/vinge>.

Warwick, Kevin. 2000. "Cyborg 1.0." *Wired.* Available from <http://wired.com>.

World Transhumanist Association. 2003. Available from <http://www.transhumanism.org>.

TRIAGE

• • •

Triage is the medical assessment of patients to establish their priority for treatment. When medical resources are limited and immediate treatment of all patients is impossible, patients are *sorted* in order to use the resources most effectively. The process of triage was first developed and refined in military medicine, and later extended to disaster and emergency medicine.

In recent years, it has become common to use the term *triage* in a wide variety of contexts where decisions are made about allocating scarce medical resources. However, triage should not be confused with more general expressions such as *allocation* or *rationing* (Childress). Triage is a process of screening patients on the basis of their immediate medical needs and the likelihood of medical success in treating those needs. Unlike the everyday practice of allocating medical resources, triage usually takes place in urgent circumstances, requiring quick decisions about the critical care of a pool of patients. Generally, these decisions are controlled by a mixture of utilitarian and egalitarian considerations.

History

Baron Dominique Jean Larrey, Napoleon's chief medical officer, is credited with organizing the first deliberate plan for classifying military casualties (Hinds, 1975). Larrey was proud of his success in treating battle casualties despite severe scarcity of medical resources. He insisted that those who were most seriously wounded be treated first, regardless of rank (Larrey). Although there is no record of Larrey's using the term *triage,* his plan for sorting casualties significantly influenced later military medicine.

The practice of systematically sorting battle casualties first became common during World War I. It was also at this time that the term *triage* entered British and U.S. military medicine from the French (Lynch, Ford, and Weed). Originally, *triage* (from the French verb *trier,* "to sort") referred to the process of sorting agricultural products such as wool and coffee. In military medicine, *triage* was first used both for the process of prioritizing casualty treatment and for the place where such screening occurred. At the *poste de triage* (casualty clearing station), casualties were assessed for the severity of their wounds and the need for rapid evacuation to hospitals in the rear. The emphasis was on determining need for immediate treatment and the feasibility of transport.

The following triage categories have become standard, even though terminology may vary:

1. *Minimal.* Those whose injuries are slight and require little or no professional care.
2. *Immediate.* Those whose injuries, such as airway obstruction or hemorrhaging, require immediate medical treatment for survival.

3. *Delayed.* Those whose injuries, such as burns or closed fractures of bones, require significant professional attention that can be delayed for some period of time without significant increase in the likelihood of death or disability.
4. *Expectant.* Those whose injuries are so extensive that there is little or no hope of survival, given the available medical resources.

First priority is given to those in the immediate group. Next, as time and resources permit, care is given to the delayed group. Little, beyond minimal efforts to provide comfort care, is given to those in the expectant category. Active euthanasia for expectant casualties has been considered but is almost never mentioned in triage proposals (British Medical Association, 1988). Those in the minimal group are sent to more distant treatment facilities or left to take care of themselves until all other medical needs are met.

From the beginning, the expressed reasons for such sorting were a blend of utilitarian and egalitarian considerations. Larrey stressed equality of care for casualties sorted into the same categories. On the other hand, one early text on military medicine advised, "The greatest good of the greatest number must be the rule" (Keen, p. 13). Over the years, it also became clear that the utilitarian principle could be interpreted in different ways. The most obvious meaning was that of limited medical utility: The good to be sought was saving the greatest number of casualties' lives.

But the principle could also be construed to mean doing the greatest good for the military effort. When interpreted this way, triage could produce very different priorities. For example, it was sometimes proposed that priority be given to the least injured in order to return them quickly to battle (Lee). An oft-cited example of the second use of the utilitarian principle for triage occurred during World War II (Beecher). Commanders of U.S. forces in North Africa had to decide how to use their extremely limited supply of penicillin. The choice was between battle casualties with infected wounds and soldiers with gonorrhea. The decision was made to give priority to those with venereal disease, on the grounds that they could most quickly be returned to battle preparedness. A similar decision was made in Great Britain to favor members of bomber crews who had contracted venereal disease, because they were deemed most valuable to the continuation of the war effort (Hinds, 1975).

As military triage has evolved during the twentieth century, the goal of maintaining fighting strength has increasingly become the dominant, stated goal. In the words of surgeons Gilbert W. Beebe and Michael E. DeBakey, "Traditionally, the military value of surgery lies in the salvage of battle casualties. This is not merely a matter of saving life; it is primarily one of returning the wounded to duty, and the earlier the better" (p. 216).

The nuclear weapons used at the end of World War II introduced unprecedented destructive power. In the nuclear age, triage plans have had to include the possibility of overwhelming numbers of hopelessly injured civilians. In earlier days, it was not uncommon to plan for 1,000 or 2,000 casualties from a single battle. Now, triage planners must consider the likelihood that a single nuclear weapon could produce a hundred times as many casualties or more. At the same time a single blast could destroy much of a community's medical capacity. Such probabilities have led some analysts to wonder if triage would be a realistic expectation following a nuclear attack (British Medical Association, 1983).

Triage has moved from military into civilian medicine in two prominent areas: the care of disaster victims and the operation of hospital emergency departments. In both areas, the categories and many of the strategies of military medicine have been adopted.

The necessity of triage in hospital emergency departments is due, in part, to the fact that a number of patients needing immediate emergency care may arrive almost simultaneously and temporarily overwhelm the hospital's emergency resources (Kipnis). More often, however, the need for triage in hospital emergency departments stems from the fact that the majority of patients are waiting for routine care and do not have emergent conditions. Thus, screening patients to determine which ones need immediate treatment has become increasingly important. Emergency-department triage is often conducted by specially-educated nurses using elaborate methods of scoring for severity of injury or illness (Purnell; Wiebe and Rosen; Grossman).

Ethical Issues

The traditional ethic of medicine obligates healthcare professionals to protect the interests of patients as individuals and to treat people equally on the basis of their medical needs. These same commitments to fidelity and equality have, at times, been prescribed for the treatment of war casualties. For example, the Geneva Conventions call for medical treatment of all casualties of war strictly on the basis of medical criteria, without regard for any other considerations (International Committee of the Red Cross; Baker and Strosberg). However, this principle of equal treatment based solely on medical needs and the likelihood of medical success has competed with utilitarian considerations in military medicine. In such triage, healthcare professionals have sometimes thought of patients as aggregates and given priority to goals such as preserving military strength; loyalty to the individual patient has, at times, been set aside in order to

accomplish the most good or prevent the most harm. The good that might have been accomplished for one has been weighed against what the same amount of effort and resources could do for others. The tension between keeping faith with the individual patient and the utilitarian goal of seeking the greatest good for the greatest number is the primary ethical issue arising from triage.

Triage generates a number of additional ethical questions. To what extent are the utilitarian goals of military or disaster triage appropriate in the more common circumstances of allocating everyday medical care, such as beds in an intensive care unit? If some casualties of war or disaster are categorized as hopeless, what care, if any, should they be accorded? Should their care include active euthanasia? Should healthcare professionals join in the triage planning for nuclear war if they are morally opposed to the policies that include the possibility of such war (Leaning, 1988)? What new issues arise for triage in a time of global terrorism (Kipnis)?

Triage is a permanent feature of contemporary medical care in military, disaster, and emergency settings. As medical research continues to produce new and costly therapies, it will continue to be tempting to import the widely accepted principles of triage for decisions about who gets what care. Indeed, whenever conditions of scarcity necessitate difficult decisions about the distribution of burdens and benefits, the language and tenets of medical triage may present an apparently attractive model. This is true for issues as far from medical care as world hunger and population control (Hardin; Hinds, 1976). The moral wisdom of appropriating the lessons of medical triage for such diverse social problems is doubtful and should be carefully questioned. Otherwise, utilitarian considerations often associated with triage may dominate issues better addressed in terms of loyalty, personal autonomy, or distributive justice (Baker and Strosberg).

GERALD R. WINSLOW (1995)
REVISED BY AUTHOR

SEE ALSO: *Healthcare Resources, Allocation Of: Microallocation; Justice; Warfare: Medicine and War*

BIBLIOGRAPHY

Baker, Robert, and Strosberg, Martin. 1992. "Triage and Equality: An Historical Reassessment of Utilitarian Analyses of Triage." *Kennedy Institute of Ethics Journal* 2: 103–123.

Beebe, Gilbert W., and DeBakey, Michael E. 1952. *Battle Casualties: Incidence, Mortality, and Logistic Considerations.* Springfield, IL: Charles C. Thomas.

Beecher, Henry K. 1970. "Scarce Resources and Medical Advancement." In *Experimentation with Human Subjects,* ed. Paul A. Freund. New York: George Braziller.

British Medical Association. 1983. *The Medical Effects of Nuclear War.* Chichester, UK: John Wiley and Sons.

British Medical Association. 1988. *Selection of Casualties for Treatment After Nuclear Attack: A Document for Discussion.* London: Author.

Burkle, Frederick M. 1984. "Triage." In *Disaster Medicine: Application for the Immediate Management and Triage of Civilian and Military Disaster Victims,* ed. Frederick M. Burkle, Jr., Patricia H. Sanner, and Barry W. Wolcott. New Hyde Park, NY: Medical Examination.

Childress, James F. 1983. "Triage in Neonatal Intensive Care: The Limitations of a Metaphor." *Virginia Law Review* 69: 547–561.

Grossman, Valerie G.A. 1999. *Quick Reference to Triage.* Philadelphia: Lippincott Williams and Wilkins.

Hardin, Garrett. 1980. *Promethean Ethics: Living with Death, Competition, and Triage.* Seattle: University of Washington Press.

Hinds, Stuart. 1975. "Triage in Medicine: A Personal History." In *Triage in Medicine and Society: Inquiries into Medical Ethics,* ed. George R. Lucas, Jr. Houston, TX: Institute of Religion and Human Development.

Hinds, Stuart. 1976. "Relations of Medical Triage to World Famine: A History." In *Lifeboat Ethics: The Moral Dilemmas of World Hunger,* ed. George R. Lucas, Jr., and Thomas W. Ogletree. New York: Harper and Row.

International Committee of the Red Cross. 1977. "Geneva Conventions: Protocol I, Additional to the Geneva Conventions of 12 August 1949, Relating to the Protection of Victims of International Armed Conflicts (1977)." In *Encyclopedia of Human Rights,* ed. Edward Lawson. New York: Taylor and Francis.

Keen, William W. 1917. *The Treatment of War Wounds.* Philadelphia: W. B. Saunders.

Kilner, John F. 1990. *Who Lives? Who Dies?: Ethical Criteria in Patient Selection.* New Haven, CT: Yale University Press.

Kipnis, Kenneth. 2003. "Overwhelming Casualties: Medical Ethics in a Time of Terror." In *After the Terror: Medicine and Morality in a Time of Crisis,* ed. Jonathan D. Moreno. Cambridge, MA: MIT Press.

Larrey, Dominique Jean. 1832. *Surgical Memoirs of the Campaign in Russia,* tr. J. Mercer. Philadelphia: Cowley and Lea.

Leaning, Jennifer. 1986. "Burn and Blast Casualties: Triage in Nuclear War." In *The Medical Implications of Nuclear War,* ed. Fredric Solomon and Robert Q. Marston. Washington, D.C.: National Academy Press.

Leaning, Jennifer. 1988. "Physicians, Triage, and Nuclear War." *Lancet* 2(8605): 269–270.

Lee, Robert I. 1917. "The Case for the More Efficient Treatment of Light Casualties in Military Hospitals." *Military Surgeon* 42: 283–286.

Lynch, Charles; Ford, J. H.; and Weed, F. W. 1925. *Field Operations: In General View of Medical Department Organization.* Vol. 8 of *The Medical Department of the United States Army in the World War.* Washington, D.C.: U.S. Government Printing Office.

O'Donnell, Thomas J. 1960. "The Morality of Triage." *Georgetown Medical Bulletin* 14(1): 68–71.

Purnell, Larry D. 1991. "A Survey of Emergency Department Triage in 185 Hospitals." *Journal of Emergency Nursing* 17(6): 402–407.

Rund, Douglas A., and Rausch, Tondra S. 1981. *Triage.* St. Louis, MO: Mosby.

Vickery, Donald M. 1975. *Triage: Problem-Oriented Sorting of Patients.* Bowie, MD: Robert J. Brady.

Wiebe, Robert A., and Rosen, Linda M. 1991. "Triage in the Emergency Department." *Emergency Medicine Clinics of North America* 9(3): 491–503.

Winslow, Gerald. 1982. *Triage and Justice.* Berkeley: University of California Press.

TRUST

• • •

Trust Between Patients and Providers

Trust between patients and providers is a central topic for bioethics. Consider the trust (or distrust) involved when someone contemplates major surgery: First of all, there is the relation between the surgeon and patient. The patient needs from the physician both a high level of competence (both judgment and skill) and a concern for the patient's well-being. For healthcare professionals to behave in a responsible or trustworthy way requires both technical competence and moral concern—specifically, a concern to achieve a good outcome in the matter covered, which is sometimes called "fiduciary responsibility," the responsibility of a person who has been entrusted in some way. The moral and technical components of professional responsibility have led sociologist Bernard Barber to speak of these as two "senses" of trust. However, if the patient trusts the surgeon, it is not in two senses; the patient trusts the surgeon simply to provide a good, or perhaps the best, outcome for the patient. To fulfill that trust, the surgeon needs to be both morally concerned for the patient's well-being (or at least health outcome) and technically competent.

Because the exercise of professional responsibility characteristically draws on a body of specialized knowledge that is brought to bear on the promotion or preservation of another's welfare, to trust someone to fulfill a professional responsibility is to trust that person to perform in a way that someone outside that profession cannot entirely specify, predict, or often even recognize. In drawing attention to this point, Trudy Govier says that trust is "open-ended." The point is not captured in the frequent suggestion that trust is necessary because the trusting party cannot control or monitor the trusted party's performance. It would do the patient little good to have full prescience of all the events in the operation, or even the ability to guide the surgeon's hand, unless the patient also happened to be a surgeon. Although a typical patient might be able to recognize some acts of gross malpractice, such as being stitched up with foreign bodies left inside, the patient would not know the implications of most of what he or she saw and would have no idea of how to improve the surgeon's performance. For this reason, from the point of view of the patient, there are no good alternatives to having trustworthy professionals. There are no good alternatives in these circumstances because the patient must rely on the discretion of the practitioner.

Philosophers like John Ladd and legal theorists like Joel Handler have drawn attention to the role of discretion in many areas of professional practice. They have argued that because of the role of discretion, the criteria for morally responsible practice cannot be specified in terms of rules or rights alone. The centrality of discretion makes it all the more difficult to separate competence (having adequate knowledge and skill) and moral elements (exercising sufficient concern for the client's well-being) in the professional's behavior.

The provider—in this case the surgeon—also must trust the patient. At a minimum, the surgeon depends on the patient to disclose all information relevant to the case so as to minimize the risks of unexpected events in the operating room. If the patient disappoints the surgeon and does not disclose all relevant information, the negative consequence for the surgeon is, at most, to impair the surgeon's professional performance. The disappointment does not carry a risk of death or disability for the surgeon. The difference in the severity of risk is one of the many aspects of a trust relationship that is counted as a difference of power in that relationship. The lesser severity of consequence for the provider—in this case the surgeon—can obscure the mutuality of trust in the patient-provider relationship.

When the provider is a nurse or physical therapist rather than a surgeon, the provider's central tasks often require an understanding of the patient's experiences, hopes, and fears. Although some nursing, such as the work of the surgical nurse who assists in the operating room, does not depend on an understanding of the patient's experience, most nursing does. Postsurgical nursing care is a good example. This care typically includes motivating the patient to do things such as coughing and breathing deeply in order to reduce the risk of postoperative lung infection. These acts are often quite uncomfortable. Such nursing requires an understanding of the individual patient's state of mind and the ability to motivate the patient—the ability to inspire confidence and hope in patients.

CHANGING THE STANDARDS OF THE PATIENT-PROVIDER RELATIONSHIP. When sociologist Talcott Parsons put forward his influential theory that professionals function as trustees, or in a "fiduciary" capacity, the standard for the so-called fiduciary aspects of the relationship between patients and physicians was that the provider furthered the patient's well-being by being entrusted to make medical decisions in the best interests of that patient.

The doctrine of informed consent for medical procedures was adopted only gradually over the next two decades as a check on provider discretion. This doctrine has been implemented to require informed consent only for a very circumscribed set of procedures. To treat competent persons against their will is considered battery, in legal terms. Therefore, there is a foundation in law for the prohibition of forced or nonconsensual treatment of all types. In practice, however, information is often given only for major procedures, and practitioners tend to assume consent for lesser interventions, including most medical tests. Although patient-oriented practitioners will offer an explanation of why they are ordering a particular test, others will explain only when explicitly asked. For procedures other than surgery, formal requests for consent are rare unless there is a significant risk of death or severe disability from the procedure.

Furthermore, most patients are well informed only about the risk of death or significant permanent injury in circumstances in which informed consent is legally or institutionally mandated. Significant risk—such as becoming temporarily psychotic as a result of the trauma of open-heart surgery, as a result of intensive-care procedures, or from the sleep deprivation that often results from those procedures—is rarely disclosed to patients. The rationale for not telling a patient about to have bypass surgery or enter intensive care is that the risk will seem so shocking that the patient will refuse needed care.

Although the standard of informed consent is enforced by law and institutional practice only for certain risks of major procedures, the U.S. President's Commission for the Study of Ethical Problems in Medicine and Biomedical and Behavioral Research (President's Commission) has urged that the informed-consent standard be replaced by another, more comprehensive standard, the standard of *shared decision making.*

The President's Commission's 1982 report, *Making Health Care Decisions,* advocated such a shift, which would presumably apply to most significant healthcare decisions. The rule of informed consent requires only the recognition of the patient's right of veto over the alternatives that the provider has presented to the patient. In contrast, shared decision making requires participation of the patient in setting the goals and methods of care and, therefore, in formulating the alternatives to be considered. This participation requires that patients and practitioners engage in complex communication, which the practitioners have a fiduciary responsibility to foster. This new standard is particularly appropriate for a pluralistic society, in which the responsible provider may have an idea of the patient's good that is significantly different from the patient's own idea.

The responsibility to foster shared decision making requires significant skill on the part of medical professionals in understanding patients of diverse backgrounds and in fostering communication with them in difficult circumstances—circumstances in which their communication may be compromised by fear and pain as well as by a lack of medical knowledge. Although some physicians, notably primary-care providers, have sought the skills to fulfill the responsibility to foster such communication, this responsibility is not one that medical education prepares physicians to accept.

IMPLEMENTING THE FIDUCIARY STANDARD. Ironically, although the fiduciary responsibility in healthcare has often been viewed primarily as the responsibility of physicians, as was noted above, it is other classes of providers, especially nurses, who are educated in a way that prepares them to understand patients' experience. Although there is much to recommend the new fiduciary standard in healthcare, its realization requires either a major change in medical education or a change in the relations among members of the healthcare team, so that those who are prepared to oversee and foster shared decision making have the authority to do so. Without such changes, the trust that one's healthcare will be shaped by one's own priorities and concerns is not well founded.

In many cases, distrust of either individual providers or medical institutions has been warranted, especially for women, people of color, and the poor, whose experience has often been discounted or who have been viewed as less rational or less competent than white males. Annette Dula argues that historical events, from the Tuskegee syphilis study to the experience with screening for sickle-cell carrier trait, confirm

that trust of the healthcare system on the part of African-Americans is often not warranted (Dula, 1992). The problem is one of the need not only for assurance but also for evidence that the former conditions no longer prevail.

Many poor or uninsured people have not even had a significant patient-provider relationship; when they are able to obtain healthcare, it is often with a provider whom they see in only a single clinical encounter. It is therefore impossible to establish a trusting relationship that would serve the patient's health interest. If society is obliged to provide decent healthcare for its citizens, this failure of the healthcare system is a betrayal of trust not by individual providers but by society and its healthcare institutions.

Trust and Family Members

Trust among family members is at least as important an issue for healthcare as is trust in the provider-patient relationship. The trustworthiness of parents and guardians to decide the care of children and other dependent family members is widely discussed, and trust among family members is beginning to receive more attention in connection with the writing of living wills and health proxy statements. The issues of the competence of family members to give various forms of care or to make technical decisions, and the sufficiency of their concern for the patient's well-being, parallel those issues for providers. The matter is further complicated by the phenomenon of psychological denial that interferes with decision making about the healthcare of a person who is important in one's own life. Denial, as well as incompetence or lack of commitment to the patient's welfare, may compromise a person's decisions or care when the health or life of a close friend or relative is gravely threatened. Therefore, warranted trust in family members to provide or decide one's care requires confidence not only in their competence and in their concern for one's well-being but also in their psychological ability to come to terms with the situation.

Other Areas of Trust in Healthcare

There is also the question of the public's trust in a class of professionals, which is distinct from the question of the public's concern that, should they become clients of these professionals, their interests will be well served. For example, Sissela Bok (1978) has examined the concern about the trustworthiness of lawyers, not by their clients but by the public. Of particular concern is lawyers' commitment to keep the crimes of their clients confidential, even certain ongoing or planned crimes. The public believes that lawyers should not violate usual ethical norms for the sake of their clients' interests. The corresponding issue in healthcare is the fear that providers will, in protecting patient confidentiality, put the public health or the safety of individuals at undue risk. The question of ethical criteria for breaking confidentiality is regularly discussed, especially in the case of a sexually transmitted disease or a patient intent on harming another person. However, there is no widespread public concern that healthcare providers may be going so far in protecting patient confidentiality that they are derelict in protecting the public.

In addition to the public's trust of providers, the trust or distrust of medical technology is often a significant factor. The risk is particularly salient in the case of artificial organs, joints, and other body parts. In place of the components of competence and concern of a trusted provider, the qualities required of a technology to warrant trust are its performance (it performs the function it was designed to perform) and its relative safety (it is relatively unlikely to cause accidents or to have other injurious side effects). Of course, with such life-critical technologies as artificial organs, the performance issue is itself a safety issue.

There are many aspects of the healthcare system on which patients rely but which most rarely consider. Many people become fully aware of their trust only when that trust is disappointed. A case in point is the discovery that research misconduct occurred in a major breast cancer study. The belated revelation of misconduct made patients aware of their trust in medical research.

The Morality of Trust

Although Sissela Bok has discussed trust as a moral resource since the 1970s, the question of the morality of trust relationships—the question of the circumstances under which, from a moral point of view, one ought to trust—was not explicitly discussed until Annette Baier's 1986 essay, "Trust and Anti-Trust." Two earlier essays were important in laying the foundation for this major turn in the discussion. In 1984, Ian Hacking provided a devastating assessment of the use of game theory to understand moral questions, such as the Prisoner's Dilemma, which will be discussed below. Baier herself argued in 1985 for broadening the focus in ethics from obligations and moral rules to the subject of who ought, as a moral matter, to be trusted and when. As Kathryn Addelson points out, Baier's change of focus establishes a general perspective on ethical legitimacy that is shared by all—both the powerful and those whom society labels *deviant*—rather than privileging the perspective of those who make, instill, and enforce moral rules.

Baier's general account of the morality of trust illuminates the strong relation between the trustworthy and the

true. A trust relationship, according to Baier, is decent to the extent that it stands the test of disclosure of the premises of each party's trust (Baier, 1986). For example, if one party trusts the other to perform as needed only because the truster believes the trusted is too timid or unimaginative to do otherwise, disclosure of these premises will tend to insult the trusted party and give him or her an incentive to prove the truster wrong. Similarly, if the trusted party fulfills the truster's expectations only through fear of detection and punishment, disclosure of these premises may lead the truster to suspect that the trusted would betray the trust, given an anonymous opportunity to do so.

Although explicit discussion of moral trustworthiness is relatively recent, both professional ethics and the philosophy of technology have given considerable attention to the concept of responsibility. Since being trustworthy is key to acting responsibly in a professional capacity, or to being a responsible person if one considers responsibility a virtue, the literature on responsibility provides at least an implicit discussion of many aspects of the morality of trust, much of which is relevant to the subject of trust in healthcare.

Conceptual Relationships

Trust involves both confidence and reliance. Annette Baier (1986) argues that if we lack other options, we may continue to rely on something even when we no longer trust it. Similarly, we may have confidence in something, or confidence in our expectations concerning it, without relying on it. To rely only on what we can trust is a fortunate circumstance.

Niklas Luhmann (1988) urges a different distinction between confidence and trust, suggesting that *trust* be used only when the truster has considered the alternatives to trusting. Such use is incompatible with unconscious trust, a phenomenon to which Baier draws attention. Luhmann's discussion of the distinction between trust and confidence highlights the element of risk in trusting. Risk or vulnerability does characterize situations in which trust is necessary, in contrast to situations in which one's control of the outcome makes trust unnecessary. However, the element of risk taking in trust is captured in the notion of reliance when trust is understood as confident reliance. Being vulnerable in one's reliance does not require that one have considered the alternatives, if any, to such reliance.

Although one often trusts people, their intentions and goodwill, there is also trust in mere circumstances or events: One may trust that a taxi will come along shortly, even if no taxi has been ordered, without believing anything about another person's reliability in providing a taxi.

The risk taken in trusting does leave the truster liable to disappointment (or worse), whether that trust is of persons or events. But only when trust is in other people, and not merely in the events involving them, can one be let down by them. Suppose that a person is awakened every weekday by another person's calling for a neighbor. If the first person has come to rely on being awakened, but one day the other person does not come for the neighbor or does so quietly, the first person's expectations will be disappointed. But the person will not have been disappointed or let down by the one who usually picks up the neighbor. To be disappointed by another person, that person must at least be aware of doing or not doing the act in question. Here the person doing the calling for the neighbor is not aware of waking up the first party, much less of being trusted to do it. As Baier mentions (1986), it is possible for there to be trust of which the trusted person is unaware, and so one might let down another without being aware of letting that person down.

Niklas Luhmann (1979) has shown how trust simplifies human life by endowing some expectations with assurance. To consider all possible disappointments, defections, and betrayals by those on whom we rely, the possible consequences of those disappointments, and any actions that one might take to prevent those disappointments or change their effect is prohibitively costly in terms of time and energy. Trust reduces that burden.

The Literature on Trust

Sociologists like Bernard Barber and Luhmann (1979, 1988) have written on many facets of the notion of trust, and legal theorists have reflected on the distinct, though related, notion of a legal trust. Until the 1980s, however, the explicit attention given to the common notion of trust, or confident reliance, in Anglo-American philosophy was largely in relation to such questions as how the "prisoners" in the so-called Prisoner's Dilemma might solve their problem of assurance with regard to one another's behavior so as to cooperate in achieving a mutually beneficial outcome. (In the Prisoner's Dilemma, each of two prisoners will receive a light sentence if neither confesses to a crime, and a more severe sentence if both confess; but if one confesses and the other does not, the latter will be freed, but the former will receive the most severe sentence of all. Without assurance about each other's behavior, and in spite of knowing that both would be better off if neither confesses, both are likely to confess and be less well off.)

Recent literature on trust has examined trust in a variety of different social circumstances, involving a wide range of objects and systems, persons in a wide variety of roles, and matters in which they might be trusted or distrusted. For example, some writers focus on cases of the breakdown of trust in war, under the influence of the Mafia, or in some other extreme situation. Differences in the domain of application of the notion of trust lead to an unusually wide range of estimates of its character and importance. They also lead to disparate distinctions between trust and such notions as reliance, faith, vulnerability, and confidence, as well as to different conclusions about the moral value and the moral risks associated with trust.

Those who write about trust in a market context often take economic rationality—according to which each person simply seeks to maximize his or her goals by the most efficient means—as their model. They then often regard trust as a way of coping with *imperfect rationality,* understood as uncertainty about the facts or about one another's behavior, and how to estimate the consequences for the achievement of one's goals. The economic model of rationality is not readily applicable in considerations of ethics because it was designed to avoid consideration of values other than efficiency, and it treats moral considerations as nonobjective *personal preferences.* Where a market context is assumed, the relatively minor risk of being a "sucker" is likely to be mentioned as a barrier to trust. (See, for example, Dasgupta.) In discussions of trust among family members or between nations (Bok, 1990a), much more is recognized to be at stake.

Feminists like Trudy Govier argue that attention to trust relationships will bring attention to other relationships, such as those between parents and children, that have been neglected when contracts are the focus of attention. Such relationships, however, together with the features of trust that are prominent in them, continue to be ignored in much of the literature on trust. For example, Geoffrey Hawthorn mentions a parent's nonegotistic motives toward his or her child, only to turn immediately to "more ordinary" instances of nonegoistic motives.

Bernard Williams, who begins his own essay with a discussion of the Prisoner's Dilemma, argues that the problem of how nonegoistic motivation is to be encouraged and legitimated does not have a general solution. He argues that the problem of trust or cooperation is not one that can be solved in a general way at the level of decision theory, social psychology, or the general theory of social institutions. To ensure cooperation in a given situation requires an understanding of the ways in which the people in that situation are motivated. Williams believes that solutions to the problem of cooperation are found only for particular historically shaped societies, rather than for society in general. He argues that investigating the sorts of combinations of motivations that make sense in that society might lead to a general perspective on the problems of cooperation in such a society.

However, as he says, "there is no one problem of cooperation: the problem is always how a given set of people cooperate" (p. 13). Those whose cooperation is of the greatest interest in bioethics are patients, their families, the healthcare providers, and the policymakers who shape the healthcare system.

CAROLINE WHITBECK (1995)
BIBLIOGRAPHY REVISED

SEE ALSO: *Beneficence; Care; Confidentiality; Family and Family Medicine; Health and Disease: The Experience of Health and Illness; Informed Consent; Malpractice, Medical; Patients' Responsibilities; Patients' Rights; Privacy and Confidentiality in Research; Privacy in Healthcare; Teams, Healthcare; Virtue and Character*

BIBLIOGRAPHY

Addelson, Kathryn. 1994. *Moral Passages: Notes Toward a Collectivist Ethics.* New York: Routledge.

Baier, Annette. 1985. "What Do Women Want in a Moral Theory?" *Nous* 19(1): 53–63. Reprinted in her *Moral Prejudices: Essays on Ethics.* Cambridge, MA: Harvard University Press, 1994.

Baier, Annette. 1986. "Trust and Antitrust." *Ethics* 96(2): 232–260. Reprinted in her *Moral Prejudices: Essays on Ethics.* Cambridge, MA: Harvard University Press, 1994.

Baier, Annette. 1993. "Trust and Distrust of Moral Theorists." In *Applied Ethics: A Reader,* eds. Earl R. Winkler and Jerrold R. Coombs. Oxford: Basil Blackwell.

Baier, Annette. 1994a. *Moral Prejudices: Essays on Ethics.* Cambridge, MA: Harvard University Press.

Baier, Annette. 1994b. "Sustaining Trust." In her *Moral Prejudices: Essays on Ethics.* Cambridge, MA: Harvard University Press.

Baier, Annette. 1994c. "Trust and Its Vulnerabilities." In her *Moral Prejudices: Essays on Ethics.* Cambridge, MA: Harvard University Press.

Baier, Annette. 1994d. "Trusting People." In her *Moral Prejudices: Essays on Ethics.* Cambridge, MA: Harvard University Press.

Balos, Beverly, and Fellows, Mary Louise. 1991. "Guilty of the Crime of Trust: Nonstranger Rape." *Minnesota Law Review* 75(3): 599–618.

Barber, Bernard. 1983. *The Logic and Limits of Trust.* New Brunswick, NJ: Rutgers University Press.

Benner, Patricia E. 1984. *From Novice to Expert: Excellence and Power in Clinical Nursing Practice.* Menlo Park, CA: Addison-Wesley.

Benner, Patricia E., and Wrubel, Judith. 1989. *The Primacy of Caring: Stress and Coping in Health and Illness.* Menlo Park, CA: Addison-Wesley.

Bok, Sissela. 1978. *Lying: Moral Choice in Public and Private Life.* New York: Pantheon.

Bok, Sissela. 1990a. *A Strategy for Peace: Human Values and the Threat of War.* New York: Pantheon.

Bok, Sissela. 1990b. "Can Lawyers Be Trusted?" *University of Pennsylvania Law Review* 138(3): 913–933.

Dasgupta, Partha. 1988. "Trust as a Commodity." In *Trust: Making and Breaking Cooperative Relations,* ed. Diego Gambetta. Oxford: Basil Blackwell.

Dula, Annette. 1991. "Toward an African-American Perspective on Bioethics." *Journal of Health Care for the Poor and Underserved* 2(2): 259–269.

Dula, Annette. 1992. "African Americans and Mistrust of the Medical Community." Address given at Harvard Medical School, Cambridge, MA, November 1992.

Gambetta, Diego, ed. 1988. *Trust: Making and Breaking Cooperative Relations.* Oxford: Basil Blackwell.

Good, David. 1988. "Individuals, Interpersonal Relations, and Trust." In *Trust: Making and Breaking Cooperative Relations,* ed. Diego Gambetta. Oxford: Basil Blackwell.

Govier, Trudy. 1992. "Trust, Distrust, and Feminist Theory." *Hypatia* 7(1): 16–33.

Hacking, Ian. 1984. "Winner Takes Less." *New York Review of Books* 31: 17–21.

Handler, Joel F. 1990. *Law and the Search for Community.* Philadelphia: University of Pennsylvania Press.

Hardin, Russell. 1991. "Trusting Persons, Trusting Institutions." In *Strategy and Choice,* ed. Richard Zeckhauser. Cambridge, MA: MIT Press.

Hardin, Russell. 1992. "The Street Level Epistemology of Trust." *Analyse und Kritik* 14:152–176.

Hawthorn, Geoffrey. 1988. "Three Ironies in Trust." In *Trust: Making and Breaking Cooperative Relations,* ed. Diego Gambetta. Oxford: Basil Blackwell.

Jackson, Jennifer. 2001. *Truth, Trust and Medicine.* New York: Routledge.

Ladd, John. 1980. "Legalism and Medical Ethics." In *Contemporary Issues in Biomedical Ethics,* eds. John W. Davis, C. Barry Hoffmaster, and Sarah Shorten. Clifton, NJ: Humana.

Ladd, John. 1982. "The Distinction Between Rights and Responsibilities: A Defense." *Linacre Quarterly* 49 (May): 121–142.

Lammers, Stephen. 1985. "Some Ethical Issues in the End-Stage Renal Disease Program." *Weaver Information and Perspectives on Technological Literacy* 3(2): 4–5.

Luhmann, Niklas. 1979. *Trust and Power.* New York: John Wiley and Sons.

Luhmann, Niklas. 1988. "Familiarity, Confidence, Trust: Problems and Alternatives." In *Trust: Making and Breaking Cooperative Relations,* ed. Diego Gambetta. Oxford: Basil Blackwell.

MacIntyre, Alasdair. 1984. "Does Applied Ethics Rest on a Mistake?" *Monist* 67(4): 498–513.

McCullough, Laurence B. 1999. "Moral Authority, Power, and Trust in Clinical Ethics." *Journal of Medicine and Philosophy* 24(1): 3–10.

Mitcham, Carl. 1987. "Responsibility and Technology: The Expanding Relationship." In *Technology and Responsibility,* ed. Paul T. Durbin. Philosophy and Technology no. 3. Boston: D. Reidel.

O'Neill, Onora. 2002. *A Question of Trust: The BBC Reith Lectures 2002.* New York: Cambridge.

Parsons, Talcott. 1951. *The Social System.* Glencoe, IL: Free Press.

Pellegrino, Edmund D.; Veatch, Robert M.; and Langan, John T. 1991. *Ethics, Trust, and the Professions: Philosophical and Cultural Aspects.* Washington, D.C.: Georgetown University Press.

Rich, Adrienne C. 1979. "Women and Honor: Some Notes on Lying (1975)." In her *On Lies, Secrets and Silence: Selected Prose, 1966–1978.* New York: W. W. Norton.

U.S. President's Commission for the Study of Ethical Problems in Medicine and Biomedical and Behavioral Research. 1982. *Making Health Care Decisions: A Report on the Ethical and Legal Implications of Informed Consent in the Patient-Practitioner Relationship.* 3 vols. Washington, D.C.: U.S. Government Printing Office.

Williams, Bernard. 1988. "Formal Structures and Social Reality." In *Trust: Making and Breaking Cooperative Relations,* ed. Diego Gambetta. Oxford: Basil Blackwell.

U

UTILITARIANISM AND BIOETHICS

• • •

In bioethics the influence of utilitarianism as an applied ethical theory is widely felt, both positively and negatively. On almost all substantive issues in the area, utilitarianism anchors one of the contending positions. Yet, it is the object of fierce criticism, nearly always to do with the challenges it poses to ordinary or conventional morality, especially in cases involving the taking of life, and to the distinctions that are supposed to carry the weight of that morality.

Classical Utilitarianism

Classical or act-utilitarianism is the view that an act is right if its consequences are at least as good as those of any alternative. In this form the view is consequentialist, welfarist, aggregative, maximizing, and impersonal, and the principle of utility that it endorses what might be called the utilitarian goal.

The view is consequentialist, in that it holds that acts are right or wrong solely in virtue of the goodness or badness of their actual consequences. This view is sometimes called act-consequentialism, or, here, for reasons of brevity, simply consequentialism. It is matters to do with consequentialism, and the conflicts that consequentialist thinking is supposed to engender with ordinary morality in bioethics (and elsewhere), that has made the present topic one of note in contemporary bioethics. The view is welfarist, in that rightness is made a function of goodness, and goodness is understood as referring certainly to human welfare but also, perhaps, to animal welfare as well. The view is impersonal

and aggregative, in that rightness is determined by considering, impersonally, the increases and diminutions in well-being of all those affected by the act and summing those increases and diminutions across persons. The view is a maximizing one: One concrete formulation of the principle of utility, framed in the light of welfarist considerations is "Always maximize net desire-satisfaction."

The act-utilitarian goal, understood in the light of the above characterization, then, is to maximize (human) welfare. The crucial question to which this goal gives rise is how best to go about achieving it, and some contemporary act-utilitarians have come to think that the best way of going about maximizing (human) welfare overall may be to forego trying to maximize it on each occasion. It is this insight, in some form or other, that has spurred the most important developments in act-utilitarianism today—developments, however, that have not for the most part featured in bioethics, where the utilitarianism discussed and criticized remains classical or act-utilitarianism, with its embedded consequentialism.

Act-Utilitarianism v. Moral Intuition: The Opposition View

What has driven and continues to drive much of the opposition to act-utilitarianism has been the thought that some alternative view can better account for a number of our moral intuitions. Our moral intuitions, it is said, frown upon murdering or torturing someone, upon enslaving people or using them as means, upon acting in certain contexts and so using people in certain ways for mere marginal increases in utility, all of which act-utilitarianism is supposed to license. It is supposed to license these things because of its constituent consequentialism: If such acts were to have better consequences than the actual consequences of any alternative, then the act-utilitarian would be compelled to call such acts right. And this, allegedly, conflicts with our moral intuitions or ordinary moral convictions or what some people think of as commonsense morality.

This is familiar territory in past debates over utilitarianism generally, though it is no more settled for all that, and it raises directly the question of whether our moral intuitions have probative force in ethics. This is an important issue in its own right, separate from the fate of any form of utilitarianism, but far too broad and complex an issue to be gone into in any detail here. For those inclined to the view that moral intuitions do have probative force in ethics and utilitarianism can be rejected if it produces clashes with those intuitions, the problem has been to make it appear that certain of our intuitions are more secure than others—so secure, in fact, that we believe them to be more *correct* or *true* than any normative ethical theory that contended otherwise could be. Obviously those who adopt this line need to identify which these crucial intuitions are, and various ways of doing this have been suggested. Today reflective equilibrium methodologies are perhaps the preferred way, though some relatively straightforward intuitionists still survive, as do some who seek for the preferred intuitions or convictions in their religion. Even with the back and forth movement between intuition and principle that reflective equilibrium methodologies involve, however, it is clear that some intuitions survive and remain intact. Thus, in *A Theory of Justice*, Rawls appears to think that, if a moral/political theory gave the result that slavery was justified, that would be enough to demand from us amendment and/or abandonment of the theory. His intuition on this score needs no revision. Other writers privilege other of their moral intuitions either about particular acts or classes of acts. Of course the more people that are found, whether in our own or another culture, to differ over these crucial intuitions, the more difficulty there is in selecting just which the crucial ones are. Thus reflective equilibrium methodologists on the one hand and straightforward intuitionists on the other seek ways to discount variation in these crucial intuitions, or, at the very least, to reduce the scope and depth of variations.

The Taking of Life: A Prime Example

Whatever the scope and depth of variations, however, the assumption that certain intuitions survive critical scrutiny has been the springboard from which assaults upon act-utilitarianism have nearly always begun. In cases involving the taking of life, this has been especially true, so that, for example, the topics of abortion, infanticide, euthanasia,

suicide, and physician-assisted suicide have become battlegrounds for the playing out of certain kinds of consequentialist reasoning over intending and causing or bringing about death. Of course, other issues in bioethics have been contentious between consequentialists and their opponents, and those involving genetic engineering and therapeutic cloning promise to become intense in the near future; but it is the cases of taking life that have pressed upon the opponents of consequentialism. Four points may be used to illustrate the clash:

(1) Can a genuine distinction be drawn between intending death and merely foreseeing death as a side-effect of one's act and, if such a distinction can be drawn, whether it can be used to mark off moral differences between cases? This issue haunts the taking-life cases; it has been one of the main bones of contention over the viability of the doctrine of double effect; and it is, when allied with a whole array of concerns having to do with whether the act/omission, acting/refraining, and active/passive distinctions are morally significant ones, part of the killing/letting die debate. On the whole, consequentialists attack the moral significance of these distinctions. Thus with a patient who has required ever larger doses of a pain-killer, a physician now proposes to administer the minimum dosage necessary to relieve pain, in the knowledge, however, that the drug at that dosage will prove fatal or at least hasten death. Is the doctor's act permissible? According to some it is permissible, since the physician intends the relief of pain, not death, and only foresees as a side effect of the act that death will ensue or be hastened. Were the doctor to intend the death, either as end or as means, the act would be, not tantamount to, but in fact murder. In this way, then, some want to distinguish morally between the doctor's intentionally killing the patient and his knowingly bringing about the patient's death. Consequentialists, on the whole, have doubts that any such moral distinction can be drawn on this basis: In both cases, the patient ends up dead as the result of causal steps that the doctor takes. Suppose the doctor chooses to administer the drug and knowingly brings about the patient's death: What is one to say about this *bringing about*? One cannot say that it was the result of negligence or recklessness or of accident or mistake. In fact the death is in part the result of choice or decision on the part of the doctor, and it is an integral part of the case that the doctor is a causal agent in the patient's death. Certainly the choice or decision by the doctor to administer the drug cannot be ignored in describing what happened in the patient's case, since that choice or decision in part determines what happened to the patient. This

is true, moreover, even if it is true that the patient's death forms no part of the doctor's intention. It is simply false that the only way morality can be injected into the doctor's case is through what is intended; for that fails to take account of the fact that the patient's death is brought about by the doctor, in the sense described. Unplugging ventilators and turning off machines, among other acts, are all things that the doctor does, in the course of bringing about the patient's death. (The causal account requires complication in a case involving an omission; but the injection of morphine is not an omission.)

(2) In this regard, withdrawing treatment or food and hydration is something the doctor does as well. It is sometimes held that a doctor may not permissibly supply the means of death to a competent, informed patient who is terminally ill, who has voluntarily requested the doctor's assistance in dying, and whose request has survived depression therapy. Yet the very same doctor, it is held, may withdraw food and hydration if, for example, the patient makes a valid refusal of further treatment. Not all withdrawal cases take this form, since things other than food and hydration can be withdrawn from a patient's treatment; but consequentialists on the whole have difficulty in seeing what the morally relevant differences are between these cases. The doctor can supply a pill and produce death, he can withdraw feeding tubes and produce death; how can one be permissible and the other impermissible? Causally he appears to be a factor in the patient's death in both cases. Nor will the consequentialist allow the case to be made out to be one in which, by his valid refusal of further treatment, the patient is to be regarded as the sole actor present, as if the doctor who will withdraw feeding tubes were not there and did not act. The patient's autonomous, voluntary decision to forego further treatment is not the only morally or causally relevant fact to the situation: Death is only produced if the doctor withdraws feeding tubes. Notice, importantly, that the case cannot be reduced to one in which it is claimed that the patient is *permitted* or *allowed* by the doctor to die and that it is the underlying disease which kills him, which is what is usually claimed in the cases of omissions; for in the withdrawal of feeding tubes, it is starvation, not the patient's underlying condition, that kills him. What one causes in the world is relevant to the issue of one's moral responsibility. One may want the doctor to take seriously the autonomous, voluntary decision of the patient to refuse further treatment, but this does not settle the issue of whether withdrawing feeding tubes helped cause death by starvation. Withdrawal of feeding tubes is not an alternative to physician-assisted suicide, so far

as causality is concerned: In both cases, the doctor takes an essential step in the production of death.

(3) In the withdrawal case, if the doctor does not withdraw feeding tubes, then he fails to honor the patient's right to refuse treatment, but if he fails to provide the pill, there is no violation of the patient's right to refuse further treatment. Nor does a right to refuse treatment entail a right to be provided with the means of death. So why is there not a moral difference between the withdrawal and pill cases, in that not prescribing the pill does not violate the patient's rights, whereas not withdrawing the feeding tubes does. But this lands the opponent of consequentialism with another problem: While to insist upon one's right to refuse treatment is one way of committing suicide, taking the pill is another way of committing suicide. Why, if suicide is permissible, is one way of committing suicide, the doctor withdrawing feeding tubes, more acceptable than another way of committing suicide, the doctor supplying a pill that the patient takes? It is necessary to identify some reason to think that, if suicide is morally permissible for terminally ill patients, having a doctor withdraw feeding tubes is acceptable but having the doctor provide a pill is not, when both are seen by the patient and by the rest of society as means of committing suicide. If one refuses to allow that suicide is permissible in such cases, then there will be no moral difference between the withdrawal and the pill cases and so the one cannot be used by way of contrast to the other. Of course, in the withdrawal case, those who want to find a difference between it and the pill case may point to the fact that the law allows the doctor to withdraw feeding tubes but not, for example, the patient's son to withdraw those tubes. But it would be a mistake to treat this as if it were identical with the claim that, if the son withdraws the tubes, the withdrawal causes death, whereas if the doctor withdraws them, the withdrawal *does not cause* death. In either case the cause of death is starvation through the removal of feeding tubes; it is just that the law frowns upon the son's act in a way that it does not the doctor's act, in the relevant circumstances.

(4) There is an issue that intersects this discussion of alleged moral differences between cases that turns the debate in another direction. Consequentialists on the whole accept a quality of life view of the value of a life. The value of a life is a function of its quality, and quality of life is a function of a life's content. In this regard, some lives lack the scope and capacities for richness of life that confer on other lives untold blessings, and this regard for content can reach the desperate levels involved in the cases of anencephalic infants and those in a

permanently vegetative state, where even the very capacities for having a rich life are impaired or missing. The result is that such lives are judged on a quality of life view to be deficient in quality, with the result that their value is less than the lives of ordinary humans. This view enrages some people, for whom the thought that all lives are equally valuable, whatever their quality, is a stance or intuition or principle that is paramount and to remain unchallenged. This view is difficult in some ways to credit; for there are some lives so deficient in quality that one would not wish to live them and would not wish those lives on even enemies. To be fully in the progressive grip of amyotrophic lateral sclerosis is to have a life the quality of which seems progressively to plummet; indeed, some of those condemned to such lives often ask for relief from them through the earlier discussed examples of physician-assisted suicide. It is not society who is judging their lives adversely that prompts them to seek help; they themselves so judge their lives. It seems hard, therefore, to think of such lives on all fours with ordinary ones, and the quality of life view of the value of life reflects this fact.

It doubtless strikes some as repugnant and offensive to think of human lives as of different values. The old view would have been that all human lives were equally valuable in the eyes of God, but today this view cannot be assumed to be prevalent in all medical contexts, even when it could be agreed that people ought to base value claims about lives on the assumption of God's existence, religious tenets, or the like. So what is to replace God in this claim about lives? One can make assumptions about, say, equal worth being apart from value, but are these more than assumptions? And does society not use quality of life judgments about lives all the time in hospitals and medical settings, to decide all kinds of issues, from who gets what resource to how much of it they get? And there all the while, of course, is the plain fact that the content of some lives inspires an overwhelming sense of tragedy, of what lives once were or could have been but of what they have become. How can this sense of tragedy and dire outcome represent equal value?

Of course, in many lives, say, where certain physical handicaps are present, there does not exist this sense of overwhelming tragedy, and people cope very well with misfortune. But where a life begins to plummet disastrously in quality, equal value appears harder to defend. Unequal

value, however, implies that some are at greater risk than others: If one could save either a life of very high quality or a life of very low quality; if in hospitals medical intervention is likely to produce in one case a life of ordinary dimensions and in another a life of radically reduced dimensions, and a doctor can only make one such intervention; which life should be choosen?

R. G. FREY

SEE ALSO: *Autonomy; Care; Casuistry; Communitarianism and Bioethics; Consensus; Contractarianism and Bioethics; Emotions; Ethics: Normative Ethical Theories; Human Rights; Obligation and Supererogation*

BIBLIOGRAPHY

Beauchamp, Tom L. 1986. "Refusals of Treatment and Requests for Death." *Kennedy Institute of Ethics Journal* 6: 371–381.

Beauchamp, Tom L., ed. 1996. *Intending Death: The Ethics of Assisted Suicide and Euthanasia.* Englewood Cliffs, NJ, Prentice-Hall.

Brock, Dan. 1993. *Life and Death: Philosophical Essays in Biomedical Ethics.* Cambridge, Eng. and New York, Cambridge University Press.

Dworkin, Gerald; Frey, R. G.; and Bok, Sissela. 1998. *Euthanasia and Physician-Assisted Suicide.* Cambridge, Eng. and New York, Cambridge University Press.

Frey, R. G., and Wellman, Christopher, eds. 2003. *The Blackwell Companion to Applied Ethics.* Oxford, Eng., and Malden, MA: Blackwell.

Glover, Jonathan. 1977. *Causing Death and Saving Lives.* Harmondsworth, Eng.: Penguin.

Harris, John. 1985. *The Value of Life.* London: Routledge Kegan Paul.

Kamm, Frances. 1993. *Morality, Mortality,* Vol. 1. New York: Oxford University Press.

Rachels, James. 1986. *The End of Life: Euthanasia and Morality.* New York: Oxford University Press.

Rawls, John. 1971. *A Theory of Justice.* Cambridge, MA: Harvard University Press.

Singer, Peter. 1993. *Practical Ethics.* Cambridge, Eng., and New York: Cambridge University Press.

Singer, Peter. 1996. *Rethinking Life and Death: The Collapse of Traditional Ethics.* New York: St. Martin's Press.

Singer, Peter, and Kuhse, Helga. 2002. *Unsanctifying Human Life.* Malden, MA: Blackwell.

V

VALUE AND HEALTHCARE

• • •

Bioethics is concerned with values insofar as they are identical to universal or objective goods (benefits) and evils (harms). There is a use of *value* such that it refers to whatever any person happens to value, but this sense of value has no normative implications. What *value* refers to in this sense is completely determined by empirical research; it is a purely descriptive sense. There is a related sense of *value* such that it refers to what a large number of people value. This is the sense that seems to be important in economics. Economically speaking, something has value or is valuable if there are many people who value it, it can be transferred from one person to another, and there is not enough of it for all of the people who value it. How valuable something is on this understanding is also a completely empirical matter with no normative implications. However, there is another sense of *valuable* where what is valuable is what leads to less harms being suffered or more benefits gained, regardless of whether or not people are aware of this. This is an instrumental sense of *valuable,* and is objective. Modern healthcare, as a whole, is valuable in this sense, but some kinds of healthcare are not valuable, even though misinformed people value them.

Basic Values

Whether something has instrumental value is determined by whether it leads to a decrease in universal or objective evils or an increase in universal or objective goods. These goods and evils are the basic values because all other values in a normative sense are derived from them. Positive basic values have been called intrinsic goods, and negative basic values, intrinsic evils, but the phrases *intrinsic goods* and *intrinsic*

evils are misleading, as they suggest that whether something is an intrinsic good or evil is independent of the attitudes of rational persons. However, an account of basic values that does not relate them to the attitudes of rational persons cannot explain why all rational persons avoid evils and do not avoid goods.

The following definition of basic evils (harms) and basic goods (benefits) acknowledges the necessary connection between basic values and rationality. "In the absence of reasons, evils or harms are what all rational persons avoid, and goods or benefits are what no rational person gives up or avoids" (Gert, 1998, ch. 4, p. 92). On this account of the basic values, there are five basic evils: death (permanent loss of consciousness), pain (including mental pains and other unpleasant feelings), disability (including loss of physical, mental, or volitional abilities), loss of freedom (including loss of freedom from being acted on as well as the freedom to act), and loss of pleasure (including loss of sources of pleasure). There are four basic goods: consciousness, ability, freedom, and pleasure.

These basic values are central to healthcare. Healthcare is primarily concerned with the prevention and cure of maladies, and with the relief of the symptoms of maladies that cannot be cured. Maladies, which include both diseases and injuries, have as an essential feature, that a person with a malady is suffering one of the basic harms, or has a significantly increased risk of suffering one of them (Gert, 1997, ch. 5). It is almost a truism that healthcare is primarily concerned with preventing, as far as possible, death, pain, and disability. Although not mentioned quite so commonly, healthcare is also concerned with treating those conditions of persons that would result in their suffering a loss of freedom or pleasure. Those in healthcare might rank the basic values differently from people outside of healthcare;

physicians generally rank preventing evils as more important than promoting goods, and view death as the worst evil. However, no one in healthcare would challenge any of the items on the list of basic goods and evils, that is, the basic values.

Values and Rationality

Given that the definition of good and evils is based on the actions of rational persons, it may seem as if, without empirical research, nothing could be said about what counts as evils or harms, or what counts as goods or benefits. However, such research is impossible to carry out, for it requires examining what *all* rational persons avoid and do not avoid. A list of the basic goods and basic evils has already been provided, however, so there is a seeming inconsistency. It is important to clarify the definition so as to remove this problem. To say "In the absence of reasons, evils or harms are what all rational persons avoid, and goods or benefits are what no rational person gives up or avoids," means "In the absence of reasons, evils or harms are what all rational persons, *insofar as they are acting rationally,* avoid, and goods or benefits are what no rational person, *insofar as he is acting rationally,* gives up or avoids." Almost all rational persons sometimes act irrationally. This happens when they are in a very frightening situation or are overcome by some other strong emotion. What they happen to avoid or not avoid at these times is not relevant to the account of objective values.

Making clear that basic values are determined only by the behavior of rational persons insofar as they are acting rationally introduces a new problem. How is it determined that a person is acting rationally? This is a crucial question. Most philosophers, as well as most economists and political scientists, answer this question by providing a formal answer, one that has no universal or objective content. With various modifications, the standard answer to the question "What is it to act rationally?" is "It is to act in a way that maximizes the overall satisfaction of your desires." On the formal account of rationality under consideration, persons are acting rationally if and only if their actions are consistent with maximizing the satisfaction of their desires, regardless of the content of those desires.

On this account of rationality, there is no particular kind of thing that all rational persons act to avoid and not avoid, and thus there are no basic values or objective goods and evils. There are only values in a sense that has no normative implications. It might be thought that, at least, pleasure and pain would remain as goods and evils, but this is not so. The formal answer cannot restrict itself to persons who are not suffering from mental disorders. When people with serious mental disorders are included, it is not true that all persons acting rationally, defined as acting in a way that maximizes the overall satisfaction of their desires, act to avoid pain and act so as not to avoid pleasure, even in the absence of reasons. The maximizing satisfaction account of rationality results in values being defined as whatever people value. So defined, values have no normative implications. People determine for themselves what is good or evil and so pain and disabilities can be goods to some people, and pleasure and abilities, evils to them.

The Inadequacy of Formal Accounts of Rationality

Many attempts have been made to handle this problem, none of them satisfactory. Insofar as rationality is defined in purely formal terms with no limit on content, it loses its normative implications. It will always be possible to come up with an example that will categorize someone as acting rationally when no one would ever recommend that any person for whom they are concerned act in that way. For example, suppose a person's desire to kill himself in the most painful possible way is stronger than all of his other desires put altogether, even after full consideration. On the maximum satisfaction of desire view, he would be acting rationally to consult *Consumer Reports,* read biology books, etc., in order to achieve his goal. Once this consequence of the maximum satisfaction of desire view is made explicit, it is clear that this account of rationality has no normative force. Given this sense of rationality, it makes perfectly good sense to ask, "Why should I act rationally?" Many people would respond that on some occasions you should not act rationally.

In the normative sense of rationality, the one with which philosophers are properly concerned, no persons who are regarded as a moral agents, i.e., who are held responsible for their actions, would ever recommend to anyone for whom they were concerned, including themselves, that they ever act irrationally. They would never seriously ask, "Why shouldn't I act irrationally?" If it makes perfectly good sense to ask, "Why shouldn't I act irrationally?" then it is not important to determine whether rationality supports morality or anything else. The normative sense of rationality, like the normative sense of values, evils (harms) and goods (benefits), requires that there be universal agreement among moral agents on what kinds of things are harms and what kinds are benefits. All persons who are regarded as responsible for their behavior agree that they would always recommend to anyone for whom they were concerned, including themselves, that they act rationally and they would never recommend acting irrationally.

This agreement is what allows for clear counter-examples to all of the formal definitions of rationality. Everyone agrees that death, pain, disability, loss of freedom and loss of pleasure are evils. In the absence of reasons, all of us would recommend to anyone for whom we are concerned that he act in such a way as to avoid these harms. Likewise, in the absence of reasons, all of us would recommend to anyone for whom we are concerned that she not act so as to avoid the goods of consciousness, ability, freedom, or pleasure. Indeed, if, in the absence of reasons, persons do not act so as to avoid any of these harms or act to avoid any of these goods, they are regarded as acting irrationally. If they act in these ways for an extended period of time, they would be classified by the *Diagnostic and Statistical Manual of Mental Disorders,* fourth edition (*DSM IV*) as suffering from a mental disorder. Having objective values (objective goods and evils), and having an account of rationality with content necessarily go together. Healthcare presupposes these objective values. Medicine aims at avoiding and relieving the basic evils that are the result of a condition of the person being treated.

Reasons

As pointed out in the previous paragraph, people are regarded as acting irrationally if, in the absence of reasons, they do not avoid the evils and do avoid the goods. This correctly suggests that the primary function of a reason is to make some otherwise irrational action rational. Since irrational actions are those in which, in the absence of reasons, a person does not act to avoid an evil or acts to avoid a good, reasons must be facts about avoiding evils or gaining goods. Only such facts can make it rational not to avoid an evil or to avoid a good. It is rational to amputate my right arm if that is necessary to avoid the spread of a cancer that will kill me. It is not rational to amputate my right arm simply because I want to do so, or because I correctly believe that doing so will make me asymmetrical. If desires are taken as reasons that can make an otherwise irrational action rational, then it could be perfectly rational not to avoid an evil or to avoid a good simply because of a desire to do so.

All reasons must involve one or more of these basic goods or evils that are involved in the account of an irrational action. Of course, not all reasons will be adequate to make all otherwise irrational actions rational. An adequate reason must be one that involves a good or an evil that is viewed by a significant number of otherwise rational persons as compensating for the evil suffered. Otherwise rational persons are persons who, in the absence of reasons, avoid evils and do not avoid goods. Rational people can, within limits, differ in their rankings of the goods and evils. What one person regards as an adequate reason for not avoiding a given evil, another person might not. But there are limits. It is irrational

to commit suicide to avoid going to the dentist. However, it is not irrational to commit suicide when suffering from an incurable illness that is sufficiently painful or disabling. Although rational persons can, within limits, differ on which good counts as better and which evil counts as worse, they do not disagree on what counts as an evil or as a good. There is complete agreement on the basic values even though there is limited disagreement concerning their ranking.

Healthcare and Values

Healthcare is primarily concerned with preventing or treating those conditions of persons that cause or significantly increase the risk of death, pain, and disability and, to a lesser extent, the loss of freedom and pleasure. Healthcare is less involved with gaining any of the goods, but still has some concern with these matters. Those in healthcare might have a unique ranking of values, with the avoidance of death, pain, and disability, being ranked higher than they might be by people not in healthcare. However, English philosopher Thomas Hobbes (1588–1679), who was primarily concerned with politics, not with healthcare, also took death, pain, and disability to be of primary importance. Indeed, like many doctors, Hobbes seemed to view death as the worst of the evils. When the rankings of individual healthcare practitioners are not the same as the rankings of their patients, patients need not accept the rankings of their healthcare practitioners. On the contrary, healthcare practitioners must accept the rational rankings of their patients, for it is the patients that will actually be suffering the evils.

In addition to the basic values, there are also moral values. Moral values are the moral virtues, such as kindness, fairness, trustworthiness, and honesty. Moral values, like the basic goods and evils, are objective values. Kindness, fairness, trustworthiness, and honesty, are traits of character that all impartial rational persons want everyone to have because having these traits of character increase the probability that less harm will be suffered by all people affected. Indeed, a trait of character counts as a moral virtue only if its general practice increases the probability that less harm will be suffered than its not being generally practiced. There are other virtues of character such as courage, prudence, and temperance that all rational persons want for themselves because they increase the probability that the person himself, or those he cares for, will suffer less harm and gain greater benefits. These are personal virtues and although they are necessary in order to have the moral virtues, they are, as Hobbes and German philosopher Immanuel Kant (1724–1804) pointed out, traits of character that make immoral persons even more dangerous.

It should now be clear that there are no unique values in healthcare, either unique basic values or unique moral values. Since the moral values in healthcare cannot conflict with the moral values in the rest of life, it is not even plausible that there are any unique moral values in healthcare. There are duties that are unique to those in health case, but there are duties that are unique to those in every profession. But none of these duties exempt those in healthcare from the requirements of common morality. As in any profession, a physician may have duties that are in conflict with some other moral rule, but in all of these cases they must be willing for everyone to know that everyone is allowed to violate this other moral rule in circumstances with the same morally relevant features.

Although it may seem that some values such as kindness take on more importance in healthcare, there is no unique ranking of moral values. There are no moral values that are unique to healthcare. The importance of recognizing that there are no values, including moral values, that are unique to healthcare is that it makes clear that, as long as two persons know the facts of a situation equally well, it makes no difference to the validity of their judgments whether or not one is a practitioner of healthcare and the other not. Of course, those involved in healthcare usually know more of the relevant facts better than someone not involved in healthcare. However, the relevant facts should be made available to people outside the field as well as to those within. The advantages in moral evaluation and moral decision making about healthcare matters that those in healthcare have over those not in healthcare, in addition to greater knowledge of the facts, is greater experience and practice. These are not insignificant advantages.

Ethical Relativism

Anthropologists investigating a society previously unknown to them are very wary of criticizing any aspect of that society, even when that aspect involves a harmful practice. At one time, this reluctance to criticize was based upon a kind of naïve ethical relativism. They believed that each society had its own morality, but they believed that their own morality required tolerance, which they took to require that they not judge any practice in another society on the basis of their own moral standards. They did not even care whether the harmful practice was based on false beliefs about the empirical world. That the people of that society, or more commonly the dominant group in that society, accepted a certain practice, was all that was important. For various reasons, these views changed. Partly this was due to a great increase in the number of women anthropologists, and the widespread practice of female circumcision or genital mutilation in many societies being studied by anthropologists. However, even though many anthropologists now consider the practice of female circumcision to be immoral, they do not thereby immediately criticize that practice and try to get the society to stop practicing it. The reason for this is that they realize that this practice is tied into many other beliefs and practices, so that it is not clear how this practice can be changed or eliminated without doing greater harm to the people of that society.

Realization that objective evaluation of a society's practices is legitimate should lead to a more careful examination of the complex interrelationships between the practices in that society. It is not appropriate to criticize a practice and attempt to change or eliminate it until reasonably sure that changing or eliminating that practice will not result in even worse consequences. Caution is in order before trying to get a society to change or eliminate any of its practices. This is true not only of the practices of other societies, but also of a person's own society. Nonetheless, when encountering a harmful practice, it is now recognized that it is morally acceptable to try to find out what can be done to lessen the amount of harm, without causing even greater harm. A harmful practice should always give rise to an investigation about what can be done to change or eliminate that practice without resulting in greater harms. Anthropologists came to realize that the basic harms were universal. They also understood that a practice could be recognized as harmful even though it might not yet be known how to eliminate that harm without causing even greater harms.

Relativism and Unique Values in Healthcare

If healthcare is thought to have unique values, then people outside of healthcare, e.g., philosophers, might be in a position like those anthropologists who held ethical relativism. Evaluation by outsiders who did not share these unique values would be inappropriate. However, if healthcare shares the same values as all other areas of life, then all that outsiders need to know is what the facts are. However, similar to the situations of anthropologists, knowing all the facts is not an easy matter. Consider the following example; a philosopher claims, with some justification, that the process of providing information as practiced by the overwhelming number of doctors, is not adequate. On an ideal or philosophical level, a patient ought to be provided with all of the information that any rational person in that situation would want to know. This would include not only any significant risks and benefits of the proposed treatment, of alternative treatments, and of no treatment at all, it would also include information about which hospitals and doctors are most successful in providing those treatments.

Everyone agrees that patients are deprived of some freedom to make rational decisions if they are not supplied with all of this information. Thus the current practice of not providing this information is a harmful practice. In the absence of adequate justification, it would seem that this failure to provide all of this information is not morally acceptable. However, it does not follow that this practice should be changed and that doctors should be required to provide all of this information. It might be that, unless many other practices are also changed, requiring doctors to provide all of that information will require so much time, with so little change in outcome, that the costs, human as well as financial, make it undesirable to require physicians to provide that information. Perhaps healthcare practitioners already know that. But if we know that a practice is harmful, we should be trying to see if something can be done to change that practice without thereby causing even more harm. There should be consideration of other methods of providing this kind of information to patients.

Summary

Healthcare accepts the same basic and moral values that are accepted by all rational persons. Death, pain, disability, loss of freedom and loss of pleasure, due to conditions of person, are the focus of healthcare. Those in health case might rank the basic values differently, they may even rank the moral values differently, but even if they do, it is quite likely not a uniform difference. It is only that more individuals in healthcare might rank avoiding death higher than avoiding pain than most people not in healthcare. Sometimes, however, as in end of life care, these differences in rankings can be very important. Although there are no unique values in healthcare, there is a unique experience. Those who are healthcare practitioners know more about what actually happens and how different practices are related to one another. Anyone not in healthcare who has not studied what actually goes on in healthcare should, like anthropologists confronting a new society, be very wary of suggesting changes in the way healthcare is practiced, even when confronted with what seem like clear cases of harmful practices. But those in healthcare should recognize that when all the facts are known and appreciated, the rankings of values by those in healthcare do not have any privileged status, rather the rankings of those who will suffer the evils carry the most weight.

BERNARD GERT

SEE ALSO: *Autonomy; Care; Casuistry; Communitarianism and Bioethics; Compassionate Love; Consensus, Role and Authority of; Contractarianism and Bioethics; Emotions; Freedom and Free Will; Human Rights; Obligation and Supererogation; Principalism; Utilitarianism and Bioethics; Value and Valuation; Virtue and Character*

BIBLIOGRAPHY

Gert, Bernard. 1998. "Goods and Evils." In *Morality: Its Nature and Justification,* p. 92. New York: Oxford University Press.

Gert, Bernard; Culver, Charles M.; and Clouser, K. Danner. 1997. "Malady." In *Bioethics: A Return to Fundamentals.* New York: Oxford University Press.

Gruzalski, Bart, and Nelson, Carl, eds. 1982. *Value Conflicts in Health Care Delivery.* Cambridge, MA: Ballinger.

Hobbes, Thomas. 1991. *Man and Citizen,* ed. Bernard Gert. Indianapolis: Hackett.

Humber, James M., and Almeder, Robert F., eds. 1997. *Biomedical Ethics Reviews: What is Disease?* Atlantic Highlands, NJ: Humana Press.

Kant, Immanuel. 1981. *Grounding for the Metaphusics of Morals,* tr. James W. Elington. Indianapolis: Hackett.

Kopelman, Loretta M., ed. 1999. *Building Bioethics, Coversations with Clouser and Friends on Medical Ethics.* Dordrecht: Kluwer.

Nathanson, Stephen. 1994. *The Ideal of Rationality: A Defense within Reason.* Chicago: Open Court.

VALUE AND VALUATION

• • •

Though values are integral to human experience, it is only in modern societies that they have gained an explicit place in ethics. In traditional societies, values generally operate as components of the common culture that are taken for granted. Their moral discourse focuses on the rules that define primary human obligations and on notions of moral excellence. Values first acquire ethical importance where individuals have wide choices about how they are to live their lives. These choices lead to a plurality of value perspectives whose competing claims may appear to express little more than subjective preferences. The challenge to ethics, then, is to devise ways of assessing values critically in relation to normative moral discourse.

In European civilizations, wide value choices were first opened up by the rise of capitalism and of liberal democratic states. In this context, value considerations are never far removed from market dynamics or from basic principles of human liberty. Although class and status factors bar many from the benefits of these modern social formations, their impact on human life remains pervasive, compelling us for the sake of social order to accommodate various value orientations.

The Concept of Values

We take note of the realities in our world that matter to us. Values are concepts we use to explain how and why various realities matter. Values are not to be confused with concrete goods. They are ideas, images, notions. Values attract us. We aspire after the good they articulate. We expect to find our own good in relation to what they offer.

Because values are linked to realities we experience, they have an objective reference. They disclose features in our everyday world to which we attach special importance. Positive values are balanced by disvalues. Disvalues express what we consider undesirable, harmful, or unworthy about particular phenomena. They identify realities that we resist or strive to avoid. Virtually everything we experience has valuative significance: objects, states of affairs, activities, processes, performances, relational networks, and so on.

Values are linked to acts of valuation (Scheler). For every value that appears, there is a corresponding valuative orientation (Husserl). This orientation may not be fully self-conscious; still less is it an expression of critical judgment. It is, nonetheless, the subjective basis for the appearance of values. Without valuing subjects, there can be no such thing as values.

In an elemental sense, values are disclosed by feelings (Ricoeur). Explicit value language comes later, if at all. How do I know that health is good? I know because I feel good when I am healthy. The positive feeling signals the presence of value. How do I know that a performance of Shakespeare's *Hamlet* is good? Even an informed aesthetic judgment has an affective basis: I was moved by it. In being moved, I apprehend value. My primal awareness of value becomes explicit as I identify the features in a phenomenon that draw me to it. Human languages furnish a rich vocabulary for conversations about values.

The correlation between values and valuative acts does not imply that values are purely subjective or that they are merely secondary embellishments of empirical fact. On the contrary, the notion of an empirical reality devoid of all valuative meaning is itself an abstraction. As our perceptions disclose an object's reality, so our affections disclose its

worth (Ricoeur). By means of perceptions and affections, we apprehend facets of the realities we encounter. Apart from corresponding acts of consciousness, however, nothing whatever can appear.

Values and Human Needs

Values are intimately related to human needs and desires (Niebuhr; Ogletree; Ricoeur). We value realities that satisfy basic needs and fulfill deeply felt aspirations. We associate disvalues with realities that threaten or diminish human well-being. Human well-being is only part of the story. With a growing environmental consciousness, value discussions embrace nonhuman life forms as well, perhaps creaturely well-being as a whole. Human life then gains its value within a natural world that has intrinsic worth. Religious communities honor a world-transcending center of values from which all lesser values derive their significance.

There are as many kinds of values as there are regions of experience where we distinguish good or bad, better or worse, beneficial or harmful: sensory values, organic values, personal values, interpersonal values, social values, cultural values, and spiritual values (Scheler). Social values can be differentiated into economic, political, legal, associational, and familial subsets. Cultural values embrace religious, moral, cognitive, and aesthetic interests (Parsons). The formal value types all contain values and disvalues. Notions of creaturely well-being are implied if not stated.

Value Issues in Biomedical Practice

Virtually all kinds of values figure in biomedical practice. Organic values are basic: life, health, vigor, bodily integrity. The purpose of medicine is to save lives and to promote healing. Yet the ill and injured are never merely "patients," organisms suffering treatable maladies; they are persons with dignity who have their own life plans (May, 1991; Ramsey). Personal values, therefore, qualify organic values. Patients as persons may in no case be subjected to medical procedures without informed consent. Ideally, they participate actively in their own healing.

Organic values are inherently problematic. Our impulses press us to strive for life, strength, and agility. Yet these strivings are limited by our vulnerability to illness, injury, disability, and, finally, certain death. Modern medicine inclines us to define the limits of organic life not as natural features of finitude but as problems to be solved. This tendency requires us to make value judgments about the boundaries of medical intervention. Medical practices inattentive to these boundaries can deprive the dying of the personal space they need to achieve closure in their life pilgrimages.

At this point, organic values are qualified by more encompassing value commitments. Such commitments can help us to accept life's limits, acknowledge goods more noble than our own survival, and endure sufferings and disappointments with grace and wisdom. Life, death, health, and illness are never purely physiological; they are moral and spiritual as well. Healthcare must also have moral and spiritual as well as physiological dimensions (Cousins; May, 1991; Nelson and Rohricht).

Professional and economic values intersect medical practice in similar ways. Physicians have specialized knowledge that equips them to provide socially valued services. They enjoy social status as professionals who maintain standards for medical practice. In this role, they are public guarantors of prized social values (May, 1983). Physicians in the United States offer services for fees, primarily through third-party payments. Accordingly, medical practice is also a market transaction, and physicians are businesspeople with economic interests. The stake in economic values qualifies professional devotion to patient well-being.

The organization of healthcare profoundly conditions its operative values. Modern medicine requires sophisticated technologies affordable only to large medical centers. These institutions, usually constituted as corporations, dominate medical practice in the United States. The technologies they use are typically produced and supplied by global corporations. The income they receive derives largely from corporate employee-benefit plans and from insurance firms that service them. Health-related industries have become a major component of the economy, perhaps inappropriately overriding the legitimate claims of other social goods. Powerful economic and political interests support the continued growth of medical enterprises with little regard for wider social ramifications.

Because the desire for quality medical services is urgent, intense public debate surrounds federal policies that bear upon the organization, regulation, and funding of healthcare. The struggle is to determine appropriate government roles for the oversight and financing of biomedical activities. In this struggle, conflicting political values intersect healthcare practices as public actors respond to constituent interests. Similar sociocultural analyses could be directed to the roles played in the healthcare system by values resident in families, religious communities, research institutes, medical colleges, the legal system, the media, and the arts. Ethical studies of the intersection between biomedical practices and social processes uncover a volatile mix of conflict-laden value issues.

Fluidity of Values

Values are not only pervasive but also fluid. Any concrete experience harbors many values and disvalues, none of which is definitive or self-contained. Illness can be a physical malady, a ruthless disruption of personal plans, an economic disaster, an opportunity for self-discovery, a moment of human bonding, an occasion for medical virtuosity, or a case study in biomedical research (May, 1991). Each of these meanings captures some of the values that belong to a particular experience. As attention shifts, one set of values continually flows into another.

Our terminology for values is similarly fluid. The word *health* can be used descriptively; it also identifies an important value. *Justice* can designate a basic moral principle; it can refer equally to a value worthy of promotion in social arrangements. The term *objective* may characterize "value-free" inquiry, but it also designates a cognitive value.

Because of their fluidity, values resist schematic classification. Attempts to construct comprehensive value schemes do, however, have heuristic significance. They heighten awareness of the range of our valuative connections with our world, and they stimulate reflections on what belongs to human well-being (Hartmann; Perry; Scheler).

Moral Values

Within the value field, we can isolate a subset of moral values. Moral values cluster around personal identity, interpersonal relationships, and the makeup of groups, associations, social institutions, whole societies, and even the global community (Scheler). Numerous values—dignity, integrity, mutual respect, loyalty, friendship, social cohesion, fairness, stability, effectiveness, inclusiveness—are moral in import. Anthropocentric values are supplemented and corrected by the moral claims of animals and, more broadly, by the moral claims of the environment, a self-sustaining ecosystem. Even religious devotion to the divine life has moral dimensions, for the faithful are obliged to honor God as the final bearer of value.

Moral values enjoy precedence within the value field because they identify the basic loci of all valuing experience— that is, valuing subjects in relationship. Where moral values are secure, we can cultivate a wide array of values. Where moral values are in danger, all values are at risk.

Even so, in our responses to concrete cases we regularly rank some nonmoral values above specifically moral ones. Faced with a health emergency, our regard for life itself, an organic value, surpasses normal preoccupations with human dignity, a moral value. We do what we can to save a life! At the same time, we know that life as such is but one value among many. Prolonging human life can never, therefore, be the primary goal.

Similarly, human beings can often best advance their own good through value commitments that transcend specifically moral considerations. Cognitive, aesthetic, and especially spiritual values finally stand *higher* than moral values in most value schemes because they bestow significance on existence in its travail and woe. Yet these values still require for their realization valuing subjects who are bearers of moral value.

We normally discuss moral values in terms of rights and duties. Rights identify claims that others properly make on us. These claims intersect our value-oriented projects and disclose our duties. A physician's professional judgment about a course of therapy is subject to the patient's informed consent. The abortion debate hinges on differing assessments of fetal rights against a pregnant woman's right to choose.

Duties consist of obligations and prohibitions. Obligations specify what we must do no matter what else we might also hope to accomplish. Hospital emergency rooms must treat seriously injured persons regardless of whether they can pay, offering such care as a part of normal operations. Prohibitions specify what we must not do regardless of larger objectives. We must not use human beings as research subjects without their consent no matter how important the research may be.

It is for the sake of moral values that basic rights and duties are binding. We may set such mandates aside only when extraordinary measures are required to safeguard the values they protect. For the sake of human dignity, physicians are normally obliged to do all they reasonably can to sustain the lives of their patients. Precisely for the sake of human dignity, however, this obligation loses its force when further medical interventions would only prolong the dying process.

Values and Human Action

Value awareness gains practical importance in terms of action (Ricoeur). We adopt courses of action that promise results favoring our prized values; we act to inhibit developments that endanger our values. Values guide decision making, disposing us to choose one course of action over another. We justify our decisions in terms of the values they are designed to promote.

Matters do not always turn out as we expect. We may lack the skill, the power, the influence, or the knowledge to achieve our objectives. In medical practice, few surprises

follow the skilled application of routine therapies proven to be effective for treating particular ills. Physicians do not stay within safe territory, however. They regularly confront medical problems that they cannot diagnose with confidence and for which there are no known clinical responses with assured results. Medical outcomes frequently fall short of human hopes. They include side effects whose disvalues outweigh desired values. "Side effects" belong to action consequences even when they do not reflect our intentions.

When our actions affect the actions of others, uncertainty increases. Other people may not react as we expect. They may misunderstand our intentions or respond carelessly. We may misread their value commitments. Perhaps the relevant network of human interactions is so vast and complex that it surpasses what we can grasp. Here, too, the outcomes may not fit our values. Prediction is most reliable for highly routine actions with widely understood purposes. It is least reliable for novel initiatives, such as new directions in policy.

Because we cannot fully control or predict the consequences of our actions, the fit between actions and values is inexact. This inexactness carries over into value assessments. We may readily name the values that attach to desired outcomes. Before we can evaluate a course of action, however, we have to consider the uncertainties. We have to weigh the disvalues that could accompany significant miscalculations. Considerations of value differ from discussions of duty by virtue of the inexact fit between values and action. Duty refers not to the likely outcomes of actions but to actions as such, which are largely in our power. It specifies ground rules that order human activity. In general, we may pursue a larger vision of the good only within constraints set by these ground rules. In its early stages, biomedical ethics properly gave precedence to the delineation of basic moral duties.

The fit between values, action, and action consequences remains close enough, however, that values must figure in the ethical examination of action. I am accountable to myself and others not simply for the conformity of my actions to rules that define my duties but also for values and disvalues that reside in the results of my actions. In decision making, I project the likely outcomes of actions I am considering and I weigh probabilities that qualify my projections. I also bring into view risks of unpleasant surprises. Practical reflection on values depends on substantial knowledge of the social dynamics that structure action.

Values in Society and Culture

In traditional societies, the most crucial value issues are largely settled. To be viable, a society requires a shared set of reasonably cohesive values. This shared value cluster composes the society's moral identity. It is expressed in many ways within the common culture: public rituals, speeches, novels, paintings, school textbooks, standard histories, and scholarly investigations.

Modern societies with market economies and liberal democracies are not able to sustain comprehensive value syntheses. At best, they promote what John Rawls calls a "thin" theory of the good—that is, elemental goods that all are presumed to need and want whatever else they might also desire (Rawls). Within the framework of basic goods, such societies host a multiplicity of concrete value orientations, reflecting the diverse priorities of individuals and groups within the society. Some question whether we can sustain even a "thin" theory of the good without a widely shared, substantive value synthesis fostered in basic social institutions (MacIntyre). The disintegration of traditional cultural values tends to undermine interest in the common good. Private preoccupations with individual advantage and "interest group" politics then displaces public discourse about the good of the society as a whole. Likewise, political battles are fought without the restraints of civility necessary to social order. Value theory becomes urgent when basic values are in dispute. Its task is not only to advance critical investigations of persistent value disputes but also to show how various value streams within a pluralistic society can contribute to the good of all.

Critical Reflection on Values

The scrutiny of values has four crucial layers: (1) the reflective identification of our operative values; (2) assessments of the fit between these operative values and considered judgments about creaturely well-being; (3) analyses of value relations in order to identify compatible and incompatible values sets; and (4) imaginative constructions of value syntheses capable of ordering life priorities in personal, communal, and social contexts.

The investigation of values begins with description. We seek to become self-conscious about the values we prize, taking note of value commitments ingrained in stable life patterns and ongoing institutional involvements. The descriptive task is informed by historical studies of normative traditions and of social developments leading to current practices. As we make our operative values explicit, we are often stimulated to reorder our priorities. We recognize that existing arrangements do not reflect our convictions about what matters most in life.

The relation that values have to basic human needs suggests a second step in value studies. British utilitarians and American pragmatists sought to test our presumptive values by empirical investigations (Bentham; Dewey). Their aim was to discover life practices and value attachments that truly accord with primary human needs. Much human-science research functions as value inquiry of this sort, shedding light on value patterns that tend to promote human well-being in contrast to those that finally prove dysfunctional. Historical, philosophical, and theological reflections can also inform such inquiry. For ethics, the challenge is to clarify the contributions empirical studies can make to the critical assessment of values and to incorporate those contributions into constructive philosophical and religious thought. The third step is an analysis of value relations. Not all values are compatible with one another, at least not in practical terms. We cannot both affirm free speech and shield people from all offensive public expressions. We cannot protect the environment without constraining market freedoms. Likewise, we cannot guarantee everyone healthcare that fully utilizes the most advanced medical technologies while also controlling aggregate healthcare costs. Critical thought examines values in terms of their fit with one another. It dramatizes the necessity of choices among different sets of values. We bypass some values and endure relative disvalues for the sake of value combinations that reflect considered priorities. The crucial step in the critical study of values is the imaginative construction of coherent value syntheses capable of guiding action. Because modern societies harbor a multiplicity of value perspectives, attempts to determine value priorities take place in several contexts.

Individuals develop a mature moral identity by clarifying the connections and priorities that order personally cherished values. Value syntheses are no less vital for families, special-interest associations, and religious bodies. These collectives gain moral, and perhaps religious, identity through shared value commitments. Organizations that give concrete form to economic, legal, political, and cultural institutions are themselves more effective when they make their defining values explicit.

Coherent sets of values are not easily achieved or sustained. They enjoy the greatest authority when they emerge as critical appropriations and transformations of normative value traditions within contemporary life settings. Because of the complexity of experience, value syntheses can never fully overcome areas of ambivalence or wholly resolve internal strains. Within limits, we can accommodate value conflicts that we acknowledge and honor. Such conflicts may even stimulate creativity. Within comprehensive value syntheses, value priorities normally run in two contrary directions. Elemental sensory, organic, and economic values enjoy priority over higher political, cultural, and spiritual values in the sense that they furnish the conditions necessary to the appearance of the higher values. Political, cultural, and spiritual values enjoy priority over more basic sensory, organic, and economic values in the sense that they bestow meaning and significance on the more elemental values. Moral values play the mediating role because they identify the loci of value experience. These contrasting modes of priority can shed light on concrete values conflicts.

Public Value Syntheses

A basic value of modern societies is the protection of private spaces for people to pursue diverse visions of the good. Social cohesion rests, then, on minimal agreements that allow individuals and groups to live together in their diversity. In the United States, the prevailing value synthesis combines liberal democratic principles and principles of free-market capitalism. Enduring controversies concern the nature and extent of appropriate government intervention in market processes. Less clearly articulated are images of a greater national community embracing many races, cultures, and religions. The latter images are countered by persisting patterns of racism, ethnocentrism, and religious intolerance.

In biomedical ethics, the most urgent challenge is to form a public value synthesis that can guide healthcare reform. Though difficult disputes remain, there is considerable agreement that a good system will guarantee basic care for all, maintain acceptable standards of quality, foster an active partnership between patients and physicians, take account of the defining values of those who give and receive care, sustain advanced biomedical research, hold total costs to manageable levels, and protect contexts for personal preferences and individual initiatives in delivering and receiving care. These values—especially the contention that all people must have access to basic medical services—all have important moral dimensions.

Any workable system will include value trade-offs. It will require a reexamination of standards of quality care, a balance between healthcare needs and other social goods, and a workable mix of economic incentives and government regulations that maintains discipline within the system while allowing space for individual initiatives. Any system will also confront limits. Moral creativity requires imaginative responses to limits in the promotion of creaturely well-being.

Because of the subtleties involved, bioethics cannot easily incorporate notions of value and valuation into deliberations about basic human duties. Yet values pervade human experience. They even shape our perceptions of the obligations and prohibitions that set constraints on our actions. As we examine more comprehensively the moral issues that reside in biomedical practice, the more we will discover the necessity of systematic value assessments. Critical value studies will tend as well to force a shift in the dominant structure of moral reasoning, from the linear logic of the syllogism to the more nuanced process of weaving multiple value considerations together into an illuminating pattern of moral understanding. While the resulting judgments may appear less precise and decisive, they will probably be more true to life.

THOMAS W. OGLETREE (1995)

SEE ALSO: *Animal Welfare and Rights: Ethical Perspectives on the Treatment and Status of Animals; Healthcare Resources, Allocation of; Health and Disease; Medicine, Art of; Research Methodology: Conceptual Issues*

BIBLIOGRAPHY

Bentham, Jeremy. 1948. *An Introduction to the Principles of Morals and Legislation,* ed. Laurence J. LaFleur. New York: Hafner.

Cousins, Norman. 1979. *Anatomy of an Illness as Perceived by the Patient: Reflections on Healing and Regeneration.* New York: Norton.

Dewey, John. 1931. *Philosophy and Civilization.* New York: Minton, Balch.

Harron, Frank; Burnside, John W.; and Beauchamp, Tom L. 1983. *Health and Human Values: A Guide to Making Your Own Decisions.* New Haven, CT: Yale University Press.

Hartmann, Nicolai. 1932. *Ethics,* vol. 2: *Moral Values,* tr. Stanton Coit. New York: Allen and Unwin.

Husserl, Edmund. 1970. *The Crisis of European Sciences and Transcendental Phenomenology: An Introduction to Phenomenological Philosophy,* tr. David Carr. Evanston, IL: Northwestern University Press.

MacIntyre, Alasdair. 1984. *After Virtue,* 2nd edition. Notre Dame, IN: University of Notre Dame Press.

May, William F. 1983. *The Physician's Covenant: Images of the Healer in Medical Ethics.* Philadelphia: Westminster.

May, William F. 1991. *The Patient's Ordeal.* Bloomington: Indiana University Press.

Nelson, James B., and Rohricht, Jo Anne Smith. 1984. *Human Medicine: Ethical Perspectives on Today's Medical Issues,* rev. edition. Minneapolis, MN: Augsburg.

Niebuhr, H. Richard. 1943. *Radical Monotheism and Western Culture.* New York: Harper & Row.

Ogletree, Thomas W. 1985. *Hospitality to the Stranger: Dimensions of Moral Understanding.* Philadelphia: Fortress.

Parsons, Talcott. 1969. *Politics and Social Structure.* New York: Free Press.

Perry, Ralph Barton. 1926. *The General Theory of Value: Its Meaning and Basic Principles Construed in Terms of Interest.* Cambridge, MA: Harvard University Press.

Ramsey, Paul. 1970. *The Patient as Person: Explorations in Medical Ethics.* New Haven, CT: Yale University Press.

Rawls, John. 1971. *A Theory of Justice.* Cambridge, MA: Harvard University Press.

Ricoeur, Paul. 1966. *Freedom and Nature: The Voluntary and the Involuntary,* tr. Erazim V. Kohák. Evanston, IL: Northwestern University Press.

Scheler, Max. 1973. *Formalism in Ethics and Non-Formal Ethics of Values: A New Attempt Toward the Foundation of an Ethical Personalism,* 5th rev. edition, tr. Manfred S. Frings and Roger L. Funk. Evanston, IL: Northwestern University Press.

Veatch, Robert M. 1991. *The Patient-Physician Relation: The Patient as Partner.* Bloomington: Indiana University Press.

VETERINARY ETHICS

• • •

Veterinary medicine, as the distinctive medical discipline we know today, emerged during the nineteenth century as an adjunct to agriculture. Animals were valued for the food or fiber they provided or for the work they performed, and the veterinarian's role in society was to keep the animals healthy so they could serve people's needs. Even after anticruelty laws had become widespread by the late 1800s, and the horse doctor became the dog doctor with the growth of companion animal practice in the mid-twentieth century, the veterinarian's ethic remained unexamined and substantive ethical issues officially unacknowledged.

Unlike medical doctors, whose engaging of ethical issues can be traced back to Hippocrates, veterinarians did not have a historic tradition of professional ethics to draw on. Until the late 1970s, the field of veterinary ethics focused primarily on issues of business etiquette and professional relations. The Code of Ethics of the American Veterinary Medical Association (AVMA) addressed such areas as referrals to other veterinarians and whether it was "ethical" to have a large insert for one's practice in the Yellow Pages. Social changes, such as the emergence of the animal-welfare/rights movement and its impact on public consciousness, helped catalyze consideration of the complex of ethical concerns that face the veterinarian.

Two people acted as gadflies to the profession in this important period: Michael W. Fox, a veterinarian with the Humane Society of the United States, and Bernard E. Rollin, a philosopher at Colorado State University. Fox and Rollin published articles in influential journals (Fox, 1983b; Rollin, 1978, 1983) that pointed out the need for systematic examination of the ethical concerns of the veterinary profession. Fox also wrote letters to the *Journal of the AVMA* on this theme (Fox, 1983a). In 1978, Rollin inaugurated the first regular, required, full-term course in veterinary ethics at the Colorado State University College of Veterinary Medicine. Both Fox and Rollin wrote books on animal welfare and rights. Rollin, in addition, had taught and published in human medical ethics, and he was sensitive to the differences between the problems of human medical ethics and those of veterinary medical ethics. In particular, owing to his extensive work in the moral status of animals, Rollin was aware that veterinary medicine had not yet addressed its moral obligation to animals. By the end of the 1980s, veterinary interest in the ethics of the profession had developed enough to warrant publication of a textbook on the subject by Jerrold Tannenbaum of Tufts University (1989).

The Veterinary Oath and Its Moral Dilemmas

When the veterinarian graduates from veterinary school, he or she is administered the veterinarian's oath, which includes a promise "to use my scientific knowledge and skills for the benefit of society through the protection of animal health, the relief of animal suffering, the conservation of livestock resources, the promotion of public health, and the advancement of medical knowledge" (see the Appendix, Volume 5). The veterinarian is immediately faced with a fundamental ethical dilemma: to whom does he or she owe primary loyalty, the owner or the animal? In a 1978 article, Rollin used the examples of a pediatrician and a car mechanic to illustrate the two possible choices. When the repairs on a car are more costly than the car's value, the owner can simply tell the mechanic to "junk" it or not do the repairs; there is no such choice in a necessary surgery or treatment of a child (Rollin, 1978). The pediatrician is ethically (and legally) obligated to act as advocate of the child's well-being. On the other hand, the basic current legal status of animals is that they are property, although their sentient qualities have been the basis of limited protection provided by so-called welfare laws (in the United States, primarily local anticruelty ordinances and federal laboratory animal laws).

In addition to the responsibilities they have to the animal and the owner, veterinarians must weigh practice judgments in light of the needs of society in general ("public health"), peers, and themselves as well. As the oath also states, "I will practice my profession conscientiously, with dignity, and in keeping with the principles of veterinary medical ethics. I accept as a lifelong obligation the continual improvement of my professional knowledge and competence" (Appendix, Volume 5). In the face of often conflicting interests of animal, owner, society, profession, and self, the individual veterinarian is often presented with situations that require complex ethical judgments (Rollin, 1988). The traditional minimalistic animal ethics proscribing cruelty, from which anticruelty laws derived, are not adequate to mid-twentieth-century uses of animals such as confinement agriculture or testing and research, which were not matters of cruelty yet caused significant suffering in pursuit of profit and scientific knowledge (Rollin, 1981). In seeking a new animal ethic, society began to apply the notion of rights, which protect human nature from being submerged for the sake of general welfare, to animals in order to protect their fundamental interests as dictated by their nature (or "telos"). The veterinarian came to be considered a natural animal advocate. As society elevated to the status of animals by applying a rights ethic, the status and effectualness of the veterinarian began to increase (Rollin, 1983).

Laboratory-Animal Legislation: Effect on the Profession

One area—laboratory-animal medicine—has had its ethical obligations to animals articulated by law because of societal concern for animal welfare. Before the 1985 Amendment to the Animal Welfare Act, which originated as a Colorado state bill written by Rollin and others, and the National Institutes of Health Reauthorization Act of 1985, which turned animal use "guidelines" into regulations, researchers enjoyed carte blanche in the use of animals. The pursuit of knowledge, or "advancement of medical knowledge," had completely trumped consideration of animal pain, suffering, or distress, and laboratory-animal veterinarians were relegated to the role of keeping animals in good enough shape to serve their research purposes. The legislation that was passed in 1985, as well as the original Animal Welfare Act of 1966 and other amendments to that act, was a direct result of societal response to well-publicized atrocities in research and testing activities and the correlative demand for assurance that animals' interests were protected.

Laboratory-animal veterinarians, because of animal-protective legislation, now fulfill the most unambiguous role of all veterinarians regarding animal well-being: They are obligated by law to act as animal advocates, to assure that pain and suffering do not occur or are minimized by proper medication, that proper animal care is provided, and that humane euthanasia is performed. The veterinarians are aided by Institutional Animal Care and Use Committees, which review research or testing protocols for humane considerations before studies may commence and provide regular monitoring of facilities.

Small-Animal-Practice Concerns

Although the role of the veterinarian has been defined by society in law for the laboratory-animal veterinarian, this has not occurred in other areas of veterinary medicine in which owner interest and animal interest may conflict. The small-animal veterinarian is often faced with ethical decisions based on these conflicts. Examples include cosmetic or behavior-altering surgery and orthodontic intervention for cosmetic reasons. In general, these procedures could be considered in the interests of the animal only if the animal were afflicted with a condition that was causing or was likely to cause it pain or distress. Dewclaw removal—dewclaws can catch and tear when dogs run through rough terrain—or repair of malocclusions like base-narrow lower canines, in which the offending tooth or teeth can drive into the upper palate, can easily be justified as in the animal's interest. Cosmetic surgery that causes the animal to conform to standards of style (e.g., ear cropping) or surgery that is used to curb "objectionable" behavior (e.g., declawing of cats, devocalizing of dogs) can be viewed as causing pain and distress to the animal for frivolous human reasons. Likewise, straightening teeth that are functional to provide a perfect bite for the show dog could be considered unnecessary.

Many veterinarians refuse to do purely cosmetic surgery, and consequently they lose clients. Other small-animal veterinarians believe they owe their major loyalty to the owner. They may argue that providing the service of cosmetic surgery enhances the animal's value, emotional as well as monetary, to the owner. Still other veterinarians will provide behavior-altering surgeries, such as declawing, after first pursuing, with an owner, honest attempts at retraining or other options. They may justify their actions by saying that the owner would otherwise get rid of the pet or that they are fostering the continuation of a rewarding relationship for both pet and owner.

Surgically neutering (spaying or castrating) dogs and cats to prevent sexual behaviors and overpopulation of pets is well accepted by North American society, but (especially for dogs) is largely rejected in other countries in favor of owner responsibility in administering contraceptives and controlling pets. Many small-animal veterinarians readily neuter cats and dogs, assuming that the discomfort of the surgery is of less import than the enhancement of the desirability of the pet to the owner (the elimination of objectionable sexual behavior, for instance) and the elimination of the chance of unwanted pregnancies; in addition, there are health advantages to neutering.

Some Equine-Practice Concerns

The equine veterinarian is under similar tension, only more so. Lameness is the most frequent complaint of horse owners, as the horse's usefulness requires a smooth and efficient gait. The equine veterinarian is often pressured to provide painkilling medication or surgery to cut the nerves to the feet of race or performance horses because of lameness. In some respects this is a compassionate action, as the animal is rendered fully or relatively free of pain. However, there are cases in which eliminating painful sensations may cause the animal to use and seriously injure a limb. Pressures to administer performance-enhancing drugs, or to look the other way when objectionable training techniques may be used, may be severe for equine veterinarians. Veterinarians may also be called on to perform purely cosmetic surgery, such as tail docking or tail "breaking" for an artificially high tail carriage. Unfortunately, horses are generally of little entertainment or economic value if they do not "go sound," or conform to an ideal of beauty.

A Look at Food-Animal Medicine

Food-animal veterinarians have always been placed in a position of tension between the interests of animals and the interests of producers. In traditional agriculture, which prevailed as an "extensive" (as opposed to "intensive") endeavor until the mid-twentieth century, the tension was mitigated to some extent because producers generally did well economically only if they provided for the health and welfare of their individual animals. With the rise of confinement agriculture, however, new considerations have entered into the picture, and producers can prosper—in fact, may make the most profits—even if numerous individual animals suffer from poor health or die. For instance, feedlots may utilize diets that cause digestive and liver disease in a certain percentage of animals, but that loss will be more than compensated economically by the weight gain in the remaining animals. Furthermore, the use of antibiotics, vaccines, growth promoters, etc., have permitted selectivity in meeting animal needs and the separation of economic productivity from animal well-being. Animals can thus suffer in areas not related to economic productivity, yet

producers can do well. Since the advent of intensive agriculture, veterinary concern for individual animals has tended to be replaced by a "herd health" philosophy to serve the livestock industry.

In confinement operations, a certain death loss is expected from the animals, whether from contagious or so-called production diseases, which are caused by handling, artificial environments, selective breeding, population density, or nutrition in the operation. Veterinary care in confinement operations usually covers only animals that are expected to recover without costing more in money and labor than the animals' market value. In sheep feedlots, a common daily chore is picking up dead or moribund animals. Discovering which animals are sick, separating them from their group, and treating or euthanizing them is often considered too expensive to support. In complete confinement houses for swine, animals are fed antibiotics because respiratory disease is so prevalent owing to high ammonia levels. To combat fighting in tight quarters among feeder pigs, their tails are amputated so the animals cannot wound each other by tail biting. Mastitis and footrot in dairy cattle are production diseases caused by the enforcement of high milk yields while the cattle are maintained on dirt lots. The average dairy cow is worn out and culled in four or five years, less than half of the expected useful lifetime fifty years ago.

Agrarian values of husbandry have been abandoned in much of present-day agriculture, affecting how the veterinarian may conduct his or her profession, because whereas a small farmer once maintained a modest lifestyle by caring for a few individual animals, a corporation now looks at profit margin only. Even in the more traditional agricultural activity of cattle ranching, economic considerations militate against veterinarians' controlling the pain of such activities as branding, dehorning, and castration. Thus the modern food-animal veterinarian faces a variety of conflicts arising out of tension between economic considerations on the one hand and animal health and welfare considerations on the other.

The Veterinarian and Euthanasia

Even if the veterinarian's inclination is to act as an animal advocate, he or she may be thwarted by the owner's wishes, because of the legal status of animals as chattel or property. Occasionally a veterinarian is faced with a situation in which a pet is suffering without hope of recovery, as in terminal cancer, but where euthanasia is not an option because an owner refuses to authorize it. Many veterinarians quietly euthanize such animals as a humane act in spite of its illegality; but a more direct approach, utilized by veterinarians who often deal with death and the consequent grief of owners, is to discuss the inevitable with clients beforehand and exercise a humane ethic by requesting the clients to agree to euthanasia if certain clinical signs, like unremitting pain or inability to eat, arise.

A more common delay of euthanasia occurs when a food animal is kept alive despite suffering to maximize income. This scenario is most often seen in large, commercial operations, where, for instance, a sow with a fractured leg or a cow with a cancerous eye could be kept alive without expensive treatment until parturition or weaning of offspring. It is interesting to note that the laboratory-animal veterinarian is required by law to euthanize when faced with hopeless animal suffering, while the private practitioner is hamstrung by laws of private property in situations that do not constitute cruelty under the law.

The most obvious and rewarding use of euthanasia—killing without causing pain or distress—is to end an animal's suffering due to unremitting illness or fatal injury. However, there are other uses of euthanasia, such as end points for research, humane slaughter for meat, and humane killing of unwanted pets by pounds, shelters, or veterinarians. The AVMA Panel on Euthanasia periodically updates and publishes its report on euthanasia. The report examines methods of killing and labels as unacceptable those that cause animals to suffer. For instance, the report accepts an overdose of anesthetic, which causes an animal to become unconscious before dying, but condemns an overdose of paralytic drug, which causes motor and respiratory paralysis and suffocation in an alert animal.

Many small-animal veterinarians are confronted with requests for "convenience" euthanasia—euthanasia of healthy pets for owners who have rejected the implied contract of care they incurred when they acquired the pet. Some veterinarians avoid these ethical dilemmas by refusing categorically to perform any "convenience" euthanasia, even though they know that the owner may choose a nonhumane alternative, such as abandonment. Others accept such animals on the condition that they be allowed to find a home for the animal as an alternative to euthanasia; this route obviously requires time, effort, and probably expense on the part of the veterinarians but helps to satisfy their obligation to the animal.

Accepting an animal for euthanasia, and then not performing it, however, is a breach of contract and indefensible on legal grounds. One interesting dilemma that has challenged equine veterinarians is insurance companies'

requirement that expensive horses be euthanized if they are rendered unfit by accident or illness for an insured purpose (e.g., racing, breeding, or showing) even if these animals are otherwise capable of a pain-free, or even useful, existence. When enormous sums of money are at stake, consideration of the animal's interests tends to disappear.

Veterinarians and Anticruelty Laws

Animal cruelty laws are notoriously lax. Most allow conviction only in cases of purposeful abuse, and in any case generally result in insignificant fines. However, the veterinarian may be able to make a difference in the lives of animals by reporting and testifying in animal abuse cases. Reporting a client for battering his dog or starving his horses or other stock, when all efforts at education and persuasion are exhausted, may be the only means of protecting animals. In taking a stand as an animal advocate, the veterinarian may experience a loss of clientele and income, thereby placing personal interest in conflict with animal and client interests.

The Veterinarian's Obligation to Society

The veterinarian's obligation to society can also be the occasion for conflicts relating to self or business interests. The most straightforward example may be the protection of society from contaminated animal-source foods. Hormonal and medicinal additives to feed, or treatments of individual animals with medications, can result in residues in meat and milk. These products, if allowed for food animals, have government-mandated withdrawal times before slaughter or milking. Sometimes products used in animal production are not approved for any food animal administration. Yet because of poor planning, inattention to withdrawal times, or attempt to defraud, producers may send contaminated animals or their products to market. The underlying motive is usually profit. If a veterinarian discovers that a producer is feeding an illegal additive, or if, for example, a heifer is sent to slaughter before the withdrawal time of the penicillin she was given, the food-animal veterinarian has a public-health obligation—an obligation to society—to report the client despite professional confidentiality concerns. The loss of one client may be the least of the financial impact of such an ethical choice; other potential or actual clients may avoid association with the veterinarian because of fear of also being turned in, as some illegal practices in the food-animal industry may be widespread, especially in a given region.

The laboratory-animal veterinarian's career can be seen as a service to society, in that he or she provides clinical support or scientific information for the advancement of scientific knowledge. Despite his or her legal mandate as animal advocate, the veterinarian may experience personal conflict in areas of pain or disease research; for example, studies that involve the most animal suffering may also provide the most useful information for the betterment of humans and animals alike. The laboratory-animal veterinarian must also come to grips with the fact that virtually all of his or her patients will be killed at the end of a study.

The zoo or wildlife veterinarian serves societal interests in areas of animal conservation and wildlife management. Incarceration, as in a zoo, is not generally in individual animals' interests, but captive breeding programs may be needed to preserve a valued species. Similarly, situations may arise in which a disease is introduced into study animals to determine pathophysiology or treatment for that species or similar groups. The use of wild animals in research, especially when capture is a part of the research design, has been severely criticized by animal welfare and rights groups because of unacceptably high numbers of "stress" losses of animals used in the studies.

Policing the Profession: Obligations to Peers

The veterinarian, like practitioners in other professions, may have to take an ethical or legal stand regarding the practices of his or her peers—as, for example, when one gives testimony in a malpractice suit. Certainly a person's choice in business practices and commitment to medical standards indicate the quality of his or her moral fiber and loyalty to the profession. It is not unusual for veterinarians to sever professional or personal ties with other veterinarians over professional standards, although it is rare for them to make allegations of malpractice or business malfeasance of other veterinarians. This course is largely left to state boards of veterinary medicine, which respond to complaints by the public. Reluctance to speak out against professional misconduct by other veterinarians is not unique to this profession. A certain degree of prudence must be exercised by professionals to avoid unfairly slandering a colleague without knowing the entire story; for instance, a client's account of a veterinarian's actions may be biased and medically naïve. Many veterinarians also believe that exposing misconduct puts the entire profession in a bad light, even if the public would likely have a positive regard for "policing the ranks." Veterinarians, like other professionals, are allowed a fair amount of leeway in regulating themselves, since they are presumed to know the issues better than laypeople. Failure to self-police can result in loss of autonomy, with rules initiated and governed by people who know little about the profession, such as legislators.

The Veterinarian's Obligation to Self and Personal Values

The veterinarian's obligation to self is best fulfilled by examination of and adherence to his or her professional and personal values. Some veterinarians believe the veterinarian's only or major loyalty should be to the animal. Most veterinarians probably enter the profession with a desire to protect animal health and relieve animal suffering, without an understanding of competing interests. A fuzzy or unexamined ethic may lead to compromising professional decisions. Veterinary schools have responded to the need for ethical training in their curricula, with the understanding that veterinary students need intellectual tools to examine their own ethics throughout their professional lives.

Veterinary Ethics Today

The profession is by no means monolithic in its attitudes, but the AVMA and other veterinary organizations have gradually begun to take official positions on animal issues. A number of practitioners' organizations, including the American Society of Laboratory Animal Practitioners, the American Association of Bovine Practitioners, the American Association of Equine Practitioners, and some state veterinary organizations, have taken animal-welfare positions or have held symposia or meetings pertaining to issues of concern to them. Advocacy groups, such as the Association of Veterinarians for Animal Rights, have emerged. The Animal Welfare Committee of the AVMA has encouraged the association to take published positions on a variety of companion animal, exhibit and performance animal, research animal, and agricultural animal issues. Although some positions are weak and tentative (mainly on agricultural issues), many are specifically protective (e.g., condemning use of the steel-jawed trap and recommending to the American Kennel Club and breed associations that ear cropping be dropped from standards and that dogs with cropped ears be prohibited from showing). The AVMA also sponsors an annual Animal Welfare Forum, in which veterinary educators, animal advocates, philosophers, and others examine the need for animal-welfare reform within the profession.

Given that the formal articulation and organized study of veterinary ethical issues are new, the field has made a good deal of progress. In the future, we can expect the emergence of more sophisticated treatments of many of the issues we have articulated. With society's expectations that the veterinarian serve as mandated animal advocate (as evidenced by the aforementioned laboratory-animal laws), veterinarians will doubtless be in the forefront of emerging social concerns about animal use and treatment.

M. LYNNE KESEL (1995)
BIBLIOGRAPHY REVISED

SEE ALSO: *Animal Research; Animal Welfare and Rights: Pet and Companion Animals; Care; Cloning: Scientific Background; Harm; Research, Unethical; Value and Valuation*

BIBLIOGRAPHY

Fox, Michael W. 1983a. Letter. *Journal of the American Veterinary Medical Association* 182(12): 1314–1315.

Fox, Michael W. 1983b. "Veterinarians and Animal Rights." *California Veterinarian* 37(1): 15.

Fox, Michael W. 1984. *Farm Animals: Husbandry, Behavior, and Veterinary Practice*. Baltimore: University Park Press.

Legood, Giles, ed. 2000. *Veterinary Ethics: An Introduction*. New York: Continuum, 2000.

Rollin, Bernard E. 1977. "Moral Philosophy and Veterinary Medical Education." *Journal of Veterinary Medical Education* 4(1): 180–182.

Rollin, Bernard E. 1978. "Updating Veterinary Medical Ethics." *Journal of the American Veterinary Medical Association* 173(8): 1015–1018.

Rollin, Bernard E. 1983. "Animal Rights and Veterinary Medical Education." *California Veterinarian* 37(1): 9–15.

Rollin, Bernard E. 1988. "Veterinary and Animal Ethics." In *Law and Ethics of the Veterinary Profession*, ed. James E. Wilson. Yardley, PA: Priority.

Rollin, Bernard E. 1991-present. "Veterinary Ethics." *Canadian Veterinary Journal.*

Rollin, Bernard E. 1992. *Animal Rights and Human Morality*, rev. ed. Buffalo, NY: Prometheus.

Rollin, Bernard E. 1998. *The Unheeded Cry: Animal Consciousness, Animal Pain, and Science*. Ames: Iowa State University Press.

Rollin, Bernard E. 1999. *An Introduction to Veterinary Medical Ethics: Theory and Cases*. Ames: Iowa State University Press.

Rollin, Bernard E. 2000. "Veterinary Ethics and Animal Welfare." *Journal of the American Animal Hospital Association* 36(6): 477–479.

Schneider, B J. 1999. "Veterinary Ethics and Conflict Resolution." *Canadian Veterinary Journal* 40(2): 111–112.

Shapiro, Leland S. 1999. *Applied Animal Ethics*. Florence, KY: Delmar Learning.

Tannenbaum, Jerrold. 1989. *Veterinary Ethics*. Baltimore: Williams and Wilkins.

Thornton, P D; Morton, D. B.; Main, D. C.; et al. 2001. "Veterinary Ethics: Filling a Gap in Undergraduate Education." *Veterinary Record* 148(7): 214–216.

VIRTUE AND CHARACTER

• • •

"Virtue" is the translation of the ancient Greek *arete*, which meant any kind of excellence. Inanimate objects could have *arete*, since they were assumed to have a *telos*, that is, a purpose. Thus, the *arete* of a knife would be its sharpness. Animals could also have *arete*; for example, the strength of an ox was seen as its virtue. Though an animal could possess *arete*, the Greeks assumed natural potentialities in men and women to be virtues requiring enhancement through habits of skill. Therefore, Aristotle defined virtue as "'a kind of second nature' that disposes us not only to do the right thing rightly but also to gain pleasure from what we do" (Aristotle, 1105b25–30).

Because there are many things that "our nature" as humans inclines us to do, Aristotle argues, there can be many human virtues. How particular virtues are constituted can vary with different understandings of "human nature" and the different social roles and their correlative skills. Yet the virtues, according to Aristotle, are distinguished from the arts, since in the latter excellence lies in results. In contrast, for the virtues it matters not only that an act itself is of a certain kind, but also that the agent "has certain characteristics as he performs it; first of all, he must know what he is doing; secondly, he must choose to act the way he does, and he must choose it for its own sake; and in the third place, the act must spring from a firm and unchangeable character" (Aristotle, 1105a25–30).

The word *hexis*, which Aristotle uses for "character," is the same word that denotes the habitual dispositions constitutive of the virtues. Character, therefore, indicates the stability that is necessary so that the various virtues are acquired in a lasting way. Character is not simply the sum of the individual virtues; rather, it names the pattern of thought and action that provides a continuity sufficient for humans to claim their lives as their own (Kupperman). However, the material form associated with character may vary from one society to another. Therefore any definition of virtue, the virtues, and character can be misleading because it can conceal the differences between various accounts of the nature and kinds of virtues as well as character.

The Role of Virtue in Recent Moral Philosophy

Ancient philosophers as well as Christian theologians, though offering quite different accounts of the virtues, assumed that any account of the well-lived life had to take virtue into consideration. Modern moral philosophy, in contrast, treats virtues—if it treats them at all—as secondary to an ethics based on principles and rules. The attempt to secure an account of morality that is not as subject to variations as an ethics of virtue certainly contributed to this displacement of virtues. The first edition of the *Encyclopedia of Bioethics*, for example, had no entry on virtue or character.

In his widely used and influential introduction to philosophical ethics, William Frankena manifests the approach to ethics that simply assumed that considerations of virtue were secondary. According to Frankena, ethical theory should be concerned primarily with justifying moral terms and clarifying the differences between appeals to duty and consequences. The virtues, to the extent they were discussed by theorists such as Frankena, were understood as supplements to the determination of right and wrong action. The virtues in such a theory were seen more as the motivational component in more basic principles, such as benevolence and justice. As Frankena put it,

> We know that we should cultivate two virtues, a disposition to be beneficial (i.e., benevolence) and a disposition to treat people equally (justice as a trait). But the point of acquiring these virtues is not further guidance or instructions; the function of the virtues in an ethics of duty is not to tell us what to do, but to insure that we will do it willingly in whatever situation we may face. (Frankena, p. 67)

Frankena's understanding of the nature and role of the virtues drew on the commonsense view that in order to know what kind of person one ought to be, one needs to know what kind of behavior is good or bad. Unless one knows what constitutes acts of truth-telling or lying, one has no way to specify what the virtue of truthfulness or honesty might entail. Ethical theories were assumed to be aids to help people make good decisions on the basis of well-justified principles or rules. Virtues were secondary for that endeavor.

This account of ethics seemed particularly well suited to the emerging field of bioethics. It was assumed that the task of medical ethics was to help physicians and other healthcare providers make decisions about difficult cases created by the technological power of modern medicine. Whether a patient could be disconnected from a respirator was analyzed in terms of the difference between such basic rules as "do no harm" and "always act that the greatest good for the greatest number be done." The case orientation of medical decision making seemed ideally suited to the case orientation of ethical theory exemplified by Frankena.

In their influential book, *Principles of Biomedical Ethics*, Tom L. Beauchamp and James F. Childress retain the structure of ethics articulated by Frankena. Their account of biomedical ethics revolves around the normative alternatives of utilitarian and deontological theories and the principles of autonomy, nonmaleficence, beneficence, and justice. Each of these fundamental principles has correlative primary virtues—that is, respect for autonomy, nonmalevolence, benevolence, and justice—but these "virtues" play no central role. Beauchamp and Childress justify leaving an account of virtue to the last chapter by saying that there are no good arguments for "making judgments about persons independent of judgments about acts or … making virtue primary or sufficient for the moral life" (p. 265).

Both philosophers (Pincoffs) and theologians (Hauerwas) have challenged the assumption that ethics in general and biomedical ethics in particular should be focused primarily on decisions and principles. It is a mistake, they argue, to separate questions of the rightness or goodness of an action from the character of the agent. To relegate the virtues to the motivation for action mistakenly assumes that the description of an action can be abstracted from the character of the agent. To abstract actions from the agent's perspective fails to account for why the agent should confront this or that situation and under what description. Those who defended the importance of virtue for ethics argued, following Aristotle, that *how* one does *what* one does is as important as what one does.

The renewed interest in the nature and significance of virtue ethics has been stimulated by the work of Alasdair MacIntyre, in particular his book *After Virtue* (1984). MacIntyre's defense of an Aristotelian virtue theory was but a part of his challenge to the presuppositions of modern moral theory. MacIntyre attacked what he called "the Enlightenment project," the attempt to ground universal ethical principles in rationality qua rationality—for example, Kant's categorical imperative (Kant). MacIntyre agrees that principles and rules are important for ethics, but he rejects any attempt to justify those principles or rules that abstracts them from their rootedness in the historical particularities of concrete communities. The narratives that make such communities morally coherent focuses attention on the virtues correlative to those narratives. For the Greeks, for example, the *Odyssey* acted as the central moral text for the display of the heroic virtues. To separate ethics from its dependence on such narratives is to lose the corresponding significance of the virtues.

MacIntyre's defense of an ethics of virtue is part of his challenge to the attempt to secure agreement among people who share nothing besides the necessity to cooperate in the interest of survival. Enlightenment theories of ethics, MacIntyre argues, falsely assume that an ahistorical ethics is possible; a historical approach tries to justify ethical principles from anyone's (that is, any rational individual's) point of view.

Renewed interest in the ethics of virtue has accompanied a renewed appreciation of the importance of community in ethics. Those commentators who emphasize the importance of community presume that morally worthy political societies are constituted by goods that shape the participants in those societies to want the right things rightly. Therefore ethics, particularly an ethics of virtue, cannot be separated from accounts of politics. Such a politics cannot be reduced to the struggle for power but, rather, is about the constitution of a community's habits for the production of a certain kind of people—that is, people who have the requisite virtues to sustain such a community.

Bioethics and the Ethics of Virtue

In the past the practice of medicine was thought to be part of the tradition of the virtues. As Gary Ferngren and Darrel Amundsen observe, "If health was, for most Greeks, the greatest of the virtues, it is not surprising that they devoted a great deal of attention to preserving it. As an essential component of *arete*, physical culture was an important part of the life of what the Greeks called *kalos kagathos*, the cultivated gentleman, who represented in classical times the ideal of the human personality" (p. 7). It should not be surprising, therefore, that not only was health seen as an analogue of virtue but medicine was understood as an activity that by its very nature was virtuous. In medical ethics, the "ethics of virtue" approach tends to focus on the doctor-patient relationship. The trust, care, and compassion that seem so essential to a therapeutic relationship are virtues intrinsic to medical care. Medicine requires attention to technical knowledge and skill, which are virtues in themselves; however, the physician must also have a capacity—compassion—to feel something of patients' experience of their illness and their perception of what is worthwhile (Pellegrino). Not only compassion but also honesty, fidelity, courage, justice, temperance, magnanimity, prudence, and wisdom are required of the physician.

Not every one of these virtues is required in every decision. What we expect of the virtuous physician is that he will exhibit them when they are required

and that he will be so habitually disposed to do so that we can depend upon it. He will place the good of the patient above his own and seek that good unless its pursuit imposes an injustice upon him, or his family, or requires a violation of his own conscience. (Pellegrino, p. 246)

The importance of virtue for medical ethics has been challenged most forcefully by Robert Veatch. According to Veatch, there is no uncontested virtue ethic. The Greeks had one set of virtues, the Christians another, the Stoics another; and there is no rational way to resolve the differences among them. This is a particularly acute problem because modern medicine must be practiced as "stranger medicine," that is,

medicine that is practiced among people who are essentially strangers. It would include medicine that is practiced on an emergency basis in emergency rooms in large cities. It would also include care delivered in a clinic setting or in an HMO that does not have physician continuity, most medicine in student health services, VA Hospitals, care from consulting specialists, and the medicine in the military as well as care that is delivered by private practice general practitioners to patients who are mobile enough not to establish long-term relationships with their physicians. (Veatch, p. 338)

Virtue theory is not suited to such medicine, Veatch argues, because "there is no reasonable basis for assuming that the stranger with whom one is randomly paired in the emergency room will hold the same theory of virtue as one's self" (p. 339). The ethics of "stranger medicine" is best construed, Veatch contends, on the presumption that the relationship between doctor and patient is contractual. Such a relationship is best characterized by impersonal principles rather than in terms of virtue. The virtues make sense only within and to particular communities, and therefore only within a "sectarian" form of medicine.

Veatch's argument exemplifies what Alasdair MacIntyre calls the Enlightenment project. Yet MacIntyre would not dispute the descriptive power of Veatch's characterization of modern medicine. He thinks medicine is increasingly becoming a form of technological competence, bureaucratically institutionalized and governed by impersonal ethical norms. MacIntyre simply wishes to challenge the presumption that this is a moral advance. Put more strongly, MacIntyre challenges the presumption that such a medicine and the morality that underlies it can be justified in the terms Veatch offers. In particular, he asks, how can one account for the trust that seems a necessary component of the doctor-patient relationship without relying on an ethic of virtue?

Contrary to Veatch, James Drane and others argue that medicine does not exist within a relationship between strangers, but in fact depends on trust and confidence, if not friendship, between doctor and patient. Ethics, they hold, is not based on principles external to medical care and then applied to medicine; rather, medicine is itself one of the essential practices characteristic of good societies. Medicine thus understood does not need so much to be supplemented by ethical considerations based on a lawlike paradigm of principles and rules; on the contrary, medical care becomes one of the last examples left in liberal cultures of what the practice of virtue actually looks like. Those who work from an ethics of virtue do not come to medicine with general principles justified in other contexts, to be applied now to "medical quandaries"; rather, they see medicine itself as an exemplification of virtuous practices. Here medicine is understood in the Aristotelian sense, as an activity—that is, as a form of behavior that produces a result intrinsic to the behavior itself (Aristotle). In MacIntyre's language, medicine is a practice in which the goods internal to the practice extend our powers in a manner that we are habituated in excellence (MacIntyre). Put simply, the practice of medicine is a form of cooperative human activity that makes us more than we otherwise could be.

MacIntyre's account of practice and Aristotle's account of activity remind us that the kinds of behavior that produce virtue are those done in and for themselves. Thus virtue is not acquired by a series of acts—even if such acts would be characterized as courageous, just, or patient—if they are done in a manner that does not render the person performing the actions just. As Aristotle says, "Acts are called just and self-controlled when they are the kinds of acts which a just and self-controlled man would perform; but the just and self-controlled man is not he who performs these acts, but he who also performs them in the way that the just and self-controlled men do" (1105B5–9).

There is an inherently circular character to this account of the virtues that cannot be avoided. We can become just only by imitating just people, but such "imitation" cannot be simply the copying of their external actions. Becoming virtuous requires apprenticeship to a master; in this way the virtues are acquired through the kind of training necessary to ensure that they will not easily be lost. How such masters are located depends on a social order that is morally coherent, so that such people exhibit what everyone knows to be good. Medicine, because it remains a craft that requires apprenticeship, exemplifies how virtue can and should be taught.

William F. May suggests that the very meaning of a profession implies that one who practices it is the kind of person who can be held accountable for the goods, and corresponding virtues, of that profession. Medicine as a profession functions well to the extent that medical training forms the character of those who are being initiated into that

practice. This does not imply that those who have gone through medical training will be virtuous in other aspects of their lives; it does imply, however, that as physicians they will exhibit the virtues necessary to practice medicine.

In *Becoming a Good Doctor: The Place of Virtue and Character in Medical Ethics*, James Drane suggests that the character of the doctor is part of the therapeutic relationship, and that there is a structure to the doctor-patient relationship that is based on the patient's trust that the physician will do what is necessary to help the patient heal. The physician's task, Drane argues, is not to cure illness but to care for patients, and such care depends on the character of the physician. Drane, in contrast to Robert Veatch, argues that medicine must remain a virtuous practice if it is to be sustained in modern societies. Paul Ramsey's insistence that the focus of medicine is not the curing of illness but the care of patients "as persons," can be interpreted as an account of medicine commensurate with an emphasis on the virtues. The particular character of the judgments clinicians must make about each patient is not unlike Aristotle's description of practical wisdom, or *phronesis*. According to Aristotle, ethics deals with those matters that can be other; a virtuous person not only must act rightly but also must do so "at the right time, toward the right objects, toward the right people, for the right reasons, and in the right manner" (1106B20–23). Similarly, physicians must know when to qualify what is usually done in light of the differences a particular patient presents. From this perspective, medicine is the training of virtuous people so they are able to make skilled but fallible judgments under conditions of uncertainty. The increasing recognition of the narrative character of medical knowledge (Hunter) reinforces this emphasis on virtue and character. That the disease entities used for diagnosis are implicit narratives means medicine is an intrinsically interpretative practice that must always be practiced under conditions of uncertainty. Accordingly, patient and physician alike bring virtues (and vices) to their interaction that are necessary for sustaining therapeutic relationships.

Continuing Problems for an Ethics of Virtue

To construe medicine as a virtue tradition establishes an agenda of issues for investigation in medical ethics. How are the virtues differentiated? Are there some virtues peculiar to medicine? How are different virtues related to one another? How is the difference between being a person of virtue and character, and the possession of the individual virtues, to be understood? Can a person possess virtues necessary for the practice of medicine without being virtuous? Can a person be courageous without being just?

Such questions have been central to the discussion of the virtues in classical ethical theory. For example, Aristotle maintained that none of the individual virtues could be rightly acquired unless they were acquired in the way that the person of practical wisdom would acquire them. Yet one could not be a person of practical wisdom unless one possessed individual virtues such as courage and temperance. Aristotle did not think the circular character of his account was problematic because he assumed that the kind of habituation commensurate with being "well brought up" is the way we were initiated into the "circle."

Yet in what sense the virtues are habits remains a complex question that involves the question of how the virtues are individuated. For Aristotle some of the virtues are "qualities" that qualify the emotions, but not all the virtues are like courage and temperance in that respect. Aristotle's resort to the artificial device of the "mean" for locating the various virtues has caused more problems than it has resolved. These matters are made even more complex by the importance Aristotle gives to friendship in the *Nicomachean Ethics*, where it is treated as a virtue even though it is not a quality but a relation.

The Christian appropriation of the virtues did little to resolve these complex issues. For Saint Augustine the virtues of the pagans were only "splendid vices" insofar as they were divorced from the worship of God. In "Of the Morals of the Catholic Church," Augustine redescribed the fourfold division of the virtues as four forms of love:

> that temperance is love giving itself entirely to that which is loved; fortitude is love readily bearing all things for the loved object; justice is love serving only the loved object, and therefore ruling rightly; prudence is love distinguishing with sagacity between what hinders it and what helps it. The object of this love is not anything, but only God, the chief good, the highest wisdom, the perfect harmony. So we may express the definition thus, that temperance is love keeping itself entire and uncorrupt for God; fortitude is love bearing everything readily for the sake of God; justice is love serving God only, and therefore ruling well all else, as subject to man; prudence is love making a right distinction between what helps it toward God and what might hinder it. (p. 115)

Thomas Aquinas, influenced profoundly by Augustine and Aristotle, provided an extraordinary account of the virtues that in many ways remains unsurpassed. According to Aquinas, charity, understood as friendship with God, is the form of all the virtues. Therefore, like Augustine, he maintained that there can be no true virtue without charity (Aquinas). Unlike Augustine, however, Aquinas grounded

the virtues in an Aristotelian account of human activity, habits, and passions. For Aquinas, therefore, the virtues are dispositions or skills necessary for human flourishing.

Aquinas's account of the virtues does present some difficulties, however. Even though he followed Augustine's (and Plato's) account of the four "cardinal" virtues—prudence, courage, temperance, and justice—neither he nor Augustine successfully argued why these four should be primary. (Aristotle does not single out these four as primary.) Indeed, it is clear from Aquinas's account that he thought of the cardinal virtues as general descriptions that required more specification through other virtues, such as truthfulness, gentleness, friendship, and magnanimity.

These issues obviously bear on medicine considered as part of the virtue tradition. Are there virtues peculiar to the practice of medicine that require particular cultivation by those who would be doctors? If the virtues are interdependent, can a bad person be a good doctor? Or, put more positively, do the virtues required to be a good doctor at least set one on the way to being a good person? If the Christian claim that the "natural virtues" must be formed by the theological virtues of faith, hope, and charity is correct, does that mean that medicine as a virtue requires theological warrant?

Some of these questions have not been explored with the kind of systematic rigor they deserve. MacIntyre, however, suggests some promising directions. For example, he has argued that practices are not sufficient in themselves to sustain a full account of the individual virtues, their interrelations, or their role in areas such as medicine. Practices must be understood within the context of those goods necessary for the display of a whole human life and within a tradition that makes the goods that shape that life intelligible (MacIntyre). Those initiated into the practice of medicine, for example, might well have their moral life distorted if medicine as a virtue was not located within a tradition that placed the goods that medicine serves within an overriding hierarchy of goods and corresponding virtues. Yet what such a hierarchy would actually consist of remains to be spelled out.

These matters are made more complex to the extent that those who stand in virtue traditions cannot draw on the distinction between the moral realm and the nonmoral realm so characteristic of Kantian inspired moral theory. Once distinctions between the moral and the nonmoral are questioned, strong distinctions between deontological ethics, consequential ethics, and the "ethics of virtue" are equally questionable. L. Gregory Jones and Richard Vance argue, for example, that to assume that the virtues are an alternative to an ethics of principles and rules simply reproduces the assumption that there is a distinct realm called "ethics" that can be separated from the practices of particular communities. It was this assumption that led to the disappearance of virtue from modern moral theory.

For example, Aristotle thought that how a person laughed said much about his or her character. Therefore, what we consider matters of personal style and/or etiquette were considered morally significant by the ancients. For the virtues to encompass such matters as part of human character makes problematic the distinction so crucial to modernity—that is, the distinction between public and private morality. Thus, from such a perspective, what physicians do in their "private time" may well prove important for how they conduct themselves morally as physicians.

Equally troubling is the role *luck* plays in an ethics of virtue. For example, Aristotle thought that a lack of physical beauty made it difficult for a person to be happy: "For a man is scarcely happy if he is very ugly to look at, or of low-birth, or solitary and childless" (1099A35–37). Modern egalitarian sensibilities find it offensive to think that luck might play a role in our being virtuous (Card), yet the Greeks thought it unavoidable for any account of the virtuous and happy life. Indeed, as Martha Nussbaum has argued, the very strength the virtues provide create a "fragility" that cannot be avoided. Illness may well be considered part of a person's "luck" that limits the ability to live virtuously. Medicine may thus be understood as the practice that can help restore a person to virtue.

How medicine and an ethics of virtue are understood differs greatly from one historical period to another as well as from one community to another. To the extent that medicine can no longer be sustained as a guild, perhaps it should no longer be construed in the language of the virtues. As Mark Wartofsky asks, "How is benevolence, as a distinctively *medical* virtue, to be interpreted in those forms of the practice where the individual patient is literally seen not as a person but only through the mediation of the records, laboratory reports, or a monitoring of data in a computer network?" (p. 194).

Yet many continue to argue that any treatment of medicine that makes the virtues of both physician and patient secondary cannot be a medicine anyone should desire or morally support. Truthfulness, for example, is a virtue intrinsic to the care of patients; without it, whatever care is given, even if it is effective in the short run, cannot sustain a morally healthy relationship between patient and physician. Good medicine requires communication and participation by the patient that can be secured only by the physician's telling the patient the truth as well as the patient's demanding truthful speech. Without such truthful communication, the patient, as Plato argued, is reduced to

the status of a slave (Drane). Ironically, in the name of freedom, the kind of medicine Veatch envisioned looks like a medicine fit for slaves—admittedly an odd conclusion since Veatch assumes that a contractual relation between physician and patient is the condition for a free exchange. Moreover, even Veatch continues to assume that truthtelling is a virtue necessary for medicine to survive as a practice between strangers.

For his part, Drane raises issues at the heart of any account of the virtues as well as of medicine as a virtue tradition. If it is true that truthfulness is a virtue intrinsic to the practice of medicine, can that virtue conflict with, for example, the virtue of benevolence? Plato and Aristotle assumed the unity of the virtues. Accordingly, the virtues would not conflict with one another if they were rightly oriented to a life of happiness. Aquinas held that the virtues might conflict during the time we are "wayfarers," but not in heaven. Drane resolves the possibility of such conflict by suggesting that medicine requires the truth to be spoken, but benevolently. One may doubt, however, whether this attractive suggestion resolves all questions about the conflict among the virtues, particularly in medical care.

If medicine is to be construed in the tradition of the virtues, the virtues and character of patients must be considered. The very term *patient* suggests a necessary virtue that is closely associated with Christian accounts of the virtues. If we must learn to live our lives patiently, then illness may appear in quite a different light than it does in those accounts of the moral life that have no patience with patience. For example, if suffering is thought to be an occasion to learn better how to be patient, then a medicine of care may be sustainable even when cure cannot be accomplished.

Karen Lebacqz suggests that the circumstances in which patients find themselves, especially the circumstance of pain and helplessness, can invite them to become accepting and obedient. These traits, which may appear virtuous, may just as likely be vices if they are not shaped by fortitude, prudence, and hope. Lebacqz suggests that these virtues are particularly relevant to the condition of being a "patient," because they provide the skills necessary to respond to illness in a "fitting" manner. No *one* way of expressing these virtues suits all patients; yet they do provide the conditions for our learning the tasks required in health and illness.

Questions of virtue also relate to issues of justice in the distribution of healthcare. For if the patient can ask medicine to supply any need abstracted from a community of virtue, then there seems no way to limit in a moral way the demands for medical care. In such a situation, those who have more economic and social power can command more than is due medically, since medicine seems committed to meeting needs irrespective of the habits that created those needs. Liberal political theory has often tried to show how a just society is possible without just people; a "medicine of strangers" may result in a maldistributed medicine.

Conclusion

There is no consensus about the nature of virtue and/or the virtues that a good person should possess. That should not be surprising: the attempt to introduce the virtues into bioethics has gone hand in hand with an emphasis on the inevitable historical character of ethical reflection. If, as MacIntyre has argued, the virtues can be described only in relation to a particular tradition and narrative, then the very assumption that a universal account of ethics—and in particular, of medical ethics—is problematic. Yet the very character of medicine as a practice whose purpose is care for the ill remains one of the richest resources for those committed to an account of the moral life in the language of the virtues.

STANLEY M. HAUERWAS (1995)

SEE ALSO: *Beneficence; Care; Compassionate Love; Ethics: Normative Ethical Theories; Justice; Medicine, Art of; Narrative; Patients' Responsibilities: Virtues of Patients; Trust*

BIBLIOGRAPHY

Aquinas, Thomas. 1952. *Summa Theologica,* tr. Fathers of the English Dominican Province. Chicago: Encyclopaedia Britannica.

Aristotle. 1962. *Nicomachean Ethics,* tr. Martin Ostwald. Indianapolis, IN: Bobbs-Merrill.

Augustine. 1955. Selections from "Of the Morals of the Catholic Church." In *Christian Ethics: Sources of the Living Tradition,* pp. 110–118, ed. Waldo Beach and H. Richard Niebuhr. New York: Ronald Press.

Beauchamp, Tom L., and Childress, James F. 1983. *Principles of Biomedical Ethics,* 2nd edition. New York: Oxford University Press.

Card, Claudia. 1990. "Gender and Moral Luck." In *Identity, Character, and Morality: Essays in Moral Psychology,* pp. 199–218, ed. Owen J. Flanagan and Amelie Oksenberg Rorty. Cambridge, MA: MIT Press.

Drane, James F. 1988. *Becoming a Good Doctor: The Place of Virtue and Character in Medical Ethics.* Kansas City, MO: Sheed & Ward.

Ferngren, Gary B., and Amundsen, Darrel W. 1985. "Virtue in Hell/Medicine in Pre-Christian Antiquity." In *Virtue and Medicine: Explorations in the Character of Medicine,* pp. 3–22, ed. Earl E. Shelp. Dordrecht, Netherlands: D. Reidel.

Flanagan, Owen J., and Rorty, Amelie Oksenberg, eds. 1990. *Identity, Character, and Morality: Essays in Moral Psychology.* Cambridge, MA: MIT Press.

Frankena, William K. 1973. *Ethics,* 2nd edition. Englewood Cliffs, NJ: Prentice-Hall.

Hauerwas, Stanley. 1985. *Character and the Christian Life,* 2nd edition. Notre Dame, IN: University of Notre Dame Press.

Hunter, Kathryn Montgomery. 1991. *Doctors' Stories: The Narrative Structure of Medical Knowledge.* Princeton, NJ: Princeton University Press.

Jones, L. Gregory, and Vance, Richard P. 1993. "Why the Virtues Are Not Another Approach to Medical Ethics: Reconceiving the Place of Ethics and Contemporary Medicine." In *Religious Methods and Resources in Bioethics,* pp. 203–225, ed. Paul F. Camenisch. Dordrecht, Netherlands: Kluwer.

Kant, Immanuel. 1959. *Foundations of the Metaphysics of Morals, and What is Enlightenment?,* tr. Lewis White Beck. New York: Liberal Arts Press.

Kupperman, Joel. 1991. *Character.* New York: Oxford University Press.

Lebacqz, Karen. 1985. "The Virtuous Patient." In *Virtue and Medicine: Explorations in the Character of Medicine,* pp. 275–288, ed. Earl E. Shelp. Dordrecht, Netherlands: D. Reidel.

MacIntyre, Alasdair. 1984. *After Virtue: A Study in Moral Theology,* 2nd edition. Notre Dame, IN: University of Notre Dame Press.

May, William F. 1992. "The Beleaguered Rulers: The Public Obligation of the Professional." *Kennedy Institute of Ethics Journal* 2(1): 25–41.

Nussbaum, Martha C. 1986. *The Fragility of Goodness: Luck and Ethics in Greek Tragedy and Philosophy.* Cambridge, Eng.: Cambridge University Press.

Pellegrino, Edmund D. 1985. "The Virtuous Physician, and the Ethics of Medicine." In *Virtue and Medicine: Explorations in the Character of Medicine,* pp. 237–256, ed. Earl E. Shelp. Dordrecht, Netherlands: D. Reidel.

Pellegrino, Edmund D., and Thomasma, David C. 1993. *The Virtues in Medical Practice.* New York: Oxford University Press.

Pincoffs, Edmund L. 1986. *Quandaries and Virtues: Against Reductivism in Ethics.* Lawrence: University Press of Kansas.

Ramsey, Paul. 1970. *The Patient as Person: Explorations in Medical Ethics.* New Haven, CT: Yale University Press.

Veatch, Robert M. 1985. "Against Virtue: A Deontological Critique of Virtue Theory and Medical Ethics." In *Virtue and Medicine: Explorations in the Character of Medicine,* pp. 329–346, ed. Earl E. Shelp. Dordrecht, Netherlands: D. Reidel.

Wartofsky, Mark. 1985. "Virtues and Vices: The Social and Historical Construction of Medical Norms." In *Virtue and Medicine: Explorations in the Character of Medicine,* pp. 175–200, ed. Earl E. Shelp. Dordrecht, Netherlands: D. Reidel.

W

WARFARE

• • •

I. INTRODUCTION

In the immortal words of General William Tecumseh Sherman, one of its better known practitioners, "war is hell." Rather than diminishing with the cessation of the superpower rivalry that dominated the international scene for nearly half a century, the incidence of warfare is increasing. As the twenty-first century began over three dozen wars were being fought around the globe, like an insidious disease with no cure is in sight.

Types of War

Warfare is generally understood as armed conflict, often prolonged, between nations or parts of nations. Civil wars are fought between sections of the population within a nation. When an armed group engages in military action against its government, the war is an insurrection or a revolution, sometimes called a war of national liberation.

Despite its abhorrent character, nations routinely prepare for armed conflict, defensively, most claim. Some actively institute it for reasons their leaders deem necessary.

After the September 11, 2001, bombings of the World Trade Center and Pentagon, a new kind of war emerged, a war against terrorism. This turned out initially to be military action by the United States and its allies against the Taliban rulers of Afghanistan and against the international organization believed to be responsible for the September 11th attacks. It was followed shortly by Israeli forces invading Palestinian cities in an attempt to stop terrorist suicide bombings.

The point of all warfare, whether international, civil, revolutionary, or against terrorism, is to cause enough damage—human, physical, psychological, social, economic— that the other side gives up, surrenders, ceases to resist, or sometimes ceases to exist as a viable society. Throughout history the tactics of warfare have always included, sometimes reluctantly, sometimes not, but whenever deemed necessary, the deliberate targeting of enemy civilians. Contemporary military tactics emphasize creating severe damage to the enemy with as little loss of life on one's own side as possible.

Weapons of War

Over the centuries ever newer and more destructive means of waging war have been designed and produced. Contemporary wars are waged with highly sophisticated and lethal weapons by those societies that have sufficient technological and economic resources. The most deadly of these are the so-called weapons of mass destruction—nuclear, chemical, and biological weapons.

NUCLEAR WEAPONS. First used by the United States on the Japanese cities of Hiroshima and Nagasaki at the end of World War II, nuclear weapons can destroy an entire urban area in one blast. Thousands of them, capable of leveling cities of potentially hostile countries, are deployed by the United States, Russia, Great Britain, France, China, Israel,

India, and Pakistan. A one-megaton hydrogen bomb, a medium-sized nuclear weapon, would instantly destroy everything within a radius of a mile and a half of where it explodes. Every building in that radius would disintegrate, and all living creatures would die in a fraction of a second, and disappear. Within a three-mile radius, the heat would be so severe that anything exposed to it would burst into flames. As far as eight miles away people would suffer second-degree burns. As much as one-third of the population of a city of 1 million people would be killed or wounded by the blast and fire of such a bomb.

Smaller weapons, sometimes called mininukes or bunker busters, are designed to destroy underground targets. These bombs also create a huge crater above the target and spew radioactive dust for miles around the center. These smaller nuclear weapons are considered "usable" by military planners, by contrast with the larger city-destroying weapons whose value consists primarily in deterrence.

CHEMICAL AND BIOLOGICAL WEAPONS. Chemical weapons, first used by both sides in World War I in the form of poison gas, were later employed by Italy against Ethiopia in the 1930s, by the United States in South Vietnam in the 1960s, and by Iraq against Iran in the 1980s. In the twenty-first century the most advanced chemical warfare agent is binary nerve gas, which consists of two chemicals of relatively low toxicity that mix when their containing munition is fired. At that point they produce a lethal gas that is odorless and can be absorbed through the skin and eyes as well as by inhalation. The gas attacks the central nervous system, and those exposed to even low concentrations of it experience sweating and vomiting, followed by paralysis, respiratory failure, and then death.

Biological weapons spread viruses that cause diseases such as anthrax, botulism, plague, and smallpox, diseases that are usually accompanied by high fevers and deadly internal bleeding. Other viruses are designed to attack the lungs, brain, spinal cord, or heart. Once dispersed, these diseases can easily spread throughout a concentrated population, causing incurable illness, panic, and death.

Because it can also be used to manufacture benign agricultural and medicinal products, the equipment for manufacturing chemical or biological weapons is considered, in military terminology, "dual use." A pharmaceutical plant making civilian medical products might become a military target because it could also be used to make weapons for warfare.

The 1975 Biological Weapons Convention prohibited the development, production, and stockpiling of such weapons. But because they are relatively easy and cheap to produce—they have been called "a poor person's nuke"—less developed countries may consider them affordable weapons of mass destruction.

CONVENTIONAL WEAPONS. Conventional weapons include supersonic aircraft, swift ships and silent submarines, precision-guided munitions, remote-controlled pilot-less aircraft, rapid all-terrain vehicles for ground troops, land mines impervious to detection, visual aids for seeing in the dark, space-based sensors to pinpoint enemy targets, assault rifles that fire dozens of rounds a second, handheld grenade and rocket launchers, and shoulder-fired antiaircraft missile launchers.

SPACE-BASED WEAPONS. Space-based lasers and antimissile systems are being developed by the United States to give what military planners call full-spectrum dominance—control of land, sea, air, and outer space.

Ethical Frameworks

War involves the inflicting of pain and suffering, and the deliberate killing of other human beings, often on a large scale. It also inflicts serious emotional trauma on those who do the killing. Because warfare is so terrible, so contrary to the best inclinations of the human character, but because it is also a fact of national and international life, concerned persons through the ages have attempted to provide ethical frameworks with which to evaluate it.

Three such frameworks are traditionally presented, with a fourth added since the middle of the twentieth century. The first, often called the realist position, is the belief that a war must be prosecuted to a successful conclusion using all available means. The second, pacifism, maintains that all killing is wrong, that war is so inhumane that no one should take part in it. The third, and most widely held, is the just war theory, which maintains that, although war is regrettable, it is sometimes necessary and should be fought under specific ethical guidelines. The fourth, relatively new since Mohandas Gandhi (1869–1948) introduced it in waging India's war of national liberation against the British, involves active nonviolence as an effective alternative to the organized killing of warfare.

REALIST APPROACH. Realism is based on the belief that the end justifies the means, necessity knows no law, that if a war must be fought it should be fought totally. This meant, according to the nineteenth-century German theoretician Carl von Clausewitz in his influential book *On War* (1832), that an enemy's military power must be destroyed, and that the country must be conquered in such a way that it cannot produce a new military power. Even the will of the enemy must be destroyed. Whatever means are necessary should be used to force the other side into submission.

The realist approach was epitomized in World War II when the Allies waged what came to be called "total war" against Germany and Japan, insisting on nothing short of unconditional surrender. Earlier President Franklin D. Roosevelt had decried the German bombing of the cities of Warsaw, Poland; Coventry and London, England; and Rotterdam, the Netherlands, calling these campaigns ruthless and shocking to the conscience of humanity. But in pursuit of the goal of unconditional surrender, the United States itself used saturation bombing on cities in Germany and Japan, culminating in the atomic bombing of Hiroshima and Nagasaki.

Those countries that possess nuclear weapons in the twenty-first century have steadily maintained their will to use them if their security is severely threatened, if deterrence fails, regardless of the consequences.

Contemporary warfare tends to absolutize one's country and the cause for which it is fighting: "My country, right or wrong"; "we're good, they're evil"; or, as President George W. Bush put it in launching the war on terrorism, "you're either with us or you're with the terrorists." Given the patriotic fervor that arises when a nation finds itself at war, the vast majority of a country's political, academic, and even religious leaders tend to support the war. Rare are the instances of religious officials questioning whether the war is right, rarer still those who put forward the great ideals of peace and common humanity as an alternative to fighting and killing.

PACIFISM. Pacifism, refusal to take part in war on religious or humanitarian grounds, is based on the belief that the deliberate taking of human life is wrong. The belief might be religious (e.g., "Thou shalt not kill," "Love your enemies"), or it could be a conviction that all human life is valuable, and that deliberately terminating it, even an enemy in warfare, violates the integrity of the human condition. A pacifist's refusal to take part in war is recognized by law in some countries as conscientious objection to military service. Where such refusal is not legal, pacifists suffer the consequences—often imprisonment, and sometimes even death.

JUST WAR THEORY. The just war position is based on the conviction that violence is sometimes necessary to stop aggression or to secure the legitimate goals of one's country. The phrase *just war* was coined by the Greek philosopher Aristotle in the fourth century B.C.E. to describe military action undertaken to enslave those designed by nature for servitude but who resisted their proper place in the social scale. The term's classical formulation in Western philosophy began, however, with the Christian theologian Augustine of Hippo in the fifth century C.E.

Augustine was convinced that humanity, corrupted by sin, was prone to violence. Although loving one's enemies was the Christian ideal and peace the goal, it was inevitable that human cruelty and desire for power would emerge. When this happened, Augustine maintained, force must be used to counteract it. But the intention must always be to restore peace.

The just war theory was later codified under two headings. The first, *jus ad bellum,* was the right to go to war. This could happen only when there was a just cause, and when going to war was a last resort. It also had to be ordered by the proper authority, responsible for the common good of the society. The damage to be inflicted must be proportionate to the good expected by taking up arms.

The second heading, *jus in bello,* concerned ethically proper conduct during a war. This involved two important restrictions: using only those military means that are sufficient to accomplish the goal (sometimes called the principal of proportionality) and a prohibition both on executing hostages and prisoners and on attacking nonmilitary targets (the principle of discrimination).

Governments in modern times have tended to reduce the *jus ad bellum* argument to having a just cause for war, expressed as a serious threat to national integrity or security. Although the Charter of the United Nations declares that all war is illegal, Article 51 allows nations to go to war in self-defense, with every nation free to define self-defense as it sees fit, including the maintenance of access to sufficient natural resources such as water or oil.

Modern weapons assure that some if not many noncombatants will be killed. The *jus in bello* part of the just war theory is increasingly focused not on avoiding such killing, but on preventing public revulsion over it. Political expediency demands that civilians not be considered as direct targets but, in military terminology, as collateral damage, regrettable side effects. Restricting the news media's access to areas of combat and limiting the media only to information derived from military briefings are ways of keeping civilian casualties from arousing negative public opinion.

ACTIVE NONVIOLENCE. Gandhi, leading the people of India in their struggle for independence against Great Britain in what would otherwise have been a war of revolution or national liberation, introduced a new tactic—active, positive, organized nonviolent resistance. For the most part the Indian war of independence disavowed armed conflict in favor of a disciplined nonviolent movement by large numbers of Indian people. This new kind of war took several decades but resulted in freedom from the British and the creation of the modern nation of India.

Gandhi's tactics were taken up in the late 1950s and 1960s by the American clergyman Martin Luther King Jr. in the struggle for the civil rights of African Americans. It has also been used in other parts of the world, such as in the liberation of South Africa from the oppression of apartheid.

Gandhian nonviolence presents a whole other range of possibilities different from the pacifist refusal to take part in war. A determination to use nonviolent means to resolve international conflicts could involve a nonviolent defense force in which people would be trained in ways of resisting an aggressor through noncooperation and direct, unarmed confrontation. In his 1971 book, *The Politics of Nonviolent Action,* peace researcher Gene Sharp identified more than 146 specific techniques of nonviolent action, ranging from general strikes and boycotts to nonpayment of taxes.

Active nonviolence offers for many a fruitful alternative to the ethical positions of realism, pacifism, and the just war. It does not aim simply at achieving a more effective national defense, but also at establishing a system of human and international relationships that would eventually do away with the need for war altogether. Active nonviolence seeks to address the underlying causes of war by working for the establishment of social justice, environmental protection, and the defense of human rights.

Personal Responsibility

In the reality of the contemporary world, where warfare remains an ongoing possibility, each individual is involved in some way. Wars are made possible not only by political leaders who launch them and military personnel who fight them but also by those who design and produce the weapons, those who arouse citizen support, those who pay for war through their taxes, and those who form a chorus of patriotic approval.

Once a decision has been made for whatever reason to go to war, leaders try to mobilize popular support through communication verging on propaganda, by attempting to withhold negative information, and by discouraging public debate. It is hard to resist the groundswell of nationalistic fervor, hard to find the truth, and hard to see what is really going on, what are the causes, and where real justice lies. Hence the importance of looking at these issues ahead of time, getting information about international trouble spots

and likely scenarios before hostilities break out, assessing it all according to what one knows and believes, and exploring realistic nonviolent alternatives.

Warfare is a troubling, vexing question. In the end, each person must make a decision about approving of, participating in, or supporting a war based on one's own personal integrity, which is to say, one's conscience.

GERARD VANDERHAAR

SEE ALSO: *Bioterrorism; Conscience, Rights of;* and other *Warfare* subentries

BIBLIOGRAPHY

Ackerman, Peter, and Duvall, Jack. 2000. *A Force More Powerful: A Century of Nonviolent Conflict.* New York: St. Martin's Press.

Bailie, Gil. 1995. *Violence Unveiled.* New York: Crossroad.

Bainton, Roland H. 1960. *Christian Attitudes toward War and Peace.* New York and Nashville, TN: Abingdon Press.

Carr, Caleb. 2002. *The Lesson of Terror.* New York: Random House.

Clausewitz, Carl von. 1984. *On War,* tr. Peter Paret, intro. Michael Howard. Princeton, NJ: Princeton University Press.

Dyer, Gwynne. 1985. *War.* New York: Crown.

Ehrenreich, Barbara. 1997. *Blood Rites: Origins and History of the Passions of War.* New York: Henry Holt, Metropolitan Books.

Ferguson, John. 1978. *War and Peace in the World's Religions.* New York: Oxford University Press.

Keegan, John. 1993. *A History of Warfare.* New York: Knopf.

Klare, Michael T. 2001. *Resource Wars: The New Landscape of Global Conflict.* New York: Henry Holt, Metropolitan Books.

Lifton, Robert J., and Markusan, Eric. 1990. *The Genocidal Mentality.* New York: Basic.

Schell, Jonathan. 1982. *The Fate of the Earth.* New York: Knopf.

Sharp, Gene. 1971. *The Politics of Nonviolent Action.* Philadelphia: Pilgrim Press.

Walzer, Michael. 1977. *Just and Unjust Wars.* New York: Basic.

II. MEDICINE AND WAR

Ethical conflicts occur whenever medicine and war intersect. This entry discusses four general types of ethical conflict: (1) conflict between the military obligation of physicians and other medical personnel to provide care to members of the military force in which they are serving and the medical obligation to serve others, such as members of opposing military forces and civilians, who need their care; (2) conflict between the obligation of military medical personnel to "conserve the fighting strength" and the medical obligation to respond to the special needs or rights of individual military personnel under their care even if that response hinders the fighting strength; (3) conflict between the combatant and noncombatant roles of medical personnel; and (4) conflict between the national obligation to serve one's country through service in a military force and the international obligation to prevent war or prevent specific actions by the military force of one's country.

The history of physicians' involvement with military forces is a long one. Homer praised the efforts of the sons of Asclepios to provide surgical care before the gates of Troy, and Hippocrates, recognizing that the battleground was an important training ground for surgeons, urged that "he who would become a surgeon should join an army and follow it" (Vastyan, 1978, p. 1695).

However, physicians and other medical personnel had relatively little aid to offer to military casualties until the eighteenth century. Since that time developments in military weaponry and concurrent advances in medical technology and techniques for the evacuation of casualties have made the deployment of medical resources increasingly important to armies and their commanders. To the armies of the czar, for example, Peter the Great brought the *feldsher,* modeled after the *feldscherer* (field barber-surgeon) of the Prussian armies. In the New World deplorable medical care during the American Revolution caused political conflicts over the management of hospitals and healthcare for soldiers. The increase in the number of military casualties during the wars of the nineteenth century and the extraordinary increase in military and civilian casualties during those of the twentieth century, together with dramatic improvements in the ability to treat casualties successfully, led to changes in the types of ethical issues that arise in the context of war and an increase in their number.

Military Obligations Versus Medical Obligations

As a member of the military forces of a nation a military physician is charged with protecting the strength of that force. As a member of the medical profession, however, a physician generally is obligated to care for all the sick and wounded who need his or her services and to set priorities for providing those services on the basis of the urgency of medical need and the effectiveness of medical care.

Hippocrates, often called the father of medicine, apparently rejected the principle that physicians have an obligation in war to succor "enemies" as well as "friends." The

evidence for this appears in Plutarch's *Lives* in a reference to "Hippocrates' reply when the Great King of Persia consulted him, with the promise of a fee of many talents, namely, that he would never put his skill at the service of Barbarians who were enemies of Greece" (Plutarch, p. 373).

Just before the start of the U.S. Civil War the American Medical Association (AMA) selected as the model for a commemorative stone carving for the Washington Monument, then being built in the District of Columbia, the painting *Hippocrates Refuses the Gifts of Artaxerxes,* portraying Hippocrates's dismissal of the emissaries of the king of Persia. The inscription the AMA selected was *Vincit Amor Patriae,* "Love of Country Prevails" (Stacey).

In a time of "unjustifiable and monstrous rebellion," a phrase used by one of its leaders, the AMA probably intended by its use of the painting and the inscription to applaud the refusal to provide medical services for enemies. Indeed, no evidence can be found that in the pre–Civil War United States there was a great deal of sympathy for even-handed medical care in time of war (Sidel, 1991b).

PHYSICIANS AS IMPARTIAL HEALERS. A physician's responsibility to treat those in medical need on both sides did not burn itself into public or medical consciousness until the late 1860s, in the aftermath of the Crimean War and the U.S. Civil War. Leadership in increasing the new consciousness was assumed by the nonphysicians Florence Nightingale, who served as a nurse in Turkey and the Crimea from 1854 to 1856, and Dorothea Dix, whose work in bringing humane care to mental patients in the United States led President Abraham Lincoln to invite her to organize the U.S. Army Nursing Corps and become the first superintendent of nurses in the U.S. Army.

Henri Dunant, a Swiss banker who was an eyewitness at the Battle of Solferino in 1859, organized medical services for the Austrian and French wounded. In 1864 he helped initiate an international conference in Geneva that led to the founding of the International Red Cross and its national affiliates. The conference adopted a Convention for the Amelioration of the Condition of the Wounded and Sick in Armed Forces in the Field. Fourteen signatory nations pledged to regard the sick and wounded, as well as personnel, facilities, and transportation for their care, as neutrals on the battlefield. For his efforts Dunant was awarded the first Nobel Peace Prize.

Two contemporaneous events in the United States influenced future codifications and applications of international law and their bearing on medicine. Francis Lieber, a German-born philosopher, lawyer, and historian, was commissioned by the Union forces to draft a code of conduct for armies in the field. The resultant Lieber Code was promulgated in May 1863 as General Order No. 100 by the Union Army. Closely related to that development was the 1865 trial of Captain Henry Wirz, a physician who served as the commandant of the infamous Confederate prison at Andersonville, Georgia. Wirz was charged with a series of offenses involving inhumane treatment of the prisoners under his charge. His plea that "superior orders" mitigated the negligence of duty with which he was charged was disallowed, and Wirz was convicted and sentenced to be hanged.

During the eighty years after the first Geneva treaty on the treatment of war casualties three other related international agreements were negotiated in the Hague and in Geneva. The Convention for the Amelioration of the Wounded, Sick, and Shipwrecked Members of Armed Forces at Sea dealt with the care of casualties of naval warfare. The Convention Relative to the Treatment of Prisoners of War regulated the treatment and repatriation of prisoners. The Convention Relative to the Protection of Civilian Persons in Time of War prohibited deportation, the taking of hostages, torture, and discrimination in treatment. Those three agreements, along with the original Geneva accord, were codified in a single formal document in Geneva in 1949; together they are called the Geneva Conventions. Agreed to at that time by sixty nations, the 1949 conventions were declared binding on all nations according to "customary law, the usages established among civilized people … the laws of humanity, and the dictates of the public conscience" (Geneva Conventions of 1949).

Under the conventions medical personnel are singled out for certain specific protections by an explicit separation of the healing role from the wounding role. Medical personnel and treatment facilities are designated as immune from attack, and captured medical personnel are to be repatriated promptly. In return for that treatment, specific obligations are required of medical personnel:

1. Because they are regarded as noncombatants, medical personnel are forbidden to engage in or be parties to acts of war.
2. The wounded and sick—soldier and civilian, friend and foe—must be respected, protected, treated humanely, and cared for by the belligerents.
3. The wounded and sick must not be left without medical assistance, and only urgent medical reasons authorize any priority in the order of their treatment.
4. Medical aid must be dispensed solely on medical grounds, "without distinctions founded on sex, race, nationality, religion, political opinions, or any other similar criteria."

5. Medical personnel shall exercise no physical or moral coercion against protected persons (civilians), in particular to obtain information from them or from third parties.

Those duties are imposed clearly with no exceptions and are given priority over all other considerations. Thus, the Geneva Conventions formalized the recognition that although professional expertise merits special privileges, it incurs very specific legal as well as moral obligations (Vastyan, 1978). That special role of physicians has been incorporated in the public expectations and the ethical training of doctors in most societies. It also is embedded in the World Medical Association's Declaration of Geneva, which is administered as a "modern Hippocratic Oath" to graduating classes at many medical schools.

There is, however, evidence of deviation from those principles. An example of the erosion of the principle of equal medical care for "enemies" occurred in the United States during the Cold War. The medical society of Maryland and the AMA refused to criticize a Maryland psychiatrist who testified voluntarily before the Un-American Activities Committee of the U.S. House of Representatives in 1960 about information he had obtained while treating an employee of the National Security Agency (NSA). His patient, together with another NSA employee with whom the patient allegedly had had a sexual relationship, later defected to the Soviet Union. The psychiatrist, clearly without his patient's permission, provided to the committee information given to him by that patient, and the material was leaked to the press by the committee. In response to a petition by a group of Maryland psychiatrists and other physicians asking that the psychiatrist be censured, the medical society stated that "the interests of the nation transcend those of the individual" (Sidel, 1961).

Obligations to Enhance Military Strength Versus Personnel Needs

Military physicians must accept priorities different from those of their civilian colleagues (Vastyan, 1974). The primary role of a military physician is expressed in the motto of the U.S. Army Medical Department: "To conserve the fighting strength" (Bellamy). In describing that role, a faculty member of the Academy of Health Sciences at Fort Sam Houston in 1988 cited as "the clear objective of all health service support operations" the goal stated in 1866 by a veteran of the Army of the Potomac in the Civil War: "[to] strengthen the hands of the commanding general by keeping his Army in the most vigorous health, thus rendering it, in the highest degree, efficient for enduring fatigue and privation [sic], and for fighting" (Rubenstein, p. 145).

Principles of triage that are unacceptable in civilian practice may be required in war, such as placing emphasis on patching up the lightly wounded so that they can be sent back to battle. For example, "overevacuation" (the presumed excessive transfer of personnel to a safe area rather than back to the military operation) is cited as "one of the cardinal sins of military medicine" (Bellamy). Violation of patient confidentiality, which is unacceptable in civilian practice, may be required. Medical personnel may be required to administer experimental drugs or immunizations to troops without their free and informed consent (Annas).

Combatant Versus Noncombatant Roles for Medical Personnel

Perhaps the most dramatic attempt to meld these conflicting obligations was made by the Knights Hospitallers of Saint John of Jerusalem, a religious order founded in the eleventh century. With a sworn fealty to "our Lords the Sick," the knights defended their hospitals against "enemies of the Faith," becoming the first organized military medical officers. They were "warring physicians who could strike the enemy mighty blows, and yet later bind up the wounds of that same enemy along with those of their own comrades" (Vastyan, 1978, pp. 1695–1696).

A more recent example of the erosion of the distinction between combatant and noncombatant roles was demonstrated in a U.S. Army exhibit at the 1967 AMA convention. It was titled "Medicine as a Weapon" and featured a photograph of a Green Beret (Special Forces) aidman handing medicine to a Vietnamese peasant (Liberman et al.). Dr. Peter Bourne, who had been an army physician working with the Special Forces in Vietnam, wrote that the primary task of Special Forces medics was "to seek and destroy the enemy and only incidentally to take care of the medical needs of others on the patrol" (Liberman et al., p. 303).

In 1967 Howard Levy, a dermatologist drafted into the U.S. Army Medical Department as a captain, refused to obey an order to train Special Forces aidmen in dermatological skills. He refused specifically on the grounds that the aidmen were being trained predominantly for a combat role and that cross-training in medical techniques would erode the distinction between combatants and noncombatants. Levy was charged with one of the most serious breaches of the Uniform Code of Military Justice: willfully disobeying a lawful order. Tried by a general court-martial in 1967, Levy admitted his disobedience, saying that he had acted in accordance with his ethical principles. The physicians who testified for the defense "argued that the political use of medicine by the Special Forces jeopardized the entire tradition of the noncombatant status of medicine" (Langer, p.

1349). They agreed with Levy that physicians are responsible for even the secondary ethical implications of their acts and that they must not only act ethically but also anticipate that those to whom they teach medicine will act ethically as well. Although Levy was a medical officer, the court-martial panel did not include a physician. Levy was given a dishonorable discharge and sentenced to three years of hard labor in a military prison. His appeals were not successful (Glasser; Langer).

Inside or outside the armed forces medical personnel may be involved in war-related research and development such as work on biological weapons or the radiation effects of nuclear weapons. In that work it is said to have been common practice to concentrate physicians into "principally or primarily defensive operations" (Rosebury). However, work on weapons and their effects can never be exclusively defensive, and at times the distinction is arbitrary. The question arises whether there is a special ethical duty for physicians, because of their medical obligation to "do no harm," to refuse to participate in such work or whether in non-patient-care situations physicians only share the ethical duties of all human beings (Sidel, 1991a).

The noncombatant role of a physician in military service is ambiguous even if frank combatant activities are eschewed. Military physicians, like all members of the armed forces, are limited by the threat of military discipline in the extent to which they can protest publicly against what they consider an unjust war. The issue of what is a just war has been debated for more than two millennia (Seabury and Codevilla; Walzer). It generally is thought that there are two elements in a just war: *jus ad bellum* (when is it just to go to war?) and *jus in bello* (what methods may be used in a just war?). Among the elements required for *jus ad bellum* are a just grievance and the exhaustion of all means short of war to settle that grievance. Among the elements required for *jus in bello* are the protection of noncombatants and the proportionality of force, including avoiding the use of weapons of mass destruction such as chemical, biological, and nuclear weapons and the massive bombing of cities. Membership in the armed forces, even in a noncombatant role, usually requires self-censorship of public doubts about the justness of a war in which the armed forces are engaged.

In 2003 the United States, with the support of the United Kingdom, initiated an attack on Iraq that those countries alleged was permissible under international law as a "preventive" or "preemptive" war. The action was not approved specifically by the Security Council of the United Nations. Many lawyers and physicians argued that because there had been no attack or imminent attack on the United States, the requirements for *jus ad bellum* had not been met and the "collateral damage" to civilians caused by the attack exceeded the ethical test of *jus in bello*. Although there were protests from Physicians for Social Responsibility and other medical groups, U.S. service members, including medical personnel, evinced no public protest.

The U.S. military used depleted uranium as a casing for armor-piercing shells in the 1991 Gulf War, its actions in Kosovo and Afghanistan, and the 2003 Gulf War. Uranium is both toxic and radioactive, and its use is seen by many experts as a violation of the United Nations Charter, the Geneva Conventions, the Conventional Weapons Convention, and the Hague Conventions. There was no public protest by military physicians.

In addition, medical personnel, like other people, may consider themselves pacifists. "Absolute pacifism" opposes the use of any force against another human being even in self-defense against a direct personal attack. The argument underlying this position for many of its adherents is that the use of force can be ended only when all people refuse to use it and that acceptance of one's own injury or even death is preferable to the use of force against another person. More limited forms of pacifism, such as "nuclear pacifism," hold that the use of certain weapons of mass destruction in war is never justified no matter how great the provocation or how terrible the consequences of failure to use them. It has been suggested ("maternal pacifism") that because of their nurturing roles women have a special responsibility to oppose the use of force (Ruddick).

When a group is threatened with genocide, which the Nazis attempted in World War II, many who otherwise might adopt a pacifist or limited pacifist position believe that force may be justified. Their shift in position is based on the threat to the survival of the group, a threat that makes the pacifist argument that current failure to resist will lead to a future diminution in violence seem untenable.

There is considerable debate whether physicians, because of a special dedication to the preservation of life and health, have a special obligation to serve or to refuse to serve in a military effort. That position is made more complex by the physician's role as a military noncombatant. Many military forces permit physicians, like other military personnel, to claim conscientious objector status. In the United States conscientious objection is defined as "a firm, fixed, and sincere objection by reason of religious training and belief to: (1) participation in war in any form; or (2) the bearing of arms." Religious training and belief is defined as "belief in an external power or being or deeply held moral or ethical belief to which all else is subordinate and … which has the power or force to affect moral well-being" (U.S.

Department of Defense). A person who claims conscientious objector status must convince a military hearing officer that the objection is sincere.

Obligations to Serve in War Versus Obligations to Prevent War

As wars kill an increasing percentage of civilians with so-called conventional weapons and as threats of the use of weapons of mass destruction continue, what form of service is appropriate for an ethical physician? One response was suggested in the late 1930s by John A. Ryle, then Regius Professor of Physic at the University of Cambridge:

> It is everywhere a recognized and humane principle that prevention should be preferred to cure. By withholding service from the Armed Forces before and during war, by declining to examine and inoculate recruits, by refusing sanitary advice and the training and command of ambulances, clearing stations, medical transport, and hospitals, the doctors could so cripple the efficiency of the staff and aggravate the difficulties of campaign and so damage the morale of the troops that war would become almost unthinkable (p. 8).

During the Vietnam War more than 300 American medical students and young physicians brought Ryle's vision a step closer to reality by signing the following pledge:

> In the name of freedom the U.S. is waging an unjustifiable war in Viet Nam and is causing incalculable suffering. It is the goal of the medical profession to prevent and relieve human suffering. My effort to pursue this goal is meaningless in the context of the war. Therefore, I refuse to serve in the Armed Forces in Viet Nam; and so that I may exercise my profession with conscience and dignity, I intend to seek means to serve my country which are compatible with the preservation and enrichment of life (Liberman et al., p. 306).

Ryle's vision is a variation on that of Aristophanes in his comedy *The Lysistrata,* which was written in 411 B.C.E., just before the probable time of Hippocrates's refusal to treat the Persians (circa 400 B.C.E.). The title character, an Athenian woman, ends the second Peloponnesian War by organizing the wives of the soldiers of both Athens and Sparta to refuse sexual intercourse with their husbands while the war lasts. The Athenians and Spartans make peace quickly and go home with their wives (Aristophanes).

Some physicians and other medical personnel have refused to support war by serving in the armed forces. In one of the most dramatic examples Yolanda Huet-Vaughn, a captain in the U.S. Army Medical Service Reserve, refused active duty in the Persian Gulf. In her statement she explained her actions:

> I am refusing orders to be an accomplice in what I consider an immoral, inhumane and unconstitutional act, namely an offensive military mobilization in the Middle East. My oath as a citizen-soldier to defend the Constitution, my oath as a physician to preserve human life and prevent disease, and my responsibility as a human being to the preservation of this planet, would be violated if I cooperate (Sidel, 1991b, p. 102).

The reasons Huet-Vaughn gave for her action were quite different from the reasons given by Levy. Levy refused to obey an order that he believed required him to perform a specific act that would violate the Geneva Conventions; Huet-Vaughn refused to obey an order that she believed required her to support a particular war that she felt to be unjust and destructive to the goals of medicine and humanity.

One of the questions Huet-Vaughn's action raises is whether physicians have a special ethical responsibility, in view of their obligation to protect the health and lives of their patients and the people in their communities, to refuse to support a war they believe will cause major destruction to the health and environment of both combatants and noncombatants (Geiger; Sidel, 1991b). If a physician considers service in support of a particular war unethical on the grounds of sworn fealty to medical ethics, may—or must—that doctor refuse to serve even if that objection does not meet the criteria for formal conscientious objector status? Is there an ethical difference if the service is required by the society—as in a "doctor draft"—or if the service obligation has been entered into voluntarily in return for military support of medical training or for other reasons? Is military service a voluntary obligation if enlistment, as it is for many poor and minority people, is prodded by lack of educational or employment opportunities or, as for many doctors, by the cost of medical education or specialty training that in other societies is provided at public expense?

Although few physicians are willing or able to take an action such as that taken by Huet-Vaughn, other actions are available to oppose acts of war that are considered unjust, oppose a specific war, or oppose war in general. One is acceptance of a service alternative consistent with an ethical obligation to care for the wounded or maimed without simultaneously supporting a war effort. Opportunities for service in an international medical corps such as Médecins du Monde and Médecins sans Frontieres are limited, but U.S. physicians may wish to demand that their nation redirect some of the billions of dollars it spends annually on preparation for war to the United Nations or the World Health Organization to help fund an international medical service to treat the casualties of war.

Other physicians may work, as individuals and particularly in groups, to help prevent war by contributing to public and professional understanding of the nature of modern war, the risks of weapons of mass destruction, and the nature and effectiveness of alternatives to war. Among the groups organized for that purpose are the International Physicians for the Prevention of Nuclear War, whose U.S. affiliate is Physicians for Social Responsibility. If the world is to survive, physicians may need to consider new forms of national service and contribute in a broader sense to their nations and their planet (1986).

In the broader context of medical ethics it is widely accepted that opposition to war does not permit an ethical physician to refuse medical care to victims of war he or she is in a position to serve and that that care does not presume the physician's support of the war being fought. Ethical dilemmas arise when a physician actively supports the war effort through membership in a military medical service or by assigning priority to patient care on the basis of military demands rather than patient needs. These issues and those associated with the role of the physician in peacemaking and peacekeeping, which often are distorted by the fervor that may accompany war and preparation for war, require dispassionate analysis and action in times of peace.

VICTOR W. SIDEL (1995)
REVISED BY AUTHOR

SEE ALSO: *Care; Conflict of Interest; Conscience; Justice; Medical Codes and Oaths: Ethical Analysis; Obligation and Supererogation; Profession and Professional Ethics; Prisoners, Healthcare Issues of; Triage;* and other *Warfare* subentries

BIBLIOGRAPHY

Annas, George J. 1992. "Changing the Consent Rules for Desert Storm." *New England Journal of Medicine* 326(1): 770–773.

Aristophanes. 1979. *The Lysistrata.* In *Aristophanes,* vol. 3, trans. Benjamin Bickley Rogers. Cambridge, MA: Harvard University Press.

Bellamy, Ronald F. 1988. "Conserve the Fighting Strength." *Military Medicine* 153(4): 185–186.

Geiger, H. Jack. 1991. "Conscience and Obligation: Physicians and Just War." *PSR Quarterly* 1: 113–116.

Geneva Conventions of 1949. 1983. In *Human Rights Documents: Compilation of Documents Pertaining to Human Rights.* Washington, D.C.: U.S. Government Printing Office.

Glasser, Ira. 1967. "Judgment at Fort Jackson: The Court-Martial of Captain Howard B. Levy." *Law in Transition Quarterly* 4: 123–156.

Homer. 1990. *The Iliad,* trans. Robert Fagles. New York: Viking.

Langer, Elinor. 1967. "The Court-Martial of Captain Levy: Medical Ethics v. Military Law." *Science* 156(3780): 1346–1350.

Liberman, Robert; Gold, Warren; and Sidel, Victor W. 1968. "Medical Ethics and the Military." *New Physician* 17(11): 299–309.

Lown, Bernard. 1986. "Nobel Peace Prize Lecture: A Prescription for Hope." *New England Journal of Medicine* 314(15): 985–987.

Plutarch. 1914. "Marcus Cato." In *Lives,* vol. 2, trans. Bernadotte Perin. Cambridge, MA: Harvard University Press.

Rosebury, Theodor. 1963. "Medical Ethics and Biological Warfare." *Perspectives in Biology and Medicine* 6: 512–523.

Rubenstein, David A. 1988. "Health Service Support and the Principles of War." *Military Medicine* 153(3): 145–146.

Ruddick, Sara. 1989. *Maternal Thinking: Toward a Politics of Peace.* Boston: Beacon Press.

Ryle, John A. 1938. "Foreword." In *The Doctor's View of War,* ed. Horace Joules. London: George Allen & Unwin.

Seabury, Paul, and Codevilla, Angelo. 1989. *War: Ends and Means.* New York: Basic Books.

Sidel, Victor W. 1961. "Confidential Information and the Physician." *New England Journal of Medicine* 264(22): 1133–1137.

Sidel, Victor W. 1991a. "Biological Weapons Research and Physicians: Historical and Ethical Analysis." *PSR Quarterly* 1(1): 31–42.

Sidel, Victor W. 1991b. "Quid Est Amor Patriae?" *PSR Quarterly* 1(1): 96–104.

Sidel, Victor W. 2003. "Earth Penetrating Nuclear Weapons, Nuclear Testing, Depleted Uranium Weapons and Medical Consequences and Implications for Compliance with the Nuclear Non-Proliferation Treaty." Testimony before the Preparatory Committee for 2005 Review Conference of the Nuclear Non-Proliferation Treaty.

Stacey, James. 1988. "The Cover." *Journal of the American Medical Association* 260: 448.

U.S. Department of Defense. 1982. Air Force Regulation 35–24. Washington, D.C.: Author.

Vastyan, E. A. 1974. "Warriors in White: Some Questions about the Nature and Mission of Military Medicine." *Texas Reports on Biology and Medicine* 32(1): 327–342.

Vastyan, E. A. 1978. "Warfare: I. Medicine and War." In *Encyclopedia of Bioethics,* vol. 4, ed. Warren T. Reich. New York: Macmillan.

Walzer, Michael. 1977. *Just and Unjust Wars: A Moral Argument with Historical Illustrations.* New York: Basic Books.

III. PUBLIC HEALTH AND WAR

During the twentieth century, an estimated 110 million people lost their lives as a result of armed conflicts (WHO).

If one includes the major episodes of "collective violence," such as the Stalinist terror of the 1930s and the famine associated with the Great Leap Forward in China (1958–1960), this figure reaches 191 million (Rummel), with approximately 60 percent of these deaths occurring among noncombatants.

Since the Second World War, approximately 190 armed conflicts have occurred affecting ninety-two countries (WHO; Federation of American Scientists). Most occurred in Asia, Africa, and Latin America; however, since 1990, four European conflicts—Chechnya, Azerbaijan, Georgia, and the former Yugoslavia—have caused more than 350,000 deaths. Some wars are still fought primarily between competing armies, such as the Iran-Iraq conflict (1980–1988), in which an estimated 450,000 military personnel died (Sivard), but the vast majority now take place within states.

Civilian populations have increasingly been the intentional targets of military actions, as can be seen in the shelling of urban centers during the conflicts in Bosnia and Herzegovina, Chechnya, Angola, Lebanon, and Somalia. In addition, modern weapons such as napalm, cluster bombs, and land mines do not discriminate between combatants and innocent civilians. In Mozambique the antigovernment forces killed approximately 100,000 civilians in 1986 and 1987 alone (Ugalde, Zwi, and Richards) and between 5 million and 6 million people were either internally displaced or fled to neighboring countries.

Since World War II there have been numerous episodes of massive human rights atrocities and genocide that defy the traditional characteristics of armed warfare. Examples include Pol Pot's killing fields in Cambodia; the Guatemalan government action against indigenous Mayan communities; the use of chemical and biological weapons against the Kurds in Halabja, Iraq; the genocide against Tutsis in Rwanda; and the civilian massacres following the referendum on independence in East Timor.

Public Health Impact of War

DIRECT IMPACT. The direct public health consequences of war include death, injury, sexual assault, disability, and psychological stress. Measuring the impact and hidden costs of conflict is complex for a variety of reasons. Even where huge numbers of people are involved, agreement on the magnitude of impact varies. Estimates of the number of victims of the Rwandan genocide are still imprecise and vary from 500,000 to one million (Murray, King, Lopez, et al.). Particularly high civilian death rates have been reported in Angola, Ethiopia, Liberia, Mozambique, Rwanda, Somalia,

Southern Sudan, El Salvador, Guatemala, Afghanistan, Cambodia, Tajikistan, and Bosnia and Herzegovina (Zwi and Ugalde; Toole, Galson, and Brady).

Rape is increasingly recognized as a feature of internal wars, and it has been present in many different types of conflicts. In some conflicts, rape has been used systematically as an attempt to undermine opposing groups. In the former Yugoslavia, for example, estimates of the number of rape survivors have ranged from 10,000 to 60,000 (Swiss and Giller).

Estimates of mine-related disabilities are also sobering: 36,000 in Cambodia (one in every 236 persons in that nation has lost at least one limb), 20,000 in Angola, 8,000 in Mozambique, and 15,000 in Uganda. The costs are both physical and social and affect all age groups. Between February 1991 and February 1992, approximately 75 percent of the land-mine injuries treated worldwide were in children five to fifteen years old (Toole, Waldman, and Zwi).

Immeasurable psychological trauma has been caused by widespread human-rights abuses, including detention, torture, and forced displacement (institutionalized in the former Yugoslavia as "ethnic cleansing"). The extent of mental health "trauma" experienced during and in the aftermath of war and conflict is controversial, with some analysts identifying significant proportions of affected populations suffering from post-traumatic stress disorder, while others argue that this term and the response to it medicalizes an essentially social phenomenon.

INDIRECT IMPACT. The indirect public health consequences of war have been mediated by hunger, mass migration, and collapsed health services, especially in impoverished developing countries where basic services and food reserves are already inadequate. The intentional use of food deprivation as a weapon has become increasingly common (MacCrae and Zwi). For example, armed factions on all sides have obstructed food-aid deliveries in southern Sudan, resulting in mass hunger and, during 1993, death rates up to fifteen times those reported in nonfamine times. In 1992 widespread looting and banditry deprived millions of Somalis of much-needed food aid.

At the end of 2002 there were more than 15 million refugees worldwide, and an additional 22 million people internally displaced in their own countries (U.S. Committee for Refugees). Crude death rates (the number of deaths per 1,000 population per month) among refugees and internally displaced persons have ranged between five and twenty-five times baseline rates. Most deaths have been caused by preventable conditions such as malnutrition, diarrhea, pneumonia, measles, and malaria (Toole, Waldman, and Zwi).

High death rates reflect the prolonged period of deprivation suffered prior to displacement, the often inadequate response to humanitarian crises by the international community, and problems of gaining access to provide relief assistance to war-affected communities. More than 50,000 refugees from Rwanda died within one month of fleeing into eastern Zaire in 1994, representing a death rate more than 25 times higher than the baseline rate in Rwanda (Goma Epidemiology Group).

Health facilities have been intentionally destroyed by armed factions in Afghanistan, Angola, Bosnia, Mozambique, and other war-stricken countries. In addition, the high costs of both maintaining military forces and treating the wounded have often led to insufficient funding for basic health services. In the Bosnian province of Zenica, for example, the proportion of surgical cases related to war injuries rose from 22 percent to 78 percent between April and November 1993, resulting in the cessation of almost all preventive health services (Toole, Galson, and Brady).

Perhaps the most significant consequence of war on public health relates to the tremendous cost of preparing for war. Military budgets throughout both the industrialized and developing worlds have diverted precious resources from public health and other social development programs. For example, in April 2002 the U.S. Congress approved $85 billion to fund the initial stages of the war in Iraq. In comparison, the total global expenditure on the fight against HIV/AIDS in low- and middle-income countries was $1.5 billion in 2001. Moreover, the destruction of environmental resources, such as water sources, agricultural land, livestock, and housing has had a major impact on public health in numerous countries affected by war.

Ethical Issues

Modern warfare has increasingly involved flagrant violations of the Geneva Conventions related to the protection of civilian persons in time of war (ICRC). Ethnic cleansing, detention of civilians, summary executions, and torture are clearly illegal under international law. The unrestricted ability of combatants to target civilians is fostered by the officially sanctioned international arms trade. The International Committee of the Red Cross (ICRC), the custodian of the Geneva Conventions, has often been deprived of access to civilians in countries such as Somalia, Sudan, and Bosnia and Herzegovina. Further, providing humanitarian assistance has become more dangerous. Between 1985 and 1998, over 380 deaths occurred among humanitarian workers (Sheil et al.).

Although violations of human rights law and international humanitarian law are crimes, the legal systems for punishing the perpetrators and compensating the victims are grossly inadequate. To date, international tribunals have been established to prosecute war criminals from the former Yugoslavia and from Rwanda. While these courts help to move the punishment of war criminals from theory to practice, they have been very slow to act and very expensive to implement. The establishment of an International Court of Justice is another step towards strengthening what has, in many respects, been a legal system without law enforcement capability.

International public opinion has increasingly supported the use of force by the United Nations to ensure delivery of humanitarian aid in situations either where governance has completely collapsed (e.g., Somalia and Liberia) or where governments consciously hinder access by relief agencies (e.g., Sudan and Bosnia and Herzegovina). However, there are no clear guidelines that might promote a consistent deployment of force to achieve humanitarian objectives (Dewey). The U.N. Charter prohibits interference in the affairs of a sovereign nation, thereby giving more weight to the rights of the state than to individual citizens.

Two contradictory examples from 1992 illustrate the ethical dilemmas inherent in the use of force to save lives from hunger and disease. In Bosnia and Herzegovina, European soldiers deployed to ensure the safe delivery of humanitarian supplies were powerless to prevent flagrant abuses of human rights committed in their presence (Jean). In contrast, the international armed contingent dispatched to Somalia in late 1992 to ensure the safe delivery of relief supplies eventually became a party to the internal conflict. This led to battles between U.N. troops and one local armed faction in heavily populated areas of the capital, Mogadishu, with high civilian casualty rates (Brauman). Thus, well-motivated intervention by the international community may inadvertently increase the risks to the intended beneficiaries.

Once access to an affected area is assured, health personnel have a critical role to play in accurately documenting the public health impact of war on civilian populations, thereby acting as effective advocates for a prompt and adequate response. Relief programs may pose a difficult choice for health workers: between the provision of individual curative care and the implementation of more effective, community-based programs such as childhood immunization.

Conclusions

Modern warfare has exacted a devastating toll on civilian populations. High mortality, morbidity, and disability rates have resulted directly from traumatic injuries and indirectly from hunger and mass displacement. Since the end of the Cold War, the potential for a more unified and coherent "international community" has emerged. The United Nations has a responsibility to carefully monitor the public health consequences of evolving conflicts and to apply aggressive diplomacy early to seek solutions. When conflicting parties obstruct access to civilians by relief agencies, the world needs to respond in a consistent and effective manner, and clearer guidelines on the use of force to deliver humanitarian aid in conflict settings need to be developed.

Relief programs will be more effective if they reflect the real needs of affected populations, rather than the availability of surplus commodities in donor countries. With a proper and timely scientific assessment of public health needs and careful monitoring of health and nutrition trends, those who are suffering are more likely to receive the aid they require. Primary prevention is the basic strategy of public health; consequently, in war settings, public health practitioners need to recognize that primary prevention means stopping the violence, as well as actively exploring methods for promoting sustainable peace.

MICHAEL J. TOOLE (1995)
REVISED BY AUTHOR

SEE ALSO: *Bioterrorism; Epidemics; Healthcare Resources, Allocation of; Health Policy; Public Health;* and other *Warfare* subentries

BIBLIOGRAPHY

Brauman, Rony. 1993. *Le Crime Humanitaire: Somalie.* Paris: Arléa.

Cahill, Kevin M., ed. 1993. *A Framework for Survival: Health, Human Rights, and Humanitarian Assistance in Conflicts and Disasters.* New York: Basic Books.

Dewey, Arthur. 1993. "The Military Role in Emergency Response." In *New Strategies for a Restless World,* ed. Harlan Cleveland. Minneapolis, MN: American Refugee Committee.

Garfield, Richard M., and Neugut, Alfred I. 1991. "Epidemiologic Analysis of Warfare: A Historical Review." *Journal of the American Medical Association* 266(5): 688–692.

Goma Epidemiology Group. 1995. "Public Health Impact of Rwandan Refugee Crisis. What Happened in Goma, Zaire, in July 1994?" *Lancet* 345: 339–344.

International Committee of the Red Cross (ICRC). 1950. *The Geneva Conventions of August 12, 1949: Analysis for the Use of National Red Cross Societies.* Geneva: Author.

Jean, François. 1992. "The Former Yugoslavia." In *Populations in Danger,* ed. François Jean. London: John Libbey.

MacCrae, Joanna, and Zwi, Anthony B. 1992. "Food as an Instrument of War in Contemporary African Famines: A Review of the Evidence." *Disasters* 16(4): 299–321.

Murray, C. J. L.; King, G.; Lopez, A. D.; et al. 2002. "Armed Conflict as a Public Health Problem." *British Medical Journal* 324: 346–349.

Rummel, R. J. 1994. *Death by Government: Genocide and Mass Murder Since 1900.* New Brunswick, NJ: Transaction.

Sheil, M., et al. 2000. "Death among Humanitarian Workers." *British Medical Journal* 321: 166–168.

Sivard, R. L. 1996. *World Military and Social Expenditures,* 14th edition. Washington D.C.: World Priorities.

Swiss, Shana, and Giller, Joan E. 1993. "Rape as a Crime of War." *Journal of the American Medical Association* 270(5): 612–615.

Toole, Michael J.; Galson, Steven; and Brady, William. 1993. "Are War and Public Health Compatible?" *Lancet* 341(8854): 1193–1196.

Toole, Michael, and Waldman, Ronald. 1993. "Refugees and Displaced Persons: War, Hunger, and Public Health." *Journal of the American Medical Association* 270(5): 600–605.

Toole, Michael J.; Waldman, R. J.; and Zwi, A. 2001. "Complex Humanitarian Emergencies." In *International Public Health,* ed. M. Merson, R. E. Black, and A. J. Mills. Gaithersburg, MD: Aspen.

Ugalde, A.; Zwi, A.; and Richards, P. 1999. "Health Consequences of War and Political Violence." In *Encyclopaedia of Violence,* ed. L. Kurtz. New York. Academic Press.

U.S. Committee for Refugees. 2002. *World Refugee Survey, 2002.* Washington, D.C.: Author.

World Health Organization (WHO). 2002. *World Report on Violence and Health.* Geneva: Author.

Zwi, Anthony, and Ugalde, Antonio. 1991. "Political Violence in the Third World: A Public Health Issue." *Health Policy and Planning* 6(3): 203–217.

INTERNET RESOURCE

Federation of American Scientists. "The World at War." Available from <http://www.fas.org/man/dod-101/ops/war>.

IV. CHEMICAL AND BIOLOGICAL WEAPONS

The development, production, storage, transfer, use, and destruction (demilitarization) of chemical and biological weapons (CBW) pose a number of ethical issues. First, those weapons, like nuclear weapons, are largely indiscriminate in their effects and are generally more effective against vulnerable noncombatants than against combatants; they therefore are known as weapons of mass destruction, and their use generally is considered a violation of the proportionality principle of a just war. Second, CBW, also like nuclear weapons, are the subject of intensive international arms-control efforts involving problems of definition, verification, and enforcement. Third, biomedical scientists and physicians may be called on to participate in research and development on more effective CBW as well as on methods for defense against them and the treatment of their victims.

Chemical Weapons

Chemical weapons (CW), which have been known since antiquity, are designed to inflict direct chemical injury on their targets, in contrast to explosive or incendiary weapons, which produce their effects through blast or heat. In the siege of Plataea in 429 B.C.E., for example, the Spartans placed enormous cauldrons of pitch, sulfur, and burning charcoal outside the city walls to harass the defenders. Although nations that signed the 1899 Hague Declaration promised not to use CW, during World War I those weapons, including in descending order of use tear gas, chlorine gas, phosgene, and mustard gas, were employed. Overall, 125,000 tons of CW were used during World War I, resulting in 1.3 million casualties. One-quarter of all casualties in the American Expeditionary Force in France were caused by them (Harris and Paxman; Sidel and Goldwyn; Sidel, 1989; United Nations; World Health Organization).

In 1925 twenty-eight nations negotiated the Geneva Protocol for the "prohibition of the use in war of asphyxiating poisonous or other gases and of all analogous liquids, materials or devices and of bacteriological methods of warfare" (Wright, p. 368). In fact, however, the protocol prohibited only the use, not the development, production, testing, or stockpiling, of those weapons. Furthermore, many of the nations that ratified the protocol reserved the right to use those weapons in retaliation, and the protocol became in effect a "no first use" treaty with no verification or enforcement provisions. The United States was one of the initial signers, but the Senate did not ratify the treaty until 1975 (Sidel, 1989; Wright).

Despite the protocol, the use of CW continued. Italy used mustard gas during its invasion of Abyssinia (Ethiopia), and Japan used mustard and tear gases in its invasion of China. Germany, with its advanced dye and pesticide industries, developed acetylcholinesterase inhibitors known as nerve gases, and the United States and Britain stockpiled CW during World War II; transportation and storage accidents caused casualties (Infield), but there was no direct military use. After World War II CW were used by Egypt in Yemen, mustard and nerve gases were used in the Iran-Iraq war in the 1980s, and Iraq used CW against Kurdish villages in its territory. CW stockpiles and production facilities in Iraq were ordered destroyed by the United Nations after the 1991 Persian Gulf War. The United States and Russia are known to have maintained CW stockpiles, and a number of other countries have stockpiles or facilities for rapid CW production (Harris and Paxman; Sidel, 1989).

Troops can be protected against those weapons for limited periods through the use of gas masks and impenetrable garments. That protective gear, however, reduces the efficiency of troops by as much as 50 percent and damages morale, and so the use or threat of use of CW may continue to be considered effective against troops. Civilian populations, in contrast, cannot be protected adequately. Israel, for example, provides every civilian with a gas mask and a self-injectable syringe filled with atropine, a temporary antidote to nerve gas. However, that protection is inadequate against weapons, such as mustard gas, that attack the skin and against longer-term exposure to nerve gas. Furthermore, poorly trained civilians are likely to injure themselves with equipment such as self-injectable syringes (Amitai et al.).

The production of CW has been associated with serious accidents to workers and high levels of pollution in the production sites and nearby communities. Tests of mustard gas, nerve agents, and psychochemicals, including lysergic acid diethylamide (LSD), during and after World War II involved thousands of military personnel, many of whom later claimed disabilities from the exposure. The records of participation and effects are so poor that only a small fraction of those who participated can be identified. Even the destruction of the weapons is dangerous because toxic ash is produced by their incineration (Sidel, 1993).

A Chemical Weapons Convention (CWC) that prohibits the development, production, storage, and transfer of those weapons and calls for their demilitarization was approved by the United Nations General Assembly in 1992. The Organization for the Prohibition of Chemical Weapons (OPCW), which is responsible for ensuring the implementation of the CWC, was established in the Hague after the entry into force of the CWC in 1997. By 2003 a total of 151 "states parties" (nations) had ratified or acceded to the BWC. The First Review Conference of the States Parties to the CWC was held in the Hague in April 2003, and Kofi Annan, secretary general of the United Nations, urged that "membership in the CWC be extended to all nations in the world and that enough funds be provided to accelerate complete chemical disarmament."

In the 1960s and 1970s the United States used both tear gas and herbicides in Vietnam. Although most nations that are parties to the Geneva Protocol considered tear gas and herbicides to be CW and thus prohibited under the provisions of the protocol, the United States until recently rejected that interpretation (Sidel and Goldwyn; Sidel, 1989). Many countries use tear gas to quell civil disorders

(Hu et al.). The signatories to the CWC have agreed not to use riot-control agents or herbicides as weapons of war.

In 2002 Russia used derivatives of fentanyl, a potent opium-based narcotic, to subdue Chechen rebels who had occupied a theater in Moscow and taken 800 hostages. Although Russia formally considered the chemical agent "nonlethal" and its use permissible under the CWC, a total of 117 people died as a result of its use ("Russia Names Moscow Siege Gas").

In 1984 members of a cult in Oregon intentionally contaminated the salad bars in local restaurants with salmonella bacteria. More than 700 people became ill, but there were no reported deaths. In 2001, shortly after the attack on the World Trade Center, anthrax spores were disseminated through the U.S. mail. Approximately twenty people became ill, and five people died.

Biological Weapons

Biological weapons (BW) depend for their effects on the ability of microorganisms to infect and multiply in the attacked organism. In this regard they differ from toxins, which, as biological products used as chemicals, are covered under CW as well as BW treaties. BW are very hard to defend against and are not as controllable and predictable in their use as are CW (Harris and Paxman; Geissler, 1986; Sidel and Goldwyn; Sidel, 1989; United Nations; World Health Organization, 1970).

The effects of BW were characterized officially by a U.S. government agency in 1959: "Biological warfare is the intentional use of living organisms or their toxic products to cause death, disability, or damage in man, animals, or plants. The target is man, either by causing sickness or death or through limitation of his food supplies or other agricultural resources.... Biological warfare has been aptly described as public health in reverse" (U.S. Department of Health, Education, and Welfare).

BW have been known since antiquity. Persia, Greece, and Rome used diseased corpses to contaminate sources of drinking water. In 1347 Mongols besieging the walled city of Caffa (now called Feodosiya), a seaport on the east coast of the Crimea, began to die of the plague. The attackers threw the corpses into the besieged city; the defenders, who were Genoans, fled back to Genoa and carried the plague farther into Europe. During the French and Indian Wars Lord Jeffrey Amherst, commander of the British forces at Fort Pitt, gave tribal emissaries blankets in which smallpox victims had slept (Harris and Paxman; Geissler).

During World War I Germany is alleged to have used the equine disease glanders against the cavalries of eastern

European countries (Harris and Paxman, p. 74). According to testimony at the Nuremberg trials, prisoners in German concentration camps were infected during tests of BW. Great Britain and the United States, fearing that the Germans would use BW in World War II, developed their own BW. The British tested anthrax spores on Gruinard Island off the coast of Scotland; the island remained uninhabitable for decades. The United States developed anthrax spores, botulism toxin, and other agents as BW but did not use them (Bernstein).

In the 1930s Japanese troops dropped rice and wheat mixed with plague-carrying fleas from planes, resulting in plague in areas of China that previously had been free of it. During World War II Japanese laboratories conducted extensive experiments on prisoners of war, using a wide variety of organisms selected for possible use as BW, including anthrax, plague, gas gangrene, encephalitis, typhus, typhoid, hemorrhagic fever, cholera, smallpox, and tularemia (Wright). Unlike the Soviet Union, which in 1949 prosecuted twelve people who had been involved in that work, the United States never prosecuted any of the participants. Instead, U.S. researchers met with Japanese biological warfare experts in Tokyo and urged that the experts be "spared embarrassment" so that the United States could benefit from their knowledge (Powell; Williams and Wallace).

DIFFICULTIES OF SURVEILLANCE. After World War II the development of BW continued. None of the numerous allegations of BW use have been substantiated or even investigated fully, but it is known that extensive BW testing was done. In the 1950s and 1960s, for example, the University of Utah conducted secret large-scale field tests of BW, including tularemia, Rocky Mountain spotted fever, plague, and Q fever, at the U.S. Army Dugway Proving Ground. In 1950 U.S. Navy ships released as simulants (materials believed to be nonpathogenic that mimic the spread of BW) large quantities of bacteria in the San Francisco Bay area to test the efficiency of their dispersal. Some analysts attributed subsequent infections and deaths to one of those organisms. During the 1950s and 1960s the United States conducted 239 top-secret open-air disseminations of simulants, involving areas such as the New York City subways and Washington National Airport (Cole). The U.S. military developed a large infrastructure of laboratories, test facilities, and production plants related to BW. By the end of the 1960s the United States had stockpiles of at least ten biological and toxin weapons (Geissler). A 1979 outbreak of pulmonary anthrax in the Soviet Union is said to have been caused by accidental release from a Soviet BW factory. Recent disclosures by Russian scientists indicate extensive environmental

contamination and medical problems caused by CW production ("Russian Experts Say Many Died Making Chemical Weapons").

In 1969 the Nixon administration, with the concurrence of the U.S. Defense Department, which declared that BW lacked "military usefulness," unconditionally renounced the development, production, stockpiling, and use of BW and announced that the United States would dismantle its BW program unilaterally. In 1972 the Soviet Union, which had urged a more comprehensive treaty that would include restrictions on CW, ended its opposition to a separate BW treaty. The United States, the Soviet Union, and other nations negotiated the Convention on the Prohibition of the Development, Prevention and Stockpiling of Bacteriological (Biological) and Toxin Weapons and on Their Destruction (BWC). The BWC prohibits, except for "prophylactic, protective and other peaceful purposes," the development or acquisition of biological agents or toxins as well as weapons carrying them and means of their production, stockpiling, transfer, and delivery. The U.S. Senate ratified the BWC in 1975, the same year it ratified the Geneva Protocol of 1925. As of 1987, 110 nations had ratified the BWC and an additional 25 had signed but not yet ratified it (Wright).

Invoking the specter of new biological weapons and unproven allegations of aggressive BW programs in other countries, the Reagan administration initiated intensive efforts to conduct "defensive research," which is permitted under the BWC. The budget for the U.S. Army Biological Defense Research Program (BDRP), which sponsors programs in a wide variety of academic, commercial, and government laboratories, increased dramatically during the 1980s. Much of that research work is medical in nature, including the development of immunizations and treatments against organisms that might be used as BW (Piller and Yamamoto; Wright).

Although research on and the development of new BW are outlawed by the BWC, it is possible that they will occur in the future. Novel dangers lie in new genetic technologies that permit the development of genetically altered organisms that are not known in nature. Stable, tailor-made organisms used as BW could travel long distances and still be infectious, rapidly infiltrate a population, cause debilitating effects very quickly, and be resistant to antibiotic treatment (Piller and Yamamoto).

Ethical Issues for Biomedical Scientists

Biologists, chemists, biomedical scientists, and physicians have played important roles in CBW research and development. Fritz Haber, who was awarded the 1918 Nobel Prize in chemistry for his synthesis of ammonia, is known as the father of Germany's chemical weapons program in World War I. In his speech accepting the Nobel Prize Haber declared poison gas "a higher form of killing" (Harris and Paxman, 1982). By contrast, during the Crimean War the British government consulted the noted physicist Michael Faraday on the feasibility of developing poison gases; Faraday responded that it was entirely feasible but that it was inhumane and he would have nothing to do with it (Russell).

Many scientists who explicitly acknowledge the ethical conflicts involved in work on weapons argue that a higher ethical principle—the imperative of defending one's country or helping to curb what is perceived as evil or destructive—permits or even requires participation in such work. Dr. Theodor Rosebury, who worked on BW during World War II, based his participation on his belief that crisis circumstances that were expected to last for only a limited time required that he act as he did. "We were fighting a fire, and it seemed necessary to risk getting dirty as well as burnt," he later wrote (Rosebury, 1963). Rosebury refused to participate in BW work after the end of the war (Rosebury, 1949).

Other scientists resolved their ethical dilemma by arguing that their work on weapons was designed to reduce the devastation of war. For example, while working on "nonlethal" CBW in the 1960s Dr. Knut Krieger argued that his research would lead to decreased fatalities: "If we do indeed succeed in creating incapacitating systems and are able to substitute incapacitation for death it appears to me that, next to stopping war, this would be an important step forward" (Reid).

Relevant ethical concerns about "defensive research" on BW by biomedical scientists include issues of content, safety, context, and locus (Lappé).

CONTENT. The Japanese laboratory established in 1933 to develop BW was called the Epidemic Prevention Laboratory. One of its activities was supplying vaccines for troops bound for Manchuria, but its major work was developing and testing BW (Powell). Military forces today could conduct research on the offensive use of BW under the cover of defensive research because offensive and defensive research are joined inextricably in at least some phases of the work (Huxsoll et al.). In the parts of the work in which offensive and defensive efforts are parallel new forms of organisms may be found or developed that would be more effective as biological weapons. The possibility that offensive work on BW is being done in the United States under the cover of defensive work has been denied by the leaders of the BDRP, who point out the areas in which the two types of research diverge (Huxsoll et al.). Critics nonetheless raise questions about the ambiguity of BDRP research, arguing that "these efforts are highly ambiguous, provocative and strongly suggestive of offensive goals" (Jacobson and Rosenberg; Piller and Yamamoto; Wright).

SAFETY. Many analysts believe that CW or BW research, even if it is truly defensive in intent, may be dangerous to surrounding communities if toxic materials or virulent infectious organisms are released accidentally.

CONTEXT. CW or BW research, even if it is defensive in intent, can be viewed by a potential military adversary as an attempt to develop protection for a nation's military forces or noncombatants against weapons that that nation might wish to use for offensive purposes, thus permitting that nation to protect its own personnel in a CW or BW first strike. In fact, the military justification for preparing altered organisms is that they are needed for the preparation of defenses. It is therefore impossible for adversaries to determine whether a nation's defensive efforts are part of preparations for the offensive use of weapons.

LOCUS. Fears in this area usually are based on military sponsorship of defensive BW research. Even if that research is relatively open, other nations may view with suspicion the intense interest of military forces rather than civilian medical researchers in vaccines and treatments against specific organisms. Those fears can feed a continuing BW arms race.

More generally, concern has been expressed about the militarization of genetic engineering and biology in general. Characterization of biological weapons as "public health in reverse" therefore may have an even broader and more sinister meaning: The entire field of biology, along with and aspects of it such as the use of human genome research to design weapons to target specific groups, may be in danger of military use for destructive ends (Piller and Yamamoto; Wright). The imprisonment of a chemist by the Russian government and the revocation of his university diploma for publishing an article describing the development of new, highly toxic CW illustrate the restrictions that are placed on scientists who do CBW research (Janowski).

Ethical Issues for Physicians

The first question that arises is whether it is constructive to view certain ethical responsibilities as unique to the physician's social role. Theodor Rosebury described the response to physician participation in work on BW during World War II: "There was much quiet but searching discussion among us regarding the place of doctors in such work ... a certain delicacy concentrated most of the physicians into principally or primarily defensive operations." Rosebury went on to point out that the modifiers *principally* and *primarily* are needed "because military operations can never be exclusively defensive" (Rosebury, 1963). What is seen as the special responsibility of physicians is based largely on an ethical responsibility not to use the power of the physician to do harm (*primum non nocere*). Although the Hippocratic oath seems to apply to the relationship of the physician to an individual patient, its meaning has been broadened by many to proscribe physician participation in actions harmful to nonpatients.

In regard to research on offensive weapons of war there seems to be a consensus that physicians participate in such research at their ethical peril even if their country demands it or they think it useful for deterrence or other preventive purposes. However, because of the ambiguity of defensive work on BW, the dilemma for the physician is not easily resolved even for those who believe that defensive efforts are ethically permissible.

Some proponents of defensive research on BW have argued that it is entirely ethical—that in fact it is obligatory—that physicians work on it. According to this perspective, not only will defenses be needed if such weapons are used against the United States, that work also may be useful in developing protection against naturally occurring diseases (Crozier; Huxsoll et al.; Orient). Other analysts believe that it is unethical for physicians to play a role in military-sponsored BW research because it has a strong potential for intensifying a BW arms race and helping to militarize the science of biology, thus increasing the risk of the use of BW and the destructiveness of their effects if they are used (Jacobson and Rosenberg; Nass, 1991; Sidel, 1991).

The question is: Where on the slippery slope of participation in preparing for the use of BW should physicians draw the line? If physicians engage in civilian-sponsored research on disease control that carries an obligation to report all findings in the open literature even if the research may have implications for BW, that participation, most analysts agree, cannot be faulted on ethical grounds. However, when physicians engage in military-sponsored research in which the openness of reporting is equivocal and the purposes are ambiguous, it is difficult to distinguish their work ethically from work on the development of weapons.

As was noted above, the BWC prohibits any "development, production, stockpiling, transfer or acquisition of biological agents or toxins" except for "prophylactic, protective and other peaceful purposes." The responsibility for government-sponsored medical research for prophylactic, protective, and other peaceful purposes in the United States

lies largely with the National Institutes of Health (NIH) and the Centers for Disease Control (CDC). The NIH or the CDC therefore might be given the responsibility and the resources for medical research of this type. The U. S. Army still may want to conduct nonmedical research and development on defense against BW, such as work on detectors, protective clothing, and other barriers to the spread of organisms. Under this proposed division of effort that research is less likely to be seen as offensive, provoke a BW race, pervert the science of biology, and involve physicians (Sidel, 1989).

A different type of ethical issue related to CBW arose during the Persian Gulf War in 1991. The United States provided protective measures such as immunization against botulinum toxin and anthrax for its military forces. Despite the fact that some of those measures were experimental, no informed consent procedures were used and compliance often was required. Furthermore, the measures were made available to military forces but not to noncombatants in the area (Annas; Howe and Martin).

In addition to the ethical dilemmas involved in these decisions it may be unethical for physicians to ignore the issues involved in CBW. One of the greatest dangers of those weapons may be the apathy of the medical profession toward them. The fact that BW are the weapons with which physicians may become engaged and the ones about which they have specialized knowledge gives physicians a special responsibility not only to refuse to work on them but also actively to work to reduce the threat of their development or use.

Conclusion

Physicians and biomedical scientists should support methods for international epidemiological surveillance to detect the use of BW and investigate incidents in which use has been alleged after an unexplained disease outbreak (Geissler, 1986; Nass, 1992a, 1992b) and support the Vaccines for Peace Programme for the control of "dual-threat" agents (Geissler and Woodall). Support also might be given for measures to strengthen the BWC through the introduction of the verification proposals that were put forth at the 1991 BWC Review Conference (Falk; Rosenberg and Burck; Rosenberg). With regard to chemical weapons, biomedical scientists and physicians might support effective implementation of the 1993 CWC (Smithson).

More broadly, physicians may wish to explore the connection between CBW and nuclear weapons. It has been argued that by refusing to reduce their vast stockpiles of nuclear weapons substantially and refusing to agree to verifiable cessation of nuclear weapons testing and production, the nuclear powers provoke nonnuclear powers to contemplate the development and production of CBW for deterrence against nuclear weapons. The U.S. Defense Intelligence Agency reported that "third world nations view chemical weapons as an attractive and inexpensive alternative to nuclear weapons" (U.S. General Accounting Office; Zilinskas, 1990a, 1990b). There is much that physicians can do, for example, through the International Physicians for the Prevention of Nuclear War, the organization that received the 1985 Nobel Peace Prize, and its affiliates in many countries to reduce the provocation and proliferation of weapons of mass destruction caused by the continuing nuclear arms race.

Individual physicians and scientists can add to the awareness of the dangers of CBW by signing the pledge sponsored by the Council for Responsible Genetics "not to engage knowingly in research and teaching that will further development of chemical and biological warfare agents." U.S. physicians also may wish to support legislation to transfer all medical aspects of biological defense from the military to the NIH or the CDC. Physicians may help awaken the medical profession to the dangers of CBW and nuclear weapons by adding a clause to the oath taken by medical students upon graduation from medical school, similar to the oath for medical students in the former Soviet Union, requiring them "to struggle tirelessly for peace and for the prevention of nuclear war" (Cassel et al., p. 652). The clause might be worded as follows: "Recognizing that nuclear, chemical, and biological arms are weapons of indiscriminate mass destruction and threaten the health of all humanity, I will refuse to play any role that might increase the risk of use of such weapons and will, as part of my professional responsibility, work actively for peace and for the prevention of their use."

VICTOR W. SIDEL (1995)
REVISED BY AUTHOR

SEE ALSO: *Bioterrorism; Conflict of Interest; Harm; Military Personnel as Research Subjects; Prisoners as Research Subjects; Research, Unethical;* and other *Warfare* subentries

BIBLIOGRAPHY

Amitai, Yona; Almog, Shlomo; Singer, Raphael; Hammer, Ruth; Bentur, Yedidia; and Danon, Yehude L. 1992. "Atropine Poisoning in Children during the Persian Gulf Crisis: A National Survey in Israel." *Journal of the American Medical Association* 268(5): 630–632.

Annas, George J. 1992. "Changing the Consent Rules for Desert Storm." *New England Journal of Medicine* 326(11): 770–773.

Barss, Peter. 1992. "Epidemic Field Investigation as Applied to Allegations of Chemical, Biological or Toxin Warfare." *Politics and the Life Sciences* 11(1): 5–22.

Bernstein, Barton J. 1987. "Churchill's Secret Biological Weapons." *Bulletin of the Atomic Scientists* 43(1): 46–50.

Cassel, Christine K.; Jameton, Andrew L.; Sidel, Victor W.; and Storey, Patrick B. 1985. "The Physician's Oath and the Prevention of Nuclear War." *Journal of the American Medical Association* 254: 652–654.

Cole, Leonard A. 1988. *Clouds of Secrecy: The Army's Germ Warfare Tests over Populated Areas.* Totowa, NJ: Rowman & Littlefield.

Crozier, Dan. 1971. "The Physician and Biologic Warfare." *New England Journal of Medicine* 284(18): 1008–1011.

Falk, Richard. 1990. "Inhibiting Reliance on Biological Weaponry: The Role and Relevance of International Law." In *Preventing a Biological Arms Race,* ed. Susan Wright. Cambridge, MA: MIT Press.

Forrow, Lachlan, and Sidel, Victor W. 1998. "Medicine and Nuclear War: From Hiroshima to Mutual Assured Destruction to Abolition 2000." *Journal of the American Medical Association* 280(5): 456–461.

Geissler, Erhard, ed. 1986. *Biological and Toxin Weapons Today.* London: Oxford University Press.

Geissler, Erhard, and Woodall, John P. 1994. *Control of Dual-Threat Agents: The Vaccines for Peace Programme.* New York: Oxford University Press.

Harris, Robert, and Paxman, Jeremy. 1982. *A Higher Form of Killing: The Secret Story of Chemical and Biological Warfare.* New York: Hill & Wang.

Howe, Edmund G., and Martin, Edward D. 1991. "Treating the Troops." *Hastings Center Report* 21(2): 21–24.

Hu, Howard; Fine, Jonathan; Epstein, Paul; et al. 1989. "Tear Gas: Harassing Agent or Toxic Chemical Weapon?" *Journal of the American Medical Association* 262(5): 660–663.

Huxsoll, David L.; Parrott, Cheryl D.; and Patrick, William C. 1989. "Medicine in Defense against Biological Warfare." *Journal of the American Medical Association* 262(5): 677–678.

Infield, Glenn B. 1971. *Disaster at Bari.* New York: Macmillan.

Jacobson, Jay A., and Rosenberg, Barbara Hatch. 1989. "Biological Defense Research: Charting a Safer Course." *Journal of the American Medical Association* 262: 675–676.

Janowski, Pat. 1993. "Speak No Evil: A Dissident Is Detained for Revealing the Existence of a Powerful Poison Gas." *Science* 33(6): 4–5.

Kawachi, Ichiro, and Kennedy, Bruce P. 2002. *The Health of Nations. Why Inequality Is Harmful to Your Health.* New York: New Press.

Lappé, Marc. 1990. "Ethics in Biological Warfare Research." In *Preventing a Biological Arms Race,* ed. Susan Wright. Cambridge, MA: MIT Press.

Nass, Meryl. 1991. "The Labyrinth of Biological Defense." *PSR Quarterly* 1: 24–30.

Nass, Meryl. 1992a. "Anthrax Epizootic in Zimbabwe, 1978–1980: Due to Deliberate Spread?" *PSR Quarterly* 2:198–209.

Nass, Meryl. 1992b. "Can Biological, Toxin, and Chemical Warfare Be Eliminated?" *Politics and the Life Sciences* 11: 30–32.

Orient, Jane M. 1989. "Chemical and Biological Warfare: Should Defenses Be Researched and Deployed?" *Journal of the American Medical Association* 262(5): 644–648.

Piller, Charles, and Yamamoto, Keith R. 1988. *Gene Wars: Military Control over the New Genetic Technologies.* New York: Beech Tree.

Powell, John W. 1981. "A Hidden Chapter in History." *Bulletin of the Atomic Scientists* 37(8): 44–52.

Reid, Robert W. 1969. *Tongues of Conscience: Weapons Research and the Scientists' Dilemma.* New York: Walker.

Rosebury, Theodor. 1949. *Peace or Pestilence: Biological Warfare and How to Avoid It.* New York: Whittlesey House.

Rosebury, Theodor. 1963. "Medical Ethics and Biological Warfare." *Perspectives in Biology and Medicine* 6: 512–523.

Rosenberg, Barbara Hatch. 1993. "Progress toward Verification of the Biological Weapons Convention." In *Verification 1993,* ed. J. B. Poole and R. Guthrie. Trowbridge, Eng.: Redmond.

Rosenberg, Barbara Hatch, and Burck, Gordon. 1990. "Verification of Compliance with the Biological Weapons Convention." In *Preventing a Biological Arms Race,* ed. Susan Wright. Cambridge, MA: MIT Press.

Russell, Bertrand. 1962. *Fact and Fiction.* New York: Simon & Schuster.

"Russian Experts Say Many Died Making Chemical Weapons." 1993. *New York Times,* December 24, p. A4.

Sidel, Victor W. 1989. "Weapons of Mass Destruction: The Greatest Threat to Public Health." *Journal of the American Medical Association* 262(5): 680–682.

Sidel, Victor M. 1991. "Biological Weapons Research and Physicians: Historical and Ethical Analysis." *PSR Quarterly* 1: 31–42.

Sidel, Victor M. 1993. "Farewell to Arms: The Impact of the Arms Race on the Human Condition." *PSR Quarterly* 3: 18–26.

Sidel, Victor W., and Goldwyn, Robert M. 1966. "Chemical and Biological Weapons—A Primer." *New England Journal of Medicine* 274(1): 21–27.

Smithson, Amy E., ed. 1993. *The Chemical Weapons Convention Handbook.* Washington, D.C.: Henry L. Stimson Center.

United Nations. 1969. *Chemical and Bacteriological (Biological) Weapons and the Effects of Their Possible Use.* Report. E.69.I.24. New York: Author.

U.S. Department of Health, Education, and Welfare. 1959. *Effects of Biological Warfare Agents: For Use in Readiness Planning.* Washington, D.C.: U.S. Government Printing Office.

U.S. General Accounting Office. 1986. *Chemical Warfare Progress and Problems in Defensive Capability: Report to the Chairman, Committee on Foreign Affairs, U.S. House of Representatives.* GAO/PEMD-86–11.

Waitzkin, Howard. 2000. *The Second Sickness: Contradictions of Capitalist Health Care,* Revised and Updated edition. Lanham, MD: Rowman & Littlefield.

Waitzkin, H; Iriart, Celia; Estrada, A; and Lamadrid, S. 2001a. "Social Medicine in Latin America: Productivity and Dangers Facing the Major National Groups." *Lancet* 358(9278): 315–323.

Waitzkin, H; Iriart, Celia; Estrada, A; and Lamadrid, S. 2001b. "Social Medicine Then and Now: Lessons from Latin America." *American Journal of Public Health.* 91(10): 1592–1601.

Williams, Peter, and Wallace, David. 1989. *Unit 731: The Japanese Army's Secret of Secrets.* London: Hodder & Stoughton.

World Health Organization. 1970. *Health Aspects of Chemical and Biological Weapons: Report of a WHO Group of Consultants.* Geneva: Author.

Wright, Susan, ed. 1990. *Preventing a Biological Arms Race.* Cambridge, MA: MIT Press.

Zilinskas, Raymond A. 1990a. "Biological Warfare and the Third World." *Politics and the Life Sciences* 9(1): 59–76.

Zilinskas, Raymond A. 1990b. "Terrorism and Biological Weapons: Inevitable Alliance?" *Perspectives in Biology and Medicine* 34(1): 44–72.

INTERNET RESOURCE

"Russia Names Moscow Siege Gas." 2002. CNN World News, October 30. Available at <http://www.cnn.com/2002/WORLD/europe/10/30/moscow.gas/>.

WHISTLEBLOWING IN HEALTHCARE

• • •

The term *whistleblowing* is a metaphor, apparently derived from a referee's use of a whistle to call a foul in a sporting event. It refers to a disclosure made by a member or former member of an organization about some practice within the organization. Whistleblowing can be internal (disclosure to someone in higher authority in the organization) or external (disclosure to outside persons or organizations such as government agencies, public-interest groups, or the news media). The term is most commonly used to describe disclosure to persons outside the organization, and it is external whistleblowing that is the focus of discussion here.

The whistleblower is a person, usually willing to be identified publicly, who makes an unauthorized disclosure regarding some action or practice within the organization that the person judges to be ethically wrong or unacceptably dangerous. Whistleblowing takes place in business, in government, and in the professions. In healthcare, the most common example in the ethics literature is whistleblowing by nurses about physician behavior. With increased attention being given to ethical issues throughout the healthcare organization, it can be expected that, in the future, the examples of potentially justified whistleblowing in healthcare will be focused nearly as frequently on the business side of the organization as on the clinical side.

Whistleblowing is unauthorized disclosure. As such, it almost always involves activity that management considers disloyal to the organization. In addition, organizations and individuals can be harmed, perhaps in an irreparable manner, by public accusations. Retractions or corrections of false or unfair allegations seldom receive the same degree of public attention as the initial accusations. These considerations of disloyalty and harm have led many ethicists to stress the conditions that must be met before individuals should feel justified in blowing the whistle. It is also important to recognize, however, that the organization has a responsibility to prevent the need for whistleblowing and to treat the whistleblower fairly.

Responsible Whistleblowing

Even when potential whistleblowers are motivated by a desire to protect other individuals or society in general, they need to be careful lest they do more harm than good. Ethical or responsible whistleblowing is usually understood to mean that all of the following conditions are met:

(1) The person has clear evidence that the organization or someone in the organization is engaged in activity that is seriously wrong or that has a high potential for doing serious harm.

(2) The charge to be made by the whistleblower is accurate and accusations against any individuals are able to be substantiated.

(3) The wrongdoing or the danger to be disclosed must be serious enough to justify risking the harm that will likely result to the organization and to some individuals once the public disclosure is made.

(4) Reasonable attempts to prevent the wrong through internal consultation and reporting have been made and have failed. Potential whistleblowers should attempt to use methods of reporting within the organization before going outside, in spite of the frustrations and delays internal mechanisms can sometimes cause. (It should be recognized, however, that in some situations internal efforts to prevent the wrong are not feasible or would simply lead to an effective cover-up.)

(5) There is a reasonable possibility that the disclosure will help prevent or mitigate the harm or wrong or that the disclosure will lessen the likelihood that similar actions will occur in the future. (This condition should not be interpreted too rigidly. In many cases, it is exceedingly difficult to calculate the potential consequences that may result from acting. Furthermore, it may sometimes be legitimate just to call attention to the reality in order to have a better-informed public.)

When these conditions are all met, blowing the whistle might best be considered an ethical responsibility, not just an ethically permissible act; all employees have some responsibility to protect the public from serious harm when possible.

The Organization: Prevention and Protection

While much of the discussion of whistleblowing in the ethics literature has focused on the responsibility of the potential whistleblower, there is also a need to recognize the responsibilities of management. Many healthcare organizations now have corporate compliance programs that have mechanisms for internal reporting of suspected wrongdoing (including anonymous reporting to the compliance officer). However, unless and until employees and medical staff see that changes are made when concerns are raised internally, they will still be faced with the question of whether to go public. Management is in a weak position to claim that an employee should not blow the whistle out of loyalty to the organization if management does not adequately attend to reported problems. One of the key reasons why some nurses believe they have a responsibility to blow the whistle publicly on physician behavior is that their experience is that internal complaints have led to no changes at all.

In addition to following up quickly and with thorough investigations when staff report what they perceive to be serious wrongdoing, management can take other steps to prevent staff from concluding that they have no alternative but to blow the whistle. Those who make internal reports or complaints should be protected from any recrimination or discipline, as long as they make the report in good faith (which should be assumed until proven otherwise). Trying to protect the organization from doing harm should be rewarded, not penalized.

Organizations also have a responsibility to deal fairly with employees who do blow the whistle. In the history of whistleblowing in business, a common outcome has been the firing of whistleblowers. This has been the case, even when there was evidence that the whistleblower did, in fact, expose a serious wrongdoing that was not being addressed internally. It is difficult, if not impossible, to justify ethically the firing of an employee because the person blew the whistle on actions that seriously threaten the public good after making reasonable internal attempts to achieve a change. The ethical healthcare organization recognizes that loyalty to the public good takes priority over loyalty to the employer.

CHARLES J. DOUGHERTY (1995)
REVISED BY LEONARD J. WEBER

SEE ALSO: *Conscience; Conscience, Rights of; Malpractice, Medical; Mistakes, Medical; Pharmaceutical Industry; Profession and Professional Ethics; Responsibility; Virtue and Character*

BIBLIOGRAPHY

Alford, C. Fred. 2001. "Whistleblowers and the Narrative of Ethics." *Journal of Social Philosophy* 32(3): 402–418.

Banja, John D. 1985. "Whistleblowing in Physical Therapy." *Physical Therapy* 65(11): 1683–1686.

Fiesta, Janine. 1990. "Whistleblowers, Part I: Heroes or Stool Pigeons?" *Nursing Management* 21(6): 16–17.

Fiesta, Janine. 1990. "Whistleblowers, Part II: Retaliation or Protection?" *Nursing Management* 21(7): 38.

Glazer, Myron, and Penina Glazer. 1989. *The Whistleblowers: Exposing Corruption in Government and Industry.* New York: Basic.

Gunsalus, C. K. 1998. "How to Blow the Whistle and Still Have a Career Afterwards." *Science and Engineering Ethics* 4(1): 51–64.

Haddad, Amy M., and Charles J. Dougherty. 1991. "Whistleblowing in the O.R.: The Ethical Implications." *Today's O.R. Nurse* 13(3): 30–33.

Johnson, Roberta Ann. 2002. *Whistleblowing: When It Works—And Why.* Boulder, CO: Lynne Rienner Publishers.

Jubb, Peter B. 1999. "Whistleblowing: A Restrictive Definition and Interpretation." *Journal of Business Ethics* 21(1): 77–94.

Lewis, David B., ed. 2001. *Whistleblowing at Work.* London: Althone Press.

McKnight, Diane M. 1998. "Scientific Societies and Whistleblowers: the Relationship between the Community and the Individual." *Science and Engineering Ethics* 4(1): 97–113.

Miethe, Terance D. 1999. *Whistleblowing at Work: Tough Choices in Exposing Fraud, Waste, and Abuse on the Job.* Boulder, CO: Westveiw.

Sieber, Joan E. 1998. "The Psychology of Whistleblowing." *Science and Engineering Ethics* 4(1): 7–23.

U.S. President's Commission for the Study of Ethical Problems in Medicine and Biomedical and Behavioral Research. 1981. *Whistleblowing in Biomedical Research: Policies and Procedures for Responding to Reports of Misconduct,* ed. Judith P. Swazey and Stephen R. Sher. Washington, D.C.: Government Printing Office.

WOMEN AS HEALTH PROFESSIONALS, CONTEMPORARY ISSUES OF

• • •

After three decades of increasing numbers of women entering previously male-dominated health professions, few academic health centers have what might be considered a "critical mass" of women full professors, much less women leaders. A brief status report on women in academic medicine introduces a discussion of recent research on why gender differences in the advancement of professionals persist. For instance, no matter how complex the technical requirements of a woman's occupation, Western culture expects her to be more nurturing and emotionally accessible than a man. At the same time, it places a low value on caretaking roles, in terms of both prestige and financial remuneration. Forward-looking institutional strategies to enhance the development of women health professionals target features of the work culture that may be "simply the norm" but that disadvantages women. The concluding section of this entry attempts responses to the questions: Is the increasing number of women entering medicine and other health professions mitigating the impact of gender? And how is gender diversity changing the profession?

Status Report on Women in Academic Medical Centers

Of all the health profession schools, the most extensive data is available on medical schools (and they are largest in terms of budget and size); therefore, this statistical report centers on women in academic medicine. Most trends and findings cited would apply as well to other health professions that were male-dominated until recently.

In 2001 women constituted 45 percent of U.S. medical students, 39 percent of dental students, and 41 percent of osteopathic students (by comparison, women are 55% of enrollees in four-year colleges/universities). The number of men applying to medical school has been declining faster than the number of women. For instance, between 1995 and 2001, the number of men applying to medical school declined by 33 percent, compared to 17 percent for women. If this rate of change continues, by 2005, half of first-year medical students nationally will be women.

The proportion of full-time medical school women faculty in 2001 was 28 percent (in dental schools, 25%, and in osteopathic schools, 39%). The proportion of medical school instructors who are women has been steadily increasing and is now 46 percent, but only 12 percent of full professors are women.

With regard to the proportion of men and women faculty at each rank, these proportions have remained remarkably stable, especially at the full professor rank (Bickel, 2001). For instance, in 2001, 10.9 percent of all women faculty and 30.9 percent of all men faculty were full professors; in the mid-1980s, these proportions were 9.9 percent and 31.5 percent, respectively.

In 2001, 14 percent of tenured medical school faculty (all ranks) were women. Between 1995 and 2001, the percent of women with tenure actually dropped from 14 percent to 12 percent, about the same proportional decline as the percent of men tenured (32% to 28%) (Bickel, 2001). Data from the Association of American Medical College's Faculty Roster System also reveal that the average annual rate of women faculty attrition (9.1%) exceeds that of men (7.7%) (Yamagata).

With regard to academic administrative roles, in 2001 women chaired approximately 214 departments (91 basic science and 123 clinical departments [including interim and acting chairs]), which is about 8 percent of all medical school chairs. This total constitutes an average of just 1.7 per medical school, and at least 20 of 125 medical schools have no women chairs (most of these have never had one). The specialties with the largest number of women chairs are microbiology, pathology, anesthesiology, family medicine, obstetrics/gynecology, and pediatrics (Bickel, Clark, and Lawson).

By 2002 the number of women assistant, associate, and senior associate deans at American medical schools totaled approximately 422 (an average of three per school); three schools had no woman in a decanal position. As of July 2002, women held deanships at eight of the 125 U.S. medical schools (two were interim positions). In osteopathic schools, women held three of nineteen deanships and in dental schools, none.

Continuing Disadvantages Related to Professional Opportunities

Numerous studies from the late 1990s and early 2000s have elucidated continuing gender differences in professional opportunities and advancement. Although these areas are highly interrelated, the findings are presented below under five headings: specialty choice, sexism and mental models of gender, acquiring mentoring, practice-related areas of career disadvantage, and the intersection of gender and ethnicity.

SPECIALTY CHOICE. The specialty choices of women physicians have changed little despite their large increases in numbers, with comparatively few women entering surgery and most subspecialties. Why are women not distributing more evenly across specialties? The weight of tradition from earlier eras when women physicians were restricted to treating women and children (Bickel, 2000) explains in part why high proportions of women physicians continue to enter obstetrics and gynecology, pediatrics, general internal medicine, and family practice. But the paucity of women entering surgery also points to characteristics of the field, including hours that may preclude having a healthy family or personal life, and a lack of positive role models (Biermann). Women who enter training, however, do not drop out of surgical residencies at a higher rate than men. The American College of Surgeons' analysis of the 1993 entering cohort found that male and female U.S. and Canadian graduates had the same attrition rate from surgical residencies (Kwakwa and Jonasson). The largest study of women physicians (U.S. medical school graduates between 1950 and 1989) found that women surgeons are less likely (43%) to have children than nonsurgeons (71%) but reported a higher level of satisfaction with their specialty than nonsurgeons (Frank, Brownstein et al., 1998).

Thus, the more prestigious (and better paid) *curing* specialties continue to be male dominated (Bickel, 1988). One issue of equity related to women physicians' concentration in what might be termed the *caring* specialties is that listening and counseling skills are sometimes viewed as qualities inherent in women rather than acknowledged as technical proficiencies that deserve recognition and recompense.

SEXISM AND MENTAL MODELS OF GENDER. Harassment and sexism continue to detract from the education and opportunities of women health professionals. Even medical school department chairs admit to witnessing inappropriate sexual behavior including pressuring women to participate in sexual relationships (Yedidia and Bickel). Almost half of American women physicians believe they have been harassed during their careers, and most cite medical school as the location. In this national study, harassment was associated with depression, suicide attempts, and a desire to switch specialties (Frank, Brogan, and Schiffman). Abused students are more likely to lack confidence in their clinical skills and in their ability to give compassionate care (Kassebaum and Cutler; Schuchert).

As troublesome as overt sexual harassment continues to be, subtler forms of bias pose a much larger challenge to women's development as professionals. U.S. society associates decisiveness, rationality, and ambition with men, and gentleness, empathy, and nurturance with women (Tong). Such stereotypes, however, deny individuals the opportunity to be appraised positively on the basis of their unique traits. Indeed, men or women who act "against type" tend to be dismissed or marginalized. The "feminine" man who displays more sensitivity or emotion than is culturally normative risks derision; the assertive woman is perceived as "uncaring" and "unfeminine."

These widely shared schemas about males and females also include expectations about their professional competence (Valian). Medical school department chairs confirm that lack of recognition and respect of women in routine interactions was prevalent (Yedidia and Bickel). Women report feeling "invisible" and frequently having their contributions at meetings ascribed to men (Valian). Both men and women asked to rate works of art, articles, and curricula vitae give lower ratings when they believe they are rating the work of a woman (Valian, 1998). An analysis of peer-review scores for postdoctoral fellowship applications revealed that women applicants had to be 2.5 times more productive than the average man to receive the same competence score (Wenneras and Wold). Students judge women faculty who are not nurturing much more harshly than they do men professors who are not nurturing (Sandler, Silverberg, and Hall).

Thus, without being conscious of their "mental models" of gender, both men and women still tend to devalue women's work and to allow women a narrower band of assertive behavior (Valian). Under such conditions, women cannot realize their full potential, nor can they care for their patients with maximum effectiveness. "Mental models" persist in part because individuals, especially dominant personalities, tend to ignore information that runs counter to their stereotypes (Fiske). Features common to clinical medicine, such as time pressures, stress, and cognitive complexity, also stimulate stereotyping and "application error"

(i.e., inappropriate application of epidemiological data to all group members) (Geiger). Nonetheless, most scientists and physicians appear to believe that they work in a meritocracy and that they are not influenced by stereotypes (Bickel, 1997). Some even conclude that women are advantaged compared to men. Apparently, while individual men do not feel powerful, power is so deeply woven into their lives that it is most invisible to those who are most empowered (Kimmel). Equity demands, however, that health professionals accept responsibility for unlearning whatever stereotypes interfere with their evaluations of patients, students, and colleagues.

ACQUIRING MENTORING. While most studies find that women faculty are as likely as men to have a mentor, women gain less benefit from the mentor relationship. One internal medicine department found that mentors more actively encouraged men than women protégés to participate in professional activities outside the institution and that women were three times more likely than men to report a mentor taking credit for their work—an unethical practice rarely discussed (Fried, Francomano, and MacDonald). Women cardiologists report their mentors to be less helpful with career planning than men do and more commonly noted that their mentor was actually a negative role model (19% of women versus 8% of men) (Limacher, Zaher, and Wolf).

These challenges in obtaining mentoring are particularly unfortunate because, for a variety of reasons, women have a greater need for mentoring than men do (Bickel, 2000).

Not only does Western culture tend to devalue women's work, women tend to be more modest than men about their achievements; they are less apt than men to see themselves as qualified for top positions even when their credentials are equivalent or superior (Austin). Moreover, women's informal networks are less extensive and less likely to include colleagues or higher-ranking people from previous institutions (Hitchcock et al.). Without the "social capital" and essential information that grow out of developmental relationships, women remain isolated. And isolation further reduces their capacity for risk-taking, often translating into a reluctance to pursue professional goals or a protective response such as niche work or perfectionism (the obverse strategy of identifying a hot topic) (Etzkowitz, Kemelgor, and Uzzi). It is significant that women experience isolation at work whereas for male health professionals work tends to be highly social and socializing. This paradox is compounded when similarly isolated women are appointed as tokens to committees and pointed to as *role models* (i.e., expected to be *solutions* to a *problem*). If women seek affiliation through a women's group, they may be labeled as needy, lesbian, or *rabble-rousers*.

Many men have difficulty effectively mentoring women because of lack of experience with career-oriented women or because they find it easier to relate to women in social than in professional roles. A contemporary approach to mentoring builds on the recognition that styles and advice that worked for the mentor may not work for a protégé (Thomas) and that advice applicable even five years earlier may no longer be helpful. Thus, many chairs and senior faculty could use assistance in techniques of active listening, avoiding assumptions, and providing supportive feedback that also stimulates the protégé's professional growth (Bickel et al, 2002).

PRACTICE-RELATED AREAS OF CAREER DISADVANTAGE. A large national study conducted in 2000 found that compared with men, women physicians have more patients with complex psychosocial problems. Women physicians also have substantially less control of their work than men— in term of patient volume, selecting physicians for referrals, and office scheduling. Women physicians also have more patients with complex psychosocial problems, adding to their time and energy requirements, in an era when physicians are being pressured to see more patients in fewer minutes. Time spent with patients is time not spent with students, writing grants, or on their many other responsibilities. Thus, it is not surprising that women were 1.6 times more likely to report burnout than men, with the odds of burnout by women increasing by at least 12 percent for each additional five hours worked per week over forty hours. This study also found a $22,000 gap in income between men and women, after controlling for age, specialty, practice type, time in current practice, uninsured status of patients, region, hours worked, and other variables (McMurray, 2000). A 1998 survey of board-certified internists in Pennsylvania found that women earned 14 percent less per hour than their male counterparts, even after adjustment for demographic, training, practice, and family characteristics (Ness et al.).

Junior faculty have been hardest hit by imperatives in academic medicine to increase clinical loads; these imperatives disproportionately affect women (67% of women are instructors or assistant professors compared to 44% of men). Women faculty have less "protected" time for research and fewer academic resources than men (Carr et al.). In addition to pressures to simultaneously complete fellowship, start a practice and a research program, and take on heavy service and administrative responsibilities, most young faculty members are raising young children. Women physicians are actually more likely to be married (and less likely to be divorced) than women in the general population (Frank et al., 1997). And about 85 percent of women physicians have children, compared to 83 percent of the general population (Potee, Gerber, and Hall, 1999).

While family-leave policies at academic medical centers are now commonplace, they rarely allow for more than three months of leave and require women to use up annual and sick leave. Some schools have introduced less-than-full-time options; in many cases, however, users sacrifice benefits and the flexibility to return to the tenure track (Socolar et al.). Even when flexible policies exist, individuals who take advantage of the flexibility allowed may be labeled "uncommitted." Thus, the relationship between medicine and parenthood can be characterized as uneasy and not well-tolerated, especially in academic careers.

Moreover, family-related decisions can escalate into moral dilemmas. The traditional obligation of physicians to set patients' needs above their own sometimes confronts physician-parents (and especially couples who are both in practice) with difficult choices between the needs of patients and those of their own children. How are they to decide when a patient must take priority over their children? While such dilemmas are common because of the lack of easily available child care, they are rarely discussed. The profession would benefit from opportunities for practitioners who are also family caretakers to dialogue about the ethics of family responsibilities as related to the ethics of medicine. Even more helpful would be institutional approaches to improving and supporting flexibility for those with family responsibilities, such as on-site day care, emergency or sick child care, and nonpunitive leave policies. All of these features are much more readily available in Canada, Britian, and Australia than in the United States (McMurray et al., 2002).

THE INTERSECTION OF GENDER AND ETHNICITY. In 2001 the 125 U.S. medical schools had a total of 1,199 African-American women faculty (4% of all female faculty); smaller numbers of Native Americans, Mexican Americans, and Puerto Rican women added up to an additional 4 percent of women faculty. A higher proportion of women faculty than men faculty are underrepresented minorities.

Faculty from ethnic minorities are no more likely to attain senior rank than are women (Palepu et al.; Fang et al.; Bright, Duefield, and Stone). Both women and minorities face stigmatization and prejudice and difficulties in obtaining career-advancing mentoring. Thus women ethnic minorities experience "double jeopardy." A study of African-American women physicians found that the majority cited racial discrimination as a major obstacle during medical school and residency and in practice. In addition they perceived gender discrimination to be a greater obstacle than did non-African-American women physicians (More).

Psychologists have described the *just world* bias: That is, people want to believe that, in the absence of special treatment, individuals generally get what they deserve and deserve what they get; they adjust their perceptions of performance to match the outcomes they observe (Valian). If women, particularly women of color, are underrepresented in positions of greatest prominence, the most psychologically convenient explanation is that they lack the necessary qualifications or commitment. Thus, women of color must frequently overcome assumptions that they owe their positions to affirmative action rather than professional qualifications. At the same time, minority women encounter severe *surplus visibility,* that is, their mistakes are more readily noticed and they are less likely to be given a "second chance."

Compounding all of the above extra challenges, minority female physicians are also at highest risk for institutional service obligations (Menges and Exum), including committee work, student counseling, and patient care (Menges and Exum; Levinson and Weiner). Thus, while increasing the number of ethnic minorities progressing in academic medicine presents different challenges than increasing women, the challenges overlap, for instance, in overcoming unconscious bias related to "what a leader looks like" (Bickel, 1997).

Forward-Looking Institutional Approaches

Most approaches to improve the advancement of women have attempted to "fix" or "equip" women with skills that they are perceived to lack and to add temporal flexibility to policies. While these efforts are necessary, organizational development experts concluded that such narrow approaches can have only limited success (Ely and Meyerson).

The research findings summarized above clearly raise fundamental questions about organizational culture and the ways in which work is organized. What is wrong with U.S. health systems that women have such a hard time succeeding in them? The faculty tenure system offers a striking example; it is a forced march in the early years, allowing a slower pace later on. Most women would prefer the opposite timing, allowing them more flexibility while their children are young. The most clinically productive decade for women physicians begins at age fifty.

Another example of organizational disadvantage is medicine's overvaluation of heroic individualism, with the largely invisible work of preventing crises and maintaining relationships going unrewarded. Because women tend to be doing the less visible, collaborative, relational work, their contributions remain underrecognized (Etzkowitz, Kemelgor, and Uzzi).

Thus strategies to promote women must target features of the work culture that may be "simply the norm" but that

disadvantage women (Ely and Meyerson). For instance, new models of cooperation are needed to recognize and reward contributions of all members of the team. And these models must avoid expectations that women will do the "relationship" work; dialogue between the sexes is required to achieve the facilitating of *caring* and *leading* on the part of both women and men.

Much of the process by which disadvantage is created and reinforced occurs at the department level (e.g., recruitment, mentoring, access to resources). Thus, department heads are key, and one avenue to stimulate their cooperation is to emphasis diversity issues in departmental reviews (Etzkowitz, Kemelgor, and Uzzi).

The most comprehensive analysis to date of initiatives to develop women medical school faculty (Morahan et al.) found that exemplary schools focus on improvements not specific to women: heightening department chairs' focus on faculty development needs, preparing educational materials on promotion and tenure procedures, improving parental-leave policies, allowing temporary stops on the tenure probationary clock and a less than full-time interval without permanent penalty, and conducting exit interviews with departing faculty. These schools regularly evaluate their initiatives by comparing recruitment, retention, and promotion of women and men faculty and by conducting faculty satisfaction and salary equity studies. Surveying faculty about their career development experiences and their perceptions of the environment, comparing the responses of men and women, and presenting the results to faculty and administrators are particularly useful strategies.

Initiatives to develop women and to improve the work culture do not lower standards or disadvantage men. Interventions on behalf of women tend to improve the environment for men as well. When the Department of Medicine at Johns Hopkins University evaluated its interventions to increase the number of women succeeding in the department (Fried et al.), the proportion of women expecting to remain in academic medicine increased by 66 percent and the proportion of men increased by 57 percent.

With regard to ensuring that students and junior faculty obtain the mentoring they need, institutions find themselves challenged by the increasing heterogeneity of new entrants, not only in terms of gender but also with regard to ethnicity, age, values, and previous life experience. In order to competently mentor students unlike themselves, the relatively homogeneous senior faculty would benefit from opportunities to improve listening and feedback skills and to overcome engrained models of gender and race. Another strategy to increase positive emphasis on mentoring is to evaluate faculty on how well they meet this responsibility. For instance, just as promotions committees count first authorships in major journals, some schools are also now counting *last* authorships with mentees as first authors (Grady-Weliky, Kettyle, and Hundert). Other schools now require that on each faculty member's annual evaluation, senior faculty list their protégés; trainees and junior faculty are asked to name their mentors and role models. An increasing number of schools and individual departments offer programs that facilitate mentor/protégé pairings; another positive strategy is mentor-of-the-year awards (Bickel, 2000).

Medical schools' approaches to eliminating sex discrimination and harassment have included sporadically distributed informational resources and occasional educational programs; by and large the effectiveness of such efforts has not been evaluated. Medical educators' increasing emphasis on professionalism in general shows more promise in drawing positive attention to responsible physicians' attitudes and behaviors (Epstein and Hundert; Wear and Bickel). However, more attention to barriers created by mental models of gender and race would strengthen most professionalism initiatives. Likewise, programs designed to improve patient communication skills should include assistance in overcoming gender stereotypes.

Finally, there are encouraging trends in medical education toward problem-based learning and toward the incorporation of women's health into the curriculum. Both require interdisciplinary bridges and teamwork, actually furthering a sense of community within academic medical centers. And adding a focus on women's health also frequently incorporates a more holistic and community orientation into the curriculum (Donoghue, Hoffman, and Magrane).

Conclusion

Gender differences in professional and leadership opportunities persist, yet perceptions of these continuing inequalities are not widespread. The number of women entering the health professions, and even becoming faculty, actually obscures the work that remains—part of which is persuading many that academic medicine still greatly favors the development of men. Actually, many male physicians and medical students are concluding not only that equal opportunity has been won but also that women tend to have an "affirmative action" advantage. Many young women entering medicine, surrounded by women peers and unaware of their predecessors' struggles, are assuming that women may be freely choosing to reap fewer rewards than men for their

work but that they themselves will not have to settle for less (McCorduck and Ramsey). Thus, impetus for change is lacking, as the women who are not realizing their potential tend to be invisible or to disappear.

Is the increasing number of women entering medicine and other health professions mitigating the impact of gender? Recent studies comparing the careers of men and women consistently show that increases in the number of women is *not* reducing gender disparities in advancement nor the power of mental models of gender. Reducing the power of gender stereotypes in medicine is a moral imperative because healthcare professionals have a duty to ensure that perceptual bias does not interfere either with the best possible patient care or with clinicians' responsibilities as role models for and teachers of students of both genders. Healthcare professionals' effectiveness depends in large part on their sensitivities to others, that is, their ability to "hear" and "see" individual patients.

Is gender diversity changing the medical profession? Too many diverse forces (e.g., technological, economic, political) are shaping modern medicine to link any one change to the increasing numbers of women providers, especially given the extent to which men and women share characteristics. But the primary difficulty in answering this question is that too few women have achieved leadership positions to allow comparison with the records of their male predecessors.

That the health professions are not realizing the full value of their investment in women is not only an injustice, it is also evidence of poor stewardship. These careers involve considerable personal and public resources, but the leadership potential of most women continues to be wasted. This is a collective loss—all the more unaffordable given the leadership challenges facing the health professions. It is highly likely that women leaders can make a positive difference: "Women have lived in *embedded* roles, roles intimately interwoven into the warp and woof of the social context … serving as links between other roles, between generations, between institutions, between the public and private domains.… Consequently women are no newcomers to the complications generated by interdependence and diversity" (Lipman-Blumen, p. 289).

Gender equity will always be an elusive concept and goal; for one thing, women are as different from each other as men are from each other. Nonetheless, leaders owe it to future generations of trainees and patients to create an environment of equal opportunity—where assumptions and judgments about individuals' competencies and preferences are not colored by their sex, where women's goals and traits are as valued as men's, and where nonpunitive options facilitate the combining of professional and family responsibilities. The future of the health professions is inextricably linked to the development of its women professionals.

JANET BICKEL
GAIL J. POVAR (1995)
REVISED BY JANET BICKEL

SEE ALSO: *Alternative Therapies: Social History; Care; Compassionate Love; Feminism; Sexism; Sexual Ethics and Professional Standards*

BIBLIOGRAPHY

Austin, Linda S. 2000. *What's Holding You Back? Eight Critical Choices for Women's Success.* New York: Basic.

Bickel, Janet. 1988. "Women in Medical Education: A Status Report." *New England Journal of Medicine* 24: 1579–1584.

Bickel, Janet. 1997. "Gender Stereotypes and Misconceptions: Unresolved Issues in Physicians' Professional Development." *Journal of the American Medical Association* 277: 1405, 1407.

Bickel, Janet. 2000. *Women in Medicine: Getting In, Growing, and Advancing.* Thousand Oaks, CA: Sage.

Bickel, Janet. 2001. "Women in Medicine: The Work That Remains." *Journal of Women's Imaging* 3: 1–2.

Bickel, Janet; Clark, Valarie; and Lawson, Renee Marshall. 2001. *Women in U.S. Academic Medicine Statistics, 2000–2001.* Washington, D.C.: Association of American Medical Colleges.

Bickel, Janet; Wara, Diane; Atkinson, Barbara F.; et al. 2002. "Increasing Women's Leadership in Academic Medicine: Report of the AAMC Project Implementation Committee." *Academic Medicine* 77:1043–61.

Biermann, Jessica S. 1998. "Women in Orthopedic Surgery Residencies in the United States." *Academic Medicine* 73: 708–709.

Bright, Charles M.; C. A. Duefield; and Valerie E. Stone. 1998. "Perceived Barriers and Biases in the Medical Education Experience by Gender and Race." *Journal of the National Medical Association* 90: 681–688.

Carr, Phyllis L.; Robert H. Friedman; Mark A. Moskowitz; et al. 1993. "Comparing the Status of Women and Men in Academic Medicine." *Annals of Internal Medicine* 119: 908–913.

Donoghue, Glenda G.; Elaine Hoffman; and Diane Magrane. 2000. "Women's Health as a Catalyst for Reform of Medical Education." *Academic Medicine* 75: 1051.

Ely, Robin J., and Debra E. Meyerson. 2000. "Theories of Gender in Organizations: A New Approach to Organizational Analysis and Change." In *Research in Organizational Behavior,* ed. B. Staw and R. Sutton. Greenwich, CT: JAI Press.

Epstein, Ronald M., and Edward M. Hundert. 2002. "Defining and Assessing Professional Competence." *Journal of the American Medical Association* 287: 226–235.

Etzkowitz, Henry; Carol Kemelgor; and Brian Uzzi. 2000. *Athena Unbound: The Advancement of Women in Science and Technology.* Cambridge, Eng.: Cambridge University Press.

Fang, Di; Ernest Moy; Lois Colburn; et al. 2000. "Racial and Ethnic Disparities in Faculty Promotion in Academic Medicine." *Journal of the American Medical Association* 284: 1085–1092.

Fiske, Susan T. 1993. "Controlling Other People: The Impact of Power on Stereotyping." *American Psychologist* 48: 621–628.

Frank, Erica; Donna Brogan; and Melissa Schiffman. 1998. "Prevalence and Correlates of Harassment among U.S. Women Physicians." *Archives of Internal Medicine* 158: 352–358.

Frank, Erica; Michelle Brownstein; Kimberly Ephgrave; et al. 1998. "Characteristics of Women Surgeons in the United States." *American Journal of Surgery* 176: 244–250.

Frank, Erica; Richard Rothenberg; Virgil Brown; et al. 1997. "Basic Demographic and Professional Characteristics of U.S. Women Physicians." *Western Journal of Medicine* 166: 179–184.

Fried, Linda P.; Clair A. Francomano; Susan M. MacDonald; et al. 1996. "Career Development for Women in Academic Medicine: Multiple Interventions in a Department of Medicine." *Journal of the American Medical Association* 276: 898–905.

Geiger, H. Jack. 2001. "Racial Stereotyping and Medicine: The Need for Cultural Competence." *Canadian Medical Association Journal* 164: 1699–1700.

Grady-Weliky; Tana A.; C. Kettyle; and Edward Hundert. 2000. "New Light on Needs in the Mentor-Mentee Relationship." In *Educating for Professionalism: Creating a Culture of Humanism in Medical Education,* ed. Delese Wear and Janet W. Bickel. Iowa City: University of Iowa Press.

Hitchcock, Maurice; Carole J. Bland; Frances P. Hekelman; et al. 1995. "Professional Networks: The Influence of Colleagues on the Academic Success of Faculty." *Academic Medicine* 70: 1108–1116.

Kassebaum, Donald G., and Ellen R. Cutler. 1998. "On the Culture of Student Abuse in Medical School." *Academic Medicine* 73: 1149–1158.

Kimmel, Michael S. 2000. *The Gendered Society.* New York: Oxford University Press.

Kwakwa, F., and Olga Jonasson. 1999. "Attrition in Graduate Surgical Education: An Analysis of the 1993 Entering Cohort of Surgical Residents." *Journal of the American College of Surgeons* 189: 602–610.

Levinson, Wendy, and J. Weiner. 1991. "Promotion and Tenure of Women and Minorities on Medical School Faculty." *Annals of Internal Medicine* 114: 63–68.

Limacher, Marian; Carolyn A. Zaher; Wendy J. Wolf; et al. "The ACC Professional Life Survey: Career Decisions of Women and Men in Cardiology." *Journal of the American College of Cardiology* 32:827–835, 1998.

Lipman-Blumen, Jean. 1996. *The Connective Edge: Leading in an Interdependent World.* San Francisco: Jossey-Bass.

McCorduck, Pamela, and Nancy Ramsey. 1996. *The Futures of Women: Scenarios for the Twenty-First Century.* New York: Warner.

McMurray, Julia E.; Angus, Graham; Cohen, May; et al."Women in Medicine: A Four-Nation Comparison." *Journal of American Medical Women's Association,* 57:185–190,002.

McMurray, Julia E.; Linzer, Mark; Konrad, T. R.; et al. 2000. "The Work Lives of Women Physicians: Results from the Physician Worklife Study." *Journal of General Internal Medicine* 15: 372–380.

Menges, Robert, and Exum, William H. 1983. "Barriers to the Progress of Women and Minority Faculty." *Journal of Higher Education* 54: 123–144.

Morahan, Page, and Bickel, Janet. 2002. "Capitalizing on Women's Intellectual Capital." *Academic Medicine* 77: 110–112.

Morahan, Page; Voytko, Mary Lou; Abbuhl, Stephanie; et al. 2001. "Ensuring Successful Women Faculty to Meet the Needs of Academic Medical Centers." *Academic Medicine* 76: 19–31.

More, Ellen S. 2000. *Restoring the Balance: Women Physicians and the Profession of Medicine, 1850–1995.* Cambridge, MA: Harvard University Press.

Ness, Roberta; Ukoll, Frances; Hunt, Stephen; et al. 2000 "Salary Equity among Male and Female Internists in Pennsylvania." *Annals of Internal Medicine* 133:104–110.

Palepu, Anna; Carr, Phyllis L.; Friedman, Robert H.; et al. 1998. "Minority Faculty and Academic Rank in Medicine." *Journal of the American Medical Association* 280: 767–771.

Potee, Ruth A.; Gerber, Andrew J.; and Ickovics, Jeannette R. 1999. "Medicine and Motherhood: Shifting Trends among Female Physicians from 1922 to 1999." *Academic Medicine* 74: 911–919.

Sandler, Bernice R.; Silverberg, L. A.; and Hall, Roberta M. 1995. *The Chilly Classroom Climate: A Guide to Improve the Education of Women.* Washington, D.C.: National Association for Women in Education.

Schuchert, Michael K. 1998. "The Relationship between Verbal Abuse of Medical Students and Their Confidence in Their Clinical Abilities." *Academic Medicine* 73: 907–909.

Socolar, Rebecca S.; Kelman, Lesley S.; Lannon, Carole M.; et al. 2000. "Institutional Policies of U.S. Medical Schools Regarding Tenure, Promotion, and Benefits for Part-Time Faculty." *Academic Medicine* 75: 846–849.

Thomas, David A. 2001. "The Truth about Mentoring Minorities: Race Matters." *Harvard Business Review* 79: 99–107.

Tong, Rosemarie. 1993. *Feminine and Feminist Ethics.* Belmont, CA: Wadsworth.

Valian, Virginia. 1998. *Why So Slow: The Advancement of Women.* Cambridge, MA: MIT Press.

Wear, Delese, and Janet Bickel. 2000. *Educating for Professionalism: Creating a Culture of Humanism in Medical Education.* Iowa City: University of Iowa Press.

Wenneras, Christine, and Wold, Agnes. 1997. "Nepotism and Sexism in Peer-Review." *Science* 387: 341–343.

Yamagata, Hisashi. 2002. "Data Shot: Medical School Faculty Attrition." *Association of American Medical Colleges Reporter* 11: 1.

Yedidia, Michael, and Bickel, Janet. 2001. "Why Aren't There More Women Leaders in Academic Medicine? The Views of Clinical Chairs." *Academic Medicine* 76: 453–465.

WOMEN AS HEALTH PROFESSIONALS, HISTORICAL ISSUES OF

• • •

Historically, women's roles in healthcare were primarily as caretakers and nurturers; as wives, mothers, and nurses; and in their responsibility for children, the sick, the aged, and the disabled. When instrumental healing roles became more technical and financially lucrative, women met resistance to their assumption of those roles. This attitude often was based on mistrust of their capacities and the departure their work in healthcare represented from their more traditional roles, especially because they might compete with men.

Early History of Women in Healthcare

Women have always been healers as well as caretakers; they have acted as pharmacists, physicians, nurses, herbalists, abortionists, counselors, midwives, and *sagae* or "wise women." They also have been called witches. In the physician role, however, society rarely permitted them to perform in the same capacities and positions as men.

THE ANCIENT WORLD. Early Egyptian steles refer to a chief woman physician, Peseshet, and in 1500 B.C.E. women studied in the Egyptian medical school in Heliopolis. In the Chinese record in 1000 B.C.E. female physicians were in positions that encompassed activities other than traditional midwifery and herb gathering. There also were medical roles for women in the Greek and Roman civilizations. In Rome physicians were often slaves or freed slaves; it is likely that many were women. Women who entered medicine were frequently members of medical families and practiced together with their family members. The physician husband of a second-century woman physician wrote for his wife's epitaph, "You guided straight the rudder of life in our home and raised high our common fame in healing—though you were a woman you were not behind me in skill" (Anderson and Zinsser, p. 61).

Throughout history women have been special attendants to other women, assisting with labor and delivery, providing advice on the functions and disorders of their bodies, and tending newborns. Because childbirth was considered a normal rather than a pathological process, it was not thought to be part of medicine. Soranus of Ephesus, a first-century C.E. physician practicing in Rome, believed that women were divinely appointed to care for sick women and children. Among the criteria he delineated for those practicing medicine, inluding women, were literacy, an understanding of anatomy, a sense of patient responsibility, and ethical concerns, particularly in regard to confidentiality.

During the first few centuries of the spread of Christianity, women ordained as deaconesses by bishops with the consent of the congregation appear to have played a significant role in healthcare. Although little is known about their work, many of those deaconesses became the first parish workers and district nurses (Shryock, 1959). Among those women were Saint Monica, the mother of Saint Augustine, and Fabiola, who founded a hospital at Ostia in Italy in 398 C.E.

After the fall of the Roman Empire, medicine continued along two paths: monastic medicine, which lost touch with older traditions, and Arabic medicine, which developed in Persia and transmitted the heritage of Greek medicine to Europe. Arabic medicine produced notable practitioners and hospitals run by male and female "nurses." During the Crusades women staffed infirmaries and clinics in Jerusalem and along the European routes to the Holy Land.

THE MIDDLE AGES. Medical scholarship flourished in the ninth century at the University of Salerno in Italy and continued to develop through the tenth and eleventh centuries (Corner). At that time women apparently studied medicine at the university. Although little is known about most of those early women physicians, eleventh-century records reveal the existence of Trotula, a woman faculty member at Salerno who is said to have written important texts on obstetrics and gynecology and to have headed a department of women's diseases. Her most important work, *De Passionibus Mulierum,* remained the major reference on that subject for several centuries. The authorship of this and other works was attributed to her husband or to other male colleagues (Corner; Achterberg). Trotula suggested that infertility could be attributed to the male as well as the female. In cooperation with the "Ladies of Salerno," a group of women physicians, Trotula established the first center of medicine that was not under Church control.

The M.D. degree was first awarded in 1180, apparently only to men. One of the notable figures of the twelfth century was Hildegard of Bingen, a scientific scholar, abbess, writer, composer, and political adviser to kings and to the pope. She wrote two medical textbooks, *Liber Simplicis Medicinae* and *Liber Compositae Medicinae,* presumably for use by the nurses who were in charge of the infirmaries at Benedictine monasteries. Her textbooks described a number of diseases, including their courses, symptoms, and treatment, as well as scientific data on the pulsation of blood and the regulation of vital activities by the nervous system. Hildegard's writings also demonstrated an understanding of normal and abnormal psychology.

In the medieval period affluent women were active in medicine, particularly in Italy, where the universities were accessible to them. In 1390 Dorotea Bocchi earned a degree in medicine from the University of Bologna and followed her father as a lecturer in medicine at that university. In 1423 Constanza Calenda, the daughter of the dean of the medical faculty at Salerno, lectured on medicine at the university in Naples. Women also were qualified and permitted to practice medicine in France, England, and Germany. They generally were limited in practice to specifically defined roles, including bleeding, administering herbs and medicines, and reducing fractures, as well as practicing midwifery. As early as 1292, however, women in Paris worked as "barber surgeons," practicing what was known of surgery. Until 1694 widows automatically were allowed to continue practicing if their specific form of medicine had been their husbands' field.

From the thirteenth to the seventeenth centuries the number of physicians was low, and the role of women healers was particularly important in meeting the healthcare needs of the population. During that period women practiced as physicians, surgeons, bone setters, eye healers, and midwives. It generally was believed that women were better suited for the treatment of women's diseases.

During the fifteenth century women obtained higher degrees by presenting medical theses, and during the fifteenth century and the early part of the sixteenth century women began to excel in innovative techniques and made important contributions to medicine. They served kings, royal families, and even armies in Europe.

Although it is assumed that the number of women in medicine was small, their healthcare work in the Middle Ages caused enough concern that by 1220 the University of Paris succeeded in preventing them from gaining admission to medical school. In 1485 Charles VIII of France decreed that women could not work as surgeons.

By the fourteenth century the licensing of physicians was well established, although women rarely were allowed to sit for licensing examinations. In 1322 university-trained male physicians brought a suit against Jacoba Felicie de

Almania in France, claiming that in practicing without appropriate training and licensing, she endangered patients. Patients testified to her skill; Jacoba argued that she was both physician and nurse to her patients. She also emphasized that many women would not seek treatment for their illnesses if they had to see a male physician. Because she did not have the correct university degree, she not only was barred from medicine but also was excommunicated from the Church. Women who practiced outside their licensed specialities, for example, midwives who functioned as physicians, also were condemned.

THE RENAISSANCE AND AFTERWARD. By the end of the fifteenth century, as medicine became an academic discipline and a more established profession in several centers in Europe, the movement to exclude women from the formal practice of medicine gained momentum. That movement coincided with the ideology of misogyny as it was articulated by Heinrich Kraemer and James Sprenger in *The Malleus Maleficarum* (1486), a treatise on identifying and dealing with witches. Witch-hunting capitalized on the widespread belief in the spiritual and mental inferiority of women, a belief that was fueled by the Church. Even when active witch-hunts subsided, their effects remained. Women were effectively eliminated from performing medical roles other than traditional caretaking and midwifery.

Before the sixteenth century it was not possible for a man to be a midwife; it was a capital offense in some places. As medicine and surgery were differentiated from each other in the fifteenth and sixteenth centuries, some male barber surgeons began to practice midwifery. By the late fifteenth century licensing examinations were given, generally by a doctor and a midwife. Increasingly, concern was expressed by physicians and the laity about whether midwives were knowledgeable enough to recognize when it was appropriate to call for a consultation with male physicians and surgeons.

The sixteenth to eighteenth centuries produced several outstanding female midwives, including Louyse Bourgeois, who in 1609 became the first midwife to publish a work on obstetrics, a book that became the basic text for midwifery in Europe. Nonetheless, with the invention of the obstetrical forceps in the seventeenth century by the Chamberlens, a family of male midwives and barber surgeons, obstetrics was pushed closer to the realm of the male practitioner. In 1634 Peter Chamberlen III attempted to establish a corporation of midwives in England with himself as the governor, a move that was resented by female midwives. Increasingly, men began to participate and compete in that profession, particularly in serving the upper classes. By the eighteenth century men controlled all areas of medicine except midwifery and

nursing, and even in those areas women increasingly were required to practice only under male supervision.

By the beginning of the seventeenth century women were denied access to medical training and then prohibited from belonging to professional associations. University training was required, and women were not admitted to universities. Despite exclusion from formal training and practice, women continued to provide for the healthcare needs of family members and others in the community, especially the poor, who had no other access to healthcare.

Women in Early American Medicine

In colonial North America the healing role of women was critical to survival, and many women assumed medical roles. Ann Hutchinson, the early seventeenth-century dissident religious leader, worked as a general practitioner and midwife. Because there were relatively few university-trained physicians and no medical schools in the colonies, medicine was practiced by those who appeared to be particularly talented, and an apprenticeship system began to evolve. Two women listed as physicians in Boston in the seventeenth century later were denounced as witches, and no other woman practiced medicine in Boston until Harriot Hunt, after apprenticeship training, opened a medical office in 1835.

Eighteenth-century American medicine had no unified concept of medical care; a variety of views of practice and training offered various programs of study and concepts of healing. In that setting the role of women was extensive and complex because the medical care of families was frequently the responsibility of women.

Most women practitioners were midwives. Many went to Europe to train, as the first school for midwives in the English colonies was not started until 1762. The early training of midwives was based on the assumption that most obstetrical practice would remain in the hands of women. This did not occur in colonial North America, although it was the case in many parts of Europe.

In 1765 John Morgan founded the first university-connected, so-called regular American medical school at the University of Pennsylvania. Its formal, scientifically based curriculum departed from the almost exclusive apprenticeship training that existed in the colonies and was more reflective of European standards of that time. By excluding women, it began a tradition of barring them from formal medical training and forcing them into "irregular" training. Many women without diplomas, however, set up flourishing practices. They were trained in the homeopathic, eclectic, or "irregular" traditions, which tended to be less prestigious.

Women in Nineteenth-Century Medicine

In 1847 Elizabeth Blackwell became the first woman to be admitted to a "regular" medical school in the United States; she graduated first in her class at Geneva (New York) Medical School in 1849. The New York State Medical Association promptly censured the school, and when her sister, Emily Blackwell, applied a few years later, she was rejected. Emily subsequently received an M.D. from Western Reserve Medical College in Cleveland after her acceptance to Rush Medical College in Chicago had been rescinded in response to pressure from the state medical society.

Ann Preston began her medical studies in 1847 as an apprentice to a Quaker physician. After two years she applied to and was rejected by four medical schools. In 1850 she established the first regular women's medical college in the world, the Women's Medical College of Pennsylvania. She and her students recalled their experiences at the Pennsylvania Hospital: "We entered in a body, amidst jeerings, groaning, whistlings, and stamping of feet by the men students. On leaving the hospital, we were actually stoned by those so-called gentlemen" (Alsop, pp. 54–55). This account was corroborated by the *Evening Bulletin* of Philadelphia.

In 1847 Harriot K. Hunt, who earlier had established an irregular practice in Boston despite her lack of an M.D. degree, applied to Harvard Medical School. Although supported by the dean, Oliver Wendell Holmes, she was rejected for admission. After hearing about Elizabeth Blackwell's acceptance, she again applied for admission and was accepted. However, she was denied a seat when the all-male class threatened to leave if women or blacks were admitted. Not until almost a hundred years later, in 1946, did Harvard Medical School begin to admit women.

By 1850 two additional all-female medical colleges were founded, one in Boston and one in Cincinnati. Both were "irregular" schools. The Boston Female Medical College was designed primarily to prevent male midwifery, which its founder, Dr. Samuel Gregory, felt trespassed on female delicacy. The school was founded in 1848 and offered a medical degree by 1853, but it was always financially troubled and did not have a good reputation. In 1856 it changed its name to the New England Female Medical College and began to recruit new faculty members, including Marie Zakrzewska, who helped develop a pioneering clinical training program. In 1873 the school merged with Boston University.

In 1855 the National Eclectic Medical Association formally approved the education of women in medicine, and in 1870 it became the first medical society to accept women as members. Traditional medical societies, however, continued to be closed to women. In his 1871 American Medical Association (AMA) presidential address Alfred Stille criticized female physicians for being women who seek to rival men, who "aim toward a higher type than their own" (Ehrenreich and English, p. 26). Negative attitudes toward the presence of women in medicine appeared to be supported by accumulating "scientific" evidence that supposedly supported the inferior status of women on biological grounds, including the idea that their brain capacity was less than men's. A book published in 1873 by Edward Hammond Clarke fueled the controversy: In *Sex in Education: or, A Fair Chance for the Girls* he stated, "Higher education for women produces monstrous brains and puny bodies" (Clarke, p. 41). It echoed Charles Meigs's 1847 statement, "She [woman] has a head almost too small for the intellect but just big enough for love."

The debate about women's intellectual capacity induced Harvard Medical School to offer the Boylston Medical Prize in 1874 for the best paper on the topic "Do women require mental and bodily rest during menstruation and to what extent?" The winning research was submitted by Mary Putnam Jacobi. When the judges discovered the sex of the author, they hesitated about awarding the prize but finally did so (Walsh). Putnam Jacobi had found, contrary to prevailing views, that the majority of women in her sample did not suffer incapacity. Her study was followed by several others, all with similar findings. Despite such work and evidence, the barriers to women did not fall.

Even women who managed to obtain medical training were refused admittance to medical societies, and hospitals denied them appointments. Female physicians in the United States began to open their own hospitals and clinics. In 1857 Elizabeth and Emily Blackwell founded the New York Infirmary for Women, where they cared largely for indigent women, and in 1865 the Women's Medical College of the New York Infirmary opened. Paternalistic attitudes coupled with the difficulty women had in obtaining hospital privileges led Marie Zakrzewska in 1862 to found the New England Hospital for Women, owned and operated entirely by women.

The role of women in medicine, including the productivity and lifestyle of female physicians, continued to be debated vigorously. In 1881 Rachel Bodley, dean of the Women's Medical College of Pennsylvania, surveyed the 244 living graduates of the school and found that despite persistent beliefs to the contrary, the overwhelming majority were in active practice. Those who had married reported that their profession had had no adverse effect on their marriages and that marriage had not interfered with their work.

By the end of the nineteenth century women physicians were being accepted into many medical societies. The Massachusetts Medical Society admitted women in 1884, and the AMA seated a woman delegate in 1876 but did not accept women formally until 1915 (Morantz-Sanchez, 1985). Women physicians began to form their own associations. There were several attempts to build a national organization of women physicians, beginning in 1867. The *Women's Medical Journal* was started in 1872. In 1915 the National Women's Medical Association was founded. It was renamed the American Medical Women's Association (AMWA) in 1919 and was condemned by many male physicians. To alleviate people's fears the AMWA required that its members also join the AMA, and it held its meetings together with that organization.

Female separatism was a double-edged sword. Although it gave women a special place in the care of women and children, it also was used to exclude women from more extensive roles in medical education and from the increasing influence and prestige of the profession.

Financial contributions from women philanthropists (such as M. Carey Thomas, Mary Elizabeth Garrett, Mary Gwinn, and Elizabeth King) forced the Johns Hopkins Medical School in 1889 to accept women on the same terms that it used for accepting men. However, this did not result in large numbers of women being admitted and did not appear to increase the number of appointments of women to faculty and leadership positions (Walsh).

Following Johns Hopkins's lead, however, 75 percent of other, already existing medical schools began to accept women as students. By 1894 over 66 percent of women medical students were enrolled in regular medical schools (Walsh). The student body at Tufts Medical School was 42 percent female. Women also received a disproportionate number of the academic honors in their graduating classes.

Women Physicians in Europe and Canada

In 1859 the American Elizabeth Blackwell was placed on the British Medical Register; in the following year the British Medical Association ruled that persons with foreign medical degrees could not practice in Great Britain. In 1865 Elizabeth Garrett Anderson became the first woman to qualify to practice medicine in that country. She did that by passing the apothecaries' examination; the regulations of that guild did not exclude women. The rules were changed shortly afterward. In France, although women were allowed to study at the Faculty of Medicine in Paris, they could not become interns and thus could not complete their training.

The Royal College of Physicians in Edinburgh attempted to exclude Sophia Jex-Blake in 1869 by stating that a single woman could not attend medical school. Jex-Blake organized a group of seven women, and together they completed the first year of training. Attacks on female students from male peers, however, prompted some public support from people who were outraged that these "indelicate and ungentlemanly" men would be seeing female patients. Four years later the university won a lawsuit allowing it to refuse to grant degrees to women. Women in other European countries also experienced hostile and even violent attacks by their male peers.

The first continental European university to accept women was the University of Zurich in 1865. By the 1870s other Swiss universities had followed its lead. In Russia women were allowed to attend medical schools in 1872, partly because a number of Russian women already had studied medicine in Zurich. Negative attitudes toward women were fueled by the assassination of Czar Alexander II by a woman. After that event, from 1881 through 1905, universities in Russia were closed to women.

Many of the women who graduated from medical schools in those countries were from middle-class or upper-class backgrounds. Often they had fathers or other family members in medicine; they entered the profession to join the family practice.

The first woman doctor to practice medicine in Canada, James Barry, a graduate of the University of Edinburgh, was a British Army medical officer who became inspector general of hospitals in Canada in 1857. She was able to practice because she was thought to be a man. After her death Dr. Barry was discovered to have been a woman (Hacker).

Nineteenth-Century Midwifery

There was considerable opposition to the practice of midwifery by women in the mid-nineteenth century, particularly in the United States. In 1820 John Ware, a Boston physician, is said to have written *Remarks on the Employment of Females as Practitioners of Midwifery,* in which he raised objections that were based on his view of women's moral qualities. He stated: "Where the responsibility in scenes of distress and danger does not fall upon them when there is someone on whom they can lean, in whose skill and judgement they have entire confidence, they retain their collection and presence of mind; but where they become the principal agents, the feelings of sympathy are too powerful for the cool exercise of judgment" (p. 7).

In addition, economic and class issues played a role in women's exclusion from medicine. Midwives came primarily from working-class, rural, and poor backgrounds. They charged less than physicians did for their services and were more likely to care for the poor. With the beginning of obstetrics as a medical discipline, physicians feared economic competition from midwives.

Some physicians objected to midwives on the basis of the allegedly lower quality of healthcare they provided. However, in the 1840s two physicians, Oliver Wendell Holmes and Ignaz Semmelweiss, reported on the spread of puerperal sepsis (childbirth infection). Semmelweiss found that there was a lower incidence of it in women who were assisted in delivery by midwives. He deduced that because medical students and physicians did not wash their hands when they moved from the autopsy room to the delivery room, they spread disease. The warnings of both doctors were ignored by most of the medical profession, and controversy continued about the adequacy of midwives.

By the turn of the twentieth century about 50 percent of all babies in the United States were delivered by midwives. Midwives were held responsible for childbirth illness and puerperal sepsis, as well as neonatal ophthalmia (inflammation of the eyes generally related to maternal gonorrhea), because it was believed by many people, especially in the medical profession, that they were not sufficiently trained to prevent those illnesses. Under mounting pressure, many states began to pass laws forbidding midwifery, many of which remain in effect.

Evolution of Nursing in the Nineteenth Century

The practice of nursing was sponsored primarily by the Church until the mid-eighteenth century, when the London Infirmary appointed a lay nurse. Nursing was seen as a low-status occupation; records show long working hours and low pay. Dickens's novel *Martin Chuzzlewit* (1844) focused attention on the quality of the nursing care given by pardoned criminals, aging prostitutes, and other women of questionable morality and interest who functioned as nurses.

At the time of the Crimean War Florence Nightingale responded to the need for nursing reform and established military and then civilian nursing. In 1860 she founded a school for nurses in London that had a rigorous curriculum and specific guidelines for nursing as a profession. She met opposition from the medical profession, many of whose members felt that "nurses are in much the same position as housemaids and need little teaching beyond poultice-making and the enforcement of cleanliness and attention to the patient's wants" (Dolan, p. 230).

The first nursing schools recruited upper-class women who were "refugees from the enforced leisure of Victorian ladyhood" (Ehrenreich and English, p. 34). Despite their aristocratic image, nursing schools began to attract more women from working-class and lower-middle-class homes. Those advocating the nursing profession saw the nurse as the embodiment of Victorian femininity and nursing as a natural vocation for women, second only to motherhood. Nightingale viewed women as instinctive nurses, not physicians: "They have only tried to be men, and they have succeeded only in being third-rate men" (Ehrenreich and English, p. 36).

Women in Twentieth-Century Medicine

By the beginning of the twentieth century women were seeking admission to medical schools in increasing numbers. Because of an oversupply of physicians, however, salaries and prestige were diminishing. Some people blamed the situation on the "feminization" of the profession, and many schools began to decrease the number of women they accepted. Women also had more difficulty obtaining internships and residencies. Because all but one of the female institutions (the Women's Medical College of Pennsylvania) had consolidated or closed, many women had nowhere to train.

The conviction that women were not able to perform effectively as physicians and the belief that women would be damaged by pursuing a difficult career intensified. Women physicians seemed to be unable to develop a consolidated and effective strategy to resist that negative attitude. In 1905 Dr. F. W. Van Dyke, the president of the Oregon State Medical Society, stated, "Hard study killed sexual desire in women, took away their beauty, brought on hysteria, neurasthenia, dyspepsia, astigmatism and dysmenorrhea. Educated women could not bear children with ease because study arrested the development of the pelvis at the same time it increased the size of the child's brain and therefore its head. This caused extensive suffering in childbirth" (Bullough and Voght, pp. 74–75).

At that time academic medical schools were developing formal medical curricula. Proprietary medical schools also were increasing in number. The education they provided was focused primarily on an apprenticeship model, and there was little monitoring of the quality of the education. Because of the oversupply of doctors produced by those two systems, with consequent competition for patients as well as a lack of mechanisms to assess quality and monitor performance, the AMA asked the Carnegie Foundation to investigate the condition of medicine and make recommendations for dealing with the situation. The foundation commissioned Abraham Flexner, a schoolteacher with no medical expertise, to perform the study. In his 1910 report Flexner stated: "Medical education is now, in the United States and Canada, open to women upon practically the same terms as men. If all institutions do not receive women, so many do, that no woman desiring an education in medicine is under any disability in finding a school to which she may gain admittance. Now that women are freely admitted to the medical profession, it is clear that they show a decreasing inclination to enter it" (Flexner, pp. 178–179, 296).

Flexner's report concluded that medical education required higher standards for training and provided an important impetus for establishing medicine as an academic discipline. It resulted in the closing of many medical schools, especially the proprietary ones; unfortunately, because women continued to have difficulty gaining admission to many of the university-affiliated and more prestigious medical schools, the schools that were closed were the ones that traditionally had admitted substantial numbers of women and members of minority groups. This had the effect of lowering the numbers of women physicians in the United States.

Women physicians gained some status as a result of their patriotism during World War I, when the AMWA campaigned to have women physicians commissioned on the same basis as men. Although that effort was rejected by the government, the AMWA urged women physicians to contribute to the war effort. Fifty-five women physicians practiced medicine by signing specific contracts with the military. They received neither military status nor benefits (Walsh). At Johns Hopkins the percentage of women medical students dropped from 33 percent in 1896 to 10 percent in 1916. At the University of Michigan the percentage of women medical students dropped from 25 percent in 1890 to 3 percent in 1910 (Walsh).

The number of female physicians in the United States continued to be low until the 1970s. Other countries continued to report greater percentages of female physicians. In 1965, for example, women accounted for 7 percent of all U.S. physicians. The Soviet Union reported 65 percent female physicians; Poland, 30 percent; the Philippines, 25 percent; the German Federal Republic, 20 percent; Italy, 19 percent; the United Kingdom and Denmark, 16 percent; and Japan, 9 percent (Lopate).

Medicine was viewed as a male profession in the United States more than it was in most other countries. Some scholars hypothesize that this occurred because medicine had higher prestige and income than did many other professions and therefore interested men more. Others believe that the dominance of men adds prestige and that men demand better compensation. The reasons for the gender stereotyping of professions, however, is complex and has cultural as well as political determinants. Many areas of work are sex-role-stereotyped. This occurs because of the perception that men or women are better at certain functions. For example, in the United States women were considered to be more suited to caretaking roles and men were considered to be better in more instrumental and technological activities. Thus, although medicine presents a melding of these stereotypes, women were not considered capable of performing in the increasingly technological aspects of the field. Even in a revolutionary society such as Cuba, where these stereotypes are disparaged, there is a persistence of traditional roles for women in healthcare; 30 to 40 percent of Cuban physicians are women, but virtually all nurses and midwives are women.

In the United States the choice of a specialty and the specific positions held by women in their fields of expertise reveal a pattern that has held since women began to be admitted to medical schools. In the 1970s the fact that women would assume primary care roles was used as an argument for increasing their numbers in medical schools. This has proved to be correct. Women characteristically have entered primary care fields including pediatrics, internal medicine, family practice, and obstetrics and gynecology, as well as psychiatry, pathology, and some medical subspecialties. There has been more diversification in the choice of medical specialties for women in recent years, but the numbers in the higher-paid technically oriented surgical fields continue to be low. (Accreditation Council on Graduate Medical Education).

In the United States and other countries academic and administrative appointments as well as other decision-making positions are held almost exclusively by men, whereas the majority of women physicians tend to be involved in direct patient care. Women continue to constitute almost 30 percent of full-time medical school faculty, but they are concentrated in the lower academic ranks and do not advance at the same rate as do their male colleagues (Bickel).

In countries where women have made significant progress in terms of their influence in the healthcare fields changes have occurred most often in times of war, physician shortages, or major cultural reorganization. In Russia midwives proved to be effective as doctors in the Russo-Turkish War of 1870, beginning the influx of women into medical schools. However, after the 1917 revolution, as the prestige of medicine declined, women were admitted in greater numbers. By 1940, 62 percent of Soviet physicians were women, and by 1970, that number had risen to 72 percent. As in the United States and other countries, however, Russian women held a disproportionately small number of senior positions. The *feldschers* (semiprofessional health workers) in the Soviet Union were primarily women.

The rise of female health professionals in China occurred along with the reorganization of the medical-care system and of Chinese society under the People's Republic after 1949. About half of Chinese physicians were women. In the countryside "barefoot doctors" (peasants, primarily women, with basic medical training) provided medical care without leaving their regular work to meet the needs of fellow workers (Sidel and Sidel).

Women's Evolving Role in Healthcare

The blurring of roles and the overlapping of areas of function in a healthcare have raised important questions about roles and responsibilities, for example, among primary care physicians, physician's assistants, and nurse practitioners as well as among psychologists, psychiatrists, psychiatric social workers, and psychiatric nurses. In the United States economic factors rather than specific expertise, experience, or skills have become important determinants of decisions about which practitioners will provide care. Less well trained practitioners may be favored by payers because their services are less costly. Many of these healthcare providers are women. There are few objective guidelines for determining the scope of practice. For example, in providing routine physical examinations, obstetrical care, anesthesia, psychotherapy, and minor medical and surgical procedures, professionals of varied backgrounds and training may provide similar services. There are insufficient data assessing the outcomes of this practice.

Since 1945 there has been more regulation of medical practice in the United States, and healthcare increasingly has been paid for or subsidized by governments and/or private insurance companies. Health maintenance organizations and other managed-care models have evolved. With this has come a diminution in physicians' authority and, more recently, income. At the same time there have been fewer white men applying to medical school and more women and minority group members; as a result, almost 50 percent of medical students are women and increasing numbers are from minority groups (Lorber).

The demands of work and family life as well as the nature of the process of attaining medical leadership positions continue to result in the presence of few women in major healthcare policy decision-making positions. As a result, less has changed and women have had less of an impact on practice, research, and education in medicine than was predicted in the 1970s, when the demographic shift began. There has been evidence of some changes in practice with the increase in the number of women physicians; for example, some preventive tests are more likely to be performed depending on the sex of the patient and the

physician, and there are differences in practice styles related to gender. Most of the changes in the practice patterns of physicians appear to be related more to economics and political factors than to gender. However, the development of a focus on women's health and an emphasis on gender biology, including an expansion of research in this area, have been fueled largely by women physicians and scientists and by the women's movement, beginning in the 1960s. This has been important for women's health and represents a substantial contribution by women to medicine.

CAROL C. NADELSON
MALKAH T. NOTMAN (1995)
REVISED BY AUTHORS

SEE ALSO: *Alternative Therapies: Social History; Care; Feminism; Medical Education; Nursing, Profession of; Paternalism; Sexism*

BIBLIOGRAPHY

Abram, Ruth J., ed. 1985. *"Send Us a Lady Physician": Women Doctors in America, 1835–1920.* New York: W. W. Norton.

Accreditation Council on Graduate Medical Education. 2002. "Graduate Medical Education." *Journal of the American Medical Association* 288: 9.

Achterberg, Jeanne. 1990. *Woman as Healer.* Boston: Shambhala.

Alsop, Gulielma Fell. 1950. *History of the Woman's Medical College, Philadelphia, Pennsylvania, 1850–1950.* Philadelphia: Lippincott.

Anderson, Bonnie S., and Zinsser, Judith P. 1988. *A History of Their Own: Women in Europe from Prehistory to the Present.* New York: Harper & Row.

Apple, Rima D., ed. 1990. *Women, Health, and Medicine in America: A Historical Handbook.* New York: Garland.

Bickel, Janet. 2000. "Women in Academic Medicine." *Journal of the American Medical Women's Association* 55(1).

Bonner, Thomas N. 1992. *To the Ends of the Earth: Women's Search for Education in Medicine.* Cambridge, MA: Harvard University Press.

Bullough, Vern, and Voght, Martha. 1973. "Women, Menstruation and Nineteenth-Century Medicine." *Bulletin of the History of Medicine* 47(1): 66–82.

Calder, Jean McKinlay. 1963. *The Story of Nursing,* 4th rev. edition. London: Methuen.

Clarke, Edward Hammond. 1873. *Sex in Education: or, A Fair Chance for the Girls.* Boston: J. R. Osgood.

Corner, George W. 1937. "The Rise of Medicine at Salerno in the Twelfth Century." In *Lectures on the History of Medicine: A Series of Lectures at the Mayo Foundation and the Universities of Minnesota, Wisconsin, Iowa, Northwestern and the Des Moines Academy of Medicine, 1926–1932,* pp. 371–399. Philadelphia: Saunders.

Cutter, Irving S., and Viets, Henry R. 1964 (1933). *A Short History of Midwifery.* Philadelphia: Saunders.

Dally, Ann G. 1991. *Women under the Knife: A History of Surgery.* New York: Routledge.

Dolan, Josephine A. 1963. *Goodnow's History of Nursing,* 11th edition. Philadelphia: Saunders.

Drachman, Virginia G. 1984. *Hospital with a Heart: Women Doctors and the Paradox of Separatism at the New England Hospital, 1862–1969.* Ithaca, NY: Cornell University Press.

Ehrenreich, Barbara, and English, Deirdre. 1967. *Witches, Midwives, and Nurses: A History of Women Healers,* 2nd edition. Glass Mountain Pamphlet no. 1. Old Westbury, NY: Feminist Press.

Flexner, Abraham. 1972 (1910). "Medical Education in the United States and Canada: A Report to the Carnegie Foundation for the Advancement of Teaching." *Bulletin of the Carnegie Foundation for the Advancement of Teaching,* no. 4. New York: Arno.

Hacker, Carlotta. 1974. *The Indomitable Lady Doctors.* Toronto: Clarke, Irwin.

Hume, Ruth Fox. 1964. *Great Women of Medicine.* New York: Random House.

Leavitt, Judith Walzer, ed. 1984. *Women and Health in America: Historical Readings.* Madison: University of Wisconsin Press.

Lederman, Muriel, and Bartsch, Ingrid. 2001. *The Gender and Science Reader.* London: Routledge.

Lopate, Carol. 1968. *Women in Medicine.* Baltimore: Johns Hopkins University Press.

Lorber, Judith. 1984. *Women Physicians: Careers, Status, and Power.* New York: Tavistock, 2000.

Lorber, Judith. 2000. "What Impact Have Women Physicians Had on Women's Health?" *Journal of the American Medical Women's Association* 55(1).

Marks, Geoffrey, and Beatty, William K. 1972. *Women in White.* New York: Charles Scribner.

McGrayne, Sharon Bertsch. 1998. *Nobel Prize Women in Science.* Secausus, NJ: Citadel Press, Carol Publishing Group.

McPherson, Mary Patterson. 1981. "'On the Same Terms Precisely': The Women's Medical Fund and the Johns Hopkins School of Medicine." *Journal of the American Medical Women's Association* 36(2): 37–40.

Mead, Kate Campbell Hurd. 1938. *A History of Women in Medicine: From the Earliest Times to the Beginning of the Nineteenth Century.* Haddam, CT: Haddam Press.

Morantz-Sanchez, Regina M. 1982. "Introduction: From Art to Science: Women Physicians in American Medicine, 1600–1980." In *In Her Own Words: Oral Histories of Women Physicians,* ed. Regina M. Sanchez-Morantz, Cynthia S. Pomerleau, and Carol H. Fenichel. New Haven, CT: Yale University Press.

Morantz-Sanchez, Regina M. 1985. *Sympathy and Science: Women Physicians in American Medicine.* New York: Oxford University Press.

More, Ellen S. 1999. *Resorting the Balance—Women Physicians and the Profession of Medicine, 1850–1995.* Cambridge, MA: Harvard University Press.

Nadelson, Carol C. 1983. "The Woman Physician: Past, Present, and Future." In *The Physician: A Professional Under Stress,* ed. John P. Callan. Norwalk, CT: Appleton-Century-Crofts.

Nadelson, Carol C. 1989. "Professional Issues for Women." *Psychiatric Clinics of North America* 3(1): 25–33.

Nadelson, Carol C., and Notman, Malkah T. 1972. "The Woman Physician." *Journal of Medical Education* 47(3): 176–183.

Notman, Malkah T., and Nadelson, Carol C. 1973. "Medicine: A Career Conflict for Women." *American Journal of Psychiatry* 130(10): 1123–1127.

Piradova, M. D. 1976. "USSR—Women Health Workers." *Women and Health* 1(3): 24–29.

Rosenberg, Charles E. 1987. *The Care of Strangers: The Rise of America's Hospital System.* New York: Basic Books.

Schiebinger, Londa. 1999. *Has Feminism Changed Science?* Cambridge, MA: Harvard University Press.

Schulman, Sam. 1958. "Basic Functional Roles in Nursing: Mother Surrogate and Healer." In *Patients, Physicians and Illness: A Sourcebook in Behavioral Science and Medicine,* ed. E. Gartly Jaco. New York: Free Press.

Selby, Cecily Canan, ed. 1999. *Women in Science and Engineering—Choices for Success.* New York: Academy of Science.

Shryock, Richard H. 1959. *The History of Nursing: An Interpretation of the Social and Medical Factors Involved.* Philadelphia: Saunders.

Shryock, Richard H. 1966. "Women in American Medicine." In *Medicine in America: Historical Essays,* ed. Richard H. Shryock. Baltimore: Johns Hopkins University Press.

Sidel, Victor W., and Sidel, Ruth. 1973. *Serve the People: Observations on Medicine in the People's Republic of China.* New York: Josiah Macy, Jr., Foundation.

Sonnert, Gerhard, and Holton, Gerald. 1995. *Who Succeeds in Science? The Gender Dimension.* Rutgers, NJ: Rutgers University Press.

Valian, Virginia. 1998. *Why So Slow?* Cambridge, MA: MIT Press.

Walsh, Mary Roth. 1977. *"Doctors Wanted: No Women Need Apply": Sexual Barriers in the Medical Profession, 1835–1975.* New Haven, CT: Yale University Press.

Ware, John. 1820. *Remarks on the Employment of Females as Practitioners in Midwifery.* American Imprints, no. 4171. Boston: Cummings & Hilliard; also ascribed to Walter Channing.

Wasserman, Elga. 2000. *The Door in the Dream.* Washington, D.C.: Joseph Henry Press.

Wells, Susan. 2001. *Out of the Dead House: 19th Century Women Physicians and the Working of Medicine.* Madison: University of Wisconsin Press.

Zuckerman, Harriet; Cole, Jonathan; and Bruer, John. 1991. *The Outer Circle.* New York: Norton.

WOMEN, HISTORICAL AND CROSS-CULTURAL PERSPECTIVES

• • •

A central problem of women's history is that women have been defined by men using concepts and terms based on men's experiences. Such androcentric thought pervades all domains of knowledge. Scholarship in women's studies, developed largely since the late 1960s across a broad range of disciplines, shows that attitudes, customs, laws, and institutions affecting women are grounded in religious and functionalist perspectives according to which "woman" is said to have been created from and after man; has been identified with her sexuality and defined by her sexual function; and has been confined to roles and relationships that are extensions of her reproductive capacity. Alongside this history stands a centuries-old feminist critique that challenges as self-serving and often misogynist the assumptions and intentions of the religions, philosophies, sciences, and familial and political institutions that have shaped the experiences of women in most eras and cultures. Moreover, both the definition of women and its critique reflect a Eurocentric bias that today is the subject of much criticism. This entry summarizes the scholarship produced since the mid-1970s by historians of women, reflecting their collective efforts to compensate for ahistorical assumptions and to constitute a written record both more inclusive of the experiences of women and more open to differences of perspective. It assumes that the history of women requires consideration of moral and ethical as well as social, economic, and political issues.

Women Defined

From ancient times it has been customary to define "woman," in relationship to man, as a limited and contingent part of a dimorphic species. Western cultures have placed heavy constraints on female lives, sometimes justifying these constraints by attributing to women, such as Pandora and Eve, responsibility for human misfortunes resulting from their allegedly weaker self-control or greater lasciviousness. Despite the existence of exceptional women in myth and history, most women in most historical societies have been confined to positions of dependency. Ultimately, whether on the basis of their capacity for pregnancy and resulting physical vulnerability or the use of women's fertility in forging relationships of social and economic value, women, like children, have been denied an independent voice. Seen as "lesser men" by the fathers of Western philosophy, women have been viewed as "Other," as not-man, through a discourse in which human being was embodied in the male sex (Beauvoir).

Deprived of political power and identified with sexual temptation, women have been subject to myriad laws and customs that have at once prescribed and enforced their secondary status. Men have termed women "the sex"; defined them primarily in terms of their sexuality; and, as masters of family and public power, created and staffed the institutions that control female sexuality. In the early fifteenth century, the Italian-born French author Christine de Pizan (1364–ca. 1430) challenged the prevailing androcentric definition of her sex, declaring that the evil attributed to women by learned men existed in men's minds and that, if permitted education, women would become as virtuous and capable as men.

Resistance and rebellion by individual women have a long history; and organized protest, termed *feminism* only since the 1890s, is traceable through a history that is continuous for at least two centuries. However, the condition of women has only occasionally been viewed as a general problem of social justice. The *woman question,* as it was phrased in the nineteenth century, was debated as a political, social, and economic, but rarely as a moral issue; women's rights and responsibilities were discussed as matters of expediency. In the great democratic revolutions of the late eighteenth century, the "inalienable rights of man" were not extended to women. Men, as heads of traditional patriarchal families, continued to speak for their dependents, women as well as children. While some Enlightenment philosophers, most notably Theodore von Hippel (1741–1796), had admitted the abstract equality of all human beings, and others, such as the Marquis de Condorcet (1743–1794), advocated women's accession to equal education and to full civic rights, social arrangements nevertheless made it expedient to ignore their claims. Ultimately, most efforts to improve women's status and condition have been justified on grounds of expediency: if women vote, said the suffragists of 1915, war would be less likely; if mothers earned fathers' wages, said the feminists of 1985, fewer children would live in poverty.

Most matters related to women, then, whether intellectual constructs or social institutions, whether constraining or enlarging women's options, whether produced by misogynists or feminists, have rested on utilitarian grounds. Woman, first of all as an individual human being, was rarely the subject of thought or decision; woman as wife and mother or potential mother has been the ideal type. Even for suffragist leaders of the nineteenth and twentieth centuries, the resort to arguments of expediency over considerations of justice or ethics has itself been an expedient (Kraditor). By the 1990s, however, following two decades of reexamination of all domains of knowledge by scholars in women's studies, feminist theorists began to challenge arguments based on expediency (while sometimes using them as well) and to demand a voice in the discourse through which both knowledge and social institutions are established. Noting injustice in the treatment of women, and the absence of concern about women at the center of most modern and contemporary philosophical systems, they criticize ethical theory itself as a hegemonic expression of the values of a dominant class or gender (Walker).

It is simpler, and historically has been more effective, to argue the needs of women in terms of their differences from men—their needs as wives and mothers, their concerns with nurturant values, their familial and social responsibilities. Women often do speak "in a different voice," reflecting different moral concerns and material circumstances (Gilligan). Women have been and remain deeply divided over their own definition of self: as individuals entitled to, and now demanding, equality of treatment with men; or as persons with gender-specific differences and resulting relationships with families, friends, and communities to whom they bear responsibilities that limit individual autonomy and rights. "Equal rights feminists" have been challenged for basing their claims on an abstract concept of personhood that denies female specificity. Rather than buttressing the claims of individualism based in nineteenth-century liberal philosophy (Fox-Genovese; Pateman), they should, according to this view, emphasize the need for men as well as women to acknowledge their dependence on and debts to the communities that are essential to their existence.

Furthermore, through failure to emphasize female differences, women may continue to be measured through a single, male-constructed lens that ignores or denigrates female-specific experiences. Yet woman along with man should be the measure of all things—and the universalizing of human experience based only on consideration of dominant cultures should be avoided. Awareness of the dimensions of this "equality vs. difference" question is critical to understanding a wide range of historical and contemporary issues regarding the status of women. Can gender-specific needs of individuals such as pregnant women be acknowledged in law that also supports equality of treatment for all individuals? Can employment preferences be granted to men if, historically, most women have not pursued a given occupation? How should a history grounded in gender distinctions be interpreted (Scott)?

Scholars today recognize that neither "man" nor "woman" has a single, fixed meaning; cross-cultural and international differences defy simple definition. The concept of separate spheres of human activity labeled public and private, political and personal, society and family, however, has a long history; the reality of women's lives was obscured by these universalizing categories of analysis often used by philosophers, politicians, and professors. In the early twenty-first century, historians of women have firmly established the historicity of women, a critical first task. Women's lives, as well as their consciousness, vary, not only by era but also by class, race, age, marital status, region, religion, education, and a host of factors peculiar to individual circumstances. Implicit in this work is a political message: that changes over time past make future change conceivable. Also implicit is an accusation of injustice against a system of societal arrangements that has suppressed women, for the questions raised in this scholarship deal often with omissions, silences, and double standards. This form of scholarship elicits new knowledge and conjectures about human possibilities.

Women in Traditional Western Societies

As the story has been reconstructed, women in history have become increasingly visible (Bridenthal et al.). New anthropological studies suggest that women may have enjoyed greater equity with men in prehistorical times (Sanday). Agrarian economies with relatively little differentiation of tasks allowed for more egalitarian relationships within families; families themselves constituted societies, and participation was not dichotomized by gender, or sex roles. The classical world, with its more advanced economies, and greater wealth and militarism, vested both property rights and citizenship only in men, as heads of households. Separated into family and polity, society became a male world of civic virtue. Relegated to the household, women became men's property, and a double standard of sexuality was constructed to assure female subjection to patriarchal family interests. A woman's honor, and that of her family, was identified with her chastity. The virtue of a woman, said Aristotle, was to obey. Differentiation by class allowed some variation of roles for women; but Plato's philosopher queens aside, no women could claim equal treatment in regard to property, citizenship, marriage, criminal law, or access to social institutions. Women existed to reproduce and to serve men's needs; rights in their progeny were assigned to men.

INFLUENCE OF CHRISTIANITY. The spread of Christianity brought new possibilities for women: for some, a role in spreading the new religion; for all, a promise of spiritual equality. Christianity created new opportunities for women's voices to be heard, especially by instituting marriage laws requiring consent and establishing, in some instances, inheritance and property rights for women. Monasteries and convents, while providing shelter for the destitute, also offered education and alternative careers for a small, often highborn, minority. The high Middle Ages saw the foundation of the first universities in the Western world, beginning in 1088 with Bologna, whose famous twelfth-century legal scholar, Gratian, incorporated into his influential study Aristotle's dualistic view of women as passive and men as active, in law as well as reproductive physiology.

This Aristotelian dualism was also advanced by the work of Thomas Aquinas in the thirteenth century; he combined his reading of Aristotle with the Christian view of creation to assert that woman was a "defective and misbegotten" man, assigned by nature to the work of procreation. The rebirth of learning thus gave new life to the hoary tradition of defining women as not-men and for men, in terms of qualities they lacked and services they provided. Renaissance thinkers transmitted across the ages classical Greece's sharp distinction between polity and household. The literature of courtly love notwithstanding, as dynastic power was reconstituted in bureaucratic and political structures, the separation of public and private arenas of human activity increased; and relative to aristocratic men, upper-class women faced new restrictions. Growth of the market economy, however, probably had a more liberating effect on rural and urban women of other classes.

Neither the Renaissance nor the Reformation, both considered watersheds in European history, brought reformed ideas about women to the fore. The advent of Protestantism meant the closing of nunneries that had allowed some women, notably those who could offer a dowry to the church, agency outside marriage. It also deprived all classes of women of the succor of the Virgin Mary and female saints. However, Protestantism did provide some literate women as well as men direct access to the word of God in the Bible. By ending clerical celibacy, it opened opportunities to ministers' wives, and ultimately, especially in the dissenting sects, it allowed women wider participation in church affairs. In the Counterreformation, some Catholic laywomen formed communities through which they provided social services for the poor, ill, and orphaned. Nuns continued to serve as teachers, nurses, and social workers. But Catholics and Protestants alike, following the biblical injunction of Paul, taught women silence in public and subjection to men in private.

URBAN VS. RURAL EXPERIENCE. Controversy over the effects of the Renaissance and Reformation on women's lives continues to fuel debate among historians of women. In an increasingly complex society, generalizations fail to satisfy: some women prospered, enjoyed education by leading humanist scholars such as Erasmus, and wielded power on behalf of dynastic lines. Urban craftsmen's wives shared in domestic production and local marketing of goods, and helped to manage artisanal workshops. City women developed professions of their own, largely in the healing arts, midwifery, and retail establishments, especially those purveying food. But most wage-earning women worked as domestic servants, frequently for a decade before marriage and sometimes for their entire lives; "maid" had become synonymous with "female servant."

However, most women, like most men, lived in rural settings, where all members of the household pooled their labor in a family economy organized to produce the goods and services essential to supporting and reproducing themselves. They lived within households and made essential contributions to the economic survival of their families. Labor needs over the family's life cycle determined the status, residence, and welfare of most people (Tilly and Scott). Only after centuries-long structural changes in agriculture and industry, in company with a demographic shift that reduced both mortality and fertility, did the employment of female productive capacity generate public debate over a "woman question." Ultimately it was a shift in the location of women's traditional work—especially making cloth and garments—from the household into the factory, and the ensuring restructuring of (especially married) women's economic contribution to the family, that created the conditions for feminist debate. Only then did the question "Should a woman work?" or "Should she have a 'right to work'?" make sense.

EFFECTS OF POLITICAL AND SCIENTIFIC DEVELOPMENTS. In addition to religious reformation and the expansion of commerce and trade, other major trends in the early modern period led to new institutions and novel ideas that affected women's lives and challenged traditional views of women's "nature." Political centralization and the rise of science also meant change in women's lives. According to one recent interpretation, the great witchcraft persecution of the sixteenth and seventeenth centuries reflected not only religious and gender conflict but also efforts to legitimize political authority by exercising new forms of social control over individual behavior (Larner). Because women's relative physical and economic weaknesses made their recourse to magic power seem plausible, and because their alleged sexual insatiability predisposed them to temptation by the devil, 80 percent of the victims of witch-hunts were female—often older, single, eccentric women lacking male protection.

Ultimately science disproved many misogynist notions about the female body. However, despite studies in embryology challenging the Aristotelian view of women's passivity in reproduction that also buttressed attitudes and customs denying them agency in society, only in the late nineteenth and early twentieth centuries were such classical and false assumptions finally displaced by scientific knowledge.

Although by the eighteenth century the economic, political, and intellectual structures that maintained traditional attitudes and institutionalized age-old practices toward women were subject to a multitude of challenges, time-honored patterns persisted. Just as in the thirteenth century Thomas Aquinas had recapitulated Aristotle, so the influential eighteenth-century philosopher Jean-Jacques Rousseau reinforced belief in woman's role as the helpmate of man. Like Adam's Eve, Rousseau's Sophie, the ideal wife of his ideal citizen, Émile, was created to serve, support, and console the chief actor on the human stage, the man to whom she was legally subject. The Napoleonic Code of 1804, and similar codes of law subsequently promulgated across Europe, required married women to obey their husbands. Voices that demanded inclusion of civil rights for women along with the "Rights of Man"—Condorcet in France, von Hippel in Germany, Mary Wollstonecraft in England—were silenced as the Age of Reason gave way to an Age of Steel. Men alone wrote and signed the new "social contract"; as "natural" dependents, women could not aspire to citizenship.

And yet women increasingly did claim civil rights. Despite the negative examples of Wollstonecraft (dead after childbirth and infamous more for her unconventional lifestyle than for her contributions to radical philosophy), Marie Antoinette, Olympe de Gouges (author of *The Declaration of the Rights of Woman and the Female Citizen,* 1791), and Jeanne Manon Roland (dead on the Jacobins' guillotine, ostensibly for having violated the boundaries of conventional femininity), and despite increasingly restrictive legal codes and an ideology of domesticity that won widespread support across class lines, new philosophic currents, based in the Enlightenment concept of human perfectibility, generated the first organized movements for women's rights.

Women in Transforming Societies

Inspired by the French Revolution, women in the nineteenth century began to form groups through which collectively to advocate improved treatment of their sex. By the mid-nineteenth century, organized groups we now call *feminist* were formed in France, England, the United States, Prussia, and even Russia, to challenge women's subject status. The new protest took place in the context of economic as well as political transformation in western and central Europe and the United States. Revolutionary changes in methods of agriculture and transportation, and the rise of an enlarged market economy, industrialization, and urbanization brought profound alteration to family structures and relationships. More young people, including women, could claim and find opportunities for social and geographic mobility and economic independence.

Especially for women, however, escape from the confines of the patriarchal family brought new vulnerabilities (Tilly and Scott, 1978). With female wages far below subsistence levels, a woman alone required assistance, and might trade sex for survival, risking dismissal from employment for her "loose morals" or extreme deprivation if deserted by her male partner.

Social reformers responded, purportedly in women's defense. Not all protesters and reformers called for *equality* for women; few, if any, entertained ideas of identical rights and responsibilities for both sexes. Utopian schemes for the total reconstruction of society aside, debate over the status of women most often focused on ways to "protect" them: to shelter traditional women's work from the intrusion of men; to safeguard women (along with children) from unsafe conditions and/or excessive hours of labor; to secure for women rights to inherited property, their own earnings, and custody of their persons as well as some share in legal authority over their children in cases of divorce. Divorce itself, largely illegal or difficult to obtain before the twentieth century, was one of many reform issues about which women themselves differed, often on the basis of class, religion, or ethnicity.

DEFINING FEMINISM. Emphasis by historians on the woman-suffrage movement, which began as a minority concern within women's groups in the mid-nineteenth century and peaked near the beginning of the twentieth, has obscured not only the larger concerns of women activists but also deep differences within feminist movements. Campaigns for "equal rights," grounded in the assumptions of liberal individualism, became dominant to a greater extent in England and the United States than elsewhere. Contemporary English-language dictionaries tend to define feminism as a movement toward political, social, educational, economic, and legal rights for women equal to those of men. This has been termed *individualistic* feminism (Offen).

The feminisms of continental Europe in that earlier era, as well as later women's movements in Third World countries, reflected a closer association with the social question—that is, with issues of class and nation—and with family relationships and community ties. This constitutes a *relational* form of feminism. Socialist feminists, while cognizant of women's needs for education and encouragement to participate fully in political struggles in support of class goals, declined to envision as their purpose access to equal—and equally exploitative—conditions with working-class men. Others, including Catholic feminists in large numbers, insisted on improvement of women's status in order to enhance their performance in traditional women's roles and relationships. In some countries, notably the United States, a "century of struggle" for women's rights grew out of religious ferment and the recognition that no subjected person, woman or slave, could be fully responsible to God as a moral being. Nineteenth-century equal-rights feminism and the concurrent movement for "protective legislation" offered contrasting answers to the "woman question."

EQUAL BUT DIFFERENT. Differentiation between "individualistic" and "relational" forms of feminism heightens current debate over the definition of feminism. It also parallels a major controversy among feminist theorists that cuts to the heart of moral issues regarding women. Must arguments undergirding a political movement on behalf of women—the various forms of feminism—be grounded in the assumption that human beings are identical? If so, equal-rights law can be used to deny pregnant women special insurance and employment benefits. Equality so defined may demand identity of treatment.

Alternatively, to emphasize women's particularity, to focus on sexual differences, may invite legislation (and buttress attitudes) restricting women's options in the guise of acknowledging their special needs. Precisely this argument was long used to justify labor laws that denied many excellent employment opportunities to all women because they required occasional work during evening hours or involved physically demanding tasks. More recently, women workers in potentially hazardous industries have faced coerced sterilization or loss of employment on grounds of their capacity for reproduction. But to deny that women on the basis of their sex constitute a special class can also deprive them of support they may need—for example, in pregnancy. It can even, some argue, destroy the very basis for a political movement in their name and interest.

This "difference versus equality" debate, often in inchoate form, has led to extended conflict over definitions of feminism and feminist demands. It also raises fundamental issues regarding individual rights, family responsibilities, and the prerogatives of government. In the nineteenth century, reformers called for legislative action to ameliorate the worst abuses of industrialization and urbanization. Reformers ranged from British industrialists who wanted to improve the quality of the labor force to French Social Catholics who sought to base solutions to societal problems on Christian principles to Prussia's "Iron Chancellor" Otto von Bismarck, who schemed to reduce the threat of socialist revolution. Whether impelled by religious, philanthropic, political, or economic motives, they shared the recognition that such innovations increased governmental powers over persons' lives. They also found that they could succeed, against strongly held liberal tenets favoring laissez-faire practice, by exposing the physical, and allegedly moral, dangers to female (and young) persons posed by the new working and living conditions. Working women rarely spoke for themselves in these debates, and even feminist voices, largely from the middle class, were little heeded.

Beginning in the 1840s with the first laws limiting women's night work, every policy of the interventionist states, acting in lieu of a patriarchal family to regulate female behavior, extended the premise that women needed special consideration and that men must provide them with protection, even against themselves. The nineteenth-century debate over short hours and the twentieth-century controversy over state regulation of reproduction share the assumption that adult women, as individual citizens, cannot or should not be empowered to make decisions affecting their own persons. Whether arguing against a woman's working outside the home at night, on behalf of keeping her husband home from the cabaret, or championing limits on abortion, advocates of restrictive legislation link women's rights with those of others: husband, child, family, state.

Similar arguments may be employed on occasion in support of male-specific measures such as military conscription, which subordinates individual freedom to national security. Such denial of personal autonomy, however, remains the exception for men and, moreover, often brings with it rights of citizenship. Women, on the other hand, are assumed to serve the interests of others at all times, and rarely gain comparable advantage. Historically, legislation concerning women has not distinguished among them by race, ethnicity, or class, by marital status, age, preference, or capacity, assuming marriage and motherhood to be the overriding obligation and destiny of all women, and conflating childbearing with child rearing. As historians have highlighted in recent books, the interests of women and their calls for "freedom" may even be seen as at odds with those of the family. This, of course, is true especially of the type of family associated primarily with the white, Western world (Bell and Offen; Degler); studies of the African-American family in the United States, and of extended families in other cultures, stress their function as sources of strength as well (Jones).

The history of women in the twentieth century reveals the centrality of the "woman question" to the social, economic, and political concerns of many nations. During wars and revolutions, traditional notions of *women's place* and struggles over woman suffrage have been eclipsed by calls for female labor and patriotic support. Apparent feminist advances, however, have frequently led to the reinstitution of traditional norms. Following both world wars, women were summarily discharged from good-paying jobs or offered less skilled and less rewarding employment. However, structural changes in commerce and industry have escalated demand for female workers, especially in clerical, teaching, and other service occupations dominated by women; expansion of educational opportunities has augmented female literacy and professional expertise; advances in public health, nutrition, and medicine have continued to increase female life expectancy and decrease infant mortality; and new technologies have reduced the need for labor-intensive household chores. All of these changes tend to free many women for long periods of productive activity outside the family. As more and more countries have been swept into the global economy and information network, women's movements, often linked (and sometimes subordinated) to nationalism, have appeared around the world. Along with efforts to improve women's health and education, Third World feminists are challenging double standards in law and culture as well as such practices as clitoridectomy, marriage by capture, and sati (Johnson-Odim and Strobel).

Unlike earlier waves of feminist protest, the mid-twentieth-century rebirth of feminism called into action sufficient numbers of educated and strategically placed women and their male supporters to successfully challenge many social priorities and institutional structures. Though feminists are sometimes wrongly perceived as a *special interest* group reflecting only the needs and desires of middle-class white women in developed nations, their pressure, especially since the 1970s, has achieved significant change in legal status, medical treatment, and workplace conditions of benefit to all women. It has opened to women professions long monopolized by men, including medicine, law, the ministry, and the professoriate, whose collective powers of definition long buttressed gender biases. In some cases, most notably medicine, this represents a restoration to women of roles they held prior to the institution of professional schools and licensure, from which they were excluded. As healthcare providers, women today often challenge the gender distinction between male doctors who *cure* and female nurses who *care*. Women's health centers tend to stress women's need to question conventional medical procedures and to encourage women to assume an active role in determining their own treatment (Jaggar).

Women Challenging Epistemology

Modeled on the *self-help* agencies for women's health that first developed in the late 1960s and influenced medical practice, this new women's liberation movement has flourished in the academy, especially in the United States but increasingly in Europe and in some instances in Africa, Asia, and Latin America. The field of women's studies, which began as a search for feminist foremothers and a female past lost to history, has expanded across the disciplines to question old methodologies, ask new questions, identify new sources, reinterpret received wisdom, develop new female perspectives, and challenge the very construction of knowledge—not only about the *nature* of women but also about all the constructs in the natural and social sciences based on androcentric experience. Grounded in advocacy for the rights of women to equality in education, culture, and society, it is a form of moral as well as scientific inquiry.

Among the earliest paradigms developed from the new scholarship in women's studies was the *social construction of feminity*. Whether psychologists rereading Sigmund Freud, sociologists reinterpreting Erik Erikson, or historians rediscovering Heinrich Kramer and James Sprenger's notorious late-fifteenth-century handbook on witchcraft, these scholars found in the sciences as well as the humanities a pervasive confusion of description with prescription. Proceeding from male-imposed definitions of female nature and proscriptions limiting female behavior as old as written records of humankind, men as philosophers, preachers, physicians, politicians, patriarchs, and professors had labeled unconventional women abnormal, criminal, ill, even pathological—or, alternatively, not "real women." The *eternal feminine* of Western mythology falsely universalized descriptions of an idealized (implicitly) white woman (Spelman; Chaudhuri and Strobel).

Historical and cross-cultural studies that belie many such interpretations have now been done. The new women's history, increasingly inclusive of women of color and international perspectives (Offen et al.; Johnson-Odim and Strobel), lays bare the many consequences of the absence of female voices and agency, and the fundamental ways in which justice has been denied to half the human species. Women's history tells a tale of misconceptions, biases, and injustices that have oppressed women and limited their freedom of choice—and, hence, their moral responsibility. It also reveals the many and differing contributions, perceptions, and struggles that constitute the female past. Although this historical perspective faces challenges, sometimes by groups of women who remain dependent on traditional sex roles for economic support and social recognition, it nevertheless offers the potential for transformation of benefit to all (Jaggar). It rests, moreover, on the principles of justice.

To the extent that ethical considerations require attribution of personhood and personal agency to every human being, ethical behavior toward women calls for disclosure and discussion of the full record of women in history. It demands that women be defined by their particular positions within specific and changing contexts and allowed choices reflecting the full range of their human attributes. It calls for major societal change. Inspired by new knowledge and the new feminisms, women have begun as never before to speak in their own voices and to claim equality despite their differences—envisioning difference without hierarchy. The "woman question," as posed by women today, can no longer be answered in terms of expediency. The ground has shifted: in the new world, women stand along with men as individuals endowed equally, if perhaps differently, with moral rights and moral responsibilities.

MARILYN J. BOXER (1995)
BIBLIOGRAPHY REVISED

SEE ALSO: *Biology, Philosophy of; Body: Cultural and Religious Perspectives; Care; Circumcision, Female Circumcision; Environmental Ethics: Ecofeminism; Ethics: Social and Political Theories; Feminism; Human Rights; Paternalism; Sexism; Social Control of Sexual Behavior*

BIBLIOGRAPHY

Anderson, Bonnie S., and Zinsser, Judith P. 1988. *A History of Their Own: Women in Europe from Prehistory to the Present.* 2 vols. New York: Harper and Row.

Beauvoir, Simone de. 1952. *The Second Sex,* tr. and ed. Howard Madison Parshley. New York: Alfred A. Knopf.

Bell, Susan Groag, and Offen, Karen M., eds. 1983. *Women, the Family, and Freedom: The Debate in Documents.* 2 vols. Stanford, CA: Stanford University Press.

Boxer, Marilyn J., and Quataert, Jean H., eds. 1987. *Connecting Spheres: Women in the Western World, 1500 to the Present.* New York: Oxford University Press.

Bridenthal, Renate; Koonz, Claudia; and Stuard, Susan M., eds. 1987. *Becoming Visible: Women in European History,* 2nd edition. Boston: Houghton Mifflin.

Chaudhuri, Nupur, and Strobel, Margaret, eds. 1992. *Western Women and Imperialism: Complicity and Resistance.* Bloomington: Indiana University Press.

Cott, Nancy F. 1977. *The Bonds of Womanhood: "Woman's Sphere" in New England, 1780–1835.* New Haven, CT: Yale University Press.

Degler, Carl N. 1980. *At Odds: Women and the Family in America from the Revolution to the Present.* Oxford: Oxford University Press.

Evans, Sara M. 1989. *Born for Liberty: A History of Women in America.* New York: Free Press.

Fox-Genovese, Elizabeth. 1991. *Feminism Without Illusions: A Critique of Individualism.* Chapel Hill: University of North Carolina Press.

Gilligan, Carol. 1982. *In a Different Voice: Psychological Theory and Women's Development.* Cambridge, MA: Harvard University Press.

Gylling, Heta Aleksandra. 2000. "Women, Culture, and Violence: Traditional Values as a Threat to Individual Well-Being" *Journal of Social Philosophy* 31(4): 439–446.

Hekman, Susan J. 1995. *Moral Voices, Moral Selves: Carol Gilligan and Feminist Moral Theory.* University Park: Pennsylvania State University Press.

Jaggar, Alison M. 1983. *Feminist Politics and Human Nature.* Totowa, NJ: Rowan Allanheld.

Johnson-Odim, Cheryl, and Strobel, Margaret, eds. 1992. *Expanding the Boundaries of Women's History: Essays on Women in the Third World.* Bloomington: Indiana University Press.

Jones, Jacqueline. 1985. *Labor of Love, Labor of Sorrow: Black Women, Work, and the Family from Slavery to the Present.* New York: Basic Books.

Kerber, Linda K. 1980. *Women of the Republic: Intellect and Ideology in Revolutionary America.* Chapel Hill: University of North Carolina Press.

Kraditor, Aileen S. 1965. *The Ideas of the Woman Suffrage Movement, 1890–1920.* New York: Columbia University Press.

Larner, Christina. 1981. *Enemies of God: The Witch-Hunt in Scotland.* Baltimore: Johns Hopkins University Press.

Mahowald, Mary B. 1997. "What Classical American Philosophers Missed: Jane Addams, Critical Pragmatism, and Cultural Feminism." *Journal of Value Inquiry* 31(1): 39–54.

McAlister, Linda Lopez. 1996. *Hypatia's Daughters: Fifteen Hundred Years of Women Philosophers.* Bloomington: Indiana University Press.

Mehuron, Kate and Percesepe, Gary. 1995. *Free Spirits: Feminist Philosophers on Culture.* Englewood Cliffs, NJ: Prentice-Hall.

Meyers, Diana Tietjens. 2002. *Gender in the Mirror: Cultural Imagery and Women's Agency.* New York: Oxford University Press.

Narayan, Uma, and Harding, Sandra, eds. 2000. *Decentering the Center: Philosophy for a Multicultural, Postcolonial, and Feminist World.* Bloomington: Indiana University Press.

Nussbaum, Martha C. 2000. "Women and Cultural Universals." In *Pluralism: The Philosophy and Politics of Diversity,* ed. Maria Baghramiau. New York: Routledge.

Offen, Karen M. 1988. "Defining Feminism: A Comparative Historical Approach." *Signs* 14(1): 119–157.

Offen, Karen; Pierson, Ruth Roach; and Rendall, Jane, eds. 1991. *Writing Women's History: International Perspectives.* Bloomington: Indiana University Press.

Okin, Susan Moller. 1979. *Women in Western Political Thought.* Princeton, NJ: Princeton University Press.

O'Neill, Eileen. 1998. "Disappearing Ink: Early Modern Women Philosophers and Their Fate in History." In *Philosophy in a*

Feminist Voice, ed. Janet A. Kourany. Princeton, NJ: Princeton University Press.

Pateman, Carole. 1987. "Feminist Critiques of the Public-Private Dichotomy." In *Feminism and Equality,* ed. Anne Phillips. New York: New York University Press.

Sanday, Peggy Reeves. 1981. *Female Power and Male Dominance: On the Origins of Sexual Inequality.* Cambridge, Eng.: Cambridge University Press.

Scott, Joan Wallach. 1988. *Gender and the Politics of History.* New York: Columbia University Press.

Spelman, Elizabeth V. 1988. *Inessential Woman: Problems of Exclusion in Feminist Thought.* Boston: Beacon Press.

Tilly, Louise A., and Scott, Joan Wallach. 1978. *Women, Work, and Family.* New York: Holt, Rinehart and Winston.

Tougas, Cecile T., and Ebenreck, Sara, eds. 2000. *Presenting Women Philosophers.* Philadelphia: Temple University Press.

Waithe, Mary Ellen, ed. 1987. *A History of Women Philosophers.* 3 vols. Dordrecht, Netherlands: Kluwer.

Walker, Margaret Urban. 1992. "Feminism, Ethics, and the Question of Theory." *Hypatia* 7(3): 23–38.

Warren, Karen J., and Erkal, Nisvan, eds. 1997. *Ecofeminism: Women, Culture, Nature.* Bloomington: Indiana University Press.

XENOTRANSPLANTATION

• • •

Xenotransplantation is the transplantation of living cells, tissues, or organs between members of different species. In the human clinical context, xenotransplantation refers to the use of living biological material from any nonhuman species in human recipients for therapeutic purposes. The practice began with attempts to develop whole animal organs as "spare parts" to replace failing human organs. Current efforts also involve cellular applications.

Xenotransplantation is currently experimental. However, some applications have progressed to clinical trials in humans and could become available therapeutic options in the early twenty-first century. Decisions about such trials must draw on areas in which science currently offers inexact guidance, raising interrelated issues of ethics and social policy. Forging consensus on appropriate public policy is multinational in scope, often pits different stakeholders against each other, and has triggered heated debate among scientists, ethicists, and the public. In this respect, the issues raised by the exercise of social policymaking for xenotransplantation provide a good case study for more general discussions of how biomedical technology should be developed and implemented.

Organ transplantation has been hailed as one of the most remarkable achievements in medical history. The original kidney transplant successes of the mid-1950s were between genetically identical human twins, whose immune systems would not recognize each other's organs as genetically foreign (and therefore would not reject them). Soon thereafter, kidneys for transplantation were obtained from non-twin siblings, from unrelated living donors, and, finally, from cadavers. These transplants between members of the same species are known as *allotransplants,* and apart from the rare identical twin transplants, all require some form of manipulation of the recipients' immune systems to prevent rejection of the donated organ.

Medical advances, particularly the discovery of powerful new immunosuppressive drugs, have greatly increased the number of transplants performed worldwide. Today, where facilities and expertise are available, it is fairly routine to transplant kidneys, hearts, livers, lungs, and other organs and tissues between human beings. However, this very success has created a disparity between the demand and supply of organs. As a result, thousands of patients die every year while waiting to receive a suitable organ for transplant. The situation is particularly severe in developing countries. Were xenotransplantation to become an effective and inexpensive method of addressing end-stage organ failure, however, the same social and economic issues that limit the ability to maintain transplant programs in developing countries today will hinder efforts to develop and maintain xenotransplantation programs. Basic healthcare needs (such as vaccination, basic diagnostics, and drugs) and accessible clean water will compete with any advanced technology for limited healthcare dollars.

Allotransplantation raised important ethical issues, many of which continue to be debated (Dossetor and Daar). While xenotransplantation raises similar issues, especially in terms of equity of access and diversion of resources, it also raises issues pertaining to human rights, animal welfare, and public health risks.

Xenotransplantation Defined

While consensus is not universal, xenotransplantation is defined as "any procedure that involves the transplantation, implantation, or infusion into a human recipient of either

TABLE 1

Summary of Clinical Organ Xenotransplantation during the 1960s, 1970s and 1980s

Organ	Year	Source Animal	Number	Investigator
Kidney	1964	Chimpanzee	12	Reemtsma
	1964	Monkey	1	Reemtsma
	1964	Baboon	1	Hitchcock
	1964	Baboon	6	Starzl
	1964	Chimpanzee	1	Hume
	1964	Chimpanzee	3	Traeger
	1965	Chimpanzee	2	Goldsmith
	1966	Chimpanzee	1	Cortesini
Heart	1964	Chimpanzee	1	Hardy
	1968	Sheep	1	Cooley
	1968	Pig	1	Ross
	1968	Pig	1	Ross
	1969	Chimpanzee	1	Marion
	1977	Baboon	1	Barnard
	1977	Chimpanzee	1	Barnard
	1984	Baboon	1	Bailey
Liver	1966	Chimpanzee	1	Starzl
	1969	Chimpanzee	2	Starzl
	1969	Baboon	1	Bertoye
	1970	Baboon	1	Leger
	1970	Baboon	1	Marion
	1971	Baboon	1	Poyet
	1971	Baboon	1	Motin
	1974	Chimpanzee	1	Starzl

SOURCE: Council of Europe Working Party on Xenotransplantation. Report on the State of the Art in the Field of Xenotransplantation, February 21, 2003.

(a) live cells, tissues, or organs from a nonhuman animal source; or (b) human body fluids, cells, tissues, or organs that have had *ex vivo* contact with live nonhuman animal cells, tissues, or organs." This is the definition adopted by the U.S. Public Health Services, and the Council of Europe has a similar one. This definition would include transplantation of an animal heart into a patient with heart failure, implantation of pancreatic islets for people with diabetes, circulation of blood from a patient with acute liver failure through a nonhuman liver or a device containing nonhuman liver cells, or the treatment of burn patients using human skin cells that have been grown *ex vivo* (outside the body) over a layer of mouse feeder cells. The transplantation of inert animal tissue (such as pig heart valves) does not fall under this definition.

Scientific and Clinical State of the Art: Continuing Challenges

Tables 1 and 2 summarize the attempts at clinical xenotransplantation since the 1960s. With the exception of the inexplicable survival for nine months of a kidney transplanted from a chimpanzee into a human recipient in the 1960s, all whole-organ xenotransplants have failed rapidly,

despite massive immunosuppression of the human recipients. In contrast, a number of preclinical trials of cellular therapies have shown enough promise to justify progressing to clinical trials. These include neural-cell transplants to treat disorders such as Parkinson's disease, intractable epilepsy, and other degenerative neurologic diseases (Fink et al.). There have also been attempts at perfusing the blood of patients in acute liver failure *ex vivo* through nonhuman animal livers until a human liver becomes available or the patient recovers (Chari et al). However, as of April 2003, no xenotransplantation application has demonstrated a high enough level of efficacy in clinical trials to allow progression to general clinical adoption.

HYPERACUTE REJECTION. The initial technical obstacle to xenotransplantation is the phenomenon of *hyperacute rejection,* which occurs when tissue is transplanted between two distant (discordant) species, for example between pigs and humans. Hyperacute rejection is swifter and more severe than the acute rejection response usually seen in transplants between individuals of the same species. Xenotransplant rejection responses are, however, also less severe in transplants between members of closely related (concordant) species, such as between rats and mice. A carbohydrate

TABLE 2

Summary of Clinical Trials on Organ and Cell Xenotransplantation during the 1990s

	Graft	Indication	Number	Country	Presently including patients
Organ transplantation	Pig heart	Heart failure, bridging procedure	1	Poland	No
	Baboon liver	Hepatitis B with liver failure	2	USA	No
	Pig liver	Liver failure, bridging procedure	1	USA	No
Cellular grafts	Neonatal bovine cromaffine cells	Pain	more than 100	Poland, Czech Republic, Switzerland & USA	No?
	Encapsulated transgenic hamster cells	ALS	6	Switzerland	No?
	Fetal porcine neurons	Parkinson	21	USA	Yes
		Huntington	12	USA	Yes
		Epilepsy	3	USA	Yes
		Stroke	3	USA	Yes
	Fetal porcine islets	Diabetes	10	Sweden	No
	Neonatal porcine islets	Diabetes	6	New Zealand	No
	Fetal rabbit islets	Diabetes	Several 100	Russia	Yes
	Baboon bone marrow	HIV	1	USA	No

SOURCE: Council of Europe Working Party on Xenotransplantation. Report on the State of the Art in the Field of Xenotransplantation, February 21, 2003.

molecule known as Gal alpha-1, 3 Gal (alpha-gal) is present on all cells of most mammalian species, including pigs, which at present are considered the most likely source-animal species. Humans and closely related old-world primates such as chimpanzees lack alpha-gal, but have naturally occurring antibodies that recognize it as foreign. In hyperacute rejection these antibodies would react against the alpha-gal on pig cells, causing the blood to clot (thrombosis) and the transplanted organ to die within minutes.

Activation of complement, a substance found in blood, is part of normal defense mechanism against foreign tissue or microbes. The presence of chemical substances that inactivate complement when its work is done normally prevents thrombosis. These complement factor regulatory proteins (CRPs) are species-specific. Thus one of the scientific responses to the challenge of hyperacute rejection has been to create transgenic pigs in which the genes for various human CRPs have been incorporated into the pig's genome, and thus prevent thrombosis. Experiments in which tissue from these transgenic pigs was transplanted into nonhuman primates have shown better graft survival rates than using tissue from unmodified pigs, raising hopes that similar improved results would be reproduced in human recipients.

Another genetic approach to dealing with hyperacute rejection has aimed to alter the expression of the alpha-gal molecule on pig tissue either by inserting genes that result in carbohydrate remodeling (Sandrin et al.,1995); by a reduction in expression of alpha-gal (Sharma et al.); or by "knocking out" (removing) the gene for the enzyme that is involved in making alpha-gal (Tearle et al). A double knock-out pig, (a pig in which both copies of the gene have been deleted from its genome) was announced in 2002 (Phelps et al.). Others have focused on reducing the massive inflammatory responses.

OTHER IMMUNOLOGICAL CHALLENGES. Hyperacute rejection is only one challenge facing xenotransplantation. Even if hyperacute rejection can be avoided, progressive phases of rejection would follow, including acute vascular rejection, cellular rejection, and chronic rejection.

Related research focuses on attempts to manipulate the immune system of higher animals in ways that would make it "tolerate" one, or a few, foreign antigens without paralyzing the whole immune system. Should immunological tolerance be achieved in humans, it would become possible to transplant organs without administering the large doses of powerful immunosuppressive drugs that leave the recipients vulnerable to dangerous infections.

PHYSIOLOGICAL BARRIERS. Physiological barriers may also stand in the way of successful xenotransplantation. For example, there is serious doubt that a pig liver will be able to sustain a human being for long. The liver is not only a detoxifying and storage organ, it is the main factory in the body for the manufacture of a large number of crucial molecules, including proteins such as albumin and clotting factors. Many of these are species-specific and will function inadequately in humans (Hammer and Thein), and some may also evoke immune reactions. In contrast, porcine insulin has successfully treated human diabetics; thus porcine pancreatic islet transplantation may offer human diabetics hope for a cure.

Xenogeneic Infections

Another reason for caution is that infections not normally encountered in humans might be transmitted from source animals to human recipients. In addition to the risk to the recipient, there is a theoretical risk that an infected recipient could transmit the infection to others. Of particular concern in this regard are infectious agents such as retroviruses that result in persistent infections and remain clinically quiescent for long periods before causing identifiable disease. During that "silent" period they can be transmitted from person to person, infecting many people before the danger is recognized.

In the past, animal viruses, such as Nipah virus and avian influenza, have been known to infect humans, resulting in outbreaks of disease of limited scope and duration (CDC, 1998, 1999). Of even greater concern is evidence that viruses once restricted to a nonhuman host species may infect and adapt to humans as a host species, as is theorized to have occurred with the HIV/AIDS pandemic (Hahn et al.). There is some controversy about whether nonhuman primates are more likely than other species to transmit

dangerous infections to humans (Chapman et al). In response to widespread concern, the U.S. Food and Drug Administration produced an advisory in April 1999 against the use of primates as source animals pending adequate demonstration of safety.

Exogenous infection (infections from agents passed among animals by contagion) can theoretically be controlled by eliminating them from the source animals. More uncertainty exists about the significance of endogenous retroviruses, which exist as part of the genetic material of humans, nonhuman primates, pigs, mice, and perhaps all animals. Endogenous retroviruses are passed from one animal to another through inheritance. Unable to cause active infection in the host animal, many can produce a virus capable of causing infection in cells from other species in the laboratory. Thus, living biological material devoid of recognized microbes has an innate infectious potential of uncertain significance for xenotransplantation. Specifically, both pigs and nonhuman primates have been shown to have endogenous retroviruses that can infect human cells in the laboratory.

Since the pig is the most likely source animal for human clinical xenotransplants, endogenous retroviruses of pigs have become a major focus of research. Porcine endogenous retroviruses (PERV) exist in the genomes of all pigs. Several variants of PERV have been characterized that vary in their infectivity. It would be difficult, but perhaps possible, to eliminate PERV through breeding or genetic manipulations (Patience et al.; Stoye).

In animal experiments, short-lived (but nonclinically obvious) replicative infections have been documented (van der Laan et al.), and PERV can be transmitted from pig cells to human cells when they are cultured together in the laboratory (Patience et al.; Wilson et al.), but there is currently no convincing evidence that PERV can cause infections leading to disease in humans. This does not, of course, exclude the possibility that it may be capable of doing so given the right circumstances.

HUMAN PATIENTS PREVIOUSLY EXPOSED TO PIG TISSUE. In the past decade or so a small but significant number of patients have been exposed to various experimental forms of xenotransplantation. Several studies of these patients have found no evidence of PERV infection, despite evidence that many of those exposed exhibited "microchimerism" (they had small numbers of pig cells in their bodies which provided ongoing exposure to PERV). While many scientists do not consider that these studies conclusively establish the absence of infectious disease risk associated with xenotransplantation, they are reassuring to some extent.

Ethical, Social and Economic Issues

Research and development costs for any major new technology, including xenotransplantation, can be high. If xenotransplantation progresses from experimentation into clinical practice, the final cost is uncertain. Even beyond the development costs, many factors will contribute to the expense of a clinical xenotransplantation program, including rearing specific infection-free source animals, laboratory tests for early diagnosis of infection, specialized staff, and maintaining monitoring and surveillance regimes. Costs will also be determined by companies owning intellectual property rights to the technologies employed, the size of the market, and so on. Whether this cost will exceed the current costs of medication and extended hospital care for patients awaiting allotransplants is uncertain. It seems likely, however, that xenotransplantation, like allotransplantation, would initially benefit only a privileged few.

It has been argued that xenotransplantation efforts could be justified only if large numbers of patients could benefit at reasonable cost and with no significant diversion of resources from the healthcare system. In this light, efforts to develop applications of porcine pancreatic islets for functional cure of type I diabetes mellitus are the most easily justified. While many applications of xenotransplantation research would benefit relatively few patients, diabetes mellitus affects a large number of people and poses substantial costs to society, both in terms of economics and in years of productive life lost.

PRECAUTIONARY PRINCIPLE VERSUS RISK-BENEFIT ANALYSIS. It is possible that the public may eventually benefit indirectly from successful widespread xenotransplantation due to a decrease in the societal burdens of healthcare costs and years of productive lives lost due to chronic diseases. The public may, however, also be put at risk of infections. As a result, although the extent of the risk is not clear, many nations have regulations that would allow xenotransplant clinical trials only when using husbandry methods that eliminate exogenous infectious agents from source animals prior to transplantation, and ensuring ongoing monitoring of recipients.

As long as uncertainty about the risk to society exists, different constituencies will perceive the same scientific data on public risk in different ways. Those basing their public-policy decisions on traditional risk-benefit analysis would tend to favor patients, perhaps at the expense of the public. Many clinicians and scientists in the transplant community do this instinctively, emphasizing the benefits in terms of a moral imperative to ameliorate suffering and save lives. This attitude is reflected by the Institute of Medicine's statement that "our own humanity is diminished if, in order to protect ourselves, we turn away from others whose suffering is both clearly visible … and … devastating in … impact … we are morally obliged, not only as individuals but as a community, to accept some risk to ourselves to save our fellow human beings from more certain harm" (Institute of Medicine, p. 71). On the other hand, those who would base decisions on the "precautionary principle" (of which there are several versions) would tend to pay more attention to the public interest, perhaps at the expense of needy patients (Daar; 2001).

The precautionary principle originated in environmental risk discourse, but has been adopted into health-policy discussions partly because of the history of infections with agents that cause AIDS, mad cow disease, and so on. It is easy to misunderstand, misquote, and misuse this concept, as there is no single definition. There are two well-known formulations. The first, from Article 15 of the United Nation's 1992 Rio Declaration on Environment and Development, states: "In order to protect the environment, the precautionary approach shall be widely applied by States according to their capabilities. Where there are threats of serious or irreversible damage, lack of full scientific certainty shall not be used as a reason for postponing cost-effective measures to prevent environmental degradation." The second, the so-called Wingspread Declaration, states: "When an activity raises threats of harm to human health or the environment, precautionary measures should be taken, even if some cause-and-effect relationships are not established scientifically."

As can be expected, the precautionary principle has become a subject of intense scholarly debate and ethical analysis (Saner). Some have argued that to be true to itself the precautionary approach requires risk-risk analysis, which would suggest an alternative formulation for the principle along the lines that "Public health and environmental policies should attempt to minimize net risks to public health and the environment based on the best available scientific information and their net anticipated cost to society" (Goklany, p. 1075).

ANIMAL ISSUES. The great British reformer Jeremy Bentham, a key figure in the development of utilitarian ethics, was also one of the earliest advocates for the humane treatment of animals. In 1780 he asked two fundamental questions: (1) "The question is not can they reason? nor can they talk? but can they suffer?" and (2) "What insuperable line prevents us from extending moral regard to animals?"

Since Bentham's time, it has become widely recognized that all vertebrates essentially perceive pain in the same way. Some argue that animals can also suffer. Animals reared in stressful conditions in captivity experience fear, boredom, isolation, and separation anxiety. Recent evidence indicates that the great apes are capable of using language, including human words (BBC), and also exhibit forms of culture. The emotional repertoire of nonhuman primates, according to ethologists Jane Goodall and Dian Fossey, includes love, sorrow and jealousy. These attributes have led some to argue that such animals are more than just sentient beings, and that they possess intrinsic value. If so, then they must have rights. To some, ignoring these rights is a form of speciesism, a term analogous to racism, and a growing minority are embracing this view.

The awareness of such qualities of animal life raises serious questions: What is it in humans that bestows on us the right of killing an animal for our own self interest? Is it our complex use of language and tools? Is it our rationality, intentionality, consciousness, conscience, or empathy? Immanuel Kant argued that all nonhuman animals can be regarded as means to ends, and that only humans, who are "rational beings," have the intrinsic right to be considered as ends in themselves. If capacity for rational thought is the basis of intrinsic rights, some have questioned whether we are justified in using organs taken from a nonhuman primate but not those taken from an anencephalic, or severely retarded, human. Philosophic justifications for the prohibition against killing incapacitated humans for such purposes have referenced their memories, if any, their potential to grow and form lasting relationships, their capacity to be mourned for long periods, and the effect that using their organs would have on relationships between humans. Others justify this distinction based on religious or metaphysical notions of the inherent elevation of humans above other creatures. These views are not convincing to many animal rights advocates, however.

NONHUMAN PRIMATES AND PIGS. Nonhuman primates are biologically close to humans, and many humans feel an emotional attachment to them. They are a concordant species, and would therefore be easier to use as sources for xenotransplantation (from an immunological and physiological perspective) than pigs, which are a discordant species. However, there are several arguments against using them for such purposes. First, the microorganisms they harbor may more easily infect and be pathogenic in humans than would be the case with pigs. Humans have a long history of contact with the pig, and the resultant physical proximity has only rarely led to the acquisition of serious infections. Second, it is not possible to raise primates under the husbandry conditions that currently allow for the production of pig herds from which exogenous infectious agents of concern have been excluded (specific-pathogen-free pigs). Third, some primate species (e.g. the chimpanzee) are endangered. While the baboon exists in large numbers and is considered a pest

in some parts of the world, it breeds slowly (and it is currently impossible to rear specific-pathogen-free baboons). Thus, a consensus to exclude nonhuman primates as source animals for xenotransplantation has emerged.

There are laws to protect research animals in many countries. Sensible guidelines include the 3 Rs of Russell and Burch (1959); namely to "reduce, replace, and refine"—to which we might now add "respect and reconsider." There are increased efforts underway to look for alternatives to animal use.

GENETIC MANIPULATION OF ANIMALS FOR HUMAN PURPOSES. The recently acquired power to manipulate the genomes of animals, including the ability to produce "double knockouts" and to clone these over several generations raises an important ethical question: Where do we draw the line? The Kennedy Report (1997) and other similar reports have concluded that the current extent of manipulating the pig's genome to incorporate human genes or other manipulations of the same magnitude raise little ethical concern provided the pig "recognizably remains a pig." Today, on balance, a case has been made that it is ethically acceptable to use pig organs, but not organs from nonhuman primates, for human xenotransplantation. At this stage of development a larger consensus exists on the importance of attending to "animal welfare" than to "animal rights."

RELIGIOUS PERSPECTIVES ON XENOTRANSPLANTATION. The views of different religions concerning xenotransplantation largely depend on the manner in which these religions consider animals and how they should be treated. From the religious perspective, it would be important that a xenotransplant not tamper with the human personality or the individual's freedom, and ability, and eligibility to bear responsibility. Minimally, all religions consider that humans have stewardship responsibilities to minimize the pain and suffering of animals being used for the benefit of humans.

Within the three major monotheistic religions (Judaism, Christianity and Islam), human beings have canonically been considered unique, with the rest of creation existing to serve humankind. The Old Testament, the first five chapters of which are canonical to both Jews and Christians, declares: "Man was made in God's image and has dominion over all other creatures and all the earth" (Genesis 1:26). In both Judaism and Islam the imperative to preserve human life overcomes many religious prohibitions.

The pig is considered to be ritually unclean in both Islam and Judaism, and it is not surprising that authorities in these two religions have been asked if the pig can be used as a source animal for organs. In Islam, the conclusion of the majority seems to be that this would not be a barrier to xenotransplantation, based on the Shariah principle that need and necessity can allow that which is forbidden—and that, in any case, the prohibition is only to eating pig tissue. F. Rosner, a physician and scholar of Jewish medical ethics, has come to the same conclusion with regard to Judaism. There is, however, a minority opinion in Islam that pigs, because they are ritually unclean, cannot be used as source animals.

A number of thoughtful Christian commentators have written about xenotransplantation. On the whole, these are generally accepting, while emphasizing that animal suffering should be minimized. The Catholic Church addressed xenotransplantation as far back as 1956, and in 2000 Pope John Paul II restated its permissive position:

It is not my intention to explore in detail the problems connected with this form of intervention. I would merely recall that already in 1956 Pope Pius XII raised the question of their legitimacy. He did so when commenting on the scientific possibility, then being presaged, of transplanting animal corneas to humans. His response in still enlightening for us today: in principle, he stated, for a xenotransplant to be licit, the transplanted organ must not impair the integrity of the psychological or genetic identity of the person receiving it; and there must also be a proven biological possibility that the transplant will be successful and will not expose the recipient to inordinate risk. (Transplantation Society)

Some Christian arguments against xenotransplantation have focused on the themes of "playing God" and "interfering with creation." These arguments have less emphasis in Judaism and Islam.

Hinduism, Buddhism, and some Animist traditions have not drawn such a sharp theological distinction between humans and other animals, seeing all as part of a hierarchy of creatures, with indistinct borders between them. Other religions supportive of xenotransplantation include Baha'i and Sikhism. Those that have religious concerns about xenotransplantation include Buddhism, Hinduism and Native American faiths (Council of Europe).

REGULATORY CHALLENGES. The uncertain potential for introducing xenogeneic pathogens has influenced many countries to develop specific policies that incorporate very stringent safety standards for clinical xenotransplantation. Some countries have initiated moratoria, while others have allowed limited and tightly monitored clinical trials. Several countries have developed policies that advocate caution with xenotransplantation clinical trials, requiring that they occur only with regulatory oversight and involve stringent standards for animal husbandry, particularly for screening and surveillance for infectious diseases. (Bloom; Tibbel; OECD).

The Council of Europe, the European Agency for Evaluation of Medicinal Products, and the United Kingdom Xenotransplantation Interim Regulatory Authority (UKXIRA, 2003) are developing specific policies on at least certain kinds of xenotransplants that incorporate the concepts of safety built around pre-xenotransplantation screening to prevent transmission of infection and post-transplantation surveillance to maximize the probability of early recognition and containment of any infections introduced through xenotransplantation. Further, the European Union has advocated multinational efforts toward consensus development and collaborative work to minimize threats from emerging infections in general.

Multinational organizations have recognized infectious disease issues associated with xenotransplantation as policy issues that transcend national boundaries. The World Health Organization (WHO) has produced recommendations for addressing and harmonizing issues related to infection control, monitoring, sharing of scientific information, consent, and human rights. Both the WHO and the Organization for Economic Co-operation and Development (OECD) have recommended that member states develop regulatory frameworks for xenotransplantation clinical trials, and they have taken leadership roles that encourage international collaborative efforts to minimize infectious risks and actively discourage expatriate xenotransplantation experiments in countries with poor regulatory environments.

Some professional societies were early critics of efforts to bring xenotransplantation clinical trials under special regulatory oversight. In recent years, however, most professional societies have been active advocates for clinical trials under regulatory oversight with stringent husbandry and infection surveillance standards. Many professionals working in xenotransplantation are concerned about "xenotourism" (the migration of patients across geopolitical boundaries to obtain unregulated xenotransplantation "therapies"). These patients may undergo risky procedures without adequate understanding, and they may bring unrecognized infections back to their home communities. Further, professionals who conduct expatriate xenotransplantation clinical trials potentially endanger the ability of the field to move forward in a systematic way. In an effort to discourage such practices, the International Xenotransplantation Society has adopted a rule that reports of such experiments will not be accepted for presentation at its meetings or for publication in its journals.

MANAGING POTENTIAL CONFLICTS OF INTEREST. The increasing participation of private interests in biomedical research is an important trend. One of the key catalysts of this change in the United States was the passage in 1980 of the Bayh-Dole act, which transferred intellectual property rights to researchers funded by federal research monies. In addition, universities in many countries must now attract more private funding to function in a very competitive environment. As a result, companies and investigators with potential conflicts of interest (COI) are testing increasingly powerful experimental therapeutic interventions.

Identifying ways to deal with potential COI while introducing innovative therapies is a complex issue and a constant source of ethical tension. Many would argue that full disclosure of financial and other COI by both institutions and investigators is adequate to manage such COI. Others have argued that disclosure alone may not suffice, and that even a pilot trial should not be conducted if an institution has a major financial interest in the outcome (Emanuel and Steiner). The Institute of Medicine has observed that "Clinical trials with cellular xenotransplants are already under way, and a real danger exists that the commercial applications of xenotransplant technology will outstrip both the research base and the national capacity to address special issues raised by xenotransplantation, including the risk of disease transmission" (Executive Summary, p. 4).

TIMING OF CLINICAL INTRODUCTION OF XENOTRANS-PLANTATION OF WHOLE ORGANS. Although small-scale experimental clinical xenotransplantation of cells and xenotransplantation involving *ex vivo* contact of human living cells with living nonhuman animal cells is underway in some countries, the question of when it would be prudent to translate laboratory successes into clinical trials remains open. The accepted standard is that before clinical trials are attempted in humans, preclinical research should provide proof of the principle hypothesis adequate to anticipate that humans may benefit from the experiment. lec. However, no consensus has been reached on what would constitute adequate graft survival in animal experiments to justify clinical trials. Attempts to define this crucial criterion have ranged from a median survival time of a minimum of three months to the suggestion that, although it is likely that hyperacute rejection can be prevented, xenotransplants should be delayed until there is a better understanding of acute vascular and cellular responses (Cooper et al.).

EPIDEMIOLOGICAL SURVEILLANCE AND POST-TRANSPLANT PATIENT MONITORING. In the past, infections transferred across species boundaries (e.g. HIV-AIDS, parvoviruses, SARS coronavirus) have spread globally. The development of international surveillance for xenotransplantation-associated infections has been proposed as a way to assist countries to manage risks associated with infections introduced through xenotransplantation performed within and beyond their borders (Rhonchi). Such recommendations raise concerns for many people. The concept of lifelong international surveillance of xenotransplant recipients is fraught with ethical complexities. International consensus has not been achieved on the definition of xenotransplantation, on what constitutes a xenogeneic infection or disease, on what events should be reported and by what methods, or on which individuals should constitute the population under surveillance. Whether a surveillance system should only report transmission of xenogeneic infections from recipients to their contacts, or should go further to collect information on the contacts themselves, is a source of controversy. All proposed national policies for monitoring xenotransplantation recipients are intrusive. Most advise against unprotected sex, donation of blood or other biological materials, and for education of intimate contacts. Some go further to require the consent of intimate partners for xenotransplantation, active surveillance of intimate contacts as well as xenotransplant recipients, and pre-transplantation agreements to avoid procreation post-xenotransplantation.

PATIENT-PHYSICIAN RELATIONSHIPS AND CONSENT. The perceived potential for xenotransplantation to benefit an individual while putting the larger community at risk complicates both the patient-physician relationship and the issue of informed consent. The Helsinki Declaration on Ethical Principles for Medical Research Involving Human Subjects states that, in medical research on human subjects, considerations related to the well-being of the human subject should take precedence over the interests of science and society. Xenotransplantation clinical trials present situations that may place the interests of recipients and the greater good of society at odds. If a doctor is required to think of the public interest rather than merely the interests of the immediate patient, the traditional role of the physician as patient advocate is altered. At best, this will create confusion, since the physicians must weigh the responsibility to individual patients against the public good. At worst, the doctor-patient relationship itself could become one of antagonism rather than of trust (Daar, 1997).

The current informed-consent requirements for patients who might receive xenotransplants exceed those required in most other research settings. A major question on which there is no consensus at present is the problem of what to do if a patient changes her or his mind about intrusive follow-up monitoring and the waiver or curtailment of confidentiality rights previously agreed to. Informed consent is not usually legally binding on the patient, who retains a right to withdraw participation at any point in the investigational process.

Given the expectations of lifelong follow-up for initial xenotransplant recipients, a different kind of consent has been discussed (Daar 1999). A specific legal contract might provide enforceability of pre-transplant agreements for lifelong monitoring. Unlike the traditional consent form, such a contract would allow specific curtailment of the patient's rights (the traditional consent procedure does not, in all cases, require that a document be signed; more often than not, the signed form protects the doctor more than the patient). Such a legal contract would be a radical departure from current accepted norms, since it would directly conflict with the present emphasis on the primacy of respect for the autonomy of the research subject. Thus, these issues are fraught with controversy.

MODELS TO BUILD ON. Are there any precedents in which a patient can decide in advance what medical treatment she or he would want to receive in the future? Both "advance directives" and the so-called "Ulysses contract" fall into this category.

Advance directives are used in medicine as a means by which patients declare their wishes in anticipation of a future day when they may not be competent to make decisions. Such an instrument has been used, for example, to establish the point at which a patient desires a "do not resuscitate" status. It could be adapted to allow a mentally competent xenotransplantation recipient to make provision for intrusive post-transplant medical monitoring (with its attendant curtailment of certain rights), to continue if the recipient changes her or his mind-a situation that might occur, if, for example, the graft fails but monitoring must continue in order to protect public health.

This would be more akin to a "Ulysses contract." In Greek, mythology Ulysses was a strong, good man. He knew he would sail near the Sirens, whose enchanting songs would overcome him and cause his ship to be destroyed. He ordered his sailors to plug their ears, and, wanting to hear the songs, had himself tied to the mast of the ship, ordering his companions not to release him regardless of his subsequent demands. A Ulysses contract, then, is used for patients who are likely to experience periods of incompetence in the future, such as patients with psychiatric disorders characterized by alternating periods of therapy-induced competence and incompetence. While they are in a competent state, they can specify treatment decisions for future occasions. In the xenotransplant setting, such a binding advance directive signed by the recipient prior to the xenotransplantation could, theoretically, be used to forcibly investigate, treat, or even confine a recipient who fails to meet responsibilities to

the public agreed to prior to the procedure (Daar 1999). A Ulysses contract usually assumes that the subject is so affected as to have their *true* judgment subordinated by some other pressure, while in this instance the xenotransplantation recipient may merely have changed her or his mind about cooperating with intrusive surveillance. Discussion of these options has raised concerns about the possibility of unacceptably eroding the human rights of research participants on the basis of hypothesis and fear rather than established or proximate risk.

PUBLIC ENGAGEMENT AND PUBLIC CONSENT. Some people have argued that since the public is going to be exposed to some level of risk of xenogeneic infections, the public must be consulted, and must consent, before xenotransplantation clinical trials proceed. Many national reports recommend that the public must in some way be consulted before proceeding with xenotransplantation. It is, however, difficult to define what would constitute *public consent*. Further, efforts at public education can easily merge over into propaganda, since the opinions formed by non-experts are completely dependent on the nature and presentation of the information they receive.

While some have advocated a moratorium pending public consent (Bach et al.) there are significant problems with adopting a moratorium. The majority of researchers and clinicians appear to be opposed to this position, mainly because moratoria remove from public discourse the very issues that ought to be addressed. Most researchers and clinicians would encourage increased capacity to evaluate the potential social consequences as the technology develops. Significantly, there have been no serious calls for reduction in xenotransplantation research.

Canada has undertaken a major public engagement exercise consisting of a series of forums involving education, discussion, and *citizen juries*. A subsequent report of the Canadian Public Health Association has recommended that Canada not proceed with xenotransplantation involving humans until several critical issues are addressed. It recommends, among other steps, that further efforts be made to inform and educate the public; that additional preclinical research be carried out; and that the risks and probability of benefit from clinical trials be more fully defined. It also calls for the development of legislation and regulations to cover all aspects of xenotransplantation clinical trials, concluding that there is a continuing need to involve the public in discussions about the future of xenotransplantation. This approach, however, has been criticized as being vulnerable to biases introduced by the information presented to the public (Wright). Nevertheless, this particular exercise reflects the current uncertainties surrounding xenotransplantation.

Conclusion

Xenotransplantation currently describes a multifaceted array of experimental biotechnological approaches to disease amelioration, some of which have progressed to small-scale clinical trials. The theoretical risk of infections spreading from source animal to recipient and then to contacts and the public has triggered debates on issues of science and on how biomedical technology should be developed, regulated and implemented. The specific ethical dilemmas discussed in the context of xenotransplantation reflect areas of ethical conflict and uncertainty relevant to other aspects of community life. These include the rights of the minority in the face of concern by the majority; conflicting values around decision making in the face of uncertain collective risk; the relative rights of humans and nonhuman animals; the relative value of safety versus of hope for progress; and the rights of, and appropriate protections afforded to, human subjects of research.

ABDALLAH S. DAAR
LOUISA E. CHAPMAN

SEE ALSO: *Animal Research: Law and Policy; Organ and Tissue Procurement; Organ Transplants; Tissue Banking and Transplantation, Ethical Issues in; Transhumanism and Posthumanism*

BIBLIOGRAPHY

Advisory Group on the Ethics of Xenotransplantation. 1997. *Kennedy Report: Advisory Group on the Ethics of Xenotransplantation: Animal Tissues into Humans.* London, HM Stationery Office.

Auchincloss, H., Jr. 2001. "In Search of the Elusive Holy Grail: The Mechanisms and Prospects for Achieving Clinical Transplantation Tolerance." *American Journal of Transplantation* 1(1): 6–12.

Bach F. H.; Fishman, J. A.; Daniels, N.; Proimos, J.; et al. 1998. "Uncertainty in Xenotransplantation: Individual Benefit versus Collective Risk." *Nature Medicine* 4(2): 141–144.

Bentham, Jeremy. 1789. *An Introduction to the Principles of Morals and Legislation.*Reissued by Prometheus Books, Amherst, New York.

Bloom, Eda T. 2001. "Regulating Xenotransplantation in the United States." *Graft* 4(2): 160–162.

Centers for Disease Control and Prevention.1998. "Update: Isolation of Avian Influenza A(H5N1) Viruses from Humans— Hong Kong, 1997–1998." *Morbidity and Mortality Weekly Report* 46(52): 1245–1247.

Centers for Disease Control and Prevention. 1999. "Update: Outbreak of Nipah Virus—Malaysia and Singapore, 1999." *Morbidity and Mortality Weekly Report* 48(16): 325–348.

Centers for Disease Control and Prevention. 2001. "U.S. Public Health Service Guideline on Infectious Disease Issues in Xenotransplantation." *MMWR Recommendations and Reports,* August 24, 2001/50(RR15): 1–46.

Chapman, L.E.; Folks, T. M.; Salomon, D. R.; Patterson, A.P.; et al. 1995. "Xenotransplantation and Xenogeneic Infections." *New England Journal of Medicine* 333(22): 1498–1501.

Chari, R. S. et al. 1994. "Treatment of Hepatic Failure with Ex Vivo Pig-Liver Perfusion followed by Liver Transplantation." *New England Journal of Medicine* 331(4): 234–237.

Cooper, D. K.; Keogh, A. M.; Brink, J.; Corris, P. A.; et al. 2000. "Report of the Xenotransplantation Advisory Committee of the International Society for Heart and Lung Transplantation: The Present Status of Xenotransplantation and Its Potential Role in the Treatment of End-Stage Cardiac and Pulmonary Diseases." *Journal of Heart and Lung Transplantation* 19(12): 1125–1165.

Collins, B. H.; Parker, W. R.; and Platt, J. L. 1994. "Characterization of Porcine Endothelial Cell Determinants Recognized by Human Natural Antibodies." *Xenotransplantation* 1: 36.

Cozzi, E.; Tucker, A. W.; Langford, G. A.; Pino-Chavez, G.; et al. 1997. "Characterization of Pigs Transgenic for Human Decay-Accelerating Factor." *Transplantation* 64(10): 1383–1392.

Daar, A. S. 1994. "Xenotransplantation and Religion: The Major Monotheistic Religions." *Xeno* 2: 61–64.

Daar, A. S. 1997. "Ethics of Xenotransplantation: Animal Issues, Consent, and Likely Transformation of Transplant Ethics." *World Journal of Surgery* 21: 975–982.

Daar, A. S. 1999. "Xenotransplantation: Informed Consent/ Contract and Patient Surveillance." *Biomedical Ethics* 4(3): 87–91.

Daar, A. S. 2001. "Choosing Risk-Benefit Analysis or Precautionary Principle as Our Approach to Clinical Xenotransplantation." *Graft* 4(2): 164–166.

Diamond, L.E.; McCurry, K. R.; Martin, M. J.; McClellan, S. B.; et al. 1996. "Characterization of Transgenic Pigs Expressing Functionally Active Human CD59 on Cardiac Endothelium." *Transplantation* 61: 1241–1249.

Diamond, L. E.; Quinn, C. M.; Martin, M. J.; Lawson, J.; et al. 2001. "A Human CD46 Transgenic Pig Model System for the Study of Discordant Xenotransplantation." *Transplantation* 71: 132–142.

Dossetor, J. B., and Daar, A. S. 2001. "Ethics of Transplantation: Allotransplantation and Xenotransplantation." In *Kidney Transplantation:Principles and Practice,* 5th edition, ed. P. J. Morris. Philadelphia: W. B. Saunders.

Emanuel, E. J., and Steiner, D. 1995. "Sounding Board: Institutional Conflict of Interest." *New England Journal of Medicine* 332(4): 262–268.

Fink, J. S., et al. 2000. "Porcine Xenografts in Parkinson's Disease and Huntington's Disease Patients: Preliminary Results." *Cell Transplantation* 9: 273–278.

Fishman, J. A. 2001. "Infection in Xenotransplantation." *Journal of Cardiac Surgery* 16(5): 363–373.

Goklany, I. M. 2002. "From Precautionary Principle to Risk-Risk Analysis." *Nature Biotechnology* 20(11): 1075.

Hahn, B.H.; Shaw, G.M.; De Cock, K. M.; and Sharp, P. M. 2000. "AIDS as a Zoonosis: Scientific and Public Health Implications." *Science* 287(5453): 607–614.

Hammer, C., and Thein, E. 2001. "Physiological Aspects of Xenotransplantation." *Xenotransplantation* 9: 303–305.

Heneine, W.; Tibell, A; Switzer, W. M.; et al. 1998. "No Evidence of Infection with Porcine Endogenous Retrovirus in Recipients of Porcine Islet-Cell Xenografts." *Lancet* 352: 695–699.

Ivinson, A. J. 1998. "Does Biomedical Research Need Another Moratorium?" *Nature Medicine* 4(2): 131.

Institute of Medicine. 1996. *Xenotransplantation: Science, Ethics, and Public Policy.* Washington, D.C.: National Academy Press.

Levinsky, N. G. 2002. "Nonfinancial Conflicts of Interest in Research." *New England Journal of Medicine* 347(10): 759–761

Michaels, Marian G. 2001. "Determining the Risk of Xenozoonoses." *Graft* 4(2): 129–130.

Moosa, M. R.; Walele, A. A.; Daar, A. S. 2001. "Renal Transplantation in Developing Countries." In *Kidney Transplantation: Principles and Practice,* 5th edition, ed. P. J. Morris. Philadelphia: W. B. Saunders.

Nuffield Council on Bioethics. 1996. *Animal-to-Human Transplants: The Ethics of Xenotransplantation.* London.

O'Riordan, T., and Jordan, A. 1995. "The Precautionary Principle in Contemporary Environmental Politics." *Environmental Values* 4: 191.

Paradis, K.; Langford, G.; Long, Z.; Heneine, W.; et al. 1999. "Search for Cross-Species Transmission of Porcine Endogenous Retrovirus in Patients Treated with Living Pig Tissue." *Science* 285: 1236–1241.

Patience, C.; Patton, G. S.; Takeuchi, Y.; Weiss, R. A.; et al. 1998. "No Evidence of Pig DNA or Retroviral Infection in Patients with Short-Term Extracorporeal Connection to Pig Kidneys." *Lancet* 352: 699–701.

Patience, C.; Takeuchi, Y.; and Weiss, R. A. 1997. "Infection of Human Cells By an Endogenous Retrovirus of Pigs." *Nature Medicine* 3: 276–282.

Phelps, C. J.; Koike, C.; Vaught, T. D.; Boone, J.; et al. 2003. "Production of Alpha1, 3-Galactosyltransferase-Deficient Pigs." *Science* 299: 411–414.

Pitkin Z., and Mullon, C. 1999. "Evidence of Absence of Porcine Endogenous Retrovirus (PERV) Infection in Patients Treated with a Bioartificial Liver System." *Artificial Organs* 23(9): 829–833.

Regan T. 1983. *The Case for Animal Rights.* Los Angeles: University of California Press.

Rosner F. 1999. "Pig Organs for Transplantation into Humans: A Jewish View."*Mount Sinai Journal of Medicine* 66(5–6): 314–319.

Russel, W. M. S., and Burch, R. L. 1959. *The Principles of Humane Experimental Technique.* London: Methuen.

Sandrin, M. S.; Fodor, W. L.; Mouhtouris, E.; Osman, N.; et al. 1995. "Enzymatic Remodeling of the Carbohydrate Surface of a Xenogenic Cell Substantially Reduces Human Antibody Binding and Complement-Mediated Cytolysis." *Nature Medicine* 1: 1261–1267.

Sandrin, M. S.; Vaughan, H. A.; Dabkowski, P. L.; and McKenzie, I. F. C. 1993. "Anti-Pig IgM Antibodies in Human Serum React Predominatly with Gala(1,3) Gal Epitopes." *Proceedings of the National Academy of Science USA* 90: 11391.

Saner, M. A. 2002. "An Ethical Analysis of the Precautionary Principle." *International Journal of Biotechnology* 4(1): 81–95.

Schumacher, J. M., Ellias, S. A.. et al. 2000. "Transplantation of Embryonic Porcine Mesencephalic Tissue in Patients with PD." *Neurology* 54(5): 1042–1050.

Sharma, A.; Okabe, J.; Birch, P.; McClellan, S. B.; et al.1996. "Reduction in the Level of Galalpha(1,3)Gal in Transgenic Mice and Pigs by the Expression of an alpha(1,2) Fucosyltransferase." *Proceedings of the National Academy of Sciences USA* 93: 7190–7195.

Shiraishi, M.; Oshiro, T.; Nozato, E.; Nagahama, M.; et al. 2002. "Adenovirus-Mediated Gene Transfer of Triple Human Complement Regulating Proteins (DAF, MCP and CD59) in the Xenogeneic Porcine-to-Human Transplantation Model." *Transplant International* 15(5): 212–219.

Singer, P. 1975. *Animal Liberation.* New York: Random House.

Soares, M. P.; Brouard, S.; Smith, R. N.; and Bach F. H. 2001. "Heme Oxygenase-1, a Protective Gene That Prevents the Rejection of Transplanted Organs." *Immunological Reviews* 184: 275–285

Stoye, J. P. 1998. "No Clear Answers on Safety of Pigs As Tissue Donor Source." *Lancet* 352(9129): 666–668.

Swedish Committee on Xenotransplantation. 1999. *From One Species to Another: Transplantation from Animals to Humans.* Swedish Government Official Report No. 1999: 120.

Tearle, R. G.; Tange, M. J.; Zanettino, Z. L.; et al. 1996 "The a-1,3-Galactosyltransferase Knockout Mouse: Implications for Xenotransplantation." *Transplantation* 61: 13.

Tibbel, Anika. 2001. "Regulating Xenotransplantation in Europe." *Graft* 4(2): 157–159.

van der Laan, J. W.; Lockey, C.; Griffeth, B. C.; Frasier, F. S.; et al. 2000. "Infection by Porcine Endogenous Retrovirus after Islet Xenotransplantation in SCID Mice." *Nature* 407: 90–94.

White, D., and Wallwork, J. 1993. "Xenografting: Probability, Possibility, or Pipe Dream?" *Lancet* 342: 879.

Wilson, C. A.; Wong, S.; Muller, J.; Davidson, C. E.; et al. 1998. "Type C Retrovirus Released from Porcine Primary Peripheral Blood Mononuclear Cells Infects Human Cells." *Journal of Virology* 72: 3082–3087.

World Health Organization. 1997. *Report of the WHO Consultation on Xenotransplantation.* Doc. No. WHO/EMC/ZOO/98.2. Geneva: WHO.

Wright, J. R., Jr. 2002. "Alternative Interpretations of the Same Data: Flaws in the Process of Consulting the Canadian Public about Xenotransplantation Issues." *Canadian Medical Association Journal* 167: 40–42.

Wu, A.; Yamada, K.; Neville, D. M.; Awwad, M.; et al. 2003. "Xenogeneic Thymus Transplantation in a Pig-to-Baboon Model." *Transplantation* 75(3): 282–291.

INTERNET RESOURCES

BBC News. 2003. "Ape 'Learns to Talk.'" Available from <http://news.bbc.co.uk/1/hi/sci/tech/2617063.stm>.

Canadian Public Health Association. 2001. "Animal-to-Human Transplantation: Should Canada Proceed?" Available from <http://www.xeno.cpha.ca>

Centers for Disease Control and Prevention. 1998. "CDC Update: Isolation of Avian Influenza A(H5N1) Viruses from Humans—Hong Kong, 1997–1998. *Morbidity and Mortality Weekly Report* 46(52): 1245–1247." Available from <http://www.cdc.gov/mmwr/PDF/wk/mm4652.pdf>.

Centers for Disease Control and Prevention. 1999. "CDC Update: Outbreak of Nipah Virus—Malaysia and Singapore, 1999." *Morbidity and Mortality Weekly Report* 48(16): 325–348. Available from <http://www.cdc.gov/mmwr/PDF/wk/mm4816.pdf>.

Centers for Disease Control and Prevention. 2001. "U.S. Public Health Service Guideline on Infectious Disease Issues in Xenotransplantation." *MMWR Recommendations and Reports,* August 24, 2001/50(RR15): 1–46. Available from <http://www.cdc.gov/mmwr/preview/mmwrhtml/rr5015a1.htm>.

Church of Scotland, Society, Religion and Technology Project. 1995. "The Ethics of Xenotransplantation." Available from <http://dspace.dial.pipex.com/srtscot/xennuf03.shtml#Contents>.

Council of Europe Working Party on Xenotransplantation. 2003. "Report on the State of the Art in the Field of Xenotransplantation." Available from <http://www.coe.int7>.

Nuffield Council on Bioethics. 1996. "Animal-to-Human Transplants: The Ethics of Xenotransplantation." London. Available from <http://www.nuffieldbioethics.org>.

Organization of Economic Co-operation and Development (OECD). Joint WHO/OECD Consultation on Xenotransplantation Surveillance, 4–6 October 2000. Available from <http://www.oecd.org>.

Rhonchi, Elettra. 2001. "OECD/WHO Consultation on Xenotransplantation Surveillance: Summary Report." Directorate for Science, Technology and Industry—Committee for Scientific and Technological Policy, Working Party on Biotechnology. Available from <http://www.olis.oecd.org/olis/2001doc.nsf>.

Transplantation Society. "Address of John Paul II to the 18th International Congress of the Transplantation Society." Available from <http://cnserver0.nkf.med.ualberta.ca/misc/Rome/Encyclical.htm>.

United Kingdom Xenotransplantation Interim Regulatory Authority (UKXIRA). Draft guidance notes on biosecurity considerations in relation to xenotransplantation. Available from <http://www.doh.gov.uk/ukxira/publications.htm>.

U.S. Food and Drug Administration. 1999. "Guidance for Industry; Public Health Issues Posed by the Use of Nonhuman Primate Xenografts in Humans." Available from <http://www.fda.gov/cber/gdlns/xenoprim.pdf>.

World Health Organization. 1997. *Report of the WHO Consultation on Xenotransplantation.* Doc. No. WHO/EMC/ZOO/98.2. Geneva: WHO. Available from <http://www.who.int/emc-documents/zoonoses/docs/whoemczoo982.pdf>.

APPENDIX CONTENTS

APPENDIX I

CODES, OATHS, AND DIRECTIVES
RELATED TO BIOETHICS

Kayhan Parsi
Neiswanger Institute for Bioethics and Health Policy
Stritch School of Medicine
Loyola University of Chicago

REVISED FROM THE WORK FOR THE 2ND EDITION OF THE
ENCYCLOPEDIA OF BIOETHICS, DONE BY

Carol Mason Spicer

CONTENTS

• • •

Section III. Ethical Directives for Other Health-Care Professions

Section IV. Ethical Directives for Human Research

Section V. Ethical Directives Pertaining to the Welfare and Use of Animals

NATURE AND ROLE OF CODES AND
OTHER ETHICS DIRECTIVES

• • •

The earliest extant documents regulating the practice of medicine are records of Egyptian laws from the sixteenth century B.C.E. and the Babylonian Code of Hammurabi, dated about 2000 B.C.E. These legal documents included guidance on what fees could be charged, what constituted competent medical care, the conditions under which a physician could be held accountable for malpractice, and what sanctions would apply. The first significant statement on medical *morality,* however, is the Hippocratic Oath (fourth century B.C.E.). Although the Oath's historical role has been critiqued by scholars such as Robert Baker, the Oath continues to play an important symbolic role in Western medical ethics.

With the notable exception of religious precepts being brought to bear on the conduct of physicians, most medical ethics documents written prior to World War II were professionally generated, that is, they were developed by physicians for physicians. Since the mid-1900s, however, a complex set of factors has challenged the professional authority of the medical profession.

The atrocities committed by Nazi physician–researchers, which led to the Nuremberg Code (Germany, 1949), and infamous cases of abuse of research subjects in the United States, such as the Tuskegee syphilis study, began to undermine trust in the profession. The various rights movements of the 1960s and 1970s and the anti-Vietnam War movement emphasized individual liberty and contributed to a general willingness to challenge authoritative traditions. At the same time, the dramatic increase in scientific knowledge and the development and use of medical technology powerfully increased the ability of health-care professionals to affect the course of people's lives and deaths. These factors, among others, contributed to an increased emphasis on respect for the autonomy and self-determination of individuals seeking health care.

With these changes came a proliferation of bioethics documents pertaining to research on human subjects, to health professionals other than physicians, and to health-care institutions. Furthermore, growing concerns over the alleged mistreatment of research animals and claims that the use of animals for any research purpose is immoral, coupled with concerns for the protection of the environment, resulted in bioethics directives that extend well beyond human medical practice. Concurrent with the increased diversity in the focus of bioethics documents, the authorship of such documents has diversified as well. Professional organizations no longer monopolize the formulation of directives governing professional behavior; religious organizations, institutions, and government agencies, for example, also set moral or legal standards for clinicians and researchers.

The resulting array of bioethics documents may be divided into three fundamental types: (1) professionally generated documents that govern behavior within the profession; (2) documents that set standards of behavior for professionals but are generated outside the profession; and (3) documents that specify values and standards of behavior for persons who are not members of a profession.

Documents Generated by and for a Profession

Although controversy exists over precisely what constitutes a profession, professions may be distinguished from occupations on several grounds (see, e.g., Barber, 1963; Greenwood, 1982; Kultgen, 1988). Professions involve a specialized body of knowledge and skill that requires lengthy education and training to acquire and provides a service to clients and to society. Once a field has achieved professional status, a trained practitioner is considered a professional regardless of employment status. Another characteristic of professions is their claim to be autonomous and self-regulating; however, with the freedom and power of self-regulation comes a concurrent obligation to establish and enforce standards of ethical behavior. Indeed, some have argued that the existence of a professional ethic is the hallmark of a profession (see, e.g., Barber, 1963; Newton, 1988; Campbell, 1982).

Professionally generated ethics documents may take the form of prayers, oaths, or codes. Prayers, such as that once attributed to the Jewish physician-philosopher Moses Maimonides, express gratitude to a deity and ask for divine assistance in developing one's skills and meeting one's responsibilities. Oaths are vows taken by individuals entering a profession to uphold specified obligations. They were frequently employed in ancient times; more recent examples include the Declaration of Geneva (World Medical Association, 1983, 1994) and the Solemn Oath of a Physician of Russia (1993), among others. In contrast to the personal, interactive nature of prayers and oaths, codes, which are often accompanied by more detailed "interpretive statements," are collective summaries of the moral ideals and conduct that are expected of the professional.

ROLES OF PROFESSIONAL ETHICS DIRECTIVES. The importance to an emerging profession of producing its own ethics directives indicates a primary role of such documents. They help to define and legitimate a profession as well as to maintain, promote, and protect its prestige. Simultaneously, the documents function as a promise to society that the profession will maintain specified standards of practice in return for the power and autonomy that society is being asked to grant the profession.

Protection of the unity, integrity, and power of the profession, which appears to be a primary goal of the rules of etiquette governing the relationship between professionals, is a "quasi-moral" role of professional ethics documents. Although maintenance of a profession has a limited moral component in that its existence promotes the well-being of society, it especially serves the interests of those within the profession who stand to lose the monopoly on their practice should society lose faith in them. In contrast, the explicitly moral role of professional ethics documents lies in the articulation of both ideal and minimal standards of character and conduct for the professional. Both the moral and some of the "quasi-moral" guidelines form the content of the profession's promise to society and serve as a guide for determining when sanctions should be brought to bear against a member of the profession.

THE NATURE OF PROFESSIONAL CODES. In professionally generated codes, the same guideline may simultaneously help to fulfill both categories of function.

"Quasi-moral" guidelines. In addition to having an ethic, professions are characterized by the possession and practice of a specialized body of knowledge. Consequently, frequently articulated requirements include: competency to practice; restriction of professional status to those who have undergone specific educational and training programs; keeping one's knowledge current; and working to advance the existing knowledge in one's field through research (see, e.g., American Nurses' Association, 1985; Canadian Nurses Association, 1991; American Dental Association, 1994; American Psychological Association, 1992; and American Chiropractic Association, 1992).

Such requirements serve a dual purpose—to maintain the profession and to serve society's well-being. By maintaining a specialized body of knowledge, the profession ensures a monopoly in providing its services. At the same time, restricting the practice of a profession to those who are qualified and requiring that they keep their skills and knowledge current are essential elements in fulfilling society's mandate to the profession: to provide a specialized service competently and safely.

Rules of professional etiquette, such as prohibitions on criticizing colleagues in the presence of clients, the proper procedures for consultation, and the process for the adjudication of disputes, constitute another characteristic of professional ethics documents. Thomas Percival's *Medical Ethics* (1803), originally commissioned to address conflicts among physicians, surgeons, and apothecaries at Manchester Infirmary, epitomizes this characteristic. Like the competency requirements, rules governing intraprofessional behavior serve the dual purpose of maintaining the profession and serving the well-being of society. Regarding the former, public criticism of colleagues could, as Percival noted, undermine the credibility of the professional and might ultimately damage the reputation of the profession. Professionally generated documents require that questions one practitioner has about another's competence or conduct be brought to the attention of the appropriate authorities, but none to my knowledge explicitly states that the client be advised of the concern. The presumption seems to be that this arrangement, at least in most cases, will protect the client from incompetent practice at the same time as it safeguards the reputation of the professional.

In addition, rules that foster harmony between members of a profession presumably promote not only the self-interest of the profession(als) but also the well-being of society. Rules of etiquette help to maintain the unity of the profession and promote teamwork, two factors that are widely perceived to optimize the quality of patient care (see, e.g., American Chiropractic Association, 1992).

Similarly, rules governing professionals' association with practitioners outside of the profession serve multiple functions. The American Medical Association, for example, proscribes the association of its physicians with "nonscientific practitioners" but permits its physicians to refer patients to nonphysician practitioners provided the referrals are believed to benefit the patients and the services "will be performed competently and in accordance with accepted scientific standards and legal requirements." In part, such rules protect the standing of a profession by not allowing a competing practice to infringe upon its professional monopoly. But if the competing practice truly is "quackery," the rules may also protect the professional's clients from harm.

Many codes include guidelines on the setting of fees as well as prohibitions of fee-splitting, deceptive advertising, and misrepresenting one's professional qualifications (see, e.g., American Dental Association, 1994; American Psychological Association, 1992). Once again, the dual purpose of protecting the profession and safeguarding its clients is evident. With regard to deceptive practices, the prohibition benefits both the consumer and the profession. Over time, deceptive practices undermine the credibility of the profession, resulting in diminished status and externally imposed sanctions. The setting of fees promotes the interests of professionals by allowing them the discretion to set fees in return for the expertise over which they hold a monopoly. However, professional codes also may admonish the professional to take into account the client's ability to pay when setting the fee in a particular case (see, e.g., Canadian Medical Association, 1990a, 1990b; International Chiropractors Association, 1990).

A common component of the "quasi-moral" elements of professional ethics codes is a description of the procedures for reviewing, adjudicating, and, if necessary, sanctioning alleged violations of professional conduct (see, e.g., American Chiropractic Association, 1992; American Psychiatric Association, 1989). There are several reasons for this often lengthy discussion. Allegations of moral impropriety can harm the reputation of the accused as well as the profession. Consequently, every effort must be made to ensure due process and the fair treatment of all parties. In addition, the potentially explosive nature of such allegations and the serious consequences if they are proved true set the stage for vehement denial and rebuttal by the professional accused. It is not unreasonable for the professional organization to protect itself, the process, and any victims, by making the rules clear in advance.

Moral guidelines. Professional ethics is best understood as a subset of ethics in general, although this might be disputed by some. The moral dictates of professional ethics documents ought to relate general moral values, duties, and virtues to the unique situations encountered in professional practice. A professional ethic cannot make a practitioner ethical; it can only hope to inform and guide a previously existing moral conscience. Lisa Newton (1988) has distinguished between the internal and external aspects of ethics in professional practice. The internal aspect is ontologically prior to the external; it is the personal conscience that each professional brings to the professional enterprise. The external aspect consists of the publicly specified moral requirements of the profession, that is, those elements of professional morality that are addressed in the profession's ethics documents. Despite the potential conflict between the internal and external aspects, both of them are important.

The external aspect may prompt professionals to reflect critically on their personal moral beliefs and values, a process that helps practitioners refine their internal ethic. The internal ethic then guides professionals when they encounter the myriad situations and conflicts of duty to which ethics documents can only allude. However, since only the external aspect is accessible to public scrutiny, the remainder of this section will explore that aspect in more detail.

The moral guidelines of ethics documents generally involve three elements: (1) values; (2) duties; and (3) virtues.

1. At the center of the professional ethic lies the value that the profession perceives to be the primary good, or its objective. Professional ethics documents often identify this value explicitly and include a pledge to promote it as their means of serving the public interest. Some professional organizations focus on general values, citing the benefit, well-being, or greatest good of their clients as the fundamental value to be pursued (see, e.g., National Federation of Societies for Clinical Social Work, 1987; American Chiropractic Association, 1992). Although including values in ethics documents helps provide a touchstone for guiding conduct when duties that are specified conflict, a problem can arise when it is the profession that articulates the value central to the client-provider relationship. An individual's well-being generally involves all aspects of his or her life, and practitioners, who might be qualified to assess and advance more specific goods, such as health, can claim no particular expertise in judging what constitutes a client's total well-being (Veatch, 1991).

Even the professional organizations that cite the health of clients as the central value encounter difficulties (see, e.g., International Council of Nurses, 1973; American Pharmaceutical Association, 1981; World Medical Association, 1983). In this case, the problem arises because a client's real goal is usually total well-being. Even if the practitioner can claim expertise in "health," it is still only one factor in the client's overall welfare. The Canadian Nurses Association (1991) takes particular care to avoid this difficulty by admonishing nurses to respect the "individual needs and values" of their clients; this injunction appears to recognize the client as the expert in judging what is in his or her own best interests.

2. The moral duties articulated in professional ethics documents may be broad (such as respecting the dignity and self-determination of one's clients) or specific (such as maintaining client confidentiality or not engaging in sexual relations with a client). The more general duties permit a certain amount of interpretation in their implementation by the individual practitioner, whereas the more specific ones

establish particular minimum standards for professional behavior.

There are, of course, gray areas, such as the duty of confidentiality. The duty to keep professional confidences secret is found in almost every professional ethic since the Hippocratic Oath. Yet exceptions to the general rule can be found. Until 1980, for example, the American Medical Association's "Principles of Medical Ethics" included an exception clause that permitted the disclosure of confidential information not only when required by law but also when "necessary in order to protect the welfare of the individual or of the community." Although most professional ethics documents allow for at least limited disclosure to ensure the safety of third parties, disclosure without consent for the benefit of the patient is suspect and subsequently has been dropped from the AMA "Principles of Medical Ethics." Also, although it is generally acceptable to disclose patient information when consulting with colleagues, there are rules governing such disclosure.

The presence of guidelines on safeguarding and disposing of written and computerized patient records emphasizes how seriously the duty to keep confidences is viewed by professions (see, e.g., British Medical Association, 1988; International Chiropractors Association, 1990). Although some discretion is permitted, the rules governing confidentiality still have the force of minimum requisite standards rather than ideals.

Some professional documents are organized around the distinction between ideal and minimalist standards (see, e.g., American Psychological Association, 1992, American College of Radiology, 1991). They begin with a set of general guidelines that are admittedly broad and explicitly not subject to sanction by the professional organization. These ideals are followed by the minimal rules of professional conduct, violations of which may be punishable by the organization.

3. Traditionally, philosophers have argued that moral behavior is governed primarily in one of two ways. Moral obligations, ideal or minimalist, may be specified, as in the documents just discussed. Alternatively, moral guidelines may focus on the character of the individual, with the assumption that moral behavior will flow naturally from a moral person.

Although the Prayer of Moses Maimonides is concerned primarily with specifying the virtues of a moral physician (Purtilo, 1977), many other professional ethics documents incorporate both basic standards of conduct and specific character traits, such as honesty, compassion, and integrity.

Even though a good or virtuous character may help a professional respond morally to a complex dilemma (in which, for example, specific duties conflict), the possession of a good character does not ensure morally right conduct. The moral character of an individual does, however, affect the way others perceive him or her. One is apt to have more regard for persons who act morally from good motives than for those who act morally simply because the rules require them to do so. Arguably a professional of good character is more trustworthy than one of poor character, and trust is an extremely important element in the relationship between client and professional.

DIFFICULTIES WITH PROFESSIONAL CODES. Professionally generated ethics documents are subject to a number of criticisms.

Monopoly and self-regulation. The most serious problems stem from the profession's power as an autonomous and self-regulating entity. The profession's monopoly on both setting and enforcing rules of conduct raises charges of elitism and opens the door to abuse of power. The presumption is that only professionals can know what constitutes ethical conduct for professionals and thus that they are the only ones who can evaluate the technical and moral quality of the services rendered.

It is true that professionals have been trained in a specialized body of knowledge that is not generally available to the layperson. That knowledge and professional judgment is part of the reason that society grants power and respect to a profession. However, professionals are neither uniquely nor the best equipped to make moral decisions (Veatch, 1973). Even if professionals were able to determine a client's best interest, they would have no special expertise in determining whether, for example, the client's interest, the client's rights, or the interests of society should take moral precedence in a given case.

Competing ethics. Historically, prayers, oaths, and certain codes have incorporated appeals to deities and/or the precepts of a broader religious or philosophical ethic into the professional mandate. Ludwig Edelstein (1943), for example, has argued that the Hippocratic Oath involves an application of Pythagorean principles to medicine. Some modern professional documents, such as the *Health Care Ethics Guide of the Catholic Health Association of Canada* (1991) and the *Islamic Code of Medical Ethics* (Islamic Organization of Medical Sciences, 1981), also explicitly place professional practice in the context of a larger ethic.

The generation of a professional ethic by modern secular professional organizations makes those organizations the functional equivalent of a religious or philosophical system and places them in direct competition with those systems, at least in their claim to know what is morally right in professional practice. In short, what the profession determines to be ethical is so, regardless of whether clients or other individuals in society agree. Of course, as illustrated by the variations between the codes authored by, for example, the medical associations of different countries (see Appendix, Section II), even secular professional ethics are influenced by the underlying values of the societies in which they are written. Furthermore, professional ethics are evolutionary and specific changes can be brought to bear from outside the profession. The significant moderation, if not obliteration, of traditional medical paternalism by societal demands for information and "informed consent" in decision making is one example of this point.

Self-policing. The self-policing of professionals raises a similar problem. If the profession does not find a practitioner to be at fault in an alleged ethics violation, there is no recourse to a general moral standard. Despite the requirement of many codes that unethical behavior by a colleague be reported, professionals may have a vested interest in not reporting or condemning violations by colleagues for fear of reprisal. They also may be deterred by the recognition that "everyone makes mistakes" and that they might be in a similar position in the future. An example of the closing of professional ranks appears in the American Academy of Orthopaedic *Surgeons' Guide to the Ethical Practice of Orthopaedic Surgery* (A.A.O.S., 1992, pp. 4–5, 9). Allegations raised by a professional against a colleague are investigated confidentially, and allegations brought by a patient, which admittedly are explicitly outside the auspices of the academy, are forwarded directly to the practitioner with a letter "urging him or her to contact the patient about the concern."

Although abuses of power can and do occur, mechanisms exist to limit them. International professional organizations, such as the World Medical Association, have arisen in part in an effort to forestall idiosyncratic, immoral practices of the sort that occurred in Nazi medicine. In addition, requiring that professionals report suspected violations, as well as maintaining, to the extent possible, the confidentiality of individuals who report them, and protecting such individuals from reprisal, helps to ensure that professionals will not be absolved of their responsibilities.

Business interests. Another criticism of professional codes is their excessive concern with nonmoral "business" interests, such as etiquette, fees, advertising, and the like, and the use of such measures to enhance professional prestige and prosperity. However, although such concerns are not specifically moral, they do have a moral component

and their presence in an ethics document can thereby be justified. Furthermore, although the potential for abuse exists, the same type of safeguards outlined above apply here as well.

Inadequate education. A persistent criticism of professional codes is that professionals themselves know very little about the content of their own codes. A survey of physicians revealed that most knew little or nothing about the contents of the AMA's Code of Medical Ethics. Few ethics educators in medical school incorporate the Code as a text in their courses. Michael Davis, an expert on professional codes of ethics at the Illinois Institute of Technology, agrees that a certain hostility to code ethics has existed in medicine for the last few decades. This can be contrasted to engineering, which generally is more receptive to code ethics, especially in the pedagogy of professional ethics. In the pre-electronic era, one could argue professional codes were inaccessible documents that gathered dust on library shelves. With the advent of the internet, however, this kind of complaint is hardly justified. Many of the professional codes in this newly revised appendix are easily accessible online and the AMA's Code of Medical Ethics is available completely online for no fee.

Generality. The remaining concerns with professional ethics documents are directed at the vagueness, conflicts, and idealism found in them. Many of the guidelines found in professional codes are intentionally vague. No document can or should pretend to foresee all eventualities and eliminate the need for individual discretion. In addition, ethics statements are "consensus documents." They reflect the general values and obligations held by most of the profession's members. The more specific such statements become, the more likely it is that there will be disagreement and loss of support for the moral authority of the document. For this reason, professional organizations address the more controversial topics in bioethics in separate documents that do not require ratification by the entire membership (Gass, 1978).

Similarly, resolutions to all conflicts of duty cannot be specified. The professional must rely on the values underlying the ethic, as well as his or her own conscience as informed by virtue, to determine the correct action when multiple duties conflict. Ethics codes may idealize the profession by suggesting that all professionals consistently possess all the virtues, uphold all the ideals, and reason through conflicts flawlessly. Holding professionals to such standards is, of course, unreasonable and may even be detrimental by undermining the motivation of those professionals who cannot, but feel they must, satisfy such expectations. Nevertheless, ideals serve as guides, as something to aspire to; if one aims high, one may land close to the goal.

As long as the difficulties with professionally generated ethics documents are recognized and accounted for both within and outside the profession, it seems that the documents do provide a standard by which questionable professional behavior can be judged. In addition, they are useful tools for generating professional awareness of the need for ethical discourse, which in turn helps to inform the internal ethic of individual practitioners.

Documents Directed Toward a Profession, but Generated Outside It

This category encompasses all bioethics documents that have direct implications for professional behavior, yet are authored by an "extraprofessional" group. The term "extraprofessional" refers to individuals who, in a specified setting, are not engaged in professional practice. Most commonly such documents are authored by an entity representing the public at large, such as a state licensing agency or other government body; a group within a field such as health care but outside of the profession(s) addressed; or a group representing a religious or philosophical ethic.

THE NATURE AND ROLES OF "EXTRAPROFESSIONAL" ETHICS DIRECTIVES. Typically, documents generated outside of a profession serve two main functions, either independently or concurrently. The first purpose is to regulate professional practice, thereby helping to limit the professional authority discussed in the previous section and addressing some of its potential abuses. Laws, regulations, and judicial decisions governing informed consent, advance directives, and research practices are examples of outside controls placed on professional practice.

Directives from outside professional organizations, such as the American Hospital Association's Patient's Bill of Rights (1973, 1992) serve a similar purpose. Rights documents are complex because they pertain not only to the individuals whose rights are being enumerated but also to the persons who are obliged to respect those rights. The American Hospital Association is, in effect, issuing guidelines governing ethical behavior for all individuals working at the facility, although in several instances the duties of physicians are singled out.

Extraprofessional documents that seek to regulate professional behavior tend to be minimalistic. Whereas professionally generated statements frequently articulate the ideals of character and behavior to which professionals should aspire, externally imposed standards are often generated in response to professional indiscretion and are designed to specify the limits to the range of acceptable professional conduct.

The second principal function of extraprofessional ethics statements is to focus attention on a broader ethic of which professional ethics is perceived by the authoring group to be a subset. Such documents derive norms for ethical practice from the values underlying a whole ethic or world view, rather than from the values underlying a specific profession. Whereas secular associations of health care professionals generally derive their ethical principles from the values of the profession, such as the health and well-being of clients, bioethics directives generated by religious bodies derive standards of practice from the values of the religion.

For example, the *Ethical and Religious Directives for Catholic Health Facilities* (United States Catholic Conference, 1975) outlines the practices that may and may not take place in Catholic facilities. Although many of the directives correspond directly to precepts already adhered to by healthcare practitioners, other directives, such as those concerning abortion and sterilization, reflect distinctly Catholic values and teaching. Although the directives are addressed to institutions, their force applies to the institutions' employees, including the professionals.

Other examples of religious or philosophical ethics being brought to bear on professional practice include the application of Jewish law to medical practice, for instance, to ascertain the moral licitness of neurological criteria for determining death, and the admonition of the old Oath of Soviet Physicians (1971) to follow the principles of communist morality in all of one's actions.

Documents that explicitly locate professional ethics within a religious or philosophical ethic tend to be idealistic in the same way that many professionally generated documents are. The goal is to provide a moral framework for professional practice. In contrast to the policing function of other extraprofessional documents, these documents attempt to define an ideal standard at which to aim.

Although some of the obligations articulated in extraprofessional documents—for example, those emphasizing duties to clients or to society—parallel those articulated in professionally generated statements, others specify the duties of professionals to an organization, institution, government, or other authority. In such cases, conflicts between the values and duties perceived by a profession and those articulated by the extraprofessional group are likely to arise.

Researchers, for example, might perceive their professional mandate to be the expansion of scientific knowledge, either generally or with the goal of aiding a specific population, such as persons with Alzheimer's disease, that might potentially benefit from the information acquired. They might further believe that the best means of advancing those goals is to violate an externally imposed ban on human fetal tissue transplantation research. Or nurses might believe that their professional mandate to care for the well-being of their client requires the violation of an institutional policy. In such cases, professionals face potential legal, monetary, or moral sanctions, on the one hand, or the loss of personal and/or professional integrity, on the other.

Such conflicts illustrate the more global problem of reconciling competing values in a pluralistic society (cf. Veatch and Mason, 1987). Professionals who simultaneously subscribe to a general religious or philosophical ethic—such as Catholicism, Islam, or libertarianism—and are members of a professional organization, or employees of an institution, that does not explicitly reflect that ethic are apt to find themselves in an untenable situation if personal values and professional duties conflict.

Some professionally generated documents attempt to address such conflicts by proscribing practices forbidden by law and by allowing, within certain confines, practitioners to withdraw from practices they find morally objectionable. The American Nurses' Association (1985) cautions its members that "neither physicians' orders nor the employing agency's policies relieve the nurse of accountability for actions taken and judgments made," implying that the precepts of the profession may outweigh the requirements of an institutional obligation. The Canadian Nurses Association (1991) advises that "prospective employers be informed of the provisions of [its] Code so that realistic and ethical expectations may be established at the beginning of the nurse-employer relationship."

Although such provisions may be of some assistance, their value may be limited by other provisions of the code. For example, a professional's right to withdraw from practices he or she deems morally offensive is conditional upon ensuring that the client is not abandoned, that is, the fundamental professional duty to care for the client ultimately takes precedence over one's personal ethic. Furthermore, even if a professional's personal morality were compatible with those of the professional association and the employing institution, the professional may still encounter conflict when a client with different values and beliefs requests a service deemed morally offensive by the professional.

Documents Directed Toward "Nonprofessionals"

The term "nonprofessional" here refers to two groups: (1) clients, for instance, patients or research subjects, and (2) persons engaged in nonprofessional work, such as orderlies,

hospital volunteers, or laboratory assistants. Since these groups do not have a self-imposed ethic other than a broad, societal one, bioethics directives pertaining to them usually are generated outside of the group by the same sources that apply to professionals. The implications, however, are rather different.

DIRECTIVES PERTAINING TO CLIENTS. Rights statements are directed at two distinct groups, those who hold rights and those who must respect them. Most of the rights documents in bioethics are not generated by individuals specifically representing the holders of the rights. For example, although groups advocating for health-care consumers helped to precipitate its establishment, the American Hospital Association's Patient's Bill of Rights (1973, 1992) was written by individuals representing member hospitals. Although the intention of protecting the interests of patients is admirable, it is not clear that the authoring group has any special expertise in determining what the rights of hospital patients actually are or should be. Similarly, the American Medical Association's Fundamental Elements of the Physician-Patient Relationship is a professionally generated document that outlines patients' rights to information, confidentiality, continuity of care, and so forth. Again, in one sense, this document sets forth the obligation of physicians to advance these rights (as such it is subject to the discussion in the first section), but in another sense, it claims authority for knowing what rights patients have, a task for which physicians are not necessarily the best suited.

In addition, rights documents, which presumably are intended to protect the rights-bearer, increasingly are accompanied by statements of the responsibilities of the rights-bearer. The American Medical Association, for example, includes among the responsibilities of patients the provision of accurate and complete information and compliance with the treatment plan and instructions of those responsible for the patient's care. It is not clear in any of the documents that issue joint statements of rights and responsibilities whether respect for the rights identified is contingent upon fulfillment of the specified responsibilities. Also not clear is why the authoring body has the moral authority to specify the responsibilities of those not members of the group.

Other bioethics documents affecting patients or research subjects are regulatory and/or governmental. Judicial and legislative actions as well as regulatory agencies and advisory bodies that represent the general populace are the closest the recipients of professional services come to a self-generated ethic. Even here, however, controversy arises over the extent to which patients and research subjects should be protected from others (and themselves). In the United States, the debates over access to experimental drugs by seriously ill patients and silicone implants by women seeking breast augmentation exemplify the dilemma.

Religious and broad philosophical ethics also affect individuals in this category. Usually individuals have elected to follow the precepts of a particular ethic in their overall existence and bring that ethic into whatever situation they encounter. As noted earlier, difficulties arise when one encounters a competing ethic. A traditional example is the difficulty faced by a Jehovah's Witness who refuses a potentially life-saving blood transfusion. On a larger scale, the imposition of one culture's beliefs upon another—for example, through regulations attached to financial assistance—poses the same problem.

DIRECTIVES PERTAINING TO NONPROFESSIONAL WORK-ERS. The final documents to be discussed are those that articulate standards for nonprofessional workers. Rights documents and other statements directed at institutions set minimal standards for all personnel, insofar as they apply, not just for professionals. Ethics directives that pertain to nonprofessionals tend to be minimalistic. They set guidelines protecting basic concerns such as respect, privacy, and competence, but unlike their professional counterparts, the job descriptions of nonprofessionals do not include a unique ethical mandate.

Nonprofessionals, like their professional counterparts, may be subject to certain duties to the institution or organization employing them. Similarly, nonprofessional workers are subject to moral standards articulated by legal and governmental bodies, as well as those stemming from religious or philosophical worldviews. The problem of conflicting duties arising from multiple moral authorities affects nonprofessionals, but not to the same degree as it plagues professionals. The conflicts faced by the nonprofessional are more analogous to those faced by any human being when the demands of law or one's employer conflict with a broader ethic that is perceived to be more fundamental. This is not to imply that these conflicts are any less difficult to resolve, only that their nature is different.

Conclusion

The number and diversity of bioethics documents reflect the pluralism of our world. When the ideologies expressed in these documents clash, controversy and conflicts may arise. In such cases, it is to be hoped that the documents will provide a basis for dialogue between the disagreeing parties.

Ethical dialogue can promote understanding and a resolution to the conflict, as well as an ongoing assessment of the precepts in question relative to their underlying ideologies.

CAROL MASON SPICER (1995)

BIBLIOGRAPHY

American Academy of Orthopaedic Surgeons. 1992. *Guide to the Ethical Practice of Orthopaedic Surgery.* 2nd ed. Park Ridge, IL: Author.

American Chiropractic Association. 1992. "Code of Ethics 1992–1993." In *1992–93 Membership Directory,* pp. B1–B11. Arlington, VA: Author.

American College of Radiology. 1991. *ACR 1991 Bylaws.* Reston, VA: Author.

American Dental Association. 1994. *ADA Principles of Ethics and Code of Professional Conduct.* Chicago: Author.

American Hospital Association. 1973, revised 1992. *A Patient's Bill of Rights.* Chicago: Author.

American Hospital Association. 1992. *A Patient's Bill of Rights Handbook.* Chicago: Author.

American Nurses' Association. 1985. *Code for Nurses with Interpretive Statements.* Kansas City, MO: Author.

American Pharmaceutical Association. 1981. *Code of Ethics.* Washington, D.C.: Author.

American Psychiatric Association. 1989. *The Principles of Medical Ethics with Annotations Especially Applicable to Psychiatry.* Washington, D.C.: Author.

American Psychological Association. 1992. "Ethical Principles of Psychologists and Code of Conduct." *American Psychologist* 47(12): 1597–1611.

Barber, Bernard. 1963. "Some Problems in the Sociology of the Professions." *Daedalus* 92(4): 669–688.

British Medical Association. 1988. *Philosophy and Practice of Medical Ethics.* London: Author.

Campbell, Dennis M. 1982. *Doctors, Lawyers, Ministers: Christian Ethics in Professional Practice.* Nashville, TN: Abingdon Press.

Canadian Medical Association. 1996 (1990). *Code of Ethics.* Ottawa: Author.

Canadian Medical Association. 1990b. *Guide to the Ethical Behaviour of Physicians.* Ottawa: Author.

Canadian Nurses Association. 1991. *Code of Ethics for Nursing.* Ottawa: Author.

Catholic Health Association of Canada. 1991. *Health Care Ethics Guide.* Ottawa: Author.

Edelstein, Ludwig. 1943. "The Hippocratic Oath: Text, Translation, and Interpretation." *Bulletin of the History of Medicine.* Suppl. no. 1: 1–64.

Freedman, Benjamin. 1989. "Bringing Codes to Newcastle: Ethics for Clinical Ethicists." In *Clinical Ethics: Theory and*

Practice, ed. Barry Hoffmaster, Benjamin Freedman, and Gwen Fraser. Clifton, NJ: Humana.

Gass, Ronald S. 1978. "Codes of the Health-Care Professions." In *Encyclopedia of Bioethics,* 2nd ed., ed. Warren T. Reich. New York: Macmillan and Free Press.

Germany (Territory Under Allied Occupation, 1945–1955: U.S. Zone). Military Tribunals. 1949. "Permissible Medical Experiments." In vol. 2 of *Trials of War Criminals before the Nuremberg Military Tribunals under Control Council Law No. 10, Nuremberg, October 1946-April 1949.* Washington D.C.: U.S. Government Printing Office.

Greenwood, Ernest. 1982. "Attributes of a Profession." In *Moral Responsibility and the Professions,* eds. Benjamin Freedman and Bernard H. Baumrin. New York: Haven.

International Chiropractors Association. 1990. "ICA Code of Professional Ethics [1987]." In *ICA Policy Handbook and Code of Ethics,* 2nd ed.. Arlington, VA.: Author.

International Council of Nurses. 1973. *Code for Nurses: Ethical Concepts Applied to Nursing.* Geneva: Author.

International Organization of Islamic Medicine. 1981. *Islamic Code of Medical Ethics: Kuwait Document.* Kuwait: Author.

Joint Commission on Accreditation of Healthcare Organizations. 1989. "Rights and Responsibilities of Patients." In *Accreditation Manual for Hospitals,* 1990. Chicago: Author.

Kultgen, John H. 1988. *Ethics and Professionalism.* Philadelphia: University of Pennsylvania Press.

Mahowald, Mary A. 1984. "Are Codes of Professional Ethics Ethical?" *Health Matrix* 8(2): 37–42.

National Federation of Societies for Clinical Social Work. Committee on Professional Standards. 1987. "National Federation of Societies for Clinical Social Work—Code of Ethics." *Clinical Social Work Journal* 15(1): 81–91.

Newton, Lisa H. 1988. "Lawgiving for Professional Life: Reflections of the Place of the Professional Code." In *Professional Ideals,* ed. Albert Flores. Belmont, CA: Wadsworth.

"Oath of Soviet Physicians." 1971. *Journal of the American Medical Association* 217(6): 834.

Percival, Thomas. 1927 (1803). *Percival's Medical Ethics, 1803.* Reprint. Edited by Chauncey D. Leake. Baltimore, MD: Williams and Wilkins.

Peterson, Susan R. 1987. "Professional Codes and Ethical Decision Making." In *Health Care Ethics: A Guide for Decision Makers,* eds. Gary R. Anderson and Valerie A. Glesnes-Anderson. Rockville, MD: Aspen Publishers.

Purtilo, Ruth B. 1977. "The American Physical Therapy Association's Code of Ethics." *Physical Therapy* 57(9): 1001–1006.

"Solemn Oath of the Physician of Russia (1992)." 1993. *Kennedy Institute of Ethics Journal* 3(4): 419.

United States Catholic Conference. 1975. *Ethical and Religious Directives for Catholic Health Facilities.* Washington, D.C.: Author.

Veatch, Robert M. 1973. "Generalization of Expertise: Scientific Expertise and Value Judgments." *Hastings Center Studies* 1(2): 29–40.

Veatch, Robert M.. 1991. "Is Trust of Professionals a Coherent Concept?" In *Ethics, Trust, and the Professions,* eds. Edmund D. Pellegrino, Robert M. Veatch, and John P. Langan. Washington, D.C.: Georgetown University Press.

Veatch, Robert M., and Mason, Carol G. 1987. "Hippocratic vs. Judeo-Christian Medical Ethics: Principles in Conflict." *Journal of Religious Ethics* 15(1): 86– 105.

World Medical Association. 1994 (1983). "Declaration of Geneva." Ferney-Voltaire, France: Author.

INTRODUCTION TO THE
CODES, OATHS, AND DIRECTIVES

• • •

The bioethics documents included in this Appendix are divided into six sections as listed in the table of contents. The first section contains documents that outline the health-related rights of individuals or address topics that are designed to implement such rights. The remaining sections contain directives that address the responsibilities of professionals, many of which can be understood as correlates of the rights of the individuals under their care or supervision.

The appendix for the third edition of the *Encyclopedia of Bioethics* has been substantially updated through online searches using the Google search engine. The internet has made many of these documents vastly more accessible. The careful researcher should use this appendix in tandem with his own online research. Frequently, these documents have their latest versions online.

Credits for the documents that appear in the Appendix can be found at the end of the Appendix.

SECTION I.

DIRECTIVES ON HEALTH-RELATED RIGHTS
AND PATIENT RESPONSIBILITIES

• • •

Constitution of the World Health Organization [1948]

Universal Declaration of Human Rights, General Assembly of the United Nations [1948]

Declaration of the Rights of the Child, General Assembly of the United Nations [1959]

Declaration on the Rights of Mentally Retarded Persons, General Assembly of the United Nations [1971]

A Patient's Bill of Rights, American Hospital Association [1973, revised 1992]

Declaration of Lisbon on the Rights of the Patient, World Medical Association [1981]

Declaration on Physician Independence and Professional Freedom, World Medical Association [1986]

Fundamental Elements of the Patient-Physician Relationship, American Medical Association [1990, updated 1993, 2001]

Patient Responsibilities, American Medical Association [1993, updated 2001]

Patient Rights, Joint Commission on Accreditation of Healthcare Organizations [1994]

The use of rights language has emerged in recent decades as a strong feature of contemporary bioethics documents. Although the language of rights cannot embrace all that must be said in bioethics, this collection of directives on health-related rights and patient responsibilities heads the Appendix both because it reinforces the common doctrine that all health care is patient-centered and because rights language has become typical of the period on which this edition is reporting.

Most of the documents in this section outline the health-related rights of specific groups of individuals, such as children, mentally retarded persons, and patients. Two documents, however, address topics that are designed to implement these rights. The World Medical Association's Declaration on Physician Independence and Professional Freedom addresses the importance of physicians' professional freedom to support patient rights. The American Medical Association (AMA) perceives patient rights and the corresponding patient responsibilities to be two elements of a mutually respectful alliance between patients and physicians. The AMA's directive on patient responsibilities elaborates upon the view expressed in the AMA's patient rights document, Fundamental Elements of the Patient-Physician Relationship, that "patients share with physicians the responsibility for their own health care."

CONSTITUTION OF THE WORLD HEALTH ORGANIZATION

1948

• • •

Originally adopted by the International Health Conference held in New York in June-July 1946 and signed by the representatives of sixty-one nations, the following statement is found in the Preamble to the Constitution of the World Health Organization, established in 1948. Especially significant elements are the controversial definition of health as "a state of complete physical, mental and social well-being and not merely the absence of disease or infirmity" and the recognition of health as a fundamental human right.

The States Parties to this Constitution declare, in conformity with the Charter of the United Nations, that the following principles are basic to the happiness, harmonious relations and security of all peoples:

Health is a state of complete physical, mental and social well-being and not merely the absence of disease or infirmity.

The enjoyment of the highest attainable standard of health is one of the fundamental rights of every human being without distinction of race, religion, political belief, economic or social condition.

The health of all peoples is fundamental to the attainment of peace and security and is dependent upon the fullest co-operation of individuals and States.

The achievement of any State in the promotion and protection of health is of value to all. Unequal

development in different countries in the promotion of health and control of disease, especially communicable disease, is a common danger.

Healthy development of the child is of basic importance; the ability to live harmoniously in a changing total environment is essential to such development.

The extension to all peoples of the benefits of medical, psychological and related knowledge is essential to the fullest attainment of health.

Informed opinion and active co-operation on the part of the public are of the utmost importance in the improvement of the health of the people.

Governments have a responsibility for the health of their peoples which can be fulfilled only by the provision of adequate health and social measures.

Accepting these principles, and for the purpose of co-operation among themselves and with others to promote and protect the health of all peoples, the Contracting parties agree to the present Constitution and hereby establish the World Health Organization as a specialized agency within the terms of Article 57 of the Charter of the United Nations.

UNIVERSAL DECLARATION OF HUMAN RIGHTS

General Assembly of the United Nations

1948

• • •

Adopted in 1948 by the General Assembly of the United Nations, the Universal Declaration of Human Rights is, as stated in its preamble, "a common standard of achievement for all peoples in all nations, to the end that every individual and every organ of society . . . shall strive by teaching and education to promote respect for these rights and freedoms and by progressive measures, national and international, to secure their universal and effective recognition and observance. . . . "

Article five should be compared to article seven of the International Covenant on Civil and Political Rights (Section IV). Article 25 directly pertains to health and healthcare.

ARTICLE 1

All human beings are born free and equal in dignity and rights. They are endowed with reason and conscience and should act towards one another in a spirit of brotherhood.

• • •

ARTICLE 3

Everyone has the right to life, liberty and the security of person.

. . .

ARTICLE 5

No one shall be subjected to torture or to cruel, inhuman or degrading treatment or punishment.

. . .

ARTICLE 16

1. Men and women of full age, without any limitation due to race, nationality or religion, have the right to marry and to found a family. They are entitled to equal rights as to marriage, during marriage and at its dissolution.
2. Marriage shall be entered into only with the free and full consent of the intending spouses.
3. The family is the natural and fundamental group unit of society and is entitled to protection by society and the State.

. . .

ARTICLE 25

1. Everyone has the right to a standard of living adequate for the health and well-being of himself and of his family, including food, clothing, housing and medical care and necessary social services, and the right to security in the event of unemployment, sickness, disability, widowhood, old age or other lack of livelihood in circumstances beyond his control.
2. Motherhood and childhood are entitled to special care and assistance. All children, whether born in or out of wedlock, shall enjoy the same social protection.

DECLARATION OF THE RIGHTS OF THE CHILD

General Assembly of the United Nations

1959

. . .

Adopted unanimously by the General Assembly of the United Nations on November 20, 1959, the Declaration of the Rights of the Child emphasizes the physical, mental, and moral health and development of children.

. . .

"Whereas the child by reason of his physical and mental immaturity, needs special safeguards and care, including appropriate legal protection, before as well as after birth.

. . .

The General Assembly

"Proclaims this Declaration of the Rights of the Child to the end that he may have a happy childhood and enjoy for his own good and for the good of society the rights and freedoms herein set forth, and calls upon parents, upon men and women as individuals, and upon voluntary organizations, local authorities and national Governments to recognize these rights and strive for their observance by legislative and other measures progressively taken in accordance with the following principles:

PRINCIPLE 1

"The child shall enjoy all the rights set forth in this Declaration. Every child, without any exception whatsoever, shall be entitled to these rights, without distinction or discrimination on account of race, colour, sex, language, religion, political or other opinion, national or social origin, property, birth or other status, whether of himself or of his family.

PRINCIPLE 2

"The child shall enjoy special protection, and shall be given opportunities and facilities, by law and by other means, to enable him to develop physically, mentally, morally, spiritually and socially in a healthy and normal manner and in conditions of freedom and dignity. In the enactment of laws for this purpose, the best interests of the child shall be the paramount considerations.

PRINCIPLE 3

"The child shall be entitled from his birth to a name and a nationality.

PRINCIPLE 4

"The child shall enjoy the benefits of social security. He shall be entitled to grow and develop in health; to this end, special care and protection shall be provided both to him and to his mother, including adequate pre-natal and post-natal care. The child shall have the right to adequate nutrition, housing, recreation and medical services.

PRINCIPLE 5

"The child who is physically, mentally or socially handicapped shall be given the special treatment, education and care required by his particular condition.

PRINCIPLE 6

"The child, for the full and harmonious development of his personality, needs love and understanding. He shall, wherever possible, grow up in the care and under the responsibility of his parents, and, in any case, in an atmosphere of affection and of moral and material security; a child of tender years shall not, save in exceptional circumstances, be separated from his mother. Society and the public authorities shall have the duty to extend particular care to children without a family and to those without adequate means of support. Payment of State and other assistance towards the maintenance of children of large families is desirable.

PRINCIPLE 7

"The child is entitled to receive education, which shall be free and compulsory, at least in the elementary stages. He shall be given an education which will promote his general culture, and enable him, on a basis of equal opportunity, to develop his abilities, his individual judgement, and his sense of moral and social responsibility, and to become a useful member of society.

"The best interests of the child shall be the guiding principle of those responsible for his education and guidance; that responsibility lies in the first place with his parents.

"The child shall have full opportunity for play and recreation, which should be directed to the same purposes as education; society and the public authorities shall endeavour to promote the enjoyment of this right.

PRINCIPLE 8

"The child shall in all circumstances be among the first to receive protection and relief.

PRINCIPLE 9

"The child shall be protected against all forms of neglect, cruelty and exploitation. He shall not be the subject of traffic, in any form.

"The child shall not be admitted to employment before an appropriate minimum age; he shall in no case be caused or permitted to engage in any occupation or employment which would prejudice his health or education, or interfere with his physical, mental or moral development.

PRINCIPLE 10

"The child shall be protected from practices which may foster racial, religious and any other form of discrimination. He shall be brought up in a spirit of understanding, tolerance, friendship among peoples, peace and universal brotherhood, and in full consciousness that his energy and talents should be devoted to the service of his fellow men."

DECLARATION ON THE RIGHTS OF MENTALLY RETARDED PERSONS

General Assembly of the United Nations

1971

. . .

The following Declaration on the Rights of Mentally Retarded Persons was adopted by the General Assembly of the United Nations on December 20, 1971. It is a revised and amended version of the Declaration of General and Special Rights of the Mentally Retarded that was adopted in 1968 by the International League of Societies for the Mentally Handicapped.

. . .

1. The mentally retarded person has, to the maximum degree of feasibility, the same rights as other human beings.
2. The mentally retarded person has a right to proper medical care and physical therapy and to such education, training, rehabilitation and guidance as will enable him to develop his ability and maximum potential.
3. The mentally retarded person has a right to economic security and to a decent standard of living. He has a right to perform productive work or to engage in any other meaningful occupation to the fullest possible extent of his capabilities.
4. Whenever possible, the mentally retarded person should live with his own family or with foster parents and participate in different forms of community life. The family with which he lives should receive assistance. If care in an institution becomes necessary, it should be provided in surroundings and other circumstances as close as possible to those of normal life.
5. The mentally retarded person has a right to a qualified guardian when this is required to protect his personal well-being and interests.
6. The mentally retarded person has a right to protection from exploitation, abuse and degrading

treatment. If prosecuted for any offence, he shall have a right to due process of law with full recognition being given to his degree of mental responsibility.

7. Whenever mentally retarded persons are unable, because of the severity of their handicap, to exercise all their rights in a meaningful way or it should become necessary to restrict or deny some or all of these rights, the procedure used for that restriction or denial of rights must contain proper legal safeguards against every form of abuse. This procedure must be based on an evaluation of the social capability of the mentally retarded person by qualified experts and must be subject to periodic review and to the right of appeal to higher authorities.

A PATIENT'S BILL OF RIGHTS

American Hospital Association

1973, REVISED 1992

• • •

In 1973, the American Hospital Association's House of Delegates adopted A Patient's Bill of Rights, which was influential in the development of similar documents in other parts of the world. The first revision of the document, and the only one to date, was approved in 1992. Some of the most notable changes from the 1973 document include: (1) deletion of the "therapeutic privilege" clause that permitted information regarding a patient's condition to be disclosed to family, rather than to the patient, when it was "not medically advisable to give such information to the patient"; (2) addition of the right to execute advance directives; (3) addition of a clause indicating that otherwise confidential information may be released when permitted or required by law for the benefit of third parties; (4) addition of the patients' right to review their medical records; (5) addition of the clarification that a patient's right to expect a hospital to reasonably respond to requests for care and services is limited to those that are "appropriate and medically indicated"; and (6) addition of a list of patient responsibilities.

Introduction

Effective health care requires collaboration between patients and physicians and other health care professionals. Open and honest communication, respect for personal and professional values, and sensitivity to differences are integral to optimal patient care. As the setting for the provision of health services, hospitals must provide a foundation for understanding and respecting the rights and responsibilities of patients, their families, physicians, and other caregivers. Hospitals must ensure a health care ethic that respects the role of patients in decision making about treatment choices

and other aspects of their care. Hospitals must be sensitive to cultural, racial, linguistic, religious, age, gender, and other differences as well as the needs of persons with disabilities.

The American Hospital Association presents A Patient's Bill of Rights with the expectation that it will contribute to more effective patient care and be supported by the hospital on behalf of the institution, its medical staff, employees, and patients. The American Hospital Association encourages health care institutions to tailor this bill of rights to their patient community by translating and/or simplifying the language of this bill of rights as may be necessary to ensure that patients and their families understand their rights and responsibilities.

Bill of Rights*

1. The patient has the right to considerate and respectful care.

2. The patient has the right to and is encouraged to obtain from physicians and other direct caregivers relevant, current, and understandable information concerning diagnosis, treatment, and prognosis.

   Except in emergencies when the patient lacks decision-making capacity and the need for treatment is urgent, the patient is entitled to the opportunity to discuss and request information related to the specific procedures and/or treatments, the risks involved, the possible length of recuperation, and the medically reasonable alternatives and their accompanying risks and benefits.

   Patients have the right to know the identity of physicians, nurses, and others involved in their care, as well as when those involved are students, residents, or other trainees. The patient also has the right to know the immediate and long-term financial implications of treatment choices, insofar as they are known.

3. The patient has the right to make decisions about the plan of care prior to and during the course of treatment and to refuse a recommended treatment or plan of care to the extent permitted by law and hospital policy and to be informed of the medical consequences of this action. In case of such refusal, the patient is entitled to other appropriate care and services that the hospital provides or transfer to another hospital. The hospital should notify patients of any policy that might affect patient choice within the institution.

4. The patient has the right to have an advance directive (such as a living will, health care proxy, or durable power of attorney for health care) concerning treatment or designating a surrogate decision

maker with the expectation that the hospital will honor the intent of that directive to the extent permitted by law and hospital policy. Health care institutions must advise patients of their rights under state law and hospital policy to make informed medical choices, ask if the patient has an advance directive, and include that information in patient records. The patient has the right to timely information about hospital policy that may limit its ability to implement fully a legally valid advance directive.

5. The patient has the right to every consideration of privacy. Case discussion, consultation, examination, and treatment should be conducted so as to protect each patient's privacy.

6. The patient has the right to expect that all communications and records pertaining to his/her care will be treated as confidential by the hospital, except in cases such as suspected abuse and public health hazards when reporting is permitted or required by law. The patient has the right to expect that the hospital will emphasize the confidentiality of this information when it releases it to any other parties entitled to review information in these records.

7. The patient has the right to review the records pertaining to his/her medical care and to have the information explained or interpreted as necessary, except when restricted by law.

8. The patient has the right to expect that, within its capacity and policies, a hospital will make reasonable response to the request of a patient for appropriate and medically indicated care and services. The hospital must provide evaluation, service, and/or referral as indicated by the urgency of the case. When medically appropriate and legally permissible, or when a patient has so requested, a patient may be transferred to another facility. The institution to which the patient is to be transferred must first have accepted the patient for transfer. The patient must also have the benefit of complete information and explanation concerning the need for, risks, benefits, and alternatives to such a transfer.

9. The patient has the right to ask and to be informed of the existence of business relationships among the hospital, educational institutions, other health care providers, or payers that may influence the patient's treatment and care.

10. The patient has the right to consent to or decline to participate in proposed research studies or human experimentation affecting care and treatment or requiring direct patient involvement, and to have those studies fully explained prior to consent. A patient who declines to participate in research or experimentation is entitled to the most effective care that the hospital can otherwise provide.

11. The patient has the right to expect reasonable continuity of care when appropriate and to be informed by physicians and other caregivers of available and realistic patient care options when hospital care is no longer appropriate.

12. The patient has the right to be informed of hospital policies and practices that relate to patient care, treatment, and responsibilities. The patient has the right to be informed of available resources for resolving disputes, grievances, and conflicts, such as ethics committees, patient representatives, or other mechanisms available in the institution. The patient has the right to be informed of the hospital's charges for services and available payment methods.

The collaborative nature of health care requires that patients, or their families/surrogates, participate in their care. The effectiveness of care and patient satisfaction with the course of treatment depend, in part, on the patient fulfilling certain responsibilities. Patients are responsible for providing information about past illnesses, hospitalizations, medications, and other matters related to health status. To participate effectively in decision making, patients must be encouraged to take responsibility for requesting additional information or clarification about their health status or treatment when they do not fully understand information and instructions. Patients are also responsible for ensuring that the health care institution has a copy of their written advance directive if they have one. Patients are responsible for informing their physicians and other caregivers if they anticipate problems in following prescribed treatment.

Patients should also be aware of the hospital's obligation to be reasonably efficient and equitable in providing care to other patients and the community. The hospital's rules and regulations are designed to help the hospital meet this obligation. Patients and their families are responsible for making reasonable accommodations to the needs of the hospital, other patients, medical staff, and hospital employees. Patients are responsible for providing necessary information for insurance claims and for working with the hospital to make payment arrangements, when necessary.

A person's health depends on much more than health care services. Patients are responsible for recognizing the impact of their life-style on their personal health.

Conclusion

Hospitals have many functions to perform, including the enhancement of health status, health promotion, and the prevention and treatment of injury and disease; the immediate and ongoing care and rehabilitation of patients; the education of health professionals, patients, and the community; and research. All these activities must be conducted with an overriding concern for the values and dignity of patients.

These rights can be exercised on the patient's behalf by a designated surrogate or proxy decision maker if the patient lacks decision-making capacity, is legally incompetent, or is a minor.

DECLARATION OF LISBON ON THE RIGHTS OF THE PATIENT

World Medical Association

1981, 1995

• • •

Whereas most of the early documents on patients' rights, such as the American Hospital Association's A Patient's Bill of Rights, focus on the rights of individuals within healthcare facilities (hospitals, nursing homes), the Declaration of Lisbon, adopted in 1981 by the 34th World Medical Assembly at Lisbon, is an international statement of the rights of patients in general. In conjunction with the International Code of Medical Ethics (Section II), it illustrates the relatively recent emphasis placed on "the rights of patients" in addition to the traditional "duties of physicians." Physicians not only "ought" to behave in certain ways, but patients also are entitled to have them do so. The Declaration of Lisbon was amended by the 47th General Assembly in Bali, Indonesia in September, 1995. This most recent version provides much more detail regarding the nature of the rights patients possess, particularly rights to quality information and health education.

Preamble

The relationship between physicians, their patients and broader society has undergone significant changes in recent times. While a physician should always act according to his/her conscience, and always in the best interests of the patient, equal effort must be made to guarantee patient autonomy and justice. The following Declaration represents some of the principal rights of the patient which the medical profession endorses and promotes. Physicians and other persons or bodies involved in the provision of health care have a joint responsibility to recognize and uphold these rights. Whenever legislation, government action or any other administration or institution denies patients these rights, physicians should pursue appropriate means to assure or to restore them.

In the context of biomedical research involving human subjects—including non therapeutic biomedical research—the subject is entitled to the same rights and consideration as any patient in a normal therapeutic situation.

Principles

1. Right to medical care of good quality
   a. Every person is entitled without discrimination to appropriate medical care.
   b. Every patient has the right to be cared for by a physician whom he/she knows to be free to make clinical and ethical judgements without any outside interference.
   c. The patient shall always be treated in accordance with his/her best interests. The treatment applied shall be in accordance with generally approved medical principles.
   d. Quality assurance always should be a part of health care. Physicians, in particular, should accept responsibility for being guardians of the quality of medical services.
   e. In circumstances where a choice must be made between potential patients for a particular treatment which is in limited supply, all such patients are entitled to a fair selection procedure for that treatment. That choice must be based on medical criteria and made without discrimination.
   f. The patient has the right of continuity of health care. The physician has an obligation to cooperate in the coordination of medically indicated care with other health care providers treating the patient. The physician may not discontinue treatment of a patient as long as further treatment is medically indicated, without giving the patient reasonable assistance and sufficient opportunity to make alternative arrangements for care.
2. Right to freedom of choice
   a. The patient has the right to choose freely and change his/her physician and hospital or health service institution, regardless of whether they are based in the private or public sector.
   b. The patient has the right to ask for the opinion of another physician at any stage.
3. Right to self-determination
   a. The patient has the right to self-determination, to make free decisions regarding himself/herself. The physician will inform the patient of the consequences of his/her decisions.
   b. A mentally competent adult patient has the right to give or withhold consent to any diagnostic

procedure or therapy. The patient has the right to the information necessary to make his/her decisions. The patient should understand clearly what is the purpose of any test or treatment, what the results would imply, and what would be the implications of withholding consent.

c. The patient has the right to refuse to participate in research or the teaching of medicine.

4. The unconscious patient

a. If the patient is unconscious or otherwise unable to express his/her will, informed consent must be obtained whenever possible, from a legally entitled representative where legally relevant.

b. If a legally entitled representative is not available, but a medical intervention is urgently needed, consent of the patient may be presumed, unless it is obvious and beyond any doubt on the basis of the patient's previous firm expression or conviction that he/she would refuse consent to the intervention in that situation.

c. However, physicians should always try to save the life of a patient unconscious due to a suicide attempt.

5. The legally incompetent patient

a. If a patient is a minor or otherwise legally incompetent the consent of a legally entitled representative, where legally relevant, is required. Nevertheless the patient must be involved in the decision making to the fullest extent allowed by his/her capacity.

b. If the legally incompetent patient can make rational decisions, his/her decisions must be respected, and he/she has the right to forbid the disclosure of information to his/her legally entitled representative.

c. If the patient's legally entitled representative, or a person authorized by the patient, forbids treatment which is, in the opinion of the physician, in the patient's best interest, the physician should challenge this decision in the relevant legal or other institution. In case of emergency, the physician will act in the patient's best interest.

6. Procedures against the patient's will

a. Diagnostic procedures or treatment against the patient's will can be carried out only in exceptional cases, if specifically permitted by law and conforming to the principles of medical ethics.

7. Right to information

a. The patient has the right to receive information about himself/herself recorded in any of his/her medical records, and to be fully informed about his/her health status including the medical facts about his/her condition. However, confidential information in the patient's records about a third party should not be given to the patient without the consent of that third party.

b. Exceptionally, information may be withheld from the patient when there is good reason to believe that this information would create a serious hazard to his/her life or health.

c. Information must be given in a way appropriate to the local culture and in such a way that the patient can understand.

d. The patient has the right not to be informed on his/her explicit request, unless required for the protection of another person's life.

e. The patient has the right to choose who, if anyone, should be informed on his/her behalf.

8. Right to confidentiality

a. All identifiable information about a patient's health status, medical condition, diagnosis, prognosis and treatment and all other information of a personal kind, must be kept confidential, even after death. Exceptionally, descendants may have a right of access to information that would inform them of their health risks.

b. Confidential information can only be disclosed if the patient gives explicit consent or if expressly provided for in the law. Information can be disclosed to other health care providers only on a strictly "need to know" basis unless the patient has given explicit consent.

c. All identifiable patient data must be protected. The protection of the data must be appropriate to the manner of its storage. Human substances from which identifiable data can be derived must be likewise protected.

9. Right to health education

a. Every person has the right to health education that will assist him/her in making informed choices about personal health and about the available health services. The education should include information about healthy lifestyles and about methods of prevention and early detection of illnesses. The personal responsibility of everybody for his/her own health should be stressed. Physicians have an obligation to participate actively in educational efforts.

10. Right to dignity

a. The patient's dignity and right to privacy shall be respected at all times in medical care and teaching, as shall his/her culture and values.

b. The patient is entitled to relief of his/her suffering according to the current state of knowledge.

  c. The patient is entitled to humane terminal care
     and to be provided with all available assistance in
     making dying as dignified and comfortable as
     possible.
11. Right to religious assistance
  a. The patient has the right to receive or to decline
     spiritual and moral comfort including the help of
     a minister of his/her chosen religion.

DECLARATION ON PHYSICIAN INDEPENDENCE AND PROFESSIONAL FREEDOM

World Medical Association

1986

• • •

Adopted in 1986 by the 38th World Medical Assembly at Rancho Mirage, California, this declaration elaborates on section (b) of the 1981 Declaration of Lisbon. Of interest is the declaration's assertion of the need for professional independence in order to ensure the rights of patients and to fulfill professional obligations to them. The document emphasizes concern over conflicts of interest in the area of cost containment and asserts that physicians must advocate for their individual patients.

The World Medical Association, Inc., recognizing the importance of the physician's independence and professional freedom, hereby adopts the following declaration of principles:

Physicians must recognize and support the rights of their patients, particularly as set forth in the World Medical Association Declaration of Lisbon (1981).

Physicians must have the professional freedom to care for their patients without interference. The exercise of the physician's professional judgement and discretion in making clinical and ethical decisions in the care and treatment of patients must be preserved and protected.

Physicians must have the professional independence to represent and defend the health needs of patients against all who would deny or restrict needed care for those who are sick or injured.

Within the context of their medical practice and the care of their patients, physicians should not be expected to administer governmental or social priorities in the allocation of scarce health resources. To do so would be to create a conflict of interest with the physician's obligation to his

patients, and would effectively destroy the physician's professional independence, upon which the patient relies.

While physicians must be conscious of the cost of medical treatment and actively participate in cost containment efforts within medicine, it is the physician's primary obligation to represent the interests of the sick and injured against demands by society for cost containment that would endanger patients' health and perhaps patients' life.

By providing independence and professional freedom for physicians to practice medicine, a community assures the best possible health care for its citizens, which in turn contributes to a strong and secure society.

FUNDAMENTAL ELEMENTS OF THE PATIENT-PHYSICIAN RELATIONSHIP

American Medical Association

1990, UPDATED 1993

• • •

This document, which constitutes one part of the American Medical Association's complete code of ethics, extends the rights language introduced in the 1980 Principles of Medical Ethics (Section II) to a separate statement listing the specific rights of patients. The opening paragraph of the Fundamental Elements also mentions the responsibilities of patients. Points of particular interest include: (1) Right #4 on confidentiality, which contains the therapeutic privilege exception dropped from the Principles of Medical Ethics in 1980 and still not restored to the principles themselves; (2) Right #5 on continuity of care, which implies that treatment may be discontinued, without making alternative arrangements for care, when further treatment is not "medically indicated"; and (3) Right #6, which establishes a basic right to adequate health care, but explicitly does not guarantee the fulfillment of such a right.

From ancient times, physicians have recognized that the health and well-being of patients depends upon a collaborative effort between physician and patient. Patients share with physicians the responsibility for their own health care. The patient-physician relationship is of greatest benefit to patients when they bring medical problems to the attention of their physicians in a timely fashion, provide information about their medical condition to the best of their ability, and work with their physicians in a mutually respectful alliance. Physicians can best contribute to this alliance by serving as their patients' advocate and by fostering these rights:

1. The patient has the right to receive information
   from physicians and to discuss the benefits, risks,

and costs of appropriate treatment alternatives. Patients should receive guidance from their physicians as to the optimal course of action. Patients are also entitled to obtain copies or summaries of their medical records, to have their questions answered, to be advised of potential conflicts of interest that their physicians might have, and to receive independent professional opinions.

2. The patient has the right to make decisions regarding the health care that is recommended by his or her physician. Accordingly, patients may accept or refuse any recommended medical treatment.

3. The patient has the right to courtesy, respect, dignity, responsiveness, and timely attention to his or her needs.

4. The patient has the right to confidentiality. The physician should not reveal confidential communications or information without the consent of the patient, unless provided for by law or by the need to protect the welfare of the individual or the public interest.

5. The patient has the right to continuity of health care. The physician has an obligation to cooperate in the coordination of medically indicated care with other health care providers treating the patient. The physician may not discontinue treatment of a patient as long as further treatment is medically indicated, without giving the patient reasonable assistance and sufficient opportunity to make alternative arrangements for care.

6. The patient has a basic right to have available adequate health care. Physicians, along with the rest of society, should continue to work toward this goal. Fulfillment of this right is dependent on society providing resources so that no patient is deprived of necessary care because of an inability to pay for the care. Physicians should continue their traditional assumption of a part of the responsibility for the medical care of those who cannot afford essential health care. Physicians should advocate for patients in dealing with third parties when appropriate.

PATIENT RESPONSIBILITIES

American Medical Association

1993, UPDATED 1998, 2000 AND 2001

• • •

The American Medical Association's (AMA) Patient Responsibilities draws upon the recognition, articulated in the preceding Fundamental

Elements of the Patient-Physician Relationship, that successful medical care depends upon a collaborative effort between physicians and patients. Originally published in July 1993 as Report 52 in the AMA Code of Medical Ethics: Reports of the Council on Ethical and Judicial Affairs, Patient Responsibilities expands upon the Fundamental Elements document by specifying the responsibilities of patients for their own health care. It has been updated three times since its creation in 1993.

The background section of the original report states: "Like patients' rights, patients' responsibilities are derived from the principle of autonomy. . . . With that exercise of self-governance and free choice comes a number of responsibilities." The list of those patient responsibilities follows.

1. Good communication is essential to a successful physician-patient relationship. To the extent possible, patients have a responsibility to be truthful and to express their concerns clearly to their physicians.

2. Patients have a responsibility to provide a complete medical history, to the extent possible, including information about past illnesses, medications, hospitalizations, family history of illness and other matters relating to present health.

3. Patients have a responsibility to request information or clarification about their health status or treatment when they do not fully understand what has been described.

4. Once patients and physicians agree upon the goals of therapy, patients have a responsibility to cooperate with the treatment plan and to keep their agreed-upon appointments. Compliance with physician instructions is often essential to public and individual safety. Patients also have a responsibility to disclose whether previously agreed upon treatments are being followed and to indicate when they would like to reconsider the treatment plan.

5. Patients generally have a responsibility to meet their financial obligations with regard to medical care or to discuss financial hardships with their physicians. Patients should be cognizant of the costs associated with using a limited resource like health care and try to use medical resources judiciously.

6. Patients should discuss end of life decisions with their physicians and make their wishes known. Such a discussion might also include writing an advance directive.

7. Patients should be committed to health maintenance through health-enhancing behavior. Illness can often be prevented by a healthy lifestyle, and patients must take personal responsibility when they are able to avert the development of disease.

8. Patients should also have an active interest in the effects of their conduct on others and refrain from behavior that unreasonably places the health of others at risk. Patients should inquire as to the

means and likelihood of infectious disease transmission and act upon that information which can best prevent further transmission.

9. Participation in medical education is to the mutual benefit of patients and the health care system. Patients are encouraged to participate in medical education by accepting care, under appropriate supervision, from medical students, residents, and other trainees. Consistent with the process of informed consent, the patient or the patient's surrogate decision maker is always free to refuse care from any member of the health care team.

10. Patients should discuss organ donation with their physicians and, if donation is desired, make applicable provisions. Patients who are part of an organ allocation system and await needed transplant should not try to go outside of or manipulate the system. A fair system of allocation should be answered with public trust and an awareness of limited resources.

11. Patients should not initiate or participate in fraudulent health care and should report illegal or unethical behavior by providers to the appropriate medical societies, licensing boards, or law enforcement authorities.

PATIENT RIGHTS

Joint Commission on Accreditation of Healthcare Organizations

1994

• • •

Patient Rights is a section of the Joint Commission on Accreditation of Healthcare Organizations' (JCAHO) Accreditation Manual for Hospitals, 1994. Although many healthcare organizations demonstrate their recognition and support of patient/client rights by issuing lists of those rights, no list can assure that the rights are respected. The standards on patient rights included in JCAHO's Accreditation Manual are designed to reflect the implementation, as well as the existence, of institutional policies and procedures for the exercise and protection of a specified set of patient rights.

The scoring of the standards in this chapter will reflect evidence of the implementation of policies and procedures as well as the existence of such policies and procedures.

RI.1 The organization supports the rights of each patient.

RI.1.1 Organizational policies and procedures describe the mechanisms by which the following rights are protected and exercised:

Intent of RI.1 and RI.1.1

The policies and procedures that guide the organization's interaction with and care of the patient demonstrate its recognition and support of patient rights.

No listing of patient rights can assure the respect of those rights. It is the intent of these standards that the organization's interaction with and care of the patient reflect concern and respect for the rights of the patient.

The organization's policies and procedures describe the mechanisms or processes established to support the following patient rights:

• Reasonable access to care;
• Considerate (and respectful) care that respects the patient's personal value and belief systems;
• Informed participation in decisions regarding his/her care;
• Participation in the consideration of ethical issues that arise in the provision of his or her care;
• Personal privacy and confidentiality of information;
• Designation of a representative decision maker in the event that the patient is incapable of understanding a proposed treatment or procedure or is unable to communicate his/her wishes regarding care.

• • •

RI.1.1.1 [Organizational policies and procedures describe the mechanisms by which the following rights are protected and exercised:] The right of the patient to the hospital's reasonable response to his/her requests and needs for treatment or service, within the hospital's capacity, its stated mission, and applicable law and regulation;

Intent of RI.1.1.1

In response to the patient's request and need, the organization provides care that is within its capacity, its stated mission and philosophy, and applicable law and regulation. When the organization cannot meet the request or need for care because of a conflict with its mission or philosophy or incapacity to meet the patient's needs or requests, the patient may be transferred to another facility when medically permissible. Such a transfer is made only after the patient has received complete information and explanation concerning the need for and alternatives to such a transfer. The transfer must be acceptable to the receiving organization.

• • •

RI.1.1.2 [Organizational policies and procedures describe the mechanisms by which the following rights are protected and exercised:] The right of the patient to considerate and respectful care;

RI1.1.2.1 The care of the patient includes consideration of the psychosocial, spiritual, and cultural variables that influence the perceptions of illness.

Intent of RI.1.1.2 and RI.1.1.2.1

The provision of patient care reflects consideration of the patient as an individual with personal values and a belief system that impact his/her attitude toward and response to the care provided by the organization. The organizational policies and procedures that guide patient care include recognition of the psychosocial, spiritual, and cultural values that affect the patient's response to the care given. Organizational policies and procedures allow the patient to express spiritual beliefs and cultural practices that do not harm others or interfere with the planned course of medical therapy for the patient.

• • •

RI.1.1.2.2 The care of the dying patient optimizes the comfort and dignity of the patient through

RI.1.1.2.2.1 treating primary and secondary symptoms that respond to treatment as desired by the patient or surrogate decision maker;

RI.1.1.2.2.2 effectively managing pain; and

RI.1.1.2.2.3 acknowledging the psychosocial and spiritual concerns of the patient and the family regarding dying and the expression of grief by the patient and family.

NOTE: *The term dying is used to refer to an incurable and irreversible condition such that death is imminent. Imminent is seen as impending or about to happen.*

Intent of RI.1.1.2.2 Through RI.1.1.2.2.3

All hospital staff are sensitized to the needs of the dying patient in an acute care hospital. Support for the psychological, social, emotional, and spiritual needs of the patient and family demonstrates respect for the patient's values, religion, and philosophy. The goal of respectful, responsive care of the dying patient is to optimize the patient's comfort and dignity by providing appropriate treatment for primary and secondary symptoms as desired by the patient or surrogate

decision maker, responding to the psychosocial, emotional, and spiritual concerns of the patient and family, and managing pain aggressively. (The management of pain is appropriate for all patients, not just dying patients. Guidelines such as those published by the Agency for Health Care Policy and Research for Acute Pain Management reflect the state of knowledge on effective and appropriate care for all patients experiencing acute pain.)

• • •

RI.1.1.3 [Organizational policies and procedures describe the mechanisms by which the following rights are protected and exercised:]The right of the patient, in collaboration with his/her physician, to make decisions involving his/her health care, including

RI.1.1.3.1 the right of the patient to accept medical care or to refuse treatment to the extent permitted by law and to be informed of the medical consequences of such refusal, and

RI.1.1.3.2 the right of the patient to formulate advance directives and appoint a surrogate to make health care decisions on his/her behalf to the extent permitted by law.

RI.1.1.3.2.1 The organization has in place a mechanism to ascertain the existence of and assist in the development of advance directives at the time of the patient's admission.

RI.1.1.3.2.2 The provision of care is not conditioned on the existence of an advance directive.

RI.1.1.3.2.3 Any advance directive(s) is in the patient's medical record and is reviewed periodically with the patient or surrogate decision maker.

Intent of RI.1.1.3 Through RI.1.1.3.2.3

The quality of patient care is enhanced when the patient's preferences are incorporated into plans for care. The process by which care and treatment decisions are made elicit respect and incorporate the patient's preferences. Sound medical judgment is provided to the patient or the patient's surrogate decision maker for informed decision making.

In hospitals providing services to neonate, child, and adolescent patients, a mechanisms exists that is designed to coordinate and facilitate the family's and/or guardian's involvement in decision making throughout the course of treatment. The patient is responsible for providing, to the best of his/her knowledge, accurate and complete information about present complaints, past illnesses, hospitalizations, medications, advance directives, and other matters relevant to his/her health or care. The patient is also responsible for reporting whether he/she clearly comprehends a contemplated course of action and what is expected of him/her.

The hospital ascertains the existence of advance directives, and health care professionals and surrogate decision makers honor them within the limits of the law and the organization's mission and philosophy. An advance directive is a document a person uses to give directions about future medical care or to designate another person to give directions about medical care should he/she lose decision-making capacity. Advance directives may include living wills, durable powers of attorney, or similar documents and contain the patient's preferences.

. . .

RI.1.1.4 [Organizational policies and procedures describe the mechanisms by which the following rights are protected and exercised:] The right of the patient to the information necessary to enable him/her to make treatment decisions that reflect his/her wishes;

RI.1.1.4.1 A policy on informed decision making is developed by the medical staff and governing body and is consistent with any legal requirements.

Intent of RI.1.1.4 and RI.1.1.4.1

The patient is given clear, concise explanation of his/her condition and of any proposed treatment(s) or procedure(s), the potential benefit(s) and the potential drawback(s) of the proposed treatment(s) or procedure(s), problems related to recuperation, and the likelihood of success. Information is also provided regarding any significant alternative treatment(s) or procedure(s).

This information includes the identity of the physician or other practitioner who has primary responsibility for the patient's care and the identity and professional status of individuals responsible for authorizing and performing procedures or treatments. The information also includes the existence of any professional relationship among individuals treating the patient, as well as the relationship to any other health care or educational institutions involved in his/her care.

. . .

RI.1.1.5 [Organizational policies and procedures describe the mechanisms by which the following rights are protected and exercised:] The right of the patient to information, at the time of admission, about the hospital's

RI.1.1.5.1 patient rights policy(ies), and

RI.1.1.5.2 mechanism designed for the initiation, review, and, when possible, resolution of patient complaints concerning the quality of care;

Intent of RI.1.1.5 through RI.1.1.5.2

The organization assists the patient in exercising his/her rights by informing the patient of those rights during the admission process. The information is given to the patient or his/her representative in a form that is understandable to the patient (for example, in a language that is understood by the patient).

The patient has the right, without recrimination, to voice complaints regarding the care received, and to have those complaints reviewed and, when possible, resolved. This right, and the mechanism(s) established by the organization to assist the patient in exercising this right, are explained to the patient during the admission process.

. . .

RI.1.1.6 [Organizational policies and procedures describe the mechanisms by which the following rights are protected and exercised:] The right of the patient or the patient's designated representative to participate in the consideration of ethical issues that arise in the care of the patient;

RI.1.1.6.1 The organization has in place a mechanism(s) for the consideration of ethical issues arising in the care of patients and to provide education to caregivers and patients on ethical issues in health care.

Intent of RI.1.1.6 and RI.1.1.6.1

Health care professionals provide patient care within an ethical framework established by their profession, the hospital, and the law. The health care professional has an obligation to respect the views of the patient or the patient's designated representative when ethical issues arise during the patient's care. Moreover, the hospital has an obligation to involve the patient or the patient's representative in the organizational mechanism for considering such issues. Such mechanisms may include community programs, education programs for patients or their representatives, and education programs for staff members. The hospital also has an obligation to provide education on important ethical issues in health care to caregivers, care recipients, and the community.

. . .

RI.1.1.7 [Organizational policies and procedures describe the mechanisms by which the following rights are protected and exercised:] The right of the patient to be informed of any human experimentation or other research/educational projects affecting his/her care or treatment;

Intent of RI.1.1.7

The patient has the right to know of any experimental, research, or educational activities involved in his/her treatment: the patient also has the right to refuse to participate in any such activity.

. . .

RI.1.1.8 [Organizational policies and procedures describe the mechanisms by which the following rights are protected and exercised:] The right of the patient, within the limits of law, to personal privacy and confidentiality of information; and

RI.1.1.8.1 The patient and/or the patient's legally designated representative has access to the information contained in the patient's medical record, within the limits of the law.

Intent of RI.1.1.8 and RI.1.1.8.1

The patient has the following rights:

- To be interviewed, examined, and treated in surroundings designed to give reasonable visual and auditory privacy;
- To have access to his/her medical record and to have his/her medical record read only by individuals directly involved in his/her care, or by individuals monitoring the quality of the patient's care, or by individuals authorized by law or regulation (other individuals may read the medical record only with the patient's written consent or that of a legally authorized or designated representative); and
- To request a transfer to a different room if another patient or a visitor in the room is unreasonably disturbing him/her and if another room equally suitable for his/her care needs is available.

. . .

RI.1.1.9 [Organizational policies and procedures describe the mechanisms by which the following rights are protected and exercised:] The right of the patient's guardian, next of kin, or a legally authorized responsible person to exercise, to the extent permitted by law, the rights delineated on behalf of the patient if

the patient has been adjudicated incompetent in accordance with the law, is found by his/her physician to be medically incapable of understanding the proposed treatment or procedure, is unable to communicate his/her wishes regarding treatment, or is a minor.

Intent of RI.1.1.9

Although the patient is recognized as having the right to participate in his/her care and treatment to the fullest extent possible, there are circumstances under which the patient may be unable to do so. In these situations, the patient's rights are to be exercised by the patient's designated representative or other legally authorized person.

. . .

RI.2 There are hospital-wide policies on the withholding of resuscitative services from patients and the forgoing or withdrawing of life-sustaining treatment.

Intent of RI.2

No single set of policies can anticipate the varied situations in which the difficult decisions about withholding resuscitative services or forgoing or withdrawing life-sustaining treatment will need to be made. However, organizations can develop the framework for a decision-making process. Such a framework would include policies designed to assist the organization in identifying its position on the initiation of resuscitative services and the use and removal of life-sustaining treatment. Policies of this nature need to conform to the legal requirements of the organization's jurisdiction.

. . .

RI.2.1 The policies are developed in consultation with the medical staff, nursing staff, and other appropriate bodies and are adopted by the medical staff and approved by the governing body.

Intent of RI.2.1

Organizational policies that provide a framework for the decision-making process for withholding resuscitative services or forgoing or withdrawing life-sustaining treatment offer guidance to health professionals on the ethical and legal issues involved in such decisions and decrease the uncertainty about the practices permitted by the organization. It is vital that the policies guiding such decisions be formally adopted by the organization's medical staff and approved by the governing body in order to assure that the process is consistent and that there is accountability for the decisions made.

• • •

RI.2.2 The policies describe

RI.2.2.1 the mechanism(s) for reaching decisions about the withholding of resuscitative services from individual patients or forgoing or withdrawing of life-sustaining treatment;

RI.2.2.2 the mechanism(s) for resolving conflicts in decision making, should they arise; and

RI.2.2.3 the roles of physicians and, when applicable, of nursing personnel, other appropriate staff, and family members in decisions to withhold resuscitative services or forgo or withdraw life-sustaining treatment.

Intent of RI.2.2 through RI.2.2.3

Organizational policies regarding the withholding of resuscitative services or the forgoing or withdrawing of life-sustaining treatment outline a process for reaching such decisions. This process protects the decision-making rights of the patient or his/her designated representative; decreases staff uncertainty about practices permitted by the organization; clarifies the roles and duties, and therefore the accountability, of health professionals; and reduces arbitrary decision-making procedures.

• • •

RI.2.3 The policies include provisions designed to assure that the rights of patients are respected.

Intent of RI.2.3

Organizational policies regarding the withholding of resuscitative services or the forgoing or withdrawing of life-sustaining treatment empower the patient or designated

representative to make such decisions and assure that such decisions made by a patient or designated representative explicitly affirm the patient's responsibility for such decision making.

• • •

RI.2.4 The policies include the requirement that appropriate orders be written by the physician primarily responsible for the patient and that documentation be made in the patient's medical record if life-sustaining treatment is to be withdrawn or resuscitative services are to be withheld.

Intent of RI.2.4

Decisions regarding the withholding of resuscitative services or the withdrawal of life-sustaining treatment are communicated to all health professionals involved in the patient's treatment to assure that the decision is implemented.

NOTE: This does not mean that for all deaths in which resuscitative services were not utilized there must be an order to withhold resuscitative services.

• • •

RI.2.5 The policies address the use of advance directives in patient care to the extent permitted by law.

Intent of RI.2.5

The organization is expected to use any advance directives prepared by the patient and known to the organization in the decision-making process surrounding the consideration of the withholding of resuscitative services or the initiation or withdrawal of life-sustaining treatment, to the extent permitted by law and supported by the organization's mission and philosophy.

• • •

SECTION II.

ETHICAL DIRECTIVES
FOR THE PRACTICE OF MEDICINE

• • •

1. **Fourth century B.C.E.-Early twentieth century C.E.**

   Oath of Hippocrates (Fourth Century B.C.E.)
   Oath of Initiation (Caraka Samhita) (First Century C.E.?)
   Oath of Asaph (Third Century-Seventh Century C.E.?)
   Advice to a Physician, Advice of Haly Abbas (Ahwazi) (Tenth Century C.E.)
   The 17 Rules of Enjuin (For Disciples of Our School) (Sixteenth Century C.E.)
   Five Commandments and Ten Requirements (1617)
   A Physician's Ethical Duties from Kholasah al Hekmah (1770)
   Daily Prayer of a Physician ("Prayer of Moses Maimonides") (1793?)
   Code of Ethics, American Medical Association (1847)
   Venezuelan Code of Medical Ethics, National Academy of Medicine (1918)

2. **Mid-twentieth century—2003**

   Declaration of Geneva, World Medical Association (1948, amended 1968, 1983, 1994)
   International Code of Medical Ethics, World Medical Association (1949, amended 1968, 1983))
   Principles of Medical Ethics (1957), American Medical Association
   Principles of Medical Ethics (2001), American Medical Association
   Current Opinions of the Council on Ethical and Judicial Affairs, American Medical Association (2002)
   Declaration of Professional Responsibility: Medicine's Social Contract with Humanity (2001), American Medical Association [2001]
   Charter on Medical Professionalism (2002), American Board of Internal Medicine Foundation, Amercian College of Physicians—American

Society of Internal Medicine Foundation, and European Foundation of Internal Medicine [2002]
The Moral and Technical Competence of the Ophthalmologist, American Academy of Ophthalmology (1995)
Code of Ethics, American Osteopathic Association (1998)
Code of Ethics and Guide to the Ethical Behaviour of Physicians, Canadian Medical Association (1996)
Code of Ethics and Guide to the Ethical Behaviour of Physicians, New Zealand Medical Association (2002)
Code of Ethics of the Chilean Medical Association, Chilean Medical Association (1983)
Code of Medical Ethics, Brazil, Federal Council of Medicine (1988)
European Code of Medical Ethics, Conférence Internationale des Ordres et des Organismes d' Attributions Similaires (1987)
Code of Ethics for Doctors, Norwegian Medical Association (amended 2000)
Final Report Concerning Brain Death and Organ Transplantation, Japan Medical Association (1988)
Summary of the Report on Information from Doctors and Consent of Patients, Japan Medical Association (1991)
Oath of Soviet Physicians (1971)
Solemn Oath of a Physician of Russia (1992)
Regulations on Criteria for Medical Ethics and Their Implementation, Ministry of Health, People's Republic of China (1988)
Ethical and Religious Directives for Catholic Health Facilities, United States Catholic Conference (1971, revised 2001)
Health Care Ethics Guide, Catholic Health Association of Canada (1991)
The Oath of a Muslim Physician, Islamic Medical Association of North America (1977)
Islamic Code of Medical Ethics, Kuwait Document, Islamic Organization for Medical Sciences (1981)

I. Fourth Century B.C.E.-Early Twentieth Century C.E.

The ethical directives for the practice of medicine included in this section are organized in two primary groups: (1) codes, oaths, prayers, and other directives from the fourth century B.C.E. through the early-twentieth century; and (2) directives from the mid-twentieth century through 2003. Documents in the first group are arranged in chronological order; those in the second group are arranged chronologically within thematic clusters, for example, by issuing body, area of the world, and philosophical or religious tradition.

Some of the documents in this section address not only physicians but also healthcare institutions and the health professions in general; they are included in this section because many medical ethics codes historically have applied not only to physicians but also to the practice of health care more generally. Ethical directives for medical specialties generally have not been included in this Appendix, due to space constraints.

OATH OF HIPPOCRATES

FOURTH CENTURY B.C.E.

• • •

Attributed to Hippocrates, the oath, which exemplifies the Pythagorean school rather than Greek thought in general, differs from other, more scientific, writings in the Hippocratic corpus. Written later than some of the other treatises in the corpus, the Oath of Hippocrates is one of the earliest and most important statements on medical ethics. Not only has the oath provided the foundation for many succeeding medical oaths, such as the Declaration of Geneva, but it is still administered to the graduating students of many medical schools, either in its original form or in an altered version.

I swear by Apollo Physician and Asclepius and Hygieia and Panaceia and all the gods and goddesses, making them my witnesses, that I will fulfil according to my ability and judgment this oath and this covenant:

To hold him who has taught me this art as equal to my parents and to live my life in partnership with him, and if he is in need of money to give him a share of mine, and to regard his offspring as equal to my brothers in male lineage and to teach them this art—if they desire to learn it—without fee and covenant; to give a share of precepts and oral instruction and all the other learning to my sons and to the sons of him who has instructed me and to pupils who have signed the covenant and have taken an oath according to the medical law, but to no one else.

I will apply dietetic measures for the benefit of the sick according to my ability and judgment; I will keep them from harm and injustice.

I will neither give a deadly drug to anybody if asked for it, nor will I make a suggestion to this effect. Similarly I will not give to a woman an abortive remedy. In purity and holiness I will guard my life and my art.

I will not use the knife, not even on sufferers from stone, but will withdraw in favor of such men as are engaged in this work.

Whatever houses I may visit, I will come for the benefit of the sick, remaining free of all intentional injustice, of all mischief and in particular of sexual relations with both female and male persons, be they free or slaves.

What I may see or hear in the course of the treatment or even outside of the treatment in regard to the life of men, which on no account one must spread abroad, I will keep to myself holding such things shameful to be spoken about.

If I fulfil this oath and do not violate it, may it be granted to me to enjoy life and art, being honored with fame among all men for all time to come; if I transgress it and swear falsely, may the opposite of all this be my lot.

OATH OF INITIATION (CARAKA SAMHITA)

FIRST CENTURY C.E.?

• • •

This ancient Indian oath for medical students appears in the Caraka Samhita (or, Charaka Samhita), a medical text written around the first century C.E. by the Indian physician Caraka. Unlike the Hippocratic Oath, which exemplifies only one, minority, school of ancient Greek thought, the Oath of the Caraka Samhita reflects concepts and beliefs found throughout ancient nonmedical Indian literature. The oath contains several uniquely Hindu elements, including the requirements to lead the life of a celibate, eat no meat, and carry no arms.

1. The teacher then should instruct the disciple in the presence of the sacred fire, Brahmanas [Brahmins] and physicians.

2. [saying] "Thou shalt lead the life of a celibate, grow thy hair and beard, speak only the truth, eat no meat, eat only pure articles of food, be free from envy and carry no arms.

3. There shall be nothing that thou should not do at my behest except hating the king, causing another's

death, or committing an act of great unrighteousness or acts leading to calamity.

4. Thou shalt dedicate thyself to me and regard me as thy chief. Thou shalt be subject to me and conduct thyself for ever for my welfare and pleasure. Thou shalt serve and dwell with me like a son or a slave or a supplicant. Thou shalt behave and act without arrogance, with care and attention and with undistracted mind, humility, constant reflection and ungrudging obedience. Acting either at my behest or otherwise, thou shalt conduct thyself for the achievement of thy teacher's purposes alone, to the best of thy abilities.

5. If thou desirest success, wealth and fame as a physician and heaven after death, thou shalt pray for the welfare of all creatures beginning with the cows and Brahmanas.

6. Day and night, however thou mayest be engaged, thou shalt endeavour for the relief of patients with all thy heart and soul. Thou shalt not desert or injure thy patient for the sake of thy life or thy living. Thou shalt not commit adultery even in thought. Even so, thou shalt not covet others' possessions. Thou shalt be modest in thy attire and appearance. Thou shouldst not be a drunkard or a sinful man nor shouldst thou associate with the abettors of crimes. Thou shouldst speak words that are gentle, pure and righteous, pleasing, worthy, true, wholesome, and moderate. Thy behaviour must be in consideration of time and place and heedful of past experience. Thou shalt act always with a view to the acquisition of knowledge and fullness of equipment.

7. No persons, who are hated by the king or who are haters of the king or who are hated by the public or who are haters of the public, shall receive treatment. Similarly, those who are extremely abnormal, wicked, and of miserable character and conduct, those who have not vindicated their honour, those who are on the point of death, and similarly women who are unattended by their husbands or guardians shall not receive treatment.

8. No offering of presents by a woman without the behest of her husband or guardian shall be accepted by thee. While entering the patient's house, thou shalt be accompanied by a man who is known to the patient and who has his permission to enter; and thou shalt be well-clad, bent of head, self-possessed, and conduct thyself only after repeated consideration. Thou shalt thus properly make thy entry. Having entered, thy speech, mind, intellect and senses shall be entirely devoted to no other thought than that of being helpful to the patient and of things concerning only him. The peculiar customs of the patient's household shall not be made public. Even knowing that the patient's span of life has come to its close, it shall not be mentioned by thee there, where if so done, it would cause shock to the patient or to others.

Though possessed of knowledge one should not boast very much of one's knowledge. Most people are offended by the boastfulness of even those who are otherwise good and authoritative.

9. There is no limit at all to the Science of Life, Medicine. So thou shouldst apply thyself to it with diligence. This is how thou shouldst act. Also thou shouldst learn the skill of practice from another without carping. The entire world is the teacher to the intelligent and the foe to the unintelligent. Hence, knowing this well, thou shouldst listen and act according to the words of instruction of even an unfriendly person, when his words are worthy and of a kind as to bring to you fame, long life, strength and prosperity."

10. Thereafter the teacher should say this—"Thou shouldst conduct thyself properly with the gods, sacred fire, Brahmanas, the guru, the aged, the scholars and the preceptors. If thou has conducted thyself well with them, the precious stones, the grains and the gods become well disposed towards thee. If thou shouldst conduct thyself otherwise, they become unfavorable to thee." To the teacher that has spoken thus, the disciple should say, "Amen."

OATH OF ASAPH

THIRD CENTURY–SEVENTH CENTURY C.E.?

• • •

The Oath of Asaph appears at the end of the Book of Asaph the Physician (Sefer Asaph ha-Rofe), which is the oldest Hebrew medical text. It was written by Asaph Judaeus, also known as Asaph ben Berachyahu, a Hebrew physician from Syria or Mesopotamia, who lived sometime between the third and seventh centuries C.E., probably in the sixth century. The oath, which in part resembles the Oath of Hippocrates, was taken by medical students when they received their diplomas.

And this is the oath adminstered by Asaph, the son of Berachyahu, and by Jochanan, the son of Zabda, to their disciples; and they adjured them in these words: Take heed that ye kill not any man with the sap of a root; and ye shall not dispense a potion to a woman with child by adultery to cause her to miscarry; and ye shall not lust after beautiful women to commit adultery with them; and ye shall not disclose secrets confided unto you; and ye shall take no bribes to cause injury and to kill; and ye shall not harden your hearts against the poor and the needy, but heal them; and ye shall not call good evil or evil good; and ye shall not walk in the way of sorcerers to cast spells, to enchant and to bewitch with intent to separate a man from the wife of his bosom or woman from the husband of her youth.

And ye shall not covet wealth or bribes to abet depraved sexual commerce.

And ye shall not make use of any manner of idol-worship to heal thereby, nor trust in the healing powers of any form of their worship. But rather must ye abhor and detest and hate all their worshippers and those that trust in them and cause others to trust in them, for all of them are but vanity and of no avail, for they are naught; and they are demons. Their own carcasses they cannot save; how, then, shall they save the living?

And now, put your trust in the Lord your God, the God of truth, the living God, for He doth kill and make alive, smite and heal. He doth teach man understanding and also to do good. He smiteth in righteousness and justice and healeth in mercy and lovingkindness. No crafty device can be concealed from Him, for naught is hidden from His sight.

He causeth healing plants to grow and doth implant in the hearts of sages skill to heal by His manifold mercies and to declare marvels to the multitude, that all that live may know that He made them, and that beside Him there is none to save. For the peoples trust in their idols to succour them from their afflictions, but they will not save them in their distress, for their hope and their trust are in the Dead. Therefore it is fitting that ye keep apart from them and hold aloof from all the abominations of their idols and cleave unto the name of the Lord God of all flesh. And every living creature is in His hand to kill and to make alive; and there is none to deliver from His hand.

Be ye mindful of Him at all times and seek Him in truth uprightness and rectitude that ye may prosper in all that ye do; then He will cause you to prosper and ye shall be praised by all men. And the peoples will leave their gods and their idols and will yearn to serve the Lord even as ye do, for they will perceive that they have put their trust in a thing of naught and that their labour is in vain; (otherwise) when they cry unto the Lord, He will not save them.

As for you, be strong and let not your hands slacken, for there is a reward for your labours. God is with you when ye

are with Him. If ye will keep His covenant and walk in His statutes to cleave unto them, ye shall be as saints in the sight of all men, and they shall say: "Happy is the people that is in such a case; happy is that people whose God is the Lord."

And their disciples answered them and said: All that ye have instructed us and commanded us, that will we do, for it is a commandment of the Torah, and it behooves us to perform it with all our heart and all our soul and all our might: to do and to obey and to turn neither to the right nor to the left. And they blessed them in the name of the Highest God, the Lord of Heaven and earth.

And they admonished them yet again and said unto them: Behold, the Lord God and His saints and His Torah be witness unto you that ye shall fear Him, turning not aside from His commandments, but walking uprightly in His statutes. Incline not to covetousness and aid not the evildoers to shed innocent blood. Neither shall ye mix poisons for a man or a woman to slay his friend therewith; nor shall ye reveal which roots be poisonous or give them into the hand of any man, or be persuaded to do evil. Ye shall not cause the shedding of blood by any manner of medical treatment. Take heed that ye do not cause a malady to any man; and ye shall not cause any man injury by hastening to cut through flesh and blood with an iron instrument or by branding, but shall first observe twice and thrice and only then shall ye give your counsel.

Let not a spirit of haughtiness cause you to lift up your eyes and your hearts in pride. Wreak not the vengeance of hatred on a sick man; and alter not your prescriptions for them that do hate the Lord our God, but keep his ordinances and commandments and walk in all His ways that ye may find favour in His sight. Be ye pure and faithful and upright.

Thus did Asaph and Jochanan instruct and adjure their disciples.

ADVICE TO A PHYSICIAN

Advice of Haly Abbas (Ahwazi)

TENTH CENTURY C.E.

• • •

A leading Persian figure in medicine and medical ethics, Haly Abbas (Ahwazi), who died in 994 C.E., devoted the first chapter of his work Liber Regius (Kamel Al Sanaah al Tibbia) to the ethics of medicine. An excerpt of his ethical admonition follows.

The first advice is to worship God and obey his commands; then be humble toward your teacher and endeavor to hold him in esteem, to serve and show gratitude to him, to hold him equally dear as you do your parents, and to share your possessions with him as with your parents.

Be kind to the children of your teachers and if one of them wants to study medicine you are to teach him without any remuneration.

You are to prohibit the unsuited and undeserving from studying medicine.

A physician is to prudently treat his patients with food and medicine out of good and spiritual motives, not for the sake of gain. He should never prescribe or use a harmful drug or abortifacient.

A physician should be chaste, pious, religious, well-spoken, and graceful, and must avoid any kind of sinfulness or impurity. He should not look upon women with lust and never go to their home except to visit a patient.

A physician should respect confidences and protect the patient's secrets. In protecting a patient's secrets, he must be more insistent than the patient himself. A physician should follow the Hippocratic counsels. He must be kind, compassionate, merciful and benevolent, and give himself unstintingly to the treatment of patients, especially the poor. He must never expect remuneration from the poor but rather provide them free medicine. If it is not impossible, he must visit them graciously whenever it is necessary, day or night, especially when they suffer from an acute disease, because the patient's condition changes very quickly with this kind of disease.

It is not proper for a physician to live luxuriously and become involved in pleasure-seeking. He must not drink alcohol because it injures the brain. He must study medical books constantly and never grow tired of research. He has to learn what he is studying and repeat and memorize what is necessary. He has to study in his youth because it is easier to memorize the subject at this age than in old age, which is the mother of oblivion.

A medical student should be constantly present in the hospital so as to study disease processes and complications under the learned professor and proficient physicians.

To be a learned and skillful physician, he has to follow this advice, develop an upright character and never hesitate to put this advice into practice so as to make his work effective, to win the patient's trust, and to receive the benefit of the patient's friendship and gratitude.

The Almighty God knows better than all....

THE 17 RULES OF ENJUIN (FOR DISCIPLES OF OUR SCHOOL)

SIXTEENTH CENTURY C.E.

• • •

The 17 Rules of Enjuin were developed for students by practitioners of the Ri-shu school, an approach to disease that was practiced in sixteenth-century Japan. The text reflects the priestly role of the physician and emphasizes the idea, also found in the Hippocratic Oath, that medical knowledge should not be disclosed outside of the school.

1. Each person should follow the path designated by Heaven (Buddha, the Gods).
2. You should always be kind to people. You should always be devoted to loving people.
3. The teaching of Medicine should be restricted to selected persons.
4. You should not tell others what you are taught, regarding treatments without permission.
5. You should not establish association with doctors who do not belong to this school.
6. All the successors and descendants of the disciples of this school shall follow the teachers' ways.
7. If any disciples cease the practice of Medicine, or, if successors are not found at the death of the disciple, all the medical books of this school should be returned to the School of Enjuin.
8. You should not kill living creatures, nor should you admire hunting or fishing.
9. In our school, teaching about poisons is prohibited, nor should you receive instructions about poisons from other physicians. Moreover, you should not give abortives to the people.
10. You should rescue even such patients as you dislike or hate. You should do virtuous acts, but in such a way that they do not become known to people. To do good deeds secretly is a mark of virtue.
11. You should not exhibit avarice and you must not strain to become famous. You should not rebuke or reprove a patient, even if he does not present you with money or goods in gratitude.
12. You should be delighted if, after treating a patient without success, the patient receives medicine from another physician, and is cured.
13. You should not speak ill of other physicians.
14. You should not tell what you have learned from the time you enter a woman's room, and, moreover, you should not have obscene or immoral feelings when examining a woman.

15. Proper or not, you should not tell others what you have learned in lectures, or what you have learned about prescribing medicine.

16. You should not like undue extravagance. If you like such living, your avarice will increase, and you will lose the ability to be kind to others.

17. If you do not keep the rules and regulations of this school, then you will be cancelled as a disciple. In more severe cases, the punishment will be greater.

FIVE COMMANDMENTS AND TEN REQUIREMENTS

1617

• • •

The Five Commandments and Ten Requirements of physicians consti-tute the most comprehensive statement on medical ethics in China. They were written by Chen Shih-kung, an early-seventeenth-century Chinese physician, and appear in his work An Orthodox Manual of Surgery.

Five Commandments

1. Physicians should be ever ready to respond to any calls of patients, high or low, rich or poor. They should treat them equally and care not for financial reward. Thus their profession will become prosper-ous naturally day by day and conscience will remain intact.

2. Physicians may visit a lady, widow or nun only in the presence of an attendant but not alone. The secret diseases of female patients should be examined with a right attitude, and should not be revealed to anybody, not even to the physician's own wife.

3. Physicians should not ask patients to send pearl, amber or other valuable substances to their home for preparing medicament. If necessary, patients should be instructed how to mix the prescriptions them-selves in order to avoid suspicion. It is also not proper to admire things which patients possess.

4. Physicians should not leave the office for excursion and drinking. Patients should be examined punctu-ally and personally. Prescriptions should be made according to the medical formulary, otherwise a dispute may arise.

5. Prostitutes should be treated just like patients from a good family and gratuitous services should not be given to the poor ones. Mocking should not be indulged for this brings loss of dignity. After examination physicians should leave the house immediately. If the case improves, drugs may be sent but physicians should not visit them again for lewd reward.

Ten Requirements

1. A physician or surgeon must first know the principles of the learned. He must study all the ancient standard medical books ceaselessly day and night, and understand them thoroughly so that the principles enlighten his eyes and are impressed on his heart. Then he will not make any mistake in the clinic.

2. Drugs must be carefully selected and prepared according to the refining process of Lei Kung. Remedies should be prepared according to the pharmaceutical formulae but may be altered to suit the patient's condition. Decoctions and powders should be freely made. Pills and distilled medicine should be prepared in advance. The older the plaster is the more effective it will be. Tampons become more effective on standing. Don't spare valuable drugs; their use is eventually advantageous.

3. A physician should not be arrogant and insult other physicians in the same district. He should be modest and careful towards his colleagues; respect his seniors, help his juniors, learn from his superiors and yield to the arrogant. Thus there will be no slander and hatred. Harmony will be es-teemed by all.

4. The managing of a family is just like the curing of a disease. If the constitution of a man is not well cared for and becomes over-exhausted, diseases will attack him. Mild ones will weaken his physique, while serious ones may result in death. Similarly, if the foundation of the family is not firmly established and extravagance be indulged in, reserves will gradually drain away and poverty will come.

5. Man receives his fate from Heaven. He should not be ungrateful to the Heavenly decree. Professional gains should be approved by the conscience and conform to the Heavenly will. If the gain is made according to the Heavenly will, natural affinity takes place. If not, offspring will be condemned. Is it not better to make light of professional gain in order to avoid the evil retribution?

6. Gifts, except in the case of weddings, funerals and for the consolation of the sick, should be simple. One dish of fish and one of vegetable will suffice for a meal. This is not only to reduce expenses but also

to save provisions. The virtue of a man lies not in grasping but rather in economy.

7. Medicine should be given free to the poor. Extra financial help should be extended to the destitute patients, if possible. Without food, medicine alone can not relieve the distress of a patient.

8. Savings should be invested in real estate but not in curios and unnecessary luxuries. The physician should also not join the drinking club and the gambling house which would hinder his practice. Hatred and slander can thus be avoided.

9. Office and dispensary should be fully equipped with necessary apparatus. The physician should improve his knowledge by studying medical books, old and new, and reading current publications. This really is the fundamental duty of a physician.

10. A physician should be ready to respond to the call of government officials with respect and sincerity. He should inform them of the cause of the disease and prescribe accordingly. After healing he should not seek for a complimentary tablet [a wooden board inscribed with complimentary words, hung in the physician's office for propaganda] or plead excuse for another's difficulty. A person who respects the law should not associate with officials.

A PHYSICIAN'S ETHICAL DUTIES

From Kholasah al Hekmah

1770

• • •

In 1770 C.E., during Persia's Islamic era, Mohamad Hosin Aghili of Shiraz wrote the work Kholasah al Hekmah. The first chapter of that work contains a list of ethical duties for the physician, which are printed here in condensed form.

1. A physician must not be conceited; he should know that the actual healer is God.

2. He should praise his teachers and professor and return thanks to them for their kindnesses.

3. He should never slander another physician. The fault of others should occasion the recognition of his own fault, not be the occasion for pride and conceit.

4. He must speak to patients with civility and good humor and never get angry at the misbehavior and insults of patients.

5. He must protect the patients' secrets and not betray them, especially to those the patients do not want to know.

6. In the case of the transmission of disease, the physician must not turn the second patient against the first.

7. He must be energetic in studying diseases and drugs and earnest in the diagnosis and treatment of a patient or disease.

8. He must never be tenacious in his opinion, and continue in his fault or mistake but, if it is possible, he is to consult with proficient physicians and ascertain the facts.

9. If someone mentions a useless or wrong idea, he must not turn it down definitely but say politely, "Maybe it is true in some cases but, in my opinion, in this case it is more probably such and such."

10. If a prior physician has a better knowledge of a patient or disease, he has to encourage the patient to return to the first physician.

11. If he is not successful in the treatment of a case or if he has found the patient did not have confidence in his work or that the patient would like to refer to another physician, it is better to offer an excuse and ask him to consult another physician.

12. He must not be prejudiced against any method of treatment and never continue any wrong practice.

13. In the treatment of disease, he must begin with simple medicine and not recommend any drug as long as the nature of the disease is resistant to it and it would not be effective.

14. If a patient has several diseases, first of all he has to cure the main disease which may be the cause of complications.

15. He should never recommend any kind of fatal, harmful or enfeebling drugs; he has to know that as a physician he has to do what is conducive to the patient's temperament, and temperament itself is an efficient corrector and protector of the body, not fatal or destructive.

16. He must not be proud of his class or his family and must not regard others with contempt.

17. He must not withhold medical knowledge; he should teach it to everyone in medicine without any discrimination between poor or rich, noble or slave.

18. He must not hold his students or his patients under his obligation.

19. He must be content, grateful, generous and magnanimous, and never be covetous, greedy, ravenous or jealous.

20. He must never covet another's property. If someone offers him a present while he himself is in need of it, he must not accept it.

21. He must never claim that he can cure an impoverished patient who has gone to many

physicians, and should not jeopardize his own reputation.

22. He should never be gluttonous and become involved in pleasure-seeking, buffoonery, drinking, and other sins.

23. He must not look upon women with lust but must look at them as he looks at his daughter, sister, or mother.

DAILY PRAYER OF A PHYSICIAN ("PRAYER OF MOSES MAIMONIDES")

1793?

• • •

Although there is considerable debate about this prayer's true authorship, it was first attributed to Moses Maimonides, a twelfth-century Jewish physician in Egypt. Many now believe it was in fact authored by Marcus Herz, a German physician, pupil of Immanuel Kant, and physician to Moses Mendelssohn. The prayer first appeared in print in 1793 as "Tägliches Gebet eines Arztes bevor er seine Kranken besucht—Aus der hebräischen Handschrift eines berühmten jüdischen Arztes in Egypten aus dem zwölften Jahrhundert" ("Daily prayer of a physician before he visits his patients—From the Hebrew manuscript of a renowned Jewish physician in Egypt from the twelfth century"). The Prayer of Moses Maimonides and the Oath of Hippocrates are probably the best known of the older statements on medical ethics.

Almighty God, Thou has created the human body with infinite wisdom. Ten thousand times ten thousand organs hast Thou combined in it that act unceasingly and harmoniously to preserve the whole in all its beauty—the body which is the envelope of the immortal soul. They are ever acting in perfect order, agreement and accord. Yet, when the frailty of matter or the unbridling of passions deranges this order or interrupts this accord, then forces clash and the body crumbles into the primal dust from which it came. Thou sendest to man diseases as beneficent messengers to foretell approaching danger and to urge him to avert it.

Thou has blest Thine earth, Thy rivers and Thy mountains with healing substances; they enable Thy creatures to alleviate their sufferings and to heal their illnesses. Thou hast endowed man with the wisdom to relieve the suffering of his brother, to recognize his disorders, to extract the healing substances, to discover their powers and to prepare and to apply them to suit every ill. In Thine Eternal Providence Thou hast chosen me to watch over the life and health of Thy creatures. I am now about to apply myself to the duties of my profession. Support me, Almighty God, in these great labors that they may benefit mankind, for without Thy help not even the least thing will succeed.

Inspire me with love for my art and for Thy creatures. Do not allow thirst for profit, ambition for renown and admiration, to interfere with my profession, for these are the enemies of truth and of love for mankind and they can lead astray in the great task of attending to the welfare of Thy creatures. Preserve the strength of my body and of my soul that they ever be ready to cheerfully help and support rich and poor, good and bad, enemy as well as friend. In the sufferer let me see only the human being. Illumine my mind that it recognize what presents itself and that it may comprehend what is absent or hidden. Let it not fail to see what is visible, but do not permit it to arrogate to itself the power to see what cannot be seen, for delicate and indefinite are the bounds of the great art of caring for the lives and health of Thy creatures. Let me never be absent-minded. May no strange thoughts divert my attention at the bedside of the sick, or disturb my mind in its silent labors, for great and sacred are the thoughtful deliberations required to preserve the lives and health of Thy creatures.

Grant that my patients have confidence in me and my art and follow my directions and my counsel. Remove from their midst all charlatans and the whole host of officious relatives and know-all nurses, cruel people who arrogantly frustrate the wisest purposes of our art and often lead Thy creatures to their death.

Should those who are wiser than I wish to improve and instruct me, let my soul gratefully follow their guidance; for vast is the extent of our art. Should conceited fools, however, censure me, then let love for my profession steel me against them, so that I remain steadfast without regard for age, for reputation, or for honor, because surrender would bring to Thy creatures sickness and death.

Imbue my soul with gentleness and calmness when older colleagues, proud of their age, wish to displace me or to scorn me or disdainfully to teach me. May even this be of advantage to me, for they know many things of which I am ignorant, but let not their arrogance give me pain. For they are old and old age is not master of the passions. I also hope to attain old age upon this earth, before Thee, Almighty God!

Let me be contented in everything except in the great science of my profession. Never allow the thought to arise in me that I have attained to sufficient knowledge, but vouchsafe to me the strength, the leisure and the ambition ever to extend my knowledge. For art is great, but the mind of man is ever expanding.

Almighty God! Thou has chosen me in Thy mercy to watch over the life and death of Thy creatures. I now apply myself to my profession. Support me in this great task so that it may benefit mankind, for without Thy help not even the least thing will succeed.

CODE OF ETHICS

American Medical Association

1847

• • •

The American Medical Association's (AMA) first code of ethics can be understood only in light of the work in medical ethics done by Thomas Percival, an eighteenth-century English physician. Percival wrote the first comprehensive modern statement of medical ethics in response to a request from the trustees of the Manchester Infirmary to draw up a "scheme of professional conduct relative to hospitals and other medical charities" that would resolve conflicts among infirmary physicians and prevent future conflicts. In 1794, after three years of writing and revising, Percival privately distributed a book titled Medical Ethics. Finally published in 1803, Percival's Medical Ethics served for many years as a model for the ethics codes of medical societies in both England and the United States.

When the AMA was founded in 1847, its first tasks were to establish standards for medical education and to formulate a code of ethics. Because most of the existing American codes of medical ethics relied heavily on Thomas Percival's work, the AMA followed suit, frequently preserving Percival's wording. The code of 1847, adopted by both the AMA and the New York Academy of Medicine, is excerpted below.

Chapter I. OF THE DUTIES OF PHYSICIANS TO THEIR PATIENTS, AND OF THE OBLIGATIONS OF PATIENTS TO THEIR PHYSICIANS

Art. I—*Duties of Physicians to Their Patients*

1. A physician should not only be ever ready to obey the calls of the sick, but his mind ought also to be imbued with the greatness of his mission, and of the responsibility he habitually incurs in its discharge. Those obligations are the more deep and enduring, because there is no tribunal other than his own conscience, to adjudge penalties for carelessness or neglect. Physicians should, therefore, minister to the sick with due impressions of the importance of their office; reflecting that the ease, the health, and the lives of those committed to their charge, depend on their skill, attention and fidelity. They should study, also, in their deportment, so to unite tenderness with firmness, and condescension with authority, as to inspire the minds of their patients with gratitude, respect and confidence.

2. Every case committed to the charge of a physician should be treated with attention, steadiness and humanity. Reasonable indulgence should be granted to the mental imbecility and caprices of the sick. Secrecy and delicacy, when required by peculiar circumstances, should be strictly observed; and the familiar and confidential intercourse to which physicians are admitted in their professional visits, should be used with discretion, and with the most scrupulous regard to fidelity and honor. The obligation of secrecy extends beyond the period of professional services;—none of the privacies of personal and domestic life, no infirmity of disposition or flaw of character observed during professional attendance, should ever be divulged by him except when he is imperatively required to do so. The force and necessity of this obligation are indeed so great, that professional men have, under certain circumstances, been protected in their observance of secrecy by courts of justice.

3. Frequent visits to the sick are in general requisite, since they enable the physician to arrive at a more perfect knowledge of the disease,—to meet promptly every change which may occur, and also tend to preserve the confidence of the patient. But unnecessary visits are to be avoided, as they give useless anxiety to the patient, tend to diminish the authority of the physician, and render him liable to be suspected of interested motives.

4. A physician should not be forward to make gloomy prognostications, because they savor of empiricism, by magnifying the importance of his services in the treatment or cure of the disease. But he should not fail, on proper occasions, to give to the friends of the patient timely notice of danger, when it really occurs; and even to the patient himself, if absolutely necessary. This office, however, is so peculiarly alarming when executed by him, that it ought to be declined whenever it can be assigned to any other person of sufficient judgment and delicacy. For, the physician should be the minister of hope and comfort to the sick; that, by such cordials to the drooping spirit, he may smooth the bed of death, revive expiring life, and counteract the depressing influence of those maladies which often disturb the tranquility of the most resigned, in their last moments. The life of a sick person can be shortened not only by the acts, but also by the words or the manner of a physician. It is, therefore, a sacred duty to guard himself carefully in this respect, and to avoid all things which have a tendency to discourage the patient and to depress his spirits.

5. A physician ought not to abandon a patient because the case is deemed incurable; for his attendance may continue to be highly useful to the patient, and comforting to the relatives around him, even to the last period of a fatal malady, by alleviating pain and other symptoms, and by soothing mental anguish. To decline attendance, under such circumstances, would be sacrificing to fanciful delicacy and mistaken liberality, that moral duty, which is independent of, and far superior to all pecuniary consideration.

6. Consultations should be promoted in difficult or protracted cases, as they give rise to confidence, energy, and more enlarged views in practice.

7. The opportunity which a physician not unfrequently enjoys of promoting and strengthening the good resolutions of his patients, suffering under the consequences of vicious conduct, ought never to be neglected. His counsels, or even remonstrances, will give satisfaction, not offence, if they be proffered with politeness, and evince a genuine love of virtue, accompanied by a sincere interest in the welfare of the person to whom they are addressed.

Art. II—*Obligations of Patients to their Physicians*

1. The members of the medical profession, upon whom are enjoined the performance of so many important and arduous duties towards the community, and who are required to make so many sacrifices of comfort, ease, and health, for the welfare of those who avail themselves of their services, certainly have a right to expect and require, that their patients should entertain a just sense of the duties which they owe to their medical attendants.

2. The first duty of a patient is, to select as his medical adviser one who has received a regular professional education. In no trade or occupation do mankind rely on the skill of an untaught artist; and in medicine, confessedly the most difficult and intricate of the sciences, the world ought not to suppose that knowledge is intuitive.

3. Patients should prefer a physician whose habits of life are regular, and who is not devoted to company, pleasure, or to any pursuit incompatible with his professional obligations. A patient should also confide the care of himself and family, as much as possible, to one physician, for a medical man who has become acquainted with the peculiarities of constitution, habits, and predispositions, of those he attends, is more likely to be successful in his treatment than one who does not possess that knowledge.

A patient who has thus selected his physician, should always apply for advice in whatever may appear to him trivial cases, for the most fatal results often supervene on the slightest accidents. It is of still more importance that he should apply for assistance in the forming stage of violent diseases; it is to a neglect of this precept that medicine owes much of the uncertainty and imperfection with which it has been reproached.

4. Patients should faithfully and unreservedly communicate to their physician the supposed cause of their disease. This is the more important, as many diseases of a mental origin simulate those depending on external causes, and yet are only to be cured by ministering to the mind diseased. A patient should never be afraid of thus making his physician his friend and adviser; he should always bear in mind that a medical man is under the strongest obligations of secrecy. Even the female sex should never allow feelings of shame and delicacy to prevent their disclosing the seat, symptoms and causes of complaints peculiar to them. However commendable a modest reserve may be in the common occurrences of life, its strict observance in medicine is often attended with the most serious consequences, and a patient may sink under a painful and loathsome disease, which might have been readily prevented had timely intimation been given to the physician.

5. A patient should never weary his physician with a tedious detail of events or matters not appertaining to his disease. Even as relates to his actual symptoms, he will convey much more real information by giving clear answers to interrogatories, than by the most minute account of his own framing. Neither should he obtrude the details of his business nor the history of his family concerns.

6. The obedience of a patient to the prescriptions of his physician should be prompt and implicit. He should never permit his own crude opinions as to their fitness, to influence his attention to them. A failure in one particular may render an otherwise judicious treatment dangerous, and even fatal. This remark is equally applicable to diet, drink, and exercise. As patients become convalescent, they are very apt to suppose that the rules prescribed for them may be disregarded, and the consequence, but too often, is a relapse. Patients should never allow themselves to be persuaded to take any medicine whatever, that may be recommended to them by the self-constituted doctors and doctoresses, who are so frequently met with, and who pretend to possess infallible remedies for the cure of every disease. However simple some of their prescriptions may

appear to be, it often happens that they are productive of much mischief, and in all cases they are injurious, by contravening the plan of treatment adopted by the physician.

7. A patient should, if possible, avoid even the friendly visits of a physician who is not attending him—and when he does receive them, he should never converse on the subject of his disease, as an observation may be made, without any intention of interference, which may destroy his confidence in the course he is pursuing, and induce him to neglect the directions prescribed to him. A patient should never send for a consulting physician without the express consent of his own medical attendant. It is of great importance that physicians should act in concert; for, although their modes of treatment may be attended with equal success when employed singly, yet conjointly they are very likely to be productive of disastrous results.

8. When a patient wishes to dismiss his physician, justice and common courtesy require that he should declare his reasons for so doing.

9. Patients should always, when practicable, send for their physician in the morning, before his usual hour of going out; for, by being early aware of the visits he has to pay during the day, the physician is able to apportion his time in such a manner as to prevent an interference of engagements. Patients should also avoid calling on their medical adviser unnecessarily during the hours devoted to meals or sleep. They should always be in readiness to receive the visits of their physician, as the detention of a few minutes is often of serious inconven- ience to him.

10. A patient should, after his recovery, entertain a just and enduring sense of the value of the services rendered him by his physician; for these are of such a character, that no mere pecuniary acknowledgment can repay or cancel them.

Chapter II. OF THE DUTIES OF PHYSICIANS TO EACH OTHER AND TO THE PROFESSION AT LARGE

Art. I—*Duties for the support of professional character*

1. Every individual, on entering the profession, as he becomes thereby entitled to all its privileges and immunities, incurs an obligation to exert his best abilities to maintain its dignity and honor, to exalt its standing, and to extend the bounds of its usefulness. He should therefore observe strictly, such laws as are instituted for the government of its members;—should avoid all contumelious and sarcastic remarks relative to the faculty, as a body; and while, by unwearied diligence, he resorts to

every honorable means of enriching the science, he should entertain a due respect for his seniors, who have, by their labors, brought it to the elevated condition in which he finds it.

2. There is no profession, from the members of which greater purity of character and a higher standard of moral excellence are required, than the medical; and to attain such eminence, is a duty every physician owes alike to his profession, and to his patients. It is due to the latter, as without it he cannot command their respect and confidence; and to both, because no scientific attainments can compensate for the want of correct moral principles. It is also incumbent upon the faculty to be temperate in all things, for the practice of physic requires the unremitting exercise of a clear and vigorous understanding; and, on emergencies for which no professional man should be unprepared, a steady hand, an acute eye, and an unclouded head, may be essential to the well-being, and even life, of a fellow creature.

3. It is derogatory to the dignity of the profession, to resort to public advertisements or private cards or handbills, inviting the attention of individuals affected with particular diseases—publicly offering advice and medicine to the poor gratis, or promising radical cures; or to publish cases and operations in the daily prints, or suffer such publications to be made;—to invite laymen to be present at op- erations—to boast of cures and remedies—to adduce certificates of skill and success, or to perform any other similar acts. These are the ordinary practices of empirics, and are highly reprehensible in a regular physician.

4. Equally derogatory to professional character is it, for a physician to hold a patent for any surgical instrument, or medicine; or to dispense a secret nostrum, whether it be the composition or exclusive property of himself or of others. For, if such nostrum be of real efficacy, any concealment regarding it is inconsistent with beneficence and professional liberality; and, if mystery alone give it value and importance, such craft implies either disgraceful ignorance, or fraudulent avarice. It is also reprehensible for physicians to give certificates attesting the efficacy of patent or secret medicines, or in any way to promote the use of them.

Art. II—*Professional services of Physicians to each other*

1. All practitioners of medicine, their wives, and their children while under the paternal care, are entitled to the gratuitous services of any one or more of the faculty residing near them, whose assistance may be desired. A physician afflicted with disease is usually

an incompetent judge of his own case; and the natural anxiety and solicitude which he experiences at the sickness of a wife, a child, or any one who by the ties of consanguinity is rendered peculiarly dear to him, tend to obscure his judgment, and produce timidity and irresolution in his practice. Under such circumstances, medical men are peculiarly dependent upon each other, and kind offices and professional aid should always be cheerfully and gratuitously afforded. Visits ought not, however, to be obtruded officiously; as such unasked civility may give rise to embarrassment, or interfere with that choice on which confidence depends. But, if a distant member of the faculty, whose circumstances are affluent, request attendance, and an honorarium be offered, it should not be declined; for no pecuniary obligation ought to be imposed, which the party receiving it would wish not to incur.

. . .

Art. IV—*Of the duties of Physicians in regard to consultations*

1. A regular medical education furnishes the only presumptive evidence of professional abilities and acquirements, and ought to be the only acknowledged right of an individual to the exercise and honors of his profession. Nevertheless, as in consultations, the good of the patient is the sole object in view, and this is often dependent on personal confidence, no intelligent regular practitioner, who has a license to practice from some medical board of known and acknowledged respectability, recognised by this association, and who is in good moral and professional standing in the place in which he resides, should be fastidiously excluded from fellowship, or his aid refused in consultation when it is requested by the patient. But no one can be considered as a regular practitioner, or fit associate in consultation, whose practice is based on an exclusive dogma, to the rejection of the accumulated experience of the profession, and of the aids actually furnished by anatomy, physiology, pathology, and organic chemistry.

2. In consultations, no rivalship or jealousy should be indulged; candor, probity, and all due respect, should be exercised towards the physician having charge of the case.

3. In consultations, the attending physician should be the first to propose the necessary questions to the sick; after which the consulting physician should have the opportunity to make such farther inquiries of the patient as may be necessary to satisfy him of the true character of the case. Both physicians should then retire to a private place for deliberation; and the one first in attendance should communicate the directions agreed upon to the patient or his friends, as well as any opinions which it may be thought proper to express. But no statement or discussion of it should take place before the patient or his friends, except in the presence of all the faculty attending, and by their common consent; and no opinions or prognostications should be delivered, which are not the result of previous deliberation and concurrence.

4. In consultations, the physician in attendance should deliver his opinion first; and when there are several consulting, they should deliver their opinions in the order in which they have been called in. No decision, however, should restrain the attending physician from making such variations in the mode of treatment, as any subsequent unexpected change in the character of the case may demand. But such variation and the reasons for it ought to be carefully detailed at the next meeting in consultation. The same privilege belongs also to the consulting physician if he is sent for in an emergency, when the regular attendant is out of the way, and similar explanations must be made by him, at the next consultation.

. . .

7. All discussions in consultation should be held as secret and confidential. Neither by words nor manner should any of the parties to a consultation assert or insinuate, that any part of the treatment pursued did not receive his assent. The responsibility must be equally divided between the medical attendants—they must equally share the credit of success as well as the blame of failure.

8. Should an irreconcilable diversity of opinion occur when several physicians are called upon to consult together, the opinion of the majority should be considered as decisive; but if the numbers be equal on each side, then the decision should rest with the attending physician. It may, moreover, sometimes happen, that two physicians cannot agree in their views of the nature of a case, and the treatment to be pursued. This is a circumstance much to be deplored, and should always be avoided, if possible, by mutual concessions, as far as they can be justified by a conscientious regard for the dictates of judgment. But in the event of its occurrence, a third physician should, if practicable, be called to act as umpire; and if circumstances prevent the adoption of this course, it must be left to the patient to select

the physician in whom he is most willing to confide. But as every physician relies upon the rectitude of his judgment, he should, when left in the minority, politely and consistently retire from any further deliberation in the consultation, or participation in the management of the case.

. . .

10. A physician who is called upon to consult, should observe the most honorable and scrupulous regard for the character and standing of the practitioner in attendance: the practice of the latter, if necessary, should be justified as far as it can be, consistently with a conscientious regard for truth, and no hint or insinuation should be thrown out, which could impair the confidence reposed in him, or affect his reputation. The consulting physician should also carefully refrain from any of those extraordinary attentions or assiduities, which are too often practiced by the dishonest for the base purpose of gaining applause, or ingratiating themselves into the favor of families and individuals.

Art. V—*Duties of Physicians in cases of interference*

1. Medicine is a liberal profession, and those admitted into its ranks should found their expectations of practice upon the extent of their qualifications, not on intrigue or artifice.

2. A physician in his intercourse with a patient under the care of another practitioner, should observe the strictest caution and reserve. No meddling inquiries should be made; no disingenuous hints given relative to the nature and treatment of his disorder; nor any course of conduct pursued that may directly or indirectly tend to diminish the trust reposed in the physician employed.

3. The same circumspection and reserve should be observed, when, from motives of business or friendship, a physician is prompted to visit an individual who is under the direction of another practitioner. Indeed, such visits should be avoided, except under peculiar circumstances; and when they are made, no particular inquiries should be instituted relative to the nature of the disease, or the remedies employed, but the topics of conversation should be as foreign to the case as circumstances will admit.

. . .

Art. VI—*Of differences between Physicians*

1. Diversity of opinion, and opposition of interest, may, in the medical, as in other professions, sometimes occasion controversy and even contention. Whenever such cases unfortunately occur, and cannot be immediately terminated, they should be referred to the arbitration of a sufficient number of physicians, or a court-medical.

As peculiar reserve must be maintained by physicians towards the public, in regard to professional matters, and as there exist numerous points in medical ethics and etiquette through which the feelings of medical men may be painfully assailed in their intercourse with each other, and which cannot be understood or appreciated by general society, neither the subject-matter of such differences nor the adjudication of the arbitrators should be made public, as publicity in a case of this nature may be personally injurious to the individuals concerned, and can hardly fail to bring discredit on the faculty.

. . .

Chapter III. OF THE DUTIES OF THE PROFESSION TO THE PUBLIC, AND OF THE OBLIGATIONS OF THE PUBLIC TO THE PROFESSION

Art. I—*Duties of the profession to the public*

1. As good citizens, it is the duty of physicians to be ever vigilant for the welfare of the community, and to bear their part in sustaining its institutions and burdens: they should also be ever ready to give counsel to the public in relation to matters especially appertaining to their profession, as on subjects of medical police, public hygiene, and legal medicine. It is their province to enlighten the public in regard to quarantine regulations,—the location, arrangement, and dietaries of hospitals, asylums, schools, prisons, and similar institutions,—in relation to the medical police of towns, as drainage, ventilation, &c.,—and in regard to measures for the prevention of epidemic and contagious diseases; and when pestilence prevails, it is their duty to face the danger, and to continue their labors for the alleviation of the suffering, even at the jeopardy of their own lives.

2. Medical men should also be always ready, when called on by the legally constituted authorities, to enlighten coroners' inquests and courts of justice, on subjects strictly medical,—such as involve questions relating to sanity, legitimacy, murder by poisons or other violent means, and in regard to the various other subjects embraced in the science of Medical Jurisprudence. But in these cases, and especially where they are required to make a post-mortem examination, it is just, in consequence of the time,

labor and skill required, and the responsibility and risk they incur, that the public should award them a proper honorarium.

3. There is no profession, by the members of which, eleemosynary services are more liberally dispensed, than the medical; but justice requires that some limits should be placed to the performance of such good offices. Poverty, professional brotherhood, and certain public duties referred to in section 1 of this chapter, should always be recognised as presenting valid claims for gratuitous services; but neither institutions endowed by the public or by rich individuals, societies for mutual benefit, for the insurance of lives or for analogous purposes, nor any profession or occupation, can be admitted to possess such privilege. Nor can it be justly expected of physicians to furnish certificates of inability to serve on juries, to perform militia duty, or to testify to the state of health of persons wishing to insure their lives, obtain pensions, or the like, without a pecuniary acknowledgment. But to individuals in indigent circumstances, such professional services should always be cheerfully and freely accorded.

4. It is the duty of physicians, who are frequent witnesses of the enormities committed by quackery, and the injury to health and even destruction of life caused by the use of quack medicines, to enlighten the public on these subjects, to expose the injuries sustained by the unwary from the devices and pretensions of artful empirics and impostors. Physicians ought to use all the influence which they may possess, as professors in Colleges of Pharmacy, and by exercising their option in regard to the shops to which their prescriptions shall be sent, to discourage druggists and apothecaries from vending quack or secret medicines, or from being in any way engaged in their manufacture and sale.

Art. II—*Obligations of the public to Physicians*

1. The benefits accruing to the public directly and indirectly from the active and unwearied beneficence of the profession, are so numerous and important, that physicians are justly entitled to the utmost consideration and respect from the community. The public ought likewise to entertain a just appreciation of medical qualifications;—to make a proper discrimination between true science and the assumption of ignorance and empiricism,—to afford every encouragement and facility for the acquisition of medical education,—and no longer to allow the statute books to exhibit the anomaly of exacting knowledge from physicians, under liability to heavy penalties, and of making them obnoxious to punishment for resorting to the only means of obtaining it.

VENEZUELAN CODE OF MEDICAL ETHICS

National Academy of Medicine

1918

• • •

The Venezuelan Code, first promulgated by the National Academy of Medicine of Venezuela in 1918, was largely the work of Dr. Luis Razetti and for this reason is sometimes called the "Razetti Code." It served as a model for other Latin American codes of medical ethics (Colombia, 1919; Peru, 1922). The Sixth Latin American Medical Congress, meeting in Havana in 1922, recommended that the Venezuelan Code (slightly revised in 1922) serve to unify medical ethical concerns in Latin America. The First Brazilian Medical Congress, held in Rio de Janeiro in 1931, was similarly influenced by the Venezuelan Code.

The Venezuelan Code of 1918 includes many elements characteristic of the codes of its day, with heavy emphasis on the protection of the dignity of the profession, the maintenance of high standards of competence and training, duties toward patients (even regarding their health habits), the rendering of professional services to other doctors, obligations regarding substitute physicians and consultants, professional discipline, fees, and the like.

There are several interesting features in the Venezuelan Code that deserve comparison with other codes:

1. *The code insists that there are "rules of medical deontology" that apply to the entire "medical guild"— physicians, surgeons, pharmacists, dentists, obstetricians, interns, and nurses.*

2. *It places emphasis on physicians' virtues and qualities of character—circumspection, honesty, honor, good faith, respect, and so forth—that serve as a basis for those practices of etiquette that support the honorable practice of medicine.*

3. *The code prohibits abortion and premature childbirth (morally and legally), except "for a therapeutic purpose in cases indicated by medical science"; but it permits embryotomy if the mother's life is in danger and no alternative medical skills are available.*

4. *The excerpt below contains an interesting and detailed set of instructions on "medical confidentiality." It combines a strong affirmation of the moral obligation of health professionals to observe confidentiality with many attenuations of that obligation in the interests of the public welfare.*

Chapter IX. On Medical Confidentiality

Article 68. Medical confidentiality is a duty inherent in the very nature of the medical profession; the public interest, the personal security of the ill, the honor of families, respect for the physician, and the dignity of the art require confidentiality. Doctors, surgeons, dentists, pharmacists, and midwives as well as interns and nurses are morally obligated to safeguard privacy of information in everything they see, hear, or discover in the practice of their profession or outside of their services and which should not be divulged.

Article 69. Confidential information may be of two forms: that which is explicitly confidential—formal, documentary information confided by the client—and that which is implicitly confidential, which is private due to the nature of things, which nobody imposes, and which governs the relations of clients with medical professionals. Both forms are inviolable, except for legally specified cases.

Article 70. Medical professionals are prohibited from revealing professionally privileged information except in those cases established by medical ethics. A revelation is an act which causes the disclosed fact to change from a private to a publicly known fact. It is not necessary to publish such a fact to make it a revealed one: it suffices to confide it to a single person.

Article 71. Professionally confidential information belongs to the client. Professionals do not incur any responsibility if they reveal the private information received by them when they are authorized to do so by the patient in complete freedom and with a knowledge of the consequences by the person or persons who have confided in them, provided always that such revelation causes no harm to a third party.

Article 72. A medical person incurs no responsibility when he reveals private information in the following cases:

1. When in his capacity as a medical expert he acts as a physician for an insurance company giving it information concerning the health of the applicant sent to him for examination; or when he is commissioned by a proper authority to identify the physical or mental health of a person; or when he has been designated to perform autopsies or give medico–legal expert knowledge of any kind, as in civil or criminal cases; or when he acts as a doctor of public health or for the city; and in general when he performs the functions of a medical expert.

2. When the treating physician declares certain diseases infectious and contagious before a health authority; and when he issues death certificates.

In any of the cases included in (1), the medical professional may be exempt from the charge of ignoring the right of privacy of a person who is the object of his examination if said person is his client at the time or if the declaration has to do with previous conditions for which the same doctor was privately consulted.

Article 73. The physician shall preserve utmost secrecy if he happens to detect a venereal disease in a married woman. Not only should he refrain from informing her of the nature of the disease but he should be very careful not to let suspicion fall on the husband as responsible for the contagion. Consequently, he shall not issue any certification or make any disclosure even if the husband gives his consent.

Article 74. If a physician knows that one of his patients in a contagious period of a venereal disease plans to be married, he shall take pains to dissuade his patient from doing so, availing himself of all possible means. If the patient ignores his advice and insists on going ahead with his plan to marry, the physician is authorized without incurring responsibility not only to give the information the bride's family asks for, but also to prevent the marriage without the bridegroom's prior consultation or authorization.

Article 75. The doctor who knows that a healthy wet-nurse is nursing a syphilitic child should warn the child's parents that they are obligated to inform the nurse. If they refuse to do so, the doctor without naming the disease will impose on the nurse the necessity of immediately ceasing to nurse the child, and he should arrange to have her remain in the house for the time needed to make sure that she has not caught the disease. If the parents do not give their consent and insist that the wet-nurse continue to nurse the child, the doctor shall offer the necessary arguments, and if they nevertheless persist he shall inform the nurse of the risk she runs of contracting a contagious disease if she continues to nurse the child.

Article 76. The doctor can without failing in his duty denounce crimes of which he may have knowledge in the exercise of his profession, in accord with article 470 of the [Venezuelan] Penal Code.

Article 77. When it is a matter of making an accusation in court in order to avoid a legal violation the doctor is permitted to disclose private information.

Article 78. When a doctor is brought before a court as a witness to testify to certain facts known to him, he may refuse to disclose professionally private facts about which he is being interrogated, but which he considers privileged.

Article 79. When a doctor finds himself obliged to claim his fees legally, he should limit himself to stating the number of visits and consultations, specifying the days and nights, the number of operations he has performed, specifying the major and minor ones, the number of trips made outside the city to attend the patient, indicating the distance and time involved in travel in each visit, etc., but in no case should he reveal the nature of the operations performed, nor the details of the care that was given to the patient. The explanation of these circumstances, if necessary, shall be referred by the doctor to the medical experts so designated by the court.

Article 80. The doctor should not answer questions concerning the nature of his patient's disease; however, he is authorized not only to tell the prognosis of the case to those closest to the patient but also the diagnosis if on occasion he considers it necessary, in view of his professional responsibility or the best treatment of his patient....

2. Mid-Twentieth Century–2003

DECLARATION OF GENEVA

World Medical Association

1948, AMENDED 1968, 1983, 1994

• • •

The Declaration of Geneva was adopted by the second General Assembly of the World Medical Association (WMA) at Geneva in 1948, and subsequently amended by the twenty-second World Medical Assembly at Sydney in 1968, the thirty-fifth World Medical Assembly at Venice in 1983, and the 46th WMA Assembly at Stockholm in 1994. The declaration, which was one of the first and most important actions of the WMA, is a declaration of physicians' dedication to the humanitarian goals of medicine, a pledge that was especially important in view of the medical crimes that had just been committed in Nazi Germany. The Declaration of Geneva was intended to update the Oath of Hippocrates, which was no longer suited to modern conditions. Of interest is the fact that the WMA considered this short declaration to be a more significant statement of medical ethics than the succeeding International Code of Medical Ethics.

Only a few changes have been made in the declaration since 1948. In 1968, the phrase "even after the patient has died" was added to the confidentiality clause. In the 1983 version, which follows, the sentence regarding respect for human life was modified. Prior to 1983, it read, "I will maintain the utmost respect for human life from the time of conception...." Finally, the 1994 version amended sexist language and added a broader range of impermissible categories of discrimination.

At the time of being admitted as a member of the medical profession:

I solemnly pledge myself to consecrate my life to the service of humanity;

I will give to my teachers the respect and gratitude which is their due;

I will practice my profession with conscience and dignity;

The health of my patient will be my first consideration;

I will respect the secrets which are confided in me, even after the patient has died;

I will maintain by all the means in my power, the honor and the noble traditions of the medical profession;

My colleagues will be my sisters and brothers;

I will not permit considerations of age, disease or disability, creed, ethnic origin, gender, nationality, political affiliation, race, sexual orientation, or social standing to intervene between my duty and my patient;

I will maintain the utmost respect for human life from its beginning even under threat and I will not use my medical knowledge contrary to the laws of humanity;

I make these promises solemnly, freely and upon my honor.

INTERNATIONAL CODE OF MEDICAL ETHICS

World Medical Association

1949, AMENDED 1968, 1983

• • •

The International Code of Medical Ethics was adopted by the third General Assembly of the World Medical Association (WMA) at London in 1949, and amended in 1968 by the twenty-second World Medical Assembly at Sydney and in 1983 by the thirty-fifth World Medical Assembly at Venice. The code, which was modeled after the Declaration of Geneva and the medical ethics codes of most modern countries, states the most general principles of ethical medical practice.

The original draft of the code included the statement, "Therapeutic abortion may only be performed if the conscience of the doctors and the national laws permit," which was deleted from the adopted version because of its controversial nature. In addition, the words "from conception" were deleted from the statement regarding the doctor's obligation to preserve human life.

The 1983 version of the code, which is still current, reflects several changes from the version originally adopted. There are numerous changes in language, for example, the phrase "A physician shall ... " replaces "A doctor must...." Substantive changes include the addition of the paragraphs on providing competent medical service; on honesty and exposing physicians deficient in character; and on respecting rights and safeguarding confidences. Also, as in the Declaration of Geneva, the duty of confidentiality is extended to "even after the patient has died." Under practices deemed unethical, collaboration "in any form of medical service in which the doctor does not have professional independence" has been deleted, but the importance of professional independence is emphasized elsewhere in the text.

Duties of Physicians in General

A physician shall always maintain the highest standards of professional conduct.

A physician shall not permit motives of profit to influence the free and independent exercise of professional judgement on behalf of patients.

A physician shall, in all types of medical practice, be dedicated to providing competent medical service in full technical and moral independence, with compassion and respect for human dignity.

A physician shall deal honestly with patients and colleagues, and strive to expose those physicians deficient in character or competence, or who engage in fraud or deception.

The following practices are deemed to be unethical conduct:

a) Self-advertising by physicians, unless permitted by the laws of the country and the Code of Ethics of the National Medical Association.

b) Paying or receiving any fee or any other consideration solely to procure the referral of a patient or for prescribing or referring a patient to any source.

A physician shall respect the rights of patients, of colleagues, and of other health professionals, and shall safeguard patient confidences.

A physician shall act only in the patient's interest when providing medical care which might have the effect of weakening the physical and mental condition of the patient.

A physician shall use great caution in divulging discoveries or new techniques or treatment through non-professional channels.

A physician shall certify only that which he has personally verified.

Duties of Physicians to the Sick

A physician shall always bear in mind the obligation of preserving human life.

A physician shall owe his patients complete loyalty and all the resources of his science. Whenever an examination or treatment is beyond the physician's capacity he should summon another physician who has the necessary ability.

A physician shall preserve absolute confidentiality on all he knows about his patient even after the patient has died.

A physician shall give emergency care as a humanitarian duty unless he is assured that others are willing and able to give such care.

Duties of Physicians to Each Other

A physician shall behave towards his colleagues as he would have them behave towards him.

A physician shall not entice patients from his colleagues.

A physician shall observe the principles of the "Declaration of Geneva" approved by the World Medical Association.

PRINCIPLES OF MEDICAL ETHICS (1957)

American Medical Association

1957

• • •

Until 1957, the American Medical Association's (AMA) Code of Ethics was basically that adopted in 1847, although there were revisions in 1903, 1912, and 1947. A major change in the code's format occurred in 1957 when the Principles of Medical Ethics printed here were adopted. The ten principles, which replaced the forty-eight sections of the older code, were intended as expressions of the fundamental concepts and requirements of the older code, unencumbered by easily outdated practical codifications. Of note are the therapeutic-privilege exception to the confidentiality clause in Section 9—confidences may be disclosed if "necessary in order to protect the welfare of the individual"—and Section 10, which highlights the tension between physicians' duties to patients and those to society.

PREAMBLE. These principles are intended to aid physicians individually and collectively in maintaining a high level of ethical conduct. They are not laws but standards by which a physician may determine the propriety of his conduct in his relationship with patients, with colleagues, with members of allied professions, and with the public.

SECTION 1. The principal objective of the medical profession is to render service to humanity with full respect for the dignity of man. Physicians should merit the confidence of patients entrusted to their care, rendering to each a full measure of service and devotion.

SECTION 2. Physicians should strive continually to improve medical knowledge and skill, and should make available to their patients and colleagues the benefits of their professional attainments.

SECTION 3. A physician should practice a method of healing founded on a scientific basis; and he should not voluntarily associate professionally with anyone who violates this principle.

SECTION 4. The medical profession should safeguard the public and itself against physicians deficient in moral character or professional competence. Physicians should observe all laws, uphold the dignity and honor of the profession and accept its self-imposed disciplines. They should expose, without hesitation, illegal or unethical conduct of fellow members of the profession.

SECTION 5. A physician may choose whom he will serve. In an emergency, however, he should render service to the best of his ability. Having undertaken the care of a patient, he may not neglect him; and unless he has been discharged he may discontinue his services only after giving adequate notice. He should not solicit patients.

SECTION 6. A physician should not dispose of his services under terms or conditions which tend to interfere with or impair the free and complete exercise of his medical judgment and skill or tend to cause a deterioration of the quality of medical care.

SECTION 7. In the practice of medicine a physician should limit the source of his professional income to medical services actually rendered by him, or under his supervision, to his patients. His fee should be commensurate with the services rendered and the patient's ability to pay. He should neither pay nor receive a commission for referral of patients. Drugs, remedies or appliances may be dispensed or supplied by the physician provided it is in the best interests of the patient.

SECTION 8. A physician should seek consultation upon request; in doubtful or difficult cases; or whenever it appears that the quality of medical service may be enhanced thereby.

SECTION 9. A physician may not reveal the confidences entrusted to him in the course of medical attendance, or the deficiencies he may observe in the character of patients, unless he is required to do so by law or unless it becomes necessary in order to protect the welfare of the individual or of the community.

SECTION 10. The honored ideals of the medical professional imply that the responsibilities of the physician extend not only to the individual, but also to society where these responsibilities deserve his interest and participation in activities which have the purpose of improving both the health and the well-being of the individual and the community.

PRINCIPLES OF MEDICAL ETHICS (2001)

• • •

The AMA adopted a new set of principles in 2001. Two completely new principles were added to the 1980 principle, making nine the total number of principles. The two new principles reinforce the primacy of the physician's responsibility to the patient and also introduce the idea of a physician's commitment to health care access for all people.

The medical profession has long subscribed to a body of ethical statements developed primarily for the benefit of the patient. As a member of this profession, a physician must recognize responsibility to patients first and foremost, as well as to society, to other health professionals, and to self. The following Principles adopted by the American Medical Association are not laws, but standards of conduct which define the essentials of honorable behavior for the physician.

<http://www.ama-assn.org/ama/pub/category/2512.html>

Principles of Medical Ethics

I. A physician shall be dedicated to providing competent medical care, with compassion and respect for human dignity and rights.

II. A physician shall uphold the standards of professionalism, be honest in all professional interactions, and strive to report physicians deficient in character or competence, or engaging in fraud or deception, to appropriate entities.

III. A physician shall respect the law and also recognize a responsibility to seek changes in those requirements which are contrary to the best interests of the patient.

IV. A physician shall respect the rights of patients, colleagues, and other health professionals, and shall safeguard patient confidences and privacy within the constraints of the law.

V. A physician shall continue to study, apply, and advance scientific knowledge, maintain a commitment to medical education, make relevant information available to patients, colleagues, and the public, obtain consultation, and use the talents of other health professionals when indicated.

VI. A physician shall, in the provision of appropriate patient care, except in emergencies, be free to choose whom to serve, with whom to associate, and the environment in which to provide medical care.

VII. A physician shall recognize a responsibility to participate in activities contributing to the improvement of the community and the betterment of public health.

VIII. A physician shall, while caring for a patient, regard responsibility to the patient as paramount.

IX. A physician shall support access to medical care for all people.

Adopted June 1957; revised June 1980; revised June 2001

CURRENT OPINIONS OF THE COUNCIL ON ETHICAL AND JUDICIAL AFFAIRS

American Medical Association

2002

• • •

The 2002 revision of the Current Opinions of the Council on Ethical and Judicial Affairs, "reflects the application of the Principles of Medical Ethics to more than 175 specific ethical issues in medicine, including health care rationing, genetic testing, withdrawal of life-sustaining treatment, and family violence." A complete list of topics of the Current Opinions and the text of selected opinions follow; the annotations of court opinions and pertinent medical, ethical, and legal literature that follow many of the opinions are not included. (For full text opinions, go to www.ama-assn.org/ceja).

E-10.00 Opinions on the Patient–Physician Relationship

· · ·

2.00 · Opinions on Social Policy Issues

2.01 **ABORTION.** The Principles of Medical Ethics of the AMA do not prohibit a physician from performing an abortion in accordance with good medical practice and under circumstances that do not violate the law. (III, IV)

Issued prior to April 1977.

2.015 **MANDATORY PARENTAL CONSENT TO ABORTION.** Physicians should ascertain the law in their state on parental involvement to ensure that their procedures are consistent with their legal obligations.

Physicians should strongly encourage minors to discuss their pregnancy with their parents. Physicians should explain how parental involvement can be helpful and that parents are generally very understanding and supportive. If a minor expresses concerns about parental involvement, the physician should ensure that the minor's reluctance is not based on any misperceptions about the likely consequences of parental involvement.

Physicians should not feel or be compelled to require minors to involve their parents before deciding whether to undergo an abortion. The patient—even an adolescent—generally must decide whether, on balance, parental involvement is advisable. Accordingly, minors should ultimately be allowed to decide whether parental involvement is appropriate. Physicians should explain under what circumstances (e.g., life-threatening, emergency) the minor's confidentiality will need to be abrogated.

Physicians should try to ensure that minor patients have made an informed decision after giving careful consideration to the issues involved. They should encourage their minor patients to consult alternative sources if parents are not going to be involved in the abortion decision. Minors should be urged to seek the advice and counsel of those adults in whom they have confidence, including professional counselors, relatives, friends, teachers, or the clergy. (III, IV)

Issued June 1994 based on the report "Mandatory Parental Consent to Abortion," issued June 1992. (JAMA. 1993; 269: 82–86)

2.02 **ABUSE OF CHILDREN, ELDERLY PERSONS, AND OTHERS AT RISK.** The following are guidelines for detecting and treating family violence:

Due to the prevalence and medical consequences of family violence, physicians should routinely inquire about physical, sexual, and psychological abuse as part of the medical history. Physicians must also consider abuse in the differential diagnosis for a number of medical complaints, particularly when treating women.

Physicians who are likely to have the opportunity to detect abuse in the course of their work have an obligation to familiarize themselves with protocols for diagnosing and treating abuse and with community resources for battered women, children, and elderly persons.

Physicians also have a duty to be aware of societal misconceptions about abuse and prevent these from affecting the diagnosis and management of abuse. Such misconceptions include the belief that abuse is a rare occurrence; that abuse does not occur in "normal" families; that abuse is a private problem best resolved without outside interference; and that victims are responsible for the abuse.

In order to improve physician knowledge of family violence, physicians must be better trained to identify signs of abuse and to work cooperatively with the range of community services currently involved. Hospitals should require additional training for those physicians who are likely to see victims of abuse. Comprehensive training on family violence should be required in medical school curricula and in residency programs for specialties in which family violence is likely to be encountered.

The following are guidelines for the reporting of abuse:

Laws that require the reporting of cases of suspected abuse of children and elderly persons often create a difficult dilemma for the physician. The parties involved, both the suspected offenders and the victims, will often plead with the physician that the matter be kept confidential and not be disclosed or reported for investigation by public authorities.

Children who have been seriously injured, apparently by their parents, may nevertheless try to protect their parents by saying that the injuries were caused by an accident, such as a fall. The reason may stem from the natural parent-child relationship or fear of further punishment. Even institutionalized elderly patients who have been physically maltreated may be concerned that disclosure of what has occurred might lead to further and more drastic maltreatment by those responsible.

The physician should comply with the laws requiring reporting of suspected cases of abuse of spouses, children, elderly persons, and others.

Public officials concerned with the welfare of children and elderly persons have expressed the opinion that the incidence of physical violence to these persons is rapidly increasing and that a very substantial percentage of such cases is unreported by hospital personnel and physicians. A child or elderly person brought to a physician with a suspicious injury is the patient whose interests require the protection of law in a particular situation, even though the physician may also provide services from time to time to parents or other members of the family.

The obligation to comply with statutory requirements is clearly stated in the Principles of Medical Ethics. Absent such legal requirement, for mentally competent, adult victims of abuse, physicians should not report to state authorities without the consent of the patient. Physicians, however, do have an ethical obligation to intervene. Actions should include, but would not be limited to: suggesting the possibility of abuse with the adult patient, discussing the safety mechanisms available to the adult patient (e.g., reporting to the police or appropriate state authority), making available to the adult patient a list of community and legal resources, providing ongoing support, and documenting the situation for future reference. Physicians must discuss possible interventions and the problem of family violence with adult patients in privacy and safety. (I, III)

Issued December 1982.

Updated June 1994 based on the report "Physicians and Family Violence: Ethical Considerations," adopted December 1991 (JAMA. 1992; 267: 3190–93); updated June 1996; and updated June 2000 based on the report "Domestic Violence Intervention," adopted June 1998.

2.03 **ALLOCATION OF LIMITED MEDICAL RESOURCES.** A physician has a duty to do all that he or she can for the benefit of the individual patient. Policies for allocating limited resources have the potential to limit the ability of physicians to fulfill this obligation to patients. Physicians have a responsibility to participate and to contribute their professional expertise in order to safeguard the interests of patients in decisions made at the societal level regarding the allocation or rationing of health resources.

Decisions regarding the allocation of limited medical resources among patients should consider only ethically appropriate criteria relating to medical need. These criteria include likelihood of benefit, urgency of need, change in quality of life, duration of benefit, and, in some cases, the amount of resources required for successful treatment. In general, only very substantial differences among patients are ethically relevant; the greater the disparities, the more justified the use of these criteria becomes. In making quality of life judgments, patients should first be prioritized so that death or extremely poor outcomes are avoided; then, patients should be prioritized according to change in quality of life, but only when there are very substantial differences among patients

Nonmedical criteria, such as ability to pay, age, social worth, perceived obstacles to treatment, patient contribution to illness, or past use of resources should not be considered.

Allocation decisions should respect the individuality of patients and the particulars of individual cases as much as possible. When very substantial differences do not exist among potential recipients of treatment on the basis of the appropriate criteria defined above, a "first-come-first-served" approach or some other equal opportunity mechanism should be employed to make final allocation decisions. Though there are several ethically acceptable strategies for- implementing these criteria, no single strategy is ethically mandated. Acceptable approaches include a three-tiered system, a minimal threshold approach, and a weighted formula. Decision-making mechanisms should be objective, flexible, and consistent to ensure that all patients are treated equally.

The treating physician must remain a patient advocate and therefore should not make allocation decisions. Patients denied access to resources have the right to be informed of the reasoning behind the decision. The allocation procedures of institutions controlling scarce resources should be disclosed to the public as well as subject to regular peer review from the medical profession. (1, VII)

Issued March 1981.

Updated June 1994 based on the report "Ethical Considerations in the Allocation of Organs and Other Scarce Medical Resources Among Patients," issued June 1993. (Archive of Internal Medicine 1995; 155: 29–40).

2.035 **FUTILE CARE.** Physicians are not ethically obligated to deliver care that, in their best professional judgment, will not have a reasonable chance of benefiting their patients. Patients should not be given treatments simply because they demand them. Denial of treatment should be justified by reliance on openly stated ethical principles and acceptable standards of care, as defined in Opinion 2.03, "Allocation of Limited Medical Resources," and Opinion 2.095, "The Provision of Adequate Health Care," not on the concept of "futility," which cannot be meaningfully defined. (I, IV)

Issued June 1994.

2.06 **CAPITAL PUNISHMENT.** An individual's opinion on capital punishment is the personal moral decision of the individual. A physician, as a member of a profession dedicated to preserving life when there is hope of doing so, should not be a participant in a legally authorized execution. Physician participation in execution is defined generally as actions which would fall into one or more of the following categories: (1) an action which would directly cause the death of the condemned; (2) an action which would assist, supervise, or contribute to the ability of another individual to directly cause the death of the condemned; (3) an action which could automatically cause an execution to be carried out on a condemned prisoner.

Physician participation in an execution includes, but is not limited to, the following actions: prescribing or administering tranquilizers and other psychotropic agents and medications that are part of the execution procedure; monitoring vital signs on site or remotely (including monitoring electrocardiograms); attending or observing an execution as a physician; and rendering of technical advice regarding execution.

In the case where the method of execution is lethal injection, the following actions by the physician would also constitute physician participation in execution: selecting injection sites; starting intravenous lines as a port for a lethal injection device; prescribing, preparing, administering, or supervising injection drugs or their doses or types; inspecting, testing, or maintaining lethal injection devices; and consulting with or supervising lethal injection personnel.

The following actions do not constitute physician participation in execution: (1) testifying as to medical history and diagnoses or mental state as they relate to competence to stand trial, testifying as to relevant medical evidence during trial, testifying as to medical aspects of aggravating or mitigating circumstances during the penalty phase of a capital case, or testifying as to medical diagnoses as they relate to the legal assessment of competence for execution; (2) certifying death, provided that the condemned has been declared dead by another person; (3) witnessing an execution in a totally nonprofessional capacity; (4) witnessing an execution at the specific voluntary request of the condemned person, provided that the physician observes the execution in a nonprofessional capacity; and (5) relieving the acute suffering of a condemned person while awaiting execution, including providing tranquilizers at the specific voluntary request of the condemned person to help relieve pain or anxiety in anticipation of the execution.

Physicians should not determine legal competence to be executed. A physician's medical opinion should be merely one aspect of the information taken into account by a legal decision maker such as a judge or hearing officer. When a condemned prisoner has been declared incompetent to be executed, physicians should not treat the prisoner for the purpose of restoring competence unless a commutation order is issued before treatment begins. The task of re-evaluating the prisoner should be performed by an independent physician examiner. If the incompetent prisoner is undergoing extreme suffering as a result of psychosis or any other illness, medical intervention intended to mitigate the level of suffering is ethically permissible. No physician should be compelled to participate in the process of establishing a prisoner's competence or be involved with treatment of an incompetent, condemned prisoner if such activity is contrary to the physician's personal beliefs. Under those circumstances, physicians should be permitted to transfer care of the prisoner to another physician.

Organ donation by condemned prisoners is permissible only if (1) the decision to donate was made before the prisoner's conviction, (2) the donated tissue is harvested after the prisoner has been pronounced dead and the body removed from the death chamber, and (3) physicians do not provide advice on modifying the method of execution for any individual to facilitate donation. (I)

Issued July 1980.

Updated June 1994 based on the report "Physician Participation in Capital Punishment," adopted December 1992, (JAMA. 1993; 270: 365–368); updated June 1996 based on the report "Physician Participation in Capital Punishment: Evaluations of Prisoner Competence to be Executed; Treatment to Restore Competence to be Executed," adopted in June 1995; Updated December 1999; and Updated June 2000 based on the report "Defining Physician Participation in State Executions," adopted June 1998.

• • •

2.077 **ETHICAL CONSIDERATIONS IN INTERNATIONAL RESEARCH.** Physicians, either in their role as investigators or as decision-makers involved in the deliberations related to the funding or the review of research, hold an ethical obligation to ensure the protection of research participants. When the research is to be conducted in countries with differing cultural traditions, health care systems, and ethical standards, and in particular in countries with developing economies and with limited health care resources, U.S. physicians should respect the following guidelines:

(1) First and foremost, physicians involved in clinical research that will be carried out internationally should be satisfied that a proposed research design has been developed according to a sound scientific design. Therefore, investigators must ascertain that there is genuine uncertainty within the clinical community about the comparative merits of the experimental treatment and the one to be offered as a control in the population among which the study is to be undertaken. In some instances, a three-pronged protocol, which offers the standard treatment in use in the U.S., a treatment that meets a level of care that is attainable and sustainable by the host country, and a placebo (see Opinion 2.075, "Surgical 'Placebo' Controls"), may be the best method to evaluate the safety and efficacy of a treatment in a given population. When U.S.

investigators participate in international research they must obtain approval for such protocols from U.S. Institutional Review Boards (IRBs).

(2) IRBs, which are responsible for ensuring the protection of research participants, must determine that risks have been minimized and that the protocol's ratio of risks to benefits is favorable to participants. In evaluating the risks and benefits that a protocol presents to a population, IRBs should obtain relevant input from representatives from the host country and from the research population. It is also appropriate for IRBs to consider the harm that is likely to result from forgoing the research.

(3) Also, IRBs are required to protect the welfare of individual participants. This can best be achieved by assuring that a suitable informed consent process is in place. Therefore, IRBs should ensure that individual potential participants will be informed of the nature of the research endeavor and that their voluntary consent will be sought. IRBs should recognize that, in some instances, information will be meaningful only if it is communicated in ways that are consistent with local customs.

(4) Overall, to ensure that the research does not exploit the population from which participants are recruited, IRBs should ensure that the research corresponds to a medical need in the region where it is undertaken. Furthermore, they should foster research with the potential for lasting benefits, especially when it is undertaken among populations that are severely deficient in health care resources. This can be achieved by facilitating the development of a health care infrastructure that will be of use during and beyond the conduct of the research. Additionally, physicians conducting studies must encourage research sponsors to continue to provide beneficial study interventions to all study participants at the conclusion of the study. (I, IV, VII, VIII, IX)

Issued December 2001 based on the report "Ethical Considerations in International Research," adopted June 2001.

2.09 **COSTS.** While physicians should be conscious of costs and not provide or prescribe unnecessary services, concern for the quality of care the patient receives should be the physician's first consideration. This does not preclude the physician, individually or through medical or other organizations, from participating in policy-making with respect to social issues affecting health care. (I, VII)

Issued March 1981.

Updated June 1994 and June 1998.

2.095 **THE PROVISION OF ADEQUATE HEALTH CARE.** Because society has an obligation to make access to an adequate level of health care available to all of its members regardless of ability to pay, physicians should contribute their expertise at a policy-making level to help achieve this goal. In determining whether particular procedures or treatments should be included in the adequate level of health care, the following ethical principles should be considered: (1) degree of benefit (the difference in outcome between treatment and no treatment), (2) likelihood of benefit, (3) duration of benefit, (4) cost, and (5) number of people who will benefit (referring to the fact that a treatment may benefit the patient and others who come into contact with the patient, as with a vaccination or antimicrobial drug).

Ethical principles require that the ethical criteria be combined with a fair process to determine the adequate level of health care. Among the many possible alternative processes, the Council recommends the following two:

(1) Democratic decision making with broad public input at both the developmental and final approval stages can be used to develop the package of benefits. With this approach, enforcement of anti-discrimination laws will be necessary to ensure that the interests of minorities and historically disadvantaged groups are protected.

(2) Equal opportunity mechanisms can also be used to determine the package of health care benefits. After applying the five ethical criteria listed above, it will be possible to designate some kinds of care as either clearly basic or clearly discretionary. However, for care that is not clearly basic or discretionary, a random selection or other equal consideration mechanism may be used to determine which kinds of care will be included in the basic benefits package.

The mechanism for providing an adequate level of health care should ensure that the health care benefits for the poor and disadvantaged will not be eroded over time. There should also be ongoing monitoring for variations in care that cannot be explained on medical grounds with special attention to evidence of discriminatory impact on historically disadvantaged groups. Finally, adjustment of the adequate level over time should be made to ensure continued and broad public acceptance.

Issued June 1994 based on the report "Ethical Issues in Health System Reform: The Provision of Adequate Health Care," issued December 1993. (JAMA. 1994; 272)

2.10 **FETAL RESEARCH GUIDELINES.** The following guidelines are offered as aids to physicians when they are engaged in fetal research:

(1) Physicians may participate in fetal research when their activities are part of a competently designed program, under accepted standards of scientific research, to produce data which are scientifically valid and significant.

(2) If appropriate, properly performed clinical studies on animals and nongravid humans should precede any particular fetal research project.

(3) In fetal research projects, the investigator should demonstrate the same care and concern for the fetus as a physician providing fetal care or treatment in a non-research setting.

(4) All valid federal or state legal requirements should be followed.

(5) There should be no monetary payment to obtain any fetal material for fetal research projects.

(6) Competent peer review committees, review boards, or advisory boards should be available, when appropriate, to protect against the possible abuses that could arise in such research.

(7) Research on the so called "dead fetus," macerated fetal material, fetal cells, fetal tissue, or fetal organs should be in accord with state laws on autopsy and state laws on organ transplantation or anatomical gifts.

(8) In fetal research primarily for treatment of the fetus:

　A. Voluntary and informed consent, in writing, should be given by the gravid woman, acting in the best interest of the fetus.

　B. Alternative treatment or methods of care, if any, should be carefully evaluated and fully explained. If simpler and safer treatment is available, it should be pursued.

(9) In research primarily for treatment of the gravid female:

　A. Voluntary and informed consent, in writing, should be given by the patient.

　B. Alternative treatment or methods of care should be carefully evaluated and fully explained to the patient. If simpler and safer treatment is available, it should be pursued.

　C. If possible, the risk to the fetus should be the least possible, consistent with the gravid female's need for treatment.

(10) In fetal research involving a fetus in utero, primarily for the accumulation of scientific knowledge:

A. Voluntary and informed consent, in writing, should be given by the gravid woman under circumstances in which a prudent and informed adult would reasonably be expected to give such consent.

B. The risk to the fetus imposed by the research should be the least possible.

C. The purpose of research is the production of data and knowledge which are scientifically significant and which cannot otherwise be obtained.

D. In this area of research, it is especially important to emphasize that care and concern for the fetus should be demonstrated. (I, III, V)

Issued March 1980.

Updated June 1994.

2.11 **GENE THERAPY.** Gene therapy involves the replacement or modification of a genetic variant to restore or enhance cellular function or to improve the reaction of non-genetic therapies.

Two types of gene therapy have been identified: (1) somatic cell therapy, in which human cells other than germ cells are genetically altered, and (2) germ line therapy, in which a replacement gene is integrated into the genome of human gametes or their precursors, resulting in expression of the new gene in the patient's offspring and subsequent generations. The fundamental difference between germ line therapy and somatic cell therapy is that germ line therapy affects the welfare of subsequent generations and may be associated with increased risk and the potential for unpredictable and irreversible results. Because of the far-reaching implications of germ line therapy, it is appropriate to limit genetic intervention to somatic cells at this time.

The goal of both somatic cell and germ line therapy is to alleviate human suffering and disease by remedying disorders for which available therapies are not satisfactory. This goal should be pursued only within the ethical tradition of medicine, which gives primacy to the welfare of the patient whose safety and well-being must be vigorously protected. To the extent possible, experience with animal studies must be sufficient to assure the effectiveness and safety of the techniques used, and the predictability of the results.

Moreover, genetic manipulation generally should be utilized only for therapeutic purposes. Efforts to enhance "desirable" characteristics through the insertion of a modified or additional gene, or efforts to "improve" complex human traits"the eugenic development of offspring"are contrary not only to the ethical tradition of medicine, but also to the egalitarian values of our society. Because of the potential for abuse, genetic manipulation to affect non-disease traits may never be acceptable and perhaps should never be pursued. If it is ever allowed, at least three conditions would have to be met before it could be deemed ethically acceptable: (1) there would have to be a clear and meaningful benefit to the person, (2) there would have to be no trade-off with other characteristics or traits, and (3) all citizens would have to have equal access to the genetic technology, irrespective of income or other socioeconomic characteristics. These criteria should be viewed as a minimal, not an exhaustive, test of the ethical propriety of non-disease-related genetic intervention. As genetic technology and knowledge of the human genome develop further, additional guidelines may be required.

As gene therapy becomes feasible for a variety of human disorders, there are several practical factors to consider to ensure safe application of this technology in society. First, any gene therapy research should meet the Council's guidelines on clinical investigation (Opinion 2.07) and investigators must adhere to the standards of medical practice and professional responsibility. The proposed procedure must be fully discussed with the patient and the written informed consent of the patient or the patient's legal representative must be voluntary.

Investigators must be thorough in their attempts to eliminate any unwanted viral agents from the viral vector containing the corrective gene. The potential for adverse effects of the viral delivery system must be disclosed to the patient. The effectiveness of gene therapy must be evaluated fully, including the determination of the natural history of the disease and follow-up examination of subsequent generations. Gene therapy should be pursued only after the availablity or effectiveness of other possible therapies is found to be insufficient. These considerations should be reviewed, as appropriate, as procedures and scientific information develop. (I, V)

Issued December 1988.

Updated June 1994 based on the report "Prenatal Genetic Screening," adopted December 1992 (Arch Fam Med. 1994; 2: 633–642), and updated June 1996.

• • •

2.147 HUMAN CLONING. "Somatic cell nuclear transfer" is the process in which the nucleus of a somatic cell of an organism is transferred into an enucleated oocyte. "Human cloning" is the application of somatic nuclear transfer technology to the creation of a human being that shares all of its nuclear genes with the person donating the implanted nucleus.

In order to clarify the many existing misconceptions about human cloning, physicians should help educate the public about the intrinsic limits of human cloning as well as the current ethical and legal protections that would prevent abuses of human cloning. These include the following: (1) using human cloning as an approach to terminal illness or mortality is a concept based on the mistaken notion that one's genotype largely determines one's individuality. A clone-child created via human cloning would not be identical to his or her clone-parent. (2) Current ethical and legal standards hold that under no circumstances should human cloning occur without an individual's permission. (3) Current ethical and legal standards hold that a human clone would be entitled to the same rights, freedoms, and protections as every other individual in society. The fact that a human clone's nuclear genes would derive from a single individual rather than two parents would not change his or her moral standing.

Physicians have an ethical obligation to consider the harms and benefits of new medical procedures and technologies. Physicians should not participate in human cloning at this time because further investigation and discussion regarding the harms and benefits of human cloning is required. Concerns include: (1) unknown physical harms introduced by cloning. Somatic cell nuclear transfer has not yet been refined and its long-term safety has not yet been proven. The risk of producing individuals with genetic anomalies gives rise to an obligation to seek better understanding of—and potential medical therapies for—the unforeseen medical consequences that could stem from human cloning. (2) Psychosocial harms introduced by cloning, including violations of privacy and autonomy. Human cloning risks limiting, at least psychologically, the seemingly unlimited potential of new human beings and thus creating enormous pressures on the clone-child to live up to expectations based on the life of the clone-parent. (3) The impact of human cloning on familial and societal relations. The family unit may be altered with the introduction of cloning, and more thought is required on a societal level regarding how to construct familial relations. (4) Potential effects on the gene pool.

Like other interventions that can change individuals' reproductive patterns and the resulting genetic characteristics of a population, human cloning has the potential to be used in a eugenic or discriminatory fashion—practices that are incompatible with the ethical norms of medical practice. Moreover, human cloning could alter irreversibly the gene pool and exacerbate genetic problems that arise from deleterious genetic mutations, resulting in harms to future generations.

Two potentially realistic and possibly appropriate medical uses of human cloning are for assisting individuals or couples to reproduce and for the generation of tissues when the donor is not harmed or sacrificed. Given the unresolved issues regarding cloning identified above, the medical profession should not undertake human cloning at this time and pursue alternative approaches that raise fewer ethical concerns.

Because cloning technology is not limited to the United States, physicians should help establish international guidelines governing human cloning. (V)

Issued December 1999 based of the report "The Ethics of Human Cloning," adopted June 1999.

. . .

2.17 QUALITY OF LIFE. In the making of decisions for the treatment of seriously disabled newborns or of other persons who are severely disabled by injury or illness, the primary consideration should be what is best for the individual patient and not the avoidance of a burden to the family or to society. Quality of life, as defined by the patient's interests and values, is a factor to be considered in determining what is best for the individual. It is permissible to consider quality of life when deciding about life-sustaining treatment in accordance with opinions 2.20, 2.215, and 2.22 (I, III, IV)

Issued March 1981.

Updated June 1994.

. . .

2.19 UNNECESSARY SERVICES. Physicians should not provide, prescribe, or seek compensation for services that are known to be unnecessary. (II, VII)

Issued prior to April 1977.

Updated June 1996.

2.20 WITHHOLDING OR WITHDRAWING LIFE-SUSTAINING MEDICAL TREATMENT. The social commitment of the physician is to sustain life and relieve suffering. Where the performance of one duty conflicts with the other, the preferences of the patient should prevail. The principle of patient autonomy requires that physicians respect the decision to forego life-sustaining treatment of a patient who possesses decision-making capacity. Life-sustaining treatment is any treatment that serves to prolong life without reversing the underlying medical condition. Life-sustaining treatment may include, but is not limited to, mechanical ventilation, renal dialysis, chemotherapy, antibiotics, and artificial nutrition and hydration.

There is no ethical distinction between withdrawing and withholding life-sustaining treatment.

A competent, adult patient may, in advance, formulate and provide a valid consent to the withholding or withdrawal of life-support systems in the event that injury or illness renders that individual incompetent to make such a decision. A patient may also appoint a surrogate decision maker in accordance with state law.

If the patient receiving life-sustaining treatment is incompetent, a surrogate decision maker should be identified. Without an advance directive that designates a proxy, the patient's family should become the surrogate decision maker. Family includes persons with whom the patient is closely associated. In the case when there is no person closely associated with the patient, but there are persons who both care about the patient and have sufficient relevant knowledge of the patient, such persons may be appropriate surrogates. Physicians should provide all relevant medical information and explain to surrogate decision makers that decisions regarding withholding or withdrawing life-sustaining treatment should be based on substituted judgment (what the patient would have decided) when there is evidence of the patient's preferences and values. In making a substituted judgment, decision makers may consider the patient's advance directive (if any); the patient's values about life and the way it should be lived; and the patient's attitudes towards sickness, suffering, medical procedures, and death. If there is not adequate evidence of the incompetent patient's preferences and values, the decision should be based on the best interests of the patient (what outcome would most likely promote the patient's well-being).

Though the surrogate's decision for the incompetent patient should almost always be accepted by the physician, there are four situations that may require either institutional or judicial review and/or intervention in the decision-making process: (1) there is no available family member willing to be the patient's surrogate decision maker, (2) there is a dispute among family members and there is no decision maker designated in an advance directive, (3) a health care provider believes that the family's decision is clearly not what the patient would have decided if competent, and (4) a health care provider believes that the decision is not a decision that could reasonably be judged to be in the patient's best interests. When there are disputes among family members or between family and health care providers, the use of ethics committees specifically designed to facilitate sound decision making is recommended before resorting to the courts.

When a permanently unconscious patient was never competent or had not left any evidence of previous preferences or values, since there is no objective way to ascertain the best interests of the patient, the surrogate's decision should not be challenged as long as the decision is based on the decision maker's true concern for what would be best for the patient.

Physicians have an obligation to relieve pain and suffering and to promote the dignity and autonomy of dying patients in their care. This includes providing effective palliative treatment even though it may foreseeably hasten death.

Even if the patient is not terminally ill or permanently unconscious, it is not unethical to discontinue all means of life-sustaining medical treatment in accordance with a proper substituted judgment or best interests analysis. (I, III, IV, V)

Issued December 1984 as Opinion 2.18, Withholding or Withdrawing Life-Prolonging Medical Treatment, and Opinion 2.19, Withholding or Withdrawing Life-Prolonging Medical Treatment—Patients' Preferences. In 1989, these Opinions were renumbered 2.20 and 2.21, respectively.

Updated June 1994 based on the reports "Decisions Near the End of Life" and "Decisions to Forego Life-Sustaining Treatment for Incompetent Patients," both adopted June 1991 (Decisions Near the End of Life. JAMA. 1992; 267: 2229–2233), and updated June 1996. [In March 1981, the Council on Ethical and Judicial Affairs issued Opinion 2.11, Terminal Illness. The Opinion was renumbered 2.15 in 1984 and was deleted in 1986.]

2.21 **EUTHANASIA.** Euthanasia is the administration of a lethal agent by another person to a patient for the purpose of relieving the patient's intolerable and incurable suffering.

It is understandable, though tragic, that some patients in extreme duress—such as those suffering from a terminal, painful, debilitating illness—may come to decide that death is preferable to life. However, permitting physicians to engage in euthanasia would ultimately cause more harm than good. Euthanasia is fundamentally incompatible with the physician's role as healer, would be difficult or impossible to control, and would pose serious societal risks.

The involvement of physicians in euthanasia heightens the significance of its ethical prohibition. The physician who performs euthanasia assumes unique responsibility for the act of ending the patient's life. Euthanasia could also readily be extended to incompetent patients and other vulnerable populations.

Instead of engaging in euthanasia, physicians must aggressively respond to the needs of patients at the end of life. Patients should not be abandoned once it is determined that cure is impossible. Patients near the end of life must continue to receive emotional support, comfort care, adequate pain control, respect for patient autonomy, and good communication. (I, IV)

Issued June 1994 based on the report "Decisions Near the End of Life," adopted June 1991 (JAMA. 1992; 267: 2229–2233).

Updated June 1996.

2.211 **PHYSICIAN ASSISTED SUICIDE.** Physician-assisted suicide occurs when a physician facilitates a patient's death by providing the necessary means and/or information to enable the patient to perform the life-ending act (e.g., the physician provides sleeping pills and information about the lethal dose, while aware that the patient may commit suicide).

It is understandable, though tragic, that some patients in extreme duress—such as those suffering from a terminal, painful, debilitating illness—may come to decide that death is preferable to life. However, allowing physicians to participate in assisted suicide would cause more harm than good. Physician-assisted suicide is fundamentally incompatible with the physician's role as healer, would be difficult or impossible to control, and would pose serious societal risks.

Instead of participating in assisted suicide, physicians must aggressively respond to the needs of patients at the end of life. Patients should not be abandoned once it is determined that cure is impossible. Multidisciplinary interventions should be sought including specialty consultation, hospice care, pastoral support, family counseling, and other modalities. Patients near the end of life must continue to receive emotional support, comfort care, adequate pain control, respect for patient autonomy, and good communication. (I, IV)

Issued June 1994 based on the reports "Decisions Near the End of Life," adopted June 1991, and "Physician-Assisted Suicide," adopted December 1993 (JAMA. 1992; 267: 2229–33).

Updated June 1996.

2.215 **TREATMENT DECISIONS FOR SERIOUSLY ILL NEWBORNS.** The primary consideration for decisions regarding life-sustaining treatment for seriously ill newborns should be what is best for the newborn. Factors that should be weighed are (1) the chance that therapy will succeed, (2) the risks involved with treatment and nontreatment, (3) the degree to which the therapy, if successful, will extend life, (4) the pain and discomfort associated with the therapy, and (5) the anticipated quality of life for the newborn with and without treatment.

Care must be taken to evaluate the newborn's expected quality of life from the child's perspective. Life-sustaining treatment may be withheld or withdrawn from a newborn when the pain and suffering expected to be endured by the child will overwhelm any potential for joy during his or her life. When an infant suffers extreme neurological damage, and is consequently not capable of experiencing either suffering or joy a decision may be made to withhold or withdraw life-sustaining treatment. When life-sustaining treatment is withheld or withdrawn, comfort care must not be discontinued.

When an infant's prognosis is largely uncertain, as is often the case with extremely premature newborns, all life-sustaining and life-enhancing treatment should be initiated. Decisions about life-sustaining treatment should be made once the prognosis becomes more certain. It is not necessary to attain absolute or near absolute prognostic certainty before life-sustaining treatment is withdrawn, since this goal is often unattainable and risks unnecessarily prolonging the infant's suffering.

Physicians must provide full information to parents of seriously ill newborns regarding the nature of treatments, therapeutic options and expected prognosis with and without therapy, so that parents can make informed decisions for their children about life-sustaining treatment. Counseling services and an opportunity to talk with persons who have had to make similar decisions should be available to parents. Ethics committees or infant review committees should also be utilized to facilitate parental decisionmaking. These committees should help mediate resolutions of conflicts that may arise among parents, physicians and others involved in the care of the infant. These committees should also be responsible for referring cases to the appropriate public agencies when it is concluded that the parents' decision is not a decision that could reasonably be judged to be in the best interests of the infant. (I, III, IV, V)

Issued June 1994 based on the report "Treatment Decisions for Seriously Ill Newborns," issued June 1992.

2.22 DO-NOT-RESUSCITATE ORDERS. Efforts should be made to resuscitate patients who suffer cardiac or respiratory arrest except when circumstances indicate that cardiopulmonary resuscitation (CPR) would be inappropriate or not in accord with the desires or best interests of the patient.

Patients at risk of cardiac or respiratory failure should be encouraged to express in advance their preferences regarding the use of CPR and this should be documented in the patient's medical record. These discussions should include a description of the procedures encompassed by CPR and, when possible, should occur in an outpatient setting when general treatment preferences are discussed, or as early as possible during hospitalization. The physician has an ethical obligation to honor the resuscitation preferences expressed by the patient. Physicians should not permit their personal value judgments about qualify of life to obstruct the implementation of a patient's preferences regarding the use of CPR.

If a patient is incapable of rendering a decision regarding the use of CPR, a decision may be made by a surrogate decisionmaker, based upon the previously expressed preferences of the patient or, if such preferences are unknown, in accordance with the patient's best interests.

If, in the judgment of the attending physician, it would be inappropriate to pursue CPR, the attending physician may enter a do-not-resuscitate order into the patient's record. Resuscitative efforts should be considered inappropriate by the attending physician only if they cannot be expected either to restore cardiac or respiratory function to the patient or to meet established ethical criteria, as defined in the Principles of Medical Ethics and Opinions 2.03 and 2.095. When there is adequate time to do so, the physician must first inform the patient, or the incompetent patient's surrogate, of the content of the DNR order, as well as the

basis for its implementation. The physician also should be prepared to discuss appropriate alternatives, such as obtaining a second opinion (e.g., consulting a bioethics committee) or arranging for transfer of care to another physician.

Do-Not-Resuscitate orders, as well as the basis for their implementation, should be entered by the attending physician in the patient's medical record.

DNR orders only preclude resuscitative efforts in the event of cardiopulmonary arrest and should not influence other therapeutic interventions that may be appropriate for the patient. (I, IV)

Issued March 1992 based on the report "Guidelines for the Appropriate Use of Do-Not-Resuscitate Orders," issued December 1990. (JAMA. 1991; 265: 1868–1871)

Updated June 1994.

2.23 HIV TESTING. HIV testing is appropriate and should be encouraged for diagnosis and treatment of HIV infection or of medical conditions that may be affected by HIV. Treatment may prolong the lives of those with AIDS and prolong the symptom-free period in those with an asymptomatic HIV infection. Wider testing is imperative to ensure that individuals in need of treatment are identified and treated.

Physicians should ensure that HIV testing is conducted in a way that respects patient autonomy and assures patient confidentiality as much as possible.

The physician should secure the patient's informed consent specific for HIV testing before testing is performed. Because of the need for pretest counseling and the potential consequences of an HIV test on an individual's job, housing, insurability, and social relationships, the consent should be specific for HIV testing. Consent for HIV testing cannot be inferred from a general consent to treatment.

When a health care provider is at risk for HIV infection because of the occurrence of puncture injury or mucosal contact with potentially infected bodily fluids, it is acceptable to test the patient for HIV infection even if the patient refuses consent. When testing without consent is performed in accordance with the law, the patient should be given the customary pretest counseling.

The confidentiality of the results of HIV testing must be maintained as much as possible and the limits of a patient's confidentiality should be known to the patient before consent is given.

Exceptions to confidentiality are appropriate when necessary to protect the public health or when necessary to protect individuals, including health care workers, who are endangered by persons infected with HIV. If a physician knows that a seropositive individual is endangering a third party, the physician should, within the constraints of the law, (1) attempt to persuade the infected patient to cease endangering the third party; (2) if persuasion fails, notify authorities; and (3) if the authorities take no action, notify the endangered third party.

In order to limit the public spread of HIV infection, physicians should encourage voluntary testing of patients at risk for infection.

It is unethical to deny treatment to HIV-infected individuals because they are HIV seropositive or because they are unwilling to undergo HIV testing, except in the instance where knowledge of the patient's HIV status is vital to the appropriate treatment of the patient. When a patient refuses to be tested after being informed of the physician's medical opinion, the physician may transfer the patient to a second physician who is willing to manage the patient's care in accordance with the patient's preferences about testing. (I, IV)

Issued March 1992 based on the report "Ethical Issues Involved in the Growing AIDS Crisis," issued December 1987. (JAMA. 1988; 259: 1360–1361)

Updated June 1994.

3.00 · Opinions on Interprofessional Relations

. . .

3.02 **NURSES.** The primary bond between the practices of medicine and nursing is mutual ethical concern for patients. One of the duties in providing reasonable care is fulfilled by a nurse who carries out the orders of the attending physician. Where orders appear to the nurse to be in error or contrary to customary medical and nursing practice, the physician has an ethical obligation to hear the nurse's concern and explain those orders to the nurse involved. The ethical physician should neither expect nor insist that nurses follow orders contrary to standards of good medical and nursing practice. In emergencies, when prompt action is necessary and the physician is not immediately available, a nurse may be justified in acting contrary to the physician's standing orders for the safety of the patient. Such occurrences

should not be considered to be a breakdown in professional relations. (IV, V)

Issued June 1983

Updated June 1994.

. . .

3.08 **SEXUAL HARASSMENT AND EXPLOITATION BETWEEN MEDICAL SUPERVISORS AND TRAINEES.** Sexual harassment may be defined as sexual advances, requests for sexual favors, and other verbal or physical conduct of a sexual nature when (1) such conduct interferes with an individual's work or academic performance or creates an intimidating, hostile, or offensive work or academic environment or (2) accepting or rejecting such conduct affects or may be perceived to affect employment decisions or academic evaluations concerning the individual. Sexual harassment is unethical.

Sexual relationships between medical supervisors and their medical trainees raise concerns because of inherent inequalities in the status and power that medical supervisors wield in relation to medical trainees and may adversely affect patient care. Sexual relationships between a medical trainee and a supervisor even when consensual are not acceptable regardless of the degree of supervision in any given situation. The supervisory role should be eliminated if the parties involved wish to pursue their relationship. (II, IV, VII)

Issued March 1992 based on the report "Sexual Harassment and Exploitation Between Medical Supervisors and Trainees," issued June 1989.

Updated June 1994

. . .

5.00 · Opinions on Confidentiality, Advertising, and Communications Media Relations

. . .

5.015 **DIRECT-TO-CONSUMER ADVERTISEMENTS OF PRESCRIPTION DRUGS.** The medical profession needs to take an active role in ensuring that proper advertising guidelines are enforced and that the care patients receive is not compromised as a result of direct-to-consumer advertising. Since the Food and Drug Administration (FDA) has a critical role in determining future directions of direct-to-consumer advertising of prescription drugs, physicians should work to ensure that the FDA remains committed to advertising standards that protect patients' health and safety. Moreover, physicians should encourage and engage in studies regarding the effect of direct-to-consumer advertising on patient health and medical care. Such studies should examine whether direct-to-consumer advertising improves the communication of health information; enhances the patient–physician relationship; and contains accurate and reasonable information on risks, precautions, adverse reactions, and costs.

Physicians must maintain professional standards of informed consent when prescribing. When a patient comes to a physician with a request for a drug he or she has seen advertised, the physician and the patient should engage in a dialogue that would assess and enhance the patient's understanding of the treatment. Although physicians should not be biased against drugs that are advertised, physicians should resist commercially induced pressure to prescribe drugs that may not be indicated. Physicians should deny requests for inappropriate prescriptions and educate patients as to why certain advertised drugs may not be suitable treatment options, providing, when available, information on the cost effectiveness of different options.

Physicians must remain vigilant to assure that direct-to-consumer advertising does not promote false expectations. Physicians should be concerned about advertisements that do not enhance consumer education; do not convey a clear, accurate, and responsible health education message; do not refer patients to their physicians for more information; do not identify the target population at risk; and fail to discourage consumer self-diagnosis and self-treatment. Physicians may choose to report these concerns directly to the pharmaceutical company that sponsored the advertisement.

To assist the FDA in enforcing existing law and tracking the effects of direct-to-consumer advertising, physicians should, whenever reasonably possible, report to them advertisements that: (1) do not provide a fair and balanced discussion of the use of the drug product for the disease, disorder, or condition; (2) do not clearly explain warnings, precautions, and potential adverse reactions associated with the drug product; (3) do not present summary information in language that can be understood by the consumer; (4) do not comply with applicable FDA rules, regulations, policies, and guidelines as provided by the FDA; or (5) do not provide collateral materials to educate both physicians and consumers. (II, III)

Issued June 1999 based on the report "Direct-to-Consumer Advertisement of Prescription Drugs," adopted December 1998 (Food and Drug Law Journal. 2000; 55: 119–24).

5.045 **FILMING PATIENTS IN HEALTH CARE SETTINGS.** The use of any medium to film, videotape, or otherwise record (hereafter film) patient interactions with their health care providers requires the utmost respect for the privacy and confidentiality of the patient. The following guidelines are offered to assure that the rights of the patient are protected. These guidelines specifically address filming with the intent of broadcast for public viewing, and do not address other uses such as in medical education, forensic or diagnostic filming, or the use of security cameras. (1) Educating the public about the health care system should be encouraged, and filming of patients may be one way to accomplish this. This educational objective is not severely compromised by filming only patients who can consent; when patients cannot consent, dramatic reenactments utilizing actors should be considered instead of violating patient privacy. (2) Filming patients without consent is a violation of the patient's privacy. Consent is therefore an ethical requirement for both initial filming and subsequent broadcast for public viewing. Because filming cannot benefit a patient medically, and moreover has the potential of causing harm to the patient, it is appropriate to limit filming to instances where the party being filmed can explicitly consent. Consent by a surrogate decision-maker is not an ethically appropriate substitute for consent by the patient because the role of surrogates is to make medically necessary decisions in the best interest of the patient. A possible exception exists when the person in question is permanently or indefinitely incompetent (e.g., permanent vegetative state or minor child). In such circumstances, if a parent or legal guardian provides consent, filming may occur. (a) Patients should have the right to have filming stopped upon request at any time and the film crew removed from the area. Also, persons involved in the direct medical care of the patient who feel that the filming may jeopardize patient care should request that the film crew be removed from the patient care area. (b) The initial granting of consent does not preclude the patient from withdrawing consent at a later time. After filming has occurred, patients who have been filmed should have the opportunity to rescind their consent up until a reasonable time period before broadcast for public viewing. The consent process should include a full disclosure of whether the tape will be destroyed if consent is rescinded, and the degree to which the patient is allowed to view and edit the final footage before broadcast for public viewing. (c) Due to the potential conflict of interest, informed consent should be obtained by a disinterested third party, and not a member of the film crew or production team. (3) Information obtained in the course of filming medical encounters between patients and physicians is confidential. Persons who are not members of the health care team, but who may be present for filming purposes, must demonstrate that they understand the confidential nature of the information and are committed to respecting it. Where possible, it is desirable for stationary cameras or health care professionals to perform the filming.

Physicians, as advocates for their patients, should not allow financial or promotional benefit to the health care institution to influence their advice to patients regarding participation in filming. Because physician compensation for participation in filming may cause an undue influence to recruit patients, physicians should not be compensated directly. To protect the best interests of patients, physicians should participate in institutional review of requests to film. (I, IV, VII, VIII)

Issued December 2001 based on the report "Filming Patients in Health Care Settings," adopted June 2001.

5.05 **CONFIDENTIALITY.** The information disclosed to a physician during the course of the relationship between physician and patient is confidential to the greatest possible degree. The patient should feel free to make a full disclosure of information to the physician in order that the physician may most effectively provide needed services. The patient should be able to make this disclosure with the knowledge that the patient will respect the confidential nature of the communication. The physician should not reveal confidential communications or information without the express consent of the patient, unless required to do so by law.

The obligation to safeguard patient confidences is subject to 2certain exceptions which are ethically and legally justified because of overriding social considerations. Where a patient threatens to inflict serious bodily harm to another person or to him or herself and there is a reasonable probability that the patient may carry out the threat, the physician should take reasonable precautions for the protection of the intended victim, including notification of law enforcement authorities. Also, communicable diseases, gun shot and knife wounds should be reported as required by applicable statutes or ordinances. (IV)

Issued December 1983.

Updated June 1994.

5.055 **CONFIDENTIAL CARE FOR MINORS.** Physicians who treat minors have an ethical duty to promote the autonomy of minor patients by involving them in the medical decision-making process to a degree commensurate with their abilities.

When minors request confidential services, physicians should encourage them to involve their parents. This includes making efforts to obtain the minor's reasons for not involving their parents and correcting misconceptions that may be motivating their objections.

Where the law does not require otherwise, physicians should permit a competent minor to consent to medical care and should not notify parents without the patient's consent. Depending on the seriousness of the decision, competence may be evaluated by physicians for most minors. When necessary, experts in adolescent medicine or child psychological development should be consulted. Use of the courts for competence determinations should be made only as a last resort.

When an immature minor requests contraceptive services, pregnancy-related care (including pregnancy testing, prenatal and postnatal care, and delivery services), or treatment for sexually transmitted disease, drug and alcohol abuse, or mental illness, physicians must recognize that requiring parental involvement may be counterproductive to the health of the patient. Physicians should encourage parental involvement in these situations. However, if the minor continues to object, his or her wishes ordinarily should be respected. If the physician is uncomfortable with providing services without parental involvement, and alternative confidential services are available, the minor may be referred to those services. In cases when the physician believes that without parental involvement and guidance, the minor will face a serious health threat, and there is reason to believe that the parents will be helpful and understanding, disclosing the problem to the parents is ethically justified. When the physician does breach confidentiality to the parents, he or she must discuss the reasons for the breach with the minor prior to the disclosure.

For minors who are mature enough to be unaccompanied by their parents for their examination, confidentiality of information disclosed during an exam, interview, or in counseling should be maintained. Such information may be disclosed to parents when the patient consents to disclosure. Confidentiality may be justifiably breached in situations for which confidentiality for adults may be breached, according to Opinion 5.05, "Confidentiality." In addition, confidentiality for immature minors may be ethically breached when necessary to enable the parent to make an informed decision about treatment for the minor or when such a breach is necessary to avert serious harm to the minor. (IV)

Issued June 1994 based on the report "Confidential Care for Minors," adopted June 1992.

Updated June 1996.

5.07 **CONFIDENTIALITY: COMPUTERS.** The utmost effort and care must be taken to protect the confidentiality of all medical records, including computerized medical records.

The guidelines below are offered to assist physicians and computer service organizations in maintaining the confidentiality of information in medical records when that information is stored in computerized data bases:

(1) Confidential medical information should be entered into the computer-based patient record only by authorized personnel. Additions to the record should be time and date stamped, and the person making the additions should be identified in the record.

(2) The patient and physician should be advised about the existence of computerized data bases in which medical information concerning the patient is stored. Such information should be communicated to the physician and patient prior to the physician's release of the medical information to the entity or entities maintaining the computer data bases. All individuals and organizations with some form of access to the computerized data bases, and the level of access permitted, should be specifically identified in advance. Full disclosure of this information to the patient is necessary in obtaining informed consent to treatment. Patient data should be assigned a security level appropriate for the data's degree of sensitivity, which should be used to control who has access to the information.

(3) The physician and patient should be notified of the distribution of all reports reflecting identifiable patient data prior to distribution of the reports by the computer facility. There should be approval by the patient and notification of the physician prior to the release of patient–identifiable clinical and administrative data to individuals or organizations external to the medical care environment. Such information should not be released without the express permission of the patient.

(4) The dissemination of confidential medical data should be limited to only those individuals or agencies with a bona fide use for the data. Only the data necessary for the bona fide use should be released. Patient identifiers should be omitted when appropriate. Release of confidential medical information from the data base should be confined to the specific purpose for which the information is requested and limited to the specific time frame requested. All such organizations or individuals should be advised that authorized release of data to them does not authorize their further release of the data to additional individuals or organizations, or subsequent use of the data for other purposes.

(5) Procedures for adding to or changing data on the computerized data base should indicate individuals authorized to make changes, time periods in which changes take place, and those individuals who will be informed about changes in the data from the medical records.

(6) Procedures for purging the computerized data base of archaic or inaccurate data should be established and the patient and physician should be notified before and after the data has been purged. There should be no mixing of a physician's computerized patient records with those of other computer service bureau clients. In addition, procedures should be developed to protect against inadvertent mixing of individual reports or segments thereof.

(7) The computerized medical data base should be on-line to the computer terminal only when authorized computer programs requiring the medical data are being used. Individuals and organizations external to the clinical facility should not be provided on-line access to a computerized data base containing identifiable data from medical records concerning patients. Access to the computerized data base should be controlled through security measures such as passwords, encryption (encoding) of information, and scannable badges or other user identification.

(8) Back-up systems and other mechanisms should be in place to prevent data loss and downtime as a result of hardware or software failure.

(9) Security:
  (a) Stringent security procedures should be in place to prevent unauthorized access to computer-based patient records. Personnel audit procedures should be developed to establish a record in the event of unauthorized disclosure of medical data. Terminated or former employees in the data processing environment should have no access to data from the medical records concerning patients.
  (b) Upon termination of computer services for a physician, those computer files maintained for

the physician should be physically turned over to the physician. They may be destroyed (erased) only if it is established that the physician has another copy (in some form). In the event of file erasure, the computer service bureau should verify in writing to the physician that the erasure has taken place. (IV) Issued prior to April 1977; Updated June 1994 and June 1998.

5.09 CONFIDENTIALITY: INDUSTRY-EMPLOYED PHYSICIANS AND INDEPENDENT MEDICAL EXAMINERS. Where a physician's services are limited to performing an isolated assessment of an individual's health or disability for an employer, business, or insurer, the information obtained by the physician as a result of such examinations is confidential and should not be communicated to a third party without the individual's prior written consent, unless required by law. If the individual authorized the release of medical information to an employer or a potential employer, the physician should release only that information which is reasonably relevant to the employer's decision regarding that individual's ability to perform the work required by the job.

When a physician renders treatment to an employee with a work-related illness or injury, the release of medical information to the employer as to the treatment provided may be subject to the provisions of worker's compensation laws. The physician must comply with the requirements of such laws, if applicable. However, the physician may not otherwise discuss the employee's health condition with the employer without the employee's consent or, in the event of the employee's incapacity, the appropriate proxy's consent.

Whenever statistical information about employees' health is released, all employee identities should be deleted. (IV)

Issued July 1983.

Updated June 1994; updated June 1996; updated December 1999 based on the report "Patient–Physician Relationship in the Context of Work-Related and Independent Medical Examinations," adopted June 1999.

• • •

6.00 · Opinions on Fees and Charges

• • •

6.11 COMPETITION. Competition between and among physicians and other health care practitioners on the basis of competitive factors such as quality of services, skill, experience, miscellaneous conveniences offered to patients, credit terms, fees charged, etc., is not only ethical but is encouraged. Ethical medical practice thrives best under free market conditions when prospective patients have adequate information and opportunity to choose freely between and among competing physicians and alternate systems of medical care. (VII)

Issued July 1983.

• • •

8.00 · Opinions on Practice Matters

• • •

8.0315 MANAGING CONFLICTS OF INTEREST IN THE CONDUCT OF CLINICAL TRIALS. As the biotechnology and pharmaceutical industries continue to expand research activities and funding of clinical trials, and as increasing numbers of physicians both within and outside academic health centers become involved in partnerships with industry to perform these activities, greater safeguards against conflicts of interest are needed to ensure the integrity of the research and to protect the welfare of human subjects. Physicians should be mindful of the conflicting roles of investigator and clinician and of the financial conflicts of interest that arise from incentives to conduct trials and to recruit subjects. In particular, physicians involved in clinical research should heed the following guidelines: (1) Physicians should agree to participate as investigators in clinical trials only when it relates to their scope of practice and area of medical expertise. They should have adequate training in the conduct of research and should participate only in protocols which they are satisfied are scientifically sound. (2) Physicians should be familiar with the ethics of research, and should agree to participate in trials only if they are satisfied that an Institutional Review Board has reviewed the protocol, that the research does not impose undue risks upon research subjects, and that the research conforms to government regulations. (3) When a physician has treated or continues to treat a patient who is eligible to enroll as a subject in a clinical trial that the physician is conducting, the informed consent process must differentiate between the physician's roles as clinician and investigator. This is best achieved when someone other than the treating physician obtains the participant's informed consent to participate in the trial. This individual should be protected from the pressures of financial incentives, as described in the following section. (4) Any financial compensation received from trial sponsors must be commensurate with the efforts of the physician performing the research. Financial compensation should be at fair market value and the rate of compensation per patient should not vary according to the volume of subjects enrolled by the physician, and should meet other existing legal requirements. Furthermore, according to Opinion 6.03, "Fee Splitting: Referral to Health Care Facilities," it is unethical for physicians to accept payment solely for referring patients to research studies. (5) Physicians should ensure that protocols include provisions for the funding of subjects' medical care in the event of complications associated with the research. Also, a physician should not bill a third-party payor when he or she has received funds from a sponsor to cover the additional expenses related to conducting the trial. (6) The nature and source of funding and financial incentives offered to the investigators must be disclosed to a potential participant as part of the informed consent process. Disclosure to participants also should include information on uncertainties that may exist regarding funding of treatment for possible complications that may arise during the course of the trial. Physicians should ensure that such disclosure is included in any written informed consent. (7) When entering into a contract to perform research, physicians should ensure themselves that the presentation or publication of results will not be unduly delayed or otherwise obstructed by the sponsoring company. (II, V)

Issued June 2001 based on the report "Managing Conflicts of Interest in the Conduct of Clinical Trials," adopted December 2000 (JAMA. 2002; 287: 78–84).

8.061 **GIFTS TO INDUSTRY FROM PHYSICIANS.** Many gifts given to physicians by companies in the pharmaceutical, device, and medical equipment industries serve an important and socially beneficial function. For example, companies have long provided funds for educational seminars and conferences. However, there has been growing concern about certain gifts from industry to physicians. Some gifts that reflect customary practices of industry may not be consistent with the Principles of Medical Ethics. To avoid the acceptance of inappropriate gifts, physicians should observe the following guidelines: (1) Any gifts accepted by physicians individually should primarily entail a benefit to patients and should not be of substantial value. Accordingly, textbooks, modest meals, and other gifts are appropriate if they serve a genuine educational function. Cash payments should not be accepted. The use of drug

samples for personal or family use is permissible as long as these practices do not interfere with patient access to drug samples. It would not be acceptable for non-retired physicians to request free pharmaceuticals for personal use or use by family members. (2) Individual gifts of minimal value are permissible as long as the gifts are related to the physician's work (e.g., pens and notepads). (3) The Council on Ethical and Judicial Affairs defines a legitimate "conference" or "meeting" as any activity, held at an appropriate location, where (a) the gathering is primarily dedicated, in both time and effort, to promoting objective scientific and educational activities and discourse (one or more educational presentation(s) should be the highlight of the gathering), and (b) the main incentive for bringing attendees together is to further their knowledge on the topic(s) being presented. An appropriate disclosure of financial support or conflict of interest should be made. (4) Subsidies to underwrite the costs of continuing medical education conferences or professional meetings can contribute to the improvement of patient care and therefore are permissible. Since the giving of a subsidy directly to a physician by a company's representative may create a relationship that could influence the use of the company's products, any subsidy should be accepted by the conference's sponsor who in turn can use the money to reduce the conference's registration fee. Payments to defray the costs of a conference should not be accepted directly from the company by the physicians attending the conference. (5) Subsidies from industry should not be accepted directly or indirectly to pay for the costs of travel, lodging, or other personal expenses of physicians attending conferences or meetings, nor should subsidies be accepted to compensate for the physicians' time. Subsidies for hospitality should not be accepted outside of modest meals or social events held as a part of a conference or meeting. It is appropriate for faculty at conferences or meetings to accept reasonable honoraria and to accept reimbursement for reasonable travel, lodging, and meal expenses. It is also appropriate for consultants who provide genuine services to receive reasonable compensation and to accept reimbursement for reasonable travel, lodging, and meal expenses. Token consulting or advisory arrangements cannot be used to justify the compensation of physicians for their time or their travel, lodging, and other out-of-pocket expenses. (6) Scholarship or other special funds to permit medical students, residents, and fellows to attend carefully selected educational conferences may be permissible as long as the selection of students, residents, or fellows who will receive the funds is made by the academic or training institution. Carefully selected educational conferences are generally defined as the major educational, scientific or policy-making meetings of national, regional, or specialty medical associations. (7) No gifts should be accepted if there are strings attached. For example, physicians should not accept gifts if they are given in relation to the physician's prescribing practices. In addition, when companies underwrite medical conferences or lectures other than their own, responsibility for and control over the selection of content, faculty, educational methods, and materials should belong to the organizers of the conferences or lectures. (II)

Issued June 1992 based on the report "Gifts to Physicians from Industry," adopted December 1990 (JAMA. 1991; 265: 501)

Updated June 1996 and June 1998.

8.08 **INFORMED CONSENT.** The patient's right of self-decision can be effectively exercised only if the patient possesses enough information to enable an intelligent choice. The patient should make his or her own determination on treatment. The physician's obligation is to present the medical facts accurately to the patient or to the individual responsible for the patient's care and to make recommendations for management in accordance with good medical practice. The physician has an ethical obligation to help the patient make choices from among the therapeutic alternatives consistent with good medical practice. Informed consent is a basic social policy for which exceptions are permitted: (1) where the patient is unconscious or otherwise incapable of consenting and harm from failure to treat is imminent; or (2) when risk-disclosure poses such a serious psychological threat of detriment to the patient as to be medically contraindicated. Social policy does not accept the paternalistic view that the physician may remain silent because divulgence might prompt the patient to forego needed therapy. Rational, informed patients should not be expected to act uniformly, even under similar circumstances, in agreeing to or refusing treatment. (I, II, III, IV, V)

Issued March 1981.

• • •

8.11 **NEGLECT OF PATIENT.** Physicians are free to choose whom they will serve. The physician should, however, respond to the best of his or her ability in cases of emergency where first aid treatment is essential. Once having undertaken a case, the physician should not neglect the patient. (I, VI)

Issued prior to April 1977.

Updated June 1996.

8.12 **PATIENT INFORMATION.** It is a fundamental ethical requirement that a physician should at all times deal honestly and openly with patients. Patients have a right to know their past and present medical status and to be free of any mistaken beliefs concerning their conditions. Situations occasionally occur in which a patient suffers significant medical complications that may have resulted from the physician's mistake or judgment. In these situations, the physician is ethically required to inform the patient of all the facts necessary to ensure understanding of what has occurred. Only through full disclosure is a patient able to make informed decisions regarding future medical care.

Ethical responsibility includes informing patients of changes in their diagnoses resulting from retrospective review of test results or any other information. This obligation holds even though the patient's medical treatment or therapeutic options may not be altered by the new information.

Concern regarding legal liability which might result following truthful disclosure should not affect the physician's honesty with a patient. (I, II, III, IV)

Issued March 1981.

Updated June 1994.

• • •

8.14 **SEXUAL MISCONDUCT IN THE PRACTICE OF MEDICINE.** Sexual contact that occurs concurrent with the physician–patient relationship constitutes sexual misconduct. Sexual or romantic interactions between physicians and patients detract from the goals of the physician–patient relationship, may exploit the vulnerability of the patient, may obscure the physician's objective judgment concerning the patient's health care, and ultimately may be detrimental to the patient's well-being.

If a physician has reason to believe that non-sexual contact with a patient may be perceived as or may lead to sexual conduct, then he or she should avoid the non-sexual contact. At a minimum, a physician's ethical duties include terminating the physician–patient relationship before initiating a dating, romantic, or sexual relationship with a patient.

Sexual or romantic relationships between a physician and a former patient may be unduly influenced by the previous physician–patient relationship. Sexual or romantic relationships with former patients are unethical if the physician uses or exploits trust, knowledge, emotions, or influence derived from the previous professional relationship. (I, II, IV)

Issued December 1986.

Updated March 1992 based on the report "Sexual Misconduct in the Practice of Medicine," issued December 1990. (JAMA. 1991; 266: 2741–2745)

8.15 **SUBSTANCE ABUSE.** It is unethical for a physician to practice medicine while under the influence of a controlled substance, alcohol, or other chemical agents which impair the ability to practice medicine. (I)

Issued December 1986.

8.181 **PERFORMING PROCEDURES ON THE NEWLY DE-CEASED FOR TRAINING PURPOSES.** Physicians should work to develop institutional policies that address the practice of performing procedures on the newly deceased for purposes of training. Any such policy should ensure that the interests of all the parties involved are respected under established and clear ethical guidelines. Such policies should consider rights of patients and their families, benefits to trainees and society, as well as potential harm to the ethical sensitivities of trainees, and risks to staff, the institution, and the profession associated with performing procedures on the newly deceased without consent. The following considerations should be addressed before medical trainees perform procedures on the newly deceased:

(1) The teaching of life-saving skills should be the culmination of a structured training sequence, rather than relying on random opportunities. Training should be performed under close supervision, in a manner and environment that takes into account the wishes and values of all involved parties.

(2) Physicians should inquire whether the deceased individual had expressed preferences regarding handling of the body or procedures performed after death. In the absence of previously expressed preferences, physicians should obtain permission from the family before performing such procedures. When reasonable efforts to discover previously expressed preferences of the deceased or to find someone with authority to grant permission for the procedure have failed, physicians must not perform procedures for training purposes on the newly deceased patient.

In the event post-mortem procedures are undertaken on the newly deceased, they must be recorded in the medical record. (I, V)

Issued December 2001 based on the report "Performing Procedures on the Newly Deceased for Training Purposes," adopted June 2001.

• • •

9.00 · Opinions on Professional Rights and Responsibilities

• • •

9.031 **REPORTING IMPAIRED, INCOMPETENT, OR UNETHICAL COLLEAGUES.** Physicians have an ethical obligation to report impaired, incompetent, and unethical colleagues in accordance with the legal requirements in each state and assisted by the following guidelines:

Impairment. Impairment should be reported to the hospital's in-house impairment program, if available. Otherwise, either the chief of an appropriate clinical service or the chief of the hospital staff should be alerted. Reports may also be made directly to an external impaired physician program. Practicing physicians who do not have hospital privileges should be reported directly to an impaired physician program, such as those run by medical societies, when appropriate. If none of these steps would facilitate the entrance of the impaired physician into an impairment program, then the impaired physician should be reported directly to the state licensing board.

Incompetence. Initial reports of incompetence should be made to the appropriate clinical authority who would be empowered to assess the potential impact on patient welfare and to facilitate remedial action. The hospital peer review body should be notified where appropriate. Incompetence which poses an immediate threat to the health of patients should be reported directly to the state licensing board. Incompetence by physicians without a hospital affiliation should be reported to the local or state medical society and/or the state licensing or disciplinary board.

Unethical conduct. With the exception of incompetence or impairment, unethical behavior should be reported in accordance with the following guidelines:

Unethical conduct that threatens patient care or welfare should be reported to the appropriate authority for a particular clinical service. Unethical behavior which violates state licensing provisions should be reported to the state licensing board or impaired physician programs, when appropriate. Unethical conduct which violates criminal statutes must be reported to the appropriate law enforcement authorities. All other unethical conduct should be reported to the local or state medical society.

Where the inappropriate behavior of a physician continues despite the initial report(s), the reporting physician should report to a higher or additional authority. The person or body receiving the initial report should notify the reporting physician when appropriate action has been taken. Physicians who receive reports of inappropriate behavior have an ethical duty to critically and objectively evaluate the reported information and to assure that identified deficiencies are either remedied or further reported to a higher or additional authority. Anonymous reports should receive appropriate review and confidential investigation. Physicians who are under scrutiny or charge should be protected by the rules of confidentiality until such charges are proven or until the physician is exonerated. (II)

Issued March 1992 based on the report "Reporting Impaired, Incompetent, or Unethical Colleagues," adopted December 1991 (J Miss St Med Assoc. 1992; 33: 176–77).

Updated June 1994 and June 1996.

• • •

9.035 GENDER DISCRIMINATION IN THE MEDICAL PROFESSION. Physician leaders in medical schools and other medical institutions should take immediate steps to increase the number of women in leadership positions as such positions become open. There is already a large enough pool of female physicians to provide strong candidates for such positions. Also, adjustments should be made to ensure that all physicians are equitably compensated for their work. Women and men in the same specialty with the same experience and doing the same work should be paid the same compensation.

Physicians in the workplace should actively develop the following: (1) Retraining or other programs which facilitate the reentry of physicians who take time away from their careers to have a family; (2) On-site child care services for dependent children; (3) Policies providing job security for physicians who are temporarily not in practice due to pregnancy or family obligations.

Physicians in the academic medical setting should strive to promote the following: (1) Extension of tenure

decisions through "stop the clock" programs, relaxation of the seven year rule, or part-time appointments that would give faculty members longer to achieve standards for promotion and tenure; (2) More reasonable guidelines regarding the appropriate quantity and timing of published material needed for promotion or tenure that would emphasize quality over quantity and that would encourage the pursuit of careers based on individual talent rather than tenure standards that undervalue teaching ability and overvalue research; (3) Fair distribution of teaching, clinical, research, administrative responsibilities, and access to tenure tracks between men and women. Also, physicians in academic institutions should consider formally structuring the mentoring process, possibly matching students or faculty with advisors through a fair and visible system.

Where such policies do not exist or have not been followed, all medical workplaces and institutions should create strict policies to deal with sexual harassment. Grievance committees should have broad representation of both sexes and other groups. Such committees should have the power to enforce harassment policies and be accessible to those persons they are meant to serve.

Grantors of research funds and editors of scientific or medical journals should consider blind peer review of grant proposals and articles for publication to help prevent bias. However, grantors and editors will be able to consider the author's identity and give it appropriate weight. (II, VII)

Issued June 1994 based on the report "Gender Discrimination in the Medical Profession," issued June 1993. (Women's Health Issues. 1994; 4:1–11)

• • •

9.045 PHYSICIANS WITH DISRUPTIVE BEHAVIOR. This Opinion is limited to the conduct of individual physicians and does not refer to physicians acting as a collective, which is considered separately in Opinion 9.025, "Collective Action and Patient Advocacy." (1) Personal conduct, whether verbal or physical, that negatively affects or that potentially may negatively affect patient care constitutes disruptive behavior. (This includes but is not limited to conduct that interferes with one's ability to work with other members of the health care team.) However, criticism that is offered in good faith with the aim of improving patient care should not be construed as disruptive behavior. (2)

Each medical staff should develop and adopt bylaw provisions or policies for intervening in situations where a physician's behavior is identified as disruptive. The medical staff bylaw provisions or policies should contain procedural safeguards that protect due process. Physicians exhibiting disruptive behavior should be referred to a medical staff wellness—or equivalent—committee. (3) In developing policies that address physicians with disruptive behavior, attention should be paid to the following elements: (a) Clearly stating principal objectives in terms that ensure high standards of patient care and promote a professional practice and work environment. (b) Describing the behavior or types of behavior that will prompt intervention. (c) Providing a channel through which disruptive behavior can be reported and appropriately recorded. A single incident may not be sufficient for action, but each individual report may help identify a pattern that requires intervention. (d) Establishing a process to review or verify reports of disruptive behavior. (e) Establishing a process to notify a physician whose behavior is disruptive that a report has been made, and providing the physician with an opportunity to respond to the report. (f) Including means of monitoring whether a physician's disruptive conduct improves after intervention. (g) Providing for evaluative and corrective actions that are commensurate with the behavior, such as self-correction and structured rehabilitation. Suspension of responsibilities or privileges should be a mechanism of final resort. Additionally, institutions should consider whether the reporting requirements of Opinion 9.031, "Reporting Impaired, Incompetent, or Unethical Colleagues," apply in particular cases. (h) Identifying which individuals will be involved in the various stages of the process, from reviewing reports to notifying physicians and monitoring conduct after intervention. (i) Providing clear guidelines for the protection of confidentiality. (j) Ensuring that individuals who report physicians with disruptive behavior are duly protected. (I, II, VIII)

Issued December 2000 based on the report "Physicians With Disruptive Behavior," adopted June 2000.

9.065 **CARING FOR THE POOR.** Each physician has an obligation to share in providing care to the indigent. The measure of what constitutes an appropriate contribution may vary with circumstances such as community characteristics, geographic location, the nature of the physician's practice and specialty, and other conditions. All physicians should work to ensure that the needs of the poor in their communities are met. Caring for the poor should be a regular part of the physician's practice schedule.

In the poorest communities, it may not be possible to meet the needs of the indigent for physicians' services by relying solely on local physicians. The local physicians should be able to turn for assistance to their colleagues in prosperous communities, particularly those in close proximity.

Physicians are meeting their obligation, and are encouraged to continue to do so, in a number of ways such as seeing indigent patients in their offices at no cost or at reduced cost, serving at freestanding or hospital clinics that treat the poor, and participating in government programs that provide health care to the poor. Physicians can also volunteer their services at weekend clinics for the poor and at shelters for battered women or the homeless.

In addition to meeting their obligations to care for the indigent, physicians can devote their energy, knowledge, and prestige to designing and lobbying at all levels for better programs to provide care for the poor. (I, VII)

Issued June 1994 based on the report "Caring for the Poor," issued December 1992. (JAMA. 1993; 269: 2533–2537)

· · ·

9.115 **ETHICS CONSULTATIONS.** Ethics consultations may be called to clarify ethical issues without reference to a particular case, facilitate discussion of an ethical dilemma in a particular case, or resolve an ethical dispute. The consultation mechanism may be through an ethics committee, a subset of the committee, individual consultants, or consultation teams. The following guidelines are offered with respect to these services: (1) All hospitals and other health care institutions should provide access to ethics consultation services. Health care facilities without ethics committees or consultation services should develop flexible, efficient mechanisms of ethics review that divide the burden of committee functioning among collaborating health care facilities. (2) Institutions offering ethics consultation services must appreciate the complexity of the task, recognizing the potential for harm as well as benefit, and act responsibly. This includes true institutional support for the service. (3) Ethics consultation services require a serious investment of time and effort by the individuals involved. Members should include either individuals with extensive formal training and experience in clinical ethics or individuals who have made a substantial commitment over several years to gain sufficient knowledge, skills, and understanding of the complexity of clinical ethics. A wide variety of background training is preferable, including such fields as philosophy, religion, medicine, and law. (4) Explicit structural standards should be developed and consistently followed. These should include developing a clear description of the consultation service's role and determining which types of cases will be addressed, how the cases will be referred to the service, whether the service will provide recommendations or simply function as a forum for discussion, and whether recommendations are binding or advisory. (5) Explicit procedural standards should be developed and consistently followed. These should include establishing who must be involved in the consultation process and how notification, informed consent, confidentiality and case write-ups will be handled. (6) In general, patient and staff informed consent may be presumed for ethics consultation. However, patients and families should be given the opportunity, not to participate in discussions either formally, through the institutional process, or informally. (7) In those cases where the patient or family has chosen not to participate in the consultation process, the final recommendations of the consultant(s) should be tempered. (8) In general, ethics consultation services, like social services, should be financed by the institution. (9) A consultation service should be careful not to take on more than it can handle, ie, the complexity of the role should correspond to the level of sophistication of the service and the resources it has available. As a result, some services may offer only information and education, others a forum for discussion but not advice, others might serve a mediation role, and some might handle even administrative or organizational ethics issues. (IV, V)

Issued June 1998 based on the report "Ethics Consultation," adopted December 1997.

9.121 **RACIAL DISPARITIES IN HEALTH CARE.** Disparities in medical care based on immutable characteristics such as race must be avoided. Whether such disparities in health care are caused by treatment decisions, differences in income and education, sociocultural factors, or failures by the medical profession, they are unjustifiable and must be eliminated. Physicians should examine their own practices to ensure that racial prejudice does not affect clinical judgment in medical care. (I, IV)

Issued March 1992 based on the report "Black-White Disparities in Health Care," issued December 1989. (JAMA. 1990; 263: 2344–2346)

Updated June 1994.

9.122 **GENDER DISPARITIES IN HEALTH CARE.** A patient's gender plays an appropriate role in medical decisionmaking when biological differences between the sexes are considered. However, some data suggest that gender bias may be playing a role in medical decisionmaking. Social attitudes, including stereotypes, prejudices and other evaluations based on gender role expectations may play themselves out in a variety of subtle ways. Physicians must ensure that gender is not used inappropriately as a consideration in clinical decisionmaking. Physicians should examine their practices and attitudes for influence of social or cultural biases which could be inadvertently affecting the delivery of medical care.

Research on health problems that affect both genders should include male and female subjects, and results of medical research done solely on males should not be generalized to females without evidence that results apply to both sexes. Medicine and society in general should ensure that resources for medical research should be distributed in a manner which promotes the health of both sexes to the greatest extent possible. (I, IV)

Issued March 1992 based on the report "Gender Disparities in Clinical Decisionmaking," issued December 1990. (JAMA. 1991; 266: 559–562)

Updated June 1994.

9.13 **PHYSICIANS AND INFECTIOUS DISEASES.** A physician who knows that he or she has an infectious disease, which if contracted by the patient would pose a significant risk to the patient, should not engage in any activity that creates a significant risk of transmission of that disease to the patient. The precautions taken to prevent the transmission of a contagious disease to a patient should be appropriate to the seriousness of the disease and must be particularly stringent in the case of a disease that is potentially fatal. (I, IV)

Issued August 1989.

Updated June 1996 and June 1999.

9.131 **HIV-INFECTED PATIENTS AND PHYSICIANS.** A physician may not ethically refuse to treat a patient whose condition is within the physician's current realm of competence solely because the patient is seropositive for HIV. Persons who are seropositive should not be subjected to discrimination based on fear or prejudice.

When physicians are unable to provide the services required by an HIV-infected patient, they should make appropriate referrals to those physicians or facilities equipped to provide such services.

A physician who knows that he or she is seropositive should not engage in any activity that creates a significant risk of transmission of the disease to others. A physician who has HIV disease or who is seropositive should consult colleagues as to which activities the physician can pursue without creating a risk to patients. (I, II, IV)

Issued March 1992 based on the report "Ethical Issues in the Growing AIDS Crisis," adopted December 1987 (JAMA. 1988; 259: 1360–1361).

Updated June 1996 and June 1998.

E-10.01 **FUNDAMENTAL ELEMENTS OF THE PATIENT-PHYSICIAN RELATIONSHIP.** From ancient times, physicians have recognized that the health and well-being of patients depends upon a collaborative effort between physician and patient. Patients share with physicians the responsibility for their own health care. The patient–physician relationship is of greatest benefit to patients when they bring medical problems to the attention of their physicians in a timely fashion, provide information about their medical condition to the best of their ability, and work with their physicians in a mutually respectful alliance. Physicians can best contribute to this alliance by serving as their patients' advocate and by fostering these rights:

(1) The patient has the right to receive information from physicians and to discuss the benefits, risks, and costs of appropriate treatment alternatives. Patients should receive guidance from their physicians as to the optimal course of action. Patients are also entitled to obtain copies or summaries of their medical records, to have their questions answered, to be advised of potential conflicts of interest that their physicians might have, and to receive independent professional opinions.

(2) The patient has the right to make decisions regarding the health care that is recommended by his or her physician. Accordingly, patients may accept or refuse any recommended medical treatment.

(3) The patient has the right to courtesy, respect, dignity, responsiveness, and timely attention to his or her needs.

(4) The patient has the right to confidentiality. The physician should not reveal confidential communications or information without the consent of the patient, unless provided for by law or by the need to protect the welfare of the individual or the public interest.

(5) The patient has the right to continuity of health care. The physician has an obligation to cooperate in the coordination of medically indicated care with other health care providers treating the patient. The physician may not discontinue treatment of a patient as long as further treatment is medically indicated, without giving the patient reasonable assistance and sufficient opportunity to make alternative arrangements for care.

(6) The patient has a basic right to have available adequate health care. Physicians, along with the rest of society, should continue to work toward this goal. Fulfillment of this right is dependent on society providing resources so that no patient is deprived of necessary care because of an inability to pay for the care. Physicians should continue their traditional assumption of a part of the responsibility for the medical care of those who cannot afford essential health care. Physicians should advocate for patients in dealing with third parties when appropriate.

Issued June 1992 based on the report, "Fundamental Elements of the Patient-Physician Relationship," adopted June 1990; Updated 1993.

• • •

E10.015 **THE PATIENT-PHYSICIAN RELATIONSHIP.** The practice of medicine, and its embodiment in the clinical encounter between a patient and a physician, is fundamentally a moral activity that arises from the imperative to care for patients and to alleviate suffering.

A patient–physician relationship exists when a physician serves a patient's medical needs, generally by mutual consent between physician and patient (or surrogate). In some instances the agreement is implied, such as in emergency care or when physicians provide services at the request of the treating physician. In rare instances, treatment without consent may be provided under court order (see Opinion 2.065). Nevertheless, the physician's obligations to the patient remain intact.

The relationship between patient and physician is based on trust and gives rise to physicians' ethical obligations to place patients' welfare above their own self-interest and above obligations to other groups, and to advocate for their patients' welfare.

Within the patient-physician relationship, a physician is ethically required to use sound medical judgment, holding the best interests of the patient as paramount.

Issued December 2001 based on the report "The Patient–Physician Relationship," adopted June 2001.

DECLARATION OF PROFESSIONAL RESPONSIBILITY MEDICINE'S SOCIAL CONTRACT WITH HUMANITY

American Medical Association

2001

• • •

This declaration was drafted by members of the Ethics Standards Group at the American Medical Association and approved by the House of Delegates of the AMA in December of 2001. Although the Declaration was drafted in part as a response to the attacks on September 11, 2001, the language of the Declaration is broad enough to be used for the world community of physicians. In addition to traditional exhortations of respecting human life and preserving confidentiality, the Declaration also states that physicians should better educate the public about health threats as well as take a more directly political role to reduce human suffering.

<http://www.ama-assn.org/ama/pub/category/7491.html>

Preamble

Never in the history of human civilization has the well being of each individual been so inextricably linked to that of every other. Plagues and pandemics respect no national borders in a world of global commerce and travel. Wars and acts of terrorism enlist innocents as combatants and mark civilians as targets. Advances in medical science and genetics, while promising great good, may also be harnessed as agents of evil. The unprecedented scope and immediacy of these universal challenges demand concerted action and response by all. As physicians, we are bound in our response by a common heritage of caring for the sick and the suffering. Through the centuries, individual physicians have fulfilled

this obligation by applying their skills and knowledge competently, selflessly and at times heroically. Today, our profession must reaffirm its historical commitment to combat natural and man-made assaults on the health and well being of humankind. Only by acting together across geographic and ideological divides can we overcome such powerful threats. Humanity is our patient.

Declaration

We, the members of the world community of physicians, solemnly commit ourselves to:

I. Respect human life and the dignity of every individual.

II. Refrain from supporting or committing crimes against humanity and condemn all such acts.

III. Treat the sick and injured with competence and compassion and without prejudice.

IV. Apply our knowledge and skills when needed, though doing so may put us at risk.

V. Protect the privacy and confidentiality of those for whom we care and breach that confidence only when keeping it would seriously threaten their health and safety or that of others.

VI. Work freely with colleagues to discover, develop, and promote advances in medicine and public health that ameliorate suffering and contribute to human well-being.

VII. Educate the public and polity about present and future threats to the health of humanity.

VIII. Advocate for social, economic, educational, and political changes that ameliorate suffering and contribute to human well-being.

IX. Teach and mentor those who follow us for they are the future of our caring profession.

We make these promises solemnly, freely, and upon our personal and professional honor.

CHARTER ON MEDICAL PROFESSIONALISM

ABIM Foundation, ACP–ASIM Foundation, and European Federation of Internal Medicine

2002

• • •

Unlike the AMA's Declaration of Professional Responsibility, which is drafted in the style of an oath, the Charter on Medical Professionalism reads more like a contract between medicine and society. The Charter outlines three principles and ten responsibilities that physicians should abide. The Charter mentions traditional ethical duties of physicians (confidentiality, avoiding sexual misconduct), as well as newer ethical duties, such as managing conflicts of interest.

Preamble

Professionalism is the basis of medicine's contract with society. It demands placing the interests of patients above those of the physician, setting and maintaining standards of competence and integrity, and providing expert advice to society on matters of health. The principles and responsibilities of medical professionalism must be clearly understood by both the profession and society. Essential to this contract is public trust in physicians, which depends on the integrity of both individual physicians and the whole profession.

At present, the medical profession is confronted by an explosion of technology, changing market forces, problems in health care delivery, bioterrorism, and globalization. As a result, physicians find it increasingly difficult to meet their responsibilities to patients and society. In these circumstances, reaffirming the fundamental and universal principles and values of medical professionalism, which remain ideals to be pursued by all physicians, becomes all the more important.

The medical profession everywhere is embedded in diverse cultures and national traditions, but its members share the role of healer, which has roots extending back to Hippocrates. Indeed, the medical profession must contend with complicated political, legal, and market forces. Moreover, there are wide variations in medical delivery and practice through which any general principles may be expressed in both complex and subtle ways. Despite these differences, common themes emerge and form the basis of this charter in the form of three fundamental principles and as a set of definitive professional responsibilities.

Fundamental Principles

Principle of primacy of patient welfare. This principle is based on a dedication to serving the interest of the patient. Altruism contributes to the trust that is central to the physician-patient relationship. Market forces, societal pressures, and administrative exigencies must not compromise this principle.

Principle of patient autonomy. Physicians must have respect for patient autonomy. Physicians must be honest with their patients and empower them to make informed decisions about their treatment. Patients' decisions about their care must be paramount, as long as those decisions are in keeping with ethical practice and do not lead to demands for inappropriate care.

Principle of social justice. The medical profession must promote justice in the health care system, including the fair distribution of health care resources. Physicians should work actively to eliminate discrimination in health care, whether based on race, gender, socioeconomic status, ethnicity, religion, or any other social category.

A Set of Professional Responsibilities

Commitment to professional competence. Physicians must be committed to lifelong learning and be responsible for maintaining the medical knowledge and clinical and team skills necessary for the provision of quality care. More broadly, the profession as a whole must strive to see that all of its members are competent and must ensure that appropriate mechanisms are available for physicians to accomplish this goal.

Commitment to honesty with patients. Physicians must ensure that patients are completely and honestly informed before the patient has consented to treatment and after treatment has occurred. This expectation does not mean that patients should be involved in every minute decision about medical care; rather, they must be empowered to decide on the course of therapy. Physicians should also acknowledge that in health care, medical errors that injure patients do sometimes occur. Whenever patients are injured as a consequence of medical care, patients should be informed promptly because failure to do so seriously compromises patient and societal trust. Reporting and analyzing medical mistakes provide the basis for appropriate prevention and improvement strategies and for appropriate compensation to injured parties.

Commitment to patient confidentiality. Earning the trust and confidence of patients requires that appropriate confidentiality safeguards be applied to disclosure of patient information. This commitment extends to discussions with persons acting on a patient's behalf when obtaining the patient's own consent is not feasible. Fulfilling the commitment to confidentiality is more pressing now than ever before, given the widespread use of electronic information systems for compiling patient data and an increasing availability of genetic information. Physicians recognize, however, that their commitment to patient confidentiality must occasionally yield to overriding considerations in the public interest (for example, when patients endanger others).

Commitment to maintaining appropriate relations with patients. Given the inherent vulnerability and dependency of patients, certain relationships between physicians and patients must be avoided. In particular, physicians should never exploit patients for any sexual advantage, personal financial gain, or other private purpose.

Commitment to improving quality of care. Physicians must be dedicated to continuous improvement in the quality of health care. This commitment entails not only maintaining clinical competence but also working collaboratively with other professionals to reduce medical error, increase patient safety, minimize overuse of health care resources, and optimize the outcomes of care. Physicians must actively participate in the development of better measures of quality of care and the application of quality measures to assess routinely the performance of all individuals, institutions, and systems responsible for health care delivery. Physicians, both individually and through their professional associations, must take responsibility for assisting in the creation and implementation of mechanisms designed to encourage continuous improvement in the quality of care.

Commitment to improving access to care. Medical professionalism demands that the objective of all health care systems be the availability of a uniform and adequate standard of care. Physicians must individually and collectively strive to reduce barriers to equitable health care. Within each system, the physician should work to eliminate barriers to access based on education, laws, finances, geography, and social discrimination. A commitment to equity entails the promotion of public health and preventive medicine, as well as public advocacy on the part of each physician, without concern for the self-interest of the physician or the profession.

Commitment to a just distribution of finite resources. While meeting the needs of individual patients, physicians are required to provide health care that is based on the wise and cost-effective management of limited clinical resources. They should be committed to working with other physicians, hospitals, and payers to develop guidelines for cost-effective care. The physician's professional responsibility for appropriate allocation of resources requires scrupulous avoidance of superfluous tests and procedures. The provision of unnecessary services not only exposes one's patients to avoidable harm and expense but also diminishes the resources available for others.

Commitment to scientific knowledge. Much of medicine's contract with society is based on the integrity and appropriate use of scientific knowledge and technology. Physicians have a duty to uphold scientific standards, to promote research, and to create new knowledge and ensure its appropriate use. The profession is responsible for the integrity of this knowledge, which is based on scientific evidence and physician experience.

Commitment to maintaining trust by managing conflicts of interest. Medical professionals and their organizations have many opportunities to compromise their professional responsibilities by pursuing private gain or personal advantage. Such compromises are especially threatening in the pursuit of personal or organizational interactions with for-profit industries, including medical equipment manufacturers, insurance companies, and pharmaceutical firms. Physicians have an obligation to recognize, disclose to the general public, and deal with conflicts of interest that arise in the course of their professional duties and activities. Relationships between industry and opinion leaders should be disclosed, especially when the latter determine the criteria for conducting and reporting clinical trials, writing editorials or therapeutic guidelines, or serving as editors of scientific journals.

Commitment to professional responsibilities. As members of a profession, physicians are expected to work collaboratively to maximize patient care, be respectful of one another, and participate in the processes of self-regulation, including remediation and discipline of members who have failed to meet professional standards. The profession should also define and organize the educational and standard-setting process for current and future members. Physicians have both individual and collective obligations to participate in these processes. These obligations include engaging in internal assessment and accepting external scrutiny of all aspects of their professional performance.

Summary

The practice of medicine in the modern era is beset with unprecedented challenges in virtually all cultures and societies. These challenges center on increasing disparities among the legitimate needs of patients, the available resources to meet those needs, the increasing dependence on market forces to transform health care systems, and the temptation for physicians to forsake their traditional commitment to the primacy of patients' interests. To maintain the fidelity of medicine's social contract during this turbulent time, we believe that physicians must reaffirm their active dedication to the principles of professionalism, which entails not only their personal commitment to the welfare of their patients but also collective efforts to improve the health care system for the welfare of society. This Charter on Medical Professionalism is intended to encourage such dedication and to promote an action agenda for the profession of medicine that is universal in scope and purpose.

THE MORAL AND TECHNICAL COMPETENCE OF THE OPHTHALMOLOGIST

American Academy of Ophthalmology

1991, REVISED 1999

The following Moral and Technial Competence material augments the AAO's Code of Ethics, which can be at http://www.aao.org/aao/ member/ethics/code_ethics.cfm.

<http://www.aao.org/aao/member/ethics/moral_competence.cfm>

• • •

Information Statement

Introduction

The overall purpose of developing ophthalmologic competency is to improve the physician–patient relationship and the medical care that accompanies that relationship. Competent ophthalmologic practice requires both moral and technical capacities. Moral capacities are demonstrated by 1) appreciation of clinical ethical problems, 2) practicing as an agent of the patient, and 3) facilitating a caring relationship with the patient. Technical capacities are comprised of the knowledge and skills required to practice medicine, and especially ophthalmology, according to current standards of care.

Background

The American Academy of Ophthalmology is dedicated to providing ophthalmologists with information and education necessary for the optimal care of the public. The quality of such care is based on competence achieved through training and continuing education. The Academy's Code of Ethics, which serves as a standard of exemplary professional conduct, requires that an ophthalmologist be competent by virtue of specific training and experience (Rule 1). However, the Rules of the Code specify neither the components of competence nor the capacities of which it is comprised. Competence for medical (ophthalmologic) practice does not occur in the abstract. Physician competence exists for the purpose of advancing the best interests of the patient as a person—with sensitivity, and with respect for and understanding of their sovereignty needs and wants.

Bioethicists generally agree that "moral" and "ethical" values are equivalent; these words are used synonymously here. Moral (and ethical) capacities are those which preserve, protect and advance the best interests of the patient through the practice (a process) of applying knowledge, skills and attitudes which resolve the human conflicts and dilemmas of clinical and scientific endeavor on principled bases.

Ophthalmologic Competence

Ophthalmologic competence is comprised of both moral and technical capacities; both are necessary to establish ophthalmologic competence. Ophthalmologic competence is thus a continuing process of self-development; of acquiring and refining the knowledge, skills, values, and expectations to provide quality patient care.

This acquisition process, of necessity, must proceed along two paths:

1. An outer-directed process of study and instruction into the vocabulary, concepts, case studies, negotiation strategies, and so on, that concern moral and technical capacities, and

2. An inner-directed process of personal experience and insight that integrates personal and professional development and moral and technical capacities.

Moral Competence

Moral competence follows from understanding the purpose of medical care and calls upon the physician to practice moral discernment, moral agency, and caring in relationships.

Moral discernment is the ability to confront, discuss, and resolve the ethical considerations in a clinical encounter. In particular, it is the ability to:

• Use the vocabulary and concepts of ethical and moral reasoning to place a moral dilemma in perspective;

• Respect the cultural, social, personal beliefs, expectations, and values that the patient brings to the therapeutic setting;

• Respect the patient's chosen lifestyle and acknowledge the conditions and events that have helped to shape that lifestyle;

• Confront one's own beliefs, expectations, and values when faced with different perspectives; and

• Reflect on the causes and consequences of one's ethical decisions.

Moral Agency is the ability to act on behalf of the patient; to act with respect for social, religious, and cultural differences that may exist between physician and patient. It is the ability to:

- Consider the possible consequences of one's actions and to act to affect consequences that are in accord with one's values and those of the patient;
- Resolve differences on the basis of principle, rather than power;
- Provide medical care that is both professionally appropriate and socially responsible;
- Genuinely engage the patient as a fellow human being; and
- Keep the confidences of the patient.

A caring and healing relationship between physician and patient is the foundation of medical care. Such a relationship is characterized by ability to:

- Acknowledge the patient's right to self-determination in the process of participating in his or her own care;
- Avoid conflicts of interests in one's own personal, professional, and financial relationships with patients, colleagues, and other members of the health care community;
- Provide the patient complete, accurate, and timely information about treatment options in the best spirit of informed consent;
- Share one's weaknesses and limits as well as one's strengths and virtues; and
- Strive for the experience of compassion through progressively deeper understandings of others' behavior.

Technical Competence

Technical competence consists of the knowledge and skills necessary to diagnose and treat disease and disability according to the precepts of medical science and especially of ophthalmology, and to assist in the maintenance of health.

In particular, technical competence consists of the ability to:

- Apply principles of ophthalmic care;
- Differentiate normal and pathological anatomy and physiology of the eyes and visual system;
- Understand the relationships between ophthalmic and systemic health and disease;
- Perform skills intrinsic to medicine in general and to ophthalmology in particular;
- Provide necessary and sufficient medical care;

- Develop, critique, and present appropriate therapeutic options;
- Provide timely, complete, and accurate documentation about patient care; and communicate appropriately with other members of the medical community and the health care system;
- Acknowledge one's limitations in skill and knowledge; and
- Make a commitment, through study, instruction, and experience, to keep one's medical skills and knowledge current.

We acknowledge the importance of these moral commitments and technical capacities to the education, practice and credentialing of ophthalmologists. Further, the curriculum of ophthalmology should specifically address each of these two competencies and the two paths to developing them and should be defined further for purposes of assessment and accountability.

Approved by: Ethics Committee, January 1991

Revised and Approved by: Secretariat for Ophthalmic Practice & Services, February 1999

CODE OF ETHICS

American Osteopathic Association

REVISED 1985, 1998, 2003

<http://www.aoa-net.org/MembersOnly/code.htm>

• • •

The 1965 revision of the American Osteopathic Association's (AOA) Code of Ethics appeared in the Appendix to the first edition of this encyclopedia. The 1985 revision of the AOA code contained standards that address the osteopathic physician's responsibilities to other health-care providers, to patients, and to society. The code serves as a guide to all AOA members; wording that denotes masculine or feminine gender has been changed to include both men and women in the latest 1998 version. The more significant changes between the 1965 and 1985 revisions included: (1) addition of the nondiscrimination clause in Section 3; (2) elimination of the earlier ban on advertising, as required by law; (3) elimination of the previous requirement that degrees be acquired only from institutions sanctioned by the AOA; and (4) elimination of the prohibition on publicly commenting on the professional services of other physicians. For the 1998 version, two new sections on sexual misconduct and sexual harassment have been added. The 2003 revision adds a section on the ethics of receiving gifts.

The American Osteopathic Association has formulated this Code to guide its member physicians in their professional lives. The standards presented are designed to address the osteopathic physician's ethical and professional responsibilities to patients, to society, to the AOA, to others involved in health care and to self.

Further, the American Osteopathic Association has adopted the position that physicians should play a major role in the development and instruction of medical ethics.

SECTION 1. The physician shall keep in confidence whatever she/he may learn about a patient in the discharge of professional duties. Information shall be divulged by the physician when required by law or when authorized by the patient.

SECTION 2. The physician shall give a candid account of the patient's condition to the patient or to those responsible for the patient's care.

SECTION 3. A physician–patient relationship must be founded on mutual trust, cooperation, and respect. The patient, therefore, must have complete freedom to choose her/his physician. The physician must have complete freedom to choose patients whom she/he will serve. However, the physician should not refuse to accept patients because of the patient's race, creed, color, sex, national origin or handicap. In emergencies, a physician should make her/his services available.

SECTION 4. A physician is never justified in abandoning a patient. The physician shall give due notice to a patient or to those responsible for the patient's care when she/he withdraws from the case so that another physician may be engaged.

SECTION 5. A physician shall practice in accordance with the body of systematized and scientific knowledge related to the healing arts. A physician shall maintain competence in such systemized and scientific knowledge through study and clinical applications.

SECTION 6. The osteopathic medical profession has an obligation to society to maintain its high standards and, therefore, to continuously regulate itself. A substantial part of such regulation is due to the efforts and influence of the recognized local, state and national associations representing the osteopathic medical profession. A physician should maintain membership in and actively support such associations and abide by their rules and regulations.

SECTION 7. Under the law a physician may advertise, but no physician shall advertise or solicit patients directly or indirectly through the use of matters or activities which are false or misleading.

SECTION 8. A physician shall not hold forth or indicate possession of any degree recognized as the basis for licensure to practice the healing arts unless she/he is actually licensed on the basis of that degree in the state in which she/he practices. A physician shall designate her/his osteopathic school of practice in all professional uses of her/his name. Indications of specialty practice, membership in professional societies, and related matters shall be governed by rules promulgated by the American Osteopathic Association.

SECTION 9. A physician should not hesitate to seek consultation whenever she/he believes it advisable for the care of the patient.

SECTION 10. In any dispute between or among physicians involving ethical or organizational matters, the matter in controversy should first be referred to the appropriate arbitrating bodies of the profession.

SECTION 11. In any dispute between or among physicians regarding the diagnosis and treatment of a patient, the attending physician has the responsibility for final decisions, consistent with any applicable osteopathic hospital rules or regulations.

SECTION 12. Any fee charged by a physician shall compensate the physician for services actually rendered. There shall be no division of professional fees for referrals of patients.

SECTION 13. A physician shall respect the law. When necessary a physician shall attempt to formulate the law by all proper means in order to improve patient care and public health.

SECTION 14. In addition to adhering to the foregoing ethical standards, a physician shall recognize a responsibility to participate in community activities and services.

SECTION 15. It is considered sexual misconduct for a physician to have sexual contact with any current patient whom the physician has interviewed and/or upon whom a medical or surgical procedure has been performed.

SECTION 16. Sexual harassment by a physician is considered unethical. Sexual harassment is defined as physical or verbal intimation of a sexual nature involving a colleague or subordinate in the workplace or academic setting, when such conduct creates an unreasonable, intimidating, hostile or offensive workplace or academic setting.

SECTION 17. The use of a product of service based solely on the receipt of a gift shall be deemed unethical.

CODE OF ETHICS AND GUIDE TO THE ETHICAL BEHAVIOUR OF PHYSICIANS

Canadian Medical Association

REVISED 1990, 1996

• • •

Most recently revised by the Canadian Medical Association (CMA) in 1996, the CMA Code of Ethics and Guide to the Ethical Behaviour of Physicians delineate standards of ethical behavior for Canadian physicians. The code offers six general responsibilities; the rest of the code pertains to the physician–patient relationship, communication, consent, confidentiality, clinical research, professional fees and responsibility to onself.

<http://www.cma.ca/cma/common/displayPage.do?pageId=/staticContent/HTML/N0/l2/where_we_stand/1996/10–15.htm>

Preface

The Canadian Medical Association accepts the responsibility for delineating the standard of ethical behaviour expected of Canadian physicians and has developed and approved this Code of Ethics as a guide for physicians.

The Code is an ethical document. Its sources are the traditional codes of medical ethics such as the Hippocratic Oath, as well as developments in human rights and recent bioethical discussion. Legislation and court decisions may also influence medical ethics. Physicians should be aware of the legal and regulatory requirements for medical practice in their jurisdiction. However, the Code may set out different standards of behaviour than does the law.

The Code has been prepared by physicians for physicians. It is based on the fundamental ethical principles of medicine, especially compassion, beneficence, nonmaleficence, respect for persons and justice. It interprets these principles with respect to the responsibilities of physicians to individual patients, family and significant others, colleagues, other health professionals, and society.

The Code is not, and cannot be, exhaustive. Its statements are general in nature, to be interpreted and applied in particular situations. Specific ethical issues such as abortion, transplantation and euthanasia are not mentioned; they are treated in appropriate detail in CMA policy statements.

Physicians may experience conflict between different ethical principles, between ethical and legal or regulatory requirements, or between their own ethical convictions and the demands of patients, proxy decision makers, other health professionals, employers or other involved parties. Training in ethical analysis and decision making during undergraduate, postgraduate and continuing medical education is recommended for physicians to develop the knowledge, skills and attitudes needed to deal with these conflicts. Consultation with colleagues, licensing authorities, ethicists, ethics committees or others who have expertise in these matters is also recommended.

The Code applies to physicians, including residents, and medical students.

General Responsibilities

1. Consider first the well-being of the patient.
2. Treat all patients with respect; do not exploit them for personal advantage.
3. Provide for appropriate care for your patient, including physical comfort and spiritual and psychosocial support even when cure is no longer possible.
4. Practise the art and science of medicine competently and without impairment.
5. Engage in lifelong learning to maintain and improve your professional knowledge, skills and attitudes.
6. Recognize your limitations and the competence of others and when indicated, recommend that additional opinions and services be sought.

Responsibilities to the Patient

Initiating and Dissolving a Patient-Physician Relationship

7. In providing medical service, do not discriminate against any patient on such grounds as age, gender, marital status, medical condition, national or ethnic origin, physical or mental disability, political affiliation, race, religion, sexual orientation, or socioeconomic status. This does not abrogate the physician's right to refuse to accept a patient for legitimate reasons.
8. Inform your patient when your personal morality would influence the recommendation or practice of any medical procedure that the patient needs or wants.
9. Provide whatever appropriate assistance you can to any person with an urgent need for medical care.
10. Having accepted professional responsibility for a patient, continue to provide services until they are no longer required or wanted; until another suitable physician has assumed responsibility for the patient;

or until the patient has been given adequate notice that you intend to terminate the relationship.

11. Limit treatment of yourself or members of your immediate family to minor or emergency services and only when another physician is not readily available; there should be no fee for such treatment.

Communication, Decision Making and Consent

12. Provide your patients with the information they need to make informed decisions about their medical care, and answer their questions to the best of your ability.

13. Make every reasonable effort to communicate with your patients in such a way that information exchanged is understood.

14. Recommend only those diagnostic and therapeutic procedures that you consider to be beneficial to your patient or to others. If a procedure is recommended for the benefit of others, as for example in matters of public health, inform your patient of this fact and proceed only with explicit informed consent or where required by law.

15. Respect the right of a competent patient to accept or reject any medical care recommended.

16. Recognize the need to balance the developing competency of children and the role of families in medical decision-making.

17. Respect your patient's reasonable request for a second opinion from a physician of the patient's choice.

18. Ascertain wherever possible and recognize your patient's wishes about the initiation, continuation or cessation of life-sustaining treatment.

19. Respect the intentions of an incompetent patient as they were expressed (e.g., through an advance directive or proxy designation) before the patient became incompetent.

20. When the intentions of an incompetent patient are unknown and when no appropriate proxy is available, render such treatment as you believe to be in accordance with the patient's values or, if these are unknown, the patient's best interests.

21. Be considerate of the patient's family and significant others and cooperate with them in the patient's interest.

Confidentiality

22. Respect the patient's right to confidentiality except when this right conflicts with your responsibility to the law, or when the maintenance of confidentiality would result in a significant risk of substantial harm to others or to the patient if the patient is incompetent; in such cases, take all reasonable steps to inform the patient that confidentiality will be breached.

23. When acting on behalf of a third party, take reasonable steps to ensure that the patient understands the nature and extent of your responsibility to the third party.

24. Upon a patient's request, provide the patient or a third party with a copy of his or her medical record, unless there is a compelling reason to believe that information contained in the record will result in substantial harm to the patient or others.

Clinical Research

25. Ensure that any research in which you participate is evaluated both scientifically and ethically, is approved by a responsible committee and is sufficiently planned and supervised that research subjects are unlikely to suffer disproportionate harm.

26. Inform the potential research subject, or proxy, about the purpose of the study, its source of funding, the nature and relative probability of harms and benefits, and the nature of your participation.

27. Before proceeding with the study, obtain the informed consent of the subject, or proxy, and advise prospective subjects that they have the right to decline or withdraw from the study at any time, without prejudice to their ongoing care.

Professional Fees

28. In determining professional fees to patients, consider both the nature of the service provided and the ability of the patient to pay, and be prepared to discuss the fee with the patient.

Responsibilities to Society

29. Recognize that community, society and the environment are important factors in the health of individual patients.

30. Accept a share of the profession's responsibility to society in matters relating to public health, health education, environmental protection, legislation affecting the health or well-being of the community, and the need for testimony at judicial proceedings.

31. Recognize the responsibility of physicians to promote fair access to health care resources.

32. Use health care resources prudently.

33. Refuse to participate in or support practices that violate basic human rights.

34. Recognize a responsibility to give the generally held opinions of the profession when interpreting scientific knowledge to the public; when presenting an opinion that is contrary to the generally held opinion of the profession, so indicate.

Responsibilities to the Profession

35. Recognize that the self-regulation of the profession is a privilege and that each physician has a continuing responsibility to merit this privilege.

36. Teach and be taught.

37. Avoid impugning the reputation of colleagues for personal motives; however, report to the appropriate authority any unprofessional conduct by colleagues.

38. Be willing to participate in peer review of other physicians and to undergo review by your peers.

39. Enter into associations only if you can maintain your professional integrity.

40. Avoid promoting, as a member of the medical profession, any service (except your own) or product for personal gain.

41. Do not keep secret from colleagues the diagnostic or therapeutic agents and procedures that you employ.

42. Collaborate with other physicians and health professionals in the care of patients and the functioning and improvement of health services.

Responsibilities to Oneself

43. Seek help from colleagues and appropriately qualified professionals for personal problems that adversely affect your service to patients, society or the profession.

CODE OF ETHICS AND GUIDE TO THE ETHICAL BEHAVIOUR OF PHYSICIANS

New Zealand Medical Association

1989, LAST AMENDED 2002

• • •

The current New Zealand Medical Association (NZMA) Code of Ethics, which includes a Guide to the Ethical Behaviour of Physicians,

was adopted in 1989, amended in December 1992, and last amended in March of 2002. There is great similarity, both in structure and content, between the NZMA code and the preceding code and guide of the Canadian Medical Association. The section of the NZMA entitled "Responsibilities to the Profession" and portions of the section entitled "Responsibilities to Society," not printed here, repeat some of the prescriptions of the Canadian code.

<http://www.nzma.org.nz/about/ethics.html>

Code of Ethics

All medical practitioners, including those who may not be engaged directly in clinical practice, will acknowledge and accept the following Principles of Ethical Behaviour:

1. Consider the health and well-being of the patient to be your first priority.

2. Respect the rights of the patient.

3. Respect the patient's autonomy and freedom of choice.

4. Avoid exploiting the patient in any manner.

5. Protect the patient's private information throughout his/her lifetime and following death, unless there are overriding public interest considerations at stake, or a patient's own safety requires a breach of confidentiality.

6. Strive to improve your knowledge and skills so that the best possible advice and treatment can be offered to the patient.

7. Adhere to the scientific basis for medical practice while acknowledging the limits of current knowledge.

8. Honour the profession and its traditions in the ways that best serve the interests of the patient.

9. Recognise your own limitations and the special skills of others in the prevention and treatment of disease.

10. Accept a responsibility for assisting in the allocation of limited resources to maximise medical benefit across the community.

11. Accept a responsibility for advocating for adequate resourcing of medical services.

Recommendations

Given the complexities of doctor–patient relationships, and the increasing difficulties brought about by the need for rationing of resources and direct intervention of third-party providers of funding, no set of guidelines can cover all situations. The following set of recommendations is designed to convey an overall pattern of professional behaviour consistent with the principles set out above in the Code of Ethics.

Responsibilities to the Patient

1. Doctors should ensure that all conduct in the practice of their profession is above reproach. Exploitation of any patient, whether it be physical, sexual, emotional, or financial, is unacceptable and the trust embodied in the doctor–patient relationship must be respected.

2. Doctors, like a number of other professionals, are involved in relationships in which there is a potential imbalance of power. Sexual relationships between doctors and their patients and students fall within this category. The NZMA is mindful of Medical Council policy in relation to sexual relationships with present and former patients, and expects doctors to be familiar with this. The NZMA considers that a sexual relationship with a current patient is unethical and that, in most instances, sexual relations with a former patient would be regarded as unethical, particularly where exploitation of patient vulnerability occurs. It is acknowledged that in some cases the patient–doctor relationship may be brief, minor in nature, or in the distant past. In such circumstances and where the sexual relationship has developed from social contact away from the professional environment, impropriety would not necessarily be inferred. Any complaints about a sexual relationship with a former patient need to be considered on an individual basis before being condemned as unethical.

3. Doctors should practise the science and art of medicine to the best of their ability in full moral independence, with compassion and respect for human dignity.

4. Doctors should ensure that every patient receives appropriate investigation into their complaint or condition, including adequate collation of information for optimal management.

5. Doctors should ensure that information is recorded accurately and is securely maintained.

6. Doctors should seek to improve their standards of medical care through continuing self education and thoughtful interaction with appropriate colleagues.

7. Doctors have the right, except in an emergency, to refuse to care for a particular patient. In any situation which is not an emergency, doctors may withdraw from or decline to provide care as long as an alternative source of care is available and that the appropriate avenue for securing this is known to the patient. Where a doctor does withdraw care from a patient, reasonable notice should be given.

8. When a patient is accepted for care, doctors will render medical service to that person without discrimination (as defined by the Human Rights Act).

9. Doctors should ensure that continuity of care is available in relation to all patients, whether seen urgently or unexpectedly, or within a long-term contractual setting, and should establish appropriate arrangements to cover absence from practice or hours off duty, informing patients of these.

10. Doctors should ensure that patients are involved, within the limits of their capacities, in understanding the nature of their problems, the range of possible solutions, as well as the likely benefits, risks, and costs, and shall assist them in making informed choices.

11. Doctors should recognise the right of patients to choose their doctors freely.

12. Doctors should recognise their own professional limitations and, when indicated, recommend to patients that additional opinions and services be obtained, and accept a patient's right to request other opinions. In making a referral to another health professional, so far as practical, the doctor shall have a basis for confidence in the competence of that practitioner.

13. Doctors should accept the right of a patient to be referred for further management in situations where there is a moral or clinical disagreement about the most appropriate course to take.

14. Doctors should keep in confidence information derived from a patient, or from a colleague regarding a patient, and divulge it only with the permission of the patient except when the law requires otherwise, or in those unusual circumstances when it is clearly in the patient's best interests or there is an overriding public good. Patients should be made aware of the information sharing which enables the delivery of good quality medical care. Where a patient expressly limits possession of particular information to one practitioner, this must ordinarily be respected. Patients should be made aware in advance, if possible, where there are limits to the confidentiality which can be provided. When it is necessary to divulge confidential patient information this must be done only to the proper authorities, and a record kept of when reporting occurred and its significance.

15. Doctors should recommend only those diagnostic procedures which seem necessary to assist in the care of the patient and only that treatment which seems necessary for the well-being of the patient.

16. When requested or when need is apparent, doctors should provide patients with information required to enable them to receive benefits to which they may be entitled.

17. Doctors shall accept those obligations to patients which are imposed by statutory provisions and the

codes of the Privacy Commissioner, the Human Rights Commissioner and the Health and Disability Commissioner, and the requirements of the Medical Council of New Zealand.

18. Doctors have a duty to explain to patients the role of doctors, patients and citizens generally in advancing medical knowledge, given that medical knowledge evolves in the light of ongoing research.

19. Doctors should accept that autonomy of patients remains important in childhood, chronic illness, ageing, and in the process of dying.

20. Doctors should bear in mind always the obligation of preserving life wherever possible and justifiable, while allowing death to occur with dignity and comfort when it appears to be inevitable. Doctors should be prepared to discuss and contribute to the content of advance directives and give effect to them. In the case of conflicts concerning management, doctors should consult widely within the profession and, if indicated, with ethicists and legal authorities.

21. In relation to transplantation and requests for organ donation, doctors should accept that when death of the brain has occurred, the cellular life of the body may be supported if some parts of the body might be used to prolong or improve the health of others. They shall recognise their responsibilities to the donor of organs that will be transplanted by disclosing fully to the donor or relatives the intent and purpose of the procedure. In the case of a living donor, the risks of the donation procedures must be fully explained. Doctors will ensure that the determination of the time of death of any donor patient is made by doctors who are in no way concerned with the transplant procedure or associated with the proposed recipient in a way that might exert any influence upon any decisions made.

22. Doctors have a responsibility to ensure that all people in their employ are fully aware of the appropriate actions to be taken in cases of medical emergency. It is strongly recommended that these procedures be included in a written policy document.

Professional Responsibilities

23. Doctors have both a right and a responsibility to maintain their own health and well-being at a standard that ensures that they are fit to practise.

24. Doctors should seek guidance and assistance from colleagues and professional or healthcare organisations whenever they are unable to function in a competent, safe and ethical manner.

25. Doctors have a general responsibility for the safety of patients and shall therefore take appropriate steps to ensure unsafe or unethical practices on the part of colleagues are curtailed and/or reported to relevant authorities without delay.

26. Doctors should make available to their colleagues, on the request of patients, a report or summary of their findings and treatment relating to that patient.

27. Doctors should recognise that an established relationship between doctor and patient has a value which dictates that this should not be disturbed without compelling reasons. Disruption of such a relationship should, wherever possible, be discussed in advance with an independent colleague.

28. Doctors should avoid impugning the reputations of other doctors with colleagues, patients or other persons.

29. Doctors should accept a share of the profession's responsibility toward society in matters relating to the health and safety of the public, health promotion and education, and legislation affecting the health or well-being of the community.

30. Doctors should not countenance, condone or participate in the practice of torture or other forms of cruel, inhuman, or degrading procedures, whatever the offence of which the victim of such procedures is suspected, accused or guilty.

31. Doctors should recognise the responsibility to assist courts, commissioners, commissions, and disciplinary bodies, in arriving at just decisions. In all circumstances doctors shall certify only that which has been personally verified when they are testifying as to circumstances of fact.

32. Doctors should not allow their standing as medical professionals to be used inappropriately in the endorsement of commercial products. When doctors are acting as agents for, or have a financial or other interest in, commercial organisations, their interest must be declared to patients.

33. Doctors should not use secret remedies.

34. Advances and innovative approaches to medical practice should be subject to review and promulgation through professional channels and medical scientific literature. Doctors should accept responsibility for providing the public with carefully considered, generally accepted opinions when presenting scientific knowledge. In presenting any personal opinion contrary to a generally held viewpoint of the profession, doctors must indicate that such is the case, and present information fairly.

35. Doctors should accept that their professional reputation must be based upon their ability, technical skills and integrity. Doctors should advertise professional services or make professional

announcements only in circumstances where the primary purpose of any notification is factual presentation of information reasonably needed by any person wishing to make an informed decision about the appropriateness and availability of services that may meet his or her medical needs. Any such announcement or advertisement must be demonstrably true in all respects and contain no testimonial material or endorsement of clinical skills. Qualifications not recognised by appropriate New Zealand statutory bodies should not be quoted.

36. Doctors should exercise careful judgement before accepting any gift, hospitality or gratuity which could be interpreted as an inducement to use or endorse any product, equipment or policy. In all cases of doubt, advice should be sought from relevant professional organisations.

Research

37. Before initiating or participating in any clinical research, doctors must assure themselves that the particular investigation is justified in the light of previous research and knowledge. Any proposed study should reasonably be expected to provide the answers to the questions raised. All studies involving patients should be subject to the scrutiny of an Ethics Committee before initiation. It is often appropriate to establish a committee independent of the primary investigators, initiators and funders of a trial to oversee ongoing ethical issues, including the evaluation of emerging results according to stated clinical, ethical and scientific criteria.

38. Doctors must be assured that the planning and conduct of any particular study is such that it minimises the risk of harm to participants. In comparative studies, the patient and control groups must receive the best available treatment.

39. Patient consent for participating in clinical research (or permission of those authorised to act on their behalf) should be obtained in writing only after a full written explanation of the purpose of that research has been made, and any foreseeable health hazards outlined. Opportunity must be given for questioning and withdrawal. When indicated, an explanation of the theory and justification for double-blind procedures should be given. Acceptance or refusal to participate in a clinical study must never interfere with the doctor–patient relationship or access to appropriate treatment. No degree of coercion is acceptable.

40. Boundaries between formalised clinical research and various types of innovation have become blurred to an increasing extent. Doctors retain the right to

recommend, and any patient has the right to receive, any new drug or treatment which, in the doctor's considered judgement, offers hope of saving life, re-establishing health or alleviating suffering. Doctors are advised to document carefully the basis for any such decisions and also record the patient's perception and basis for a decision. In all such cases the doctors must fully inform the patient about the drug or treatment, including the fact that such treatment is new or unorthodox, if that is so.

41. In situations where a doctor is undertaking an innovative or unusual procedure on his or her own initiative, it is wise to consult colleagues. This recommendation applies particularly in relation to care of the dying.

42. It is the duty of doctors to ensure that the first communication of research results be through recognised scientific channels, including journals and meetings of professional bodies, to ensure appropriate peer review. Participants in the research should also be informed of the results as soon as is practicable after completion.

43. Doctors should not participate in clinical research involving control by the funder over the release of information or results, and must retain the right to publish or otherwise release any findings they have made. Any dispute or ethical issue which may arise in the course of research should be considered openly, e.g. by consultation with the Ethics Committee of the NZMA and/or Regional Ethics Committees.

Teaching

44. Clinical teaching is the basis on which sound clinical practice is based. It is the duty of doctors to share information and promote education within the profession. Education of colleagues and medical students should be regarded as a responsibility for all doctors.

45. Teaching involving direct patient contact must be undertaken with sensitivity, compassion, respect for privacy, and, whenever possible, with the consent of the patient, guardian or appropriate agent. Particular sensitivity is required when patients are disabled or disempowered, e.g. children. If teaching involves a patient in a permanent vegetative state, the teacher should, if at all possible, consult with a nursing or medical colleague and a relative before commencing the session.

46. Wherever possible, patients should be given sufficient information on the form and content of the teaching, and adequate time for consideration,

before consenting or declining to participate in clinical teaching. Refusal by a patient to participate in a study or teaching session must not interfere with other aspects of the doctor–patient relationship or access to appropriate treatment.

47. Patients' understanding of, or perspective on, their medical problems may be influenced by involvement in clinical teaching. Doctors must be sensitive to this possibility and ensure that information is provided in an unbiased manner, and that any questions receive adequate answers. It may be appropriate for the doctor to return later to address these issues.

Medicine and Commerce

48. Commercial interests of an employer, health provider, or doctor must not interfere with the free exercise of clinical judgement in determining the best ways of meeting the needs of individual patients or the community, nor with the capacities of individual doctors to co-operate with other health providers in the interests of their patients, nor compromise standards of care in order to meet financial or commercial targets.

49. Where potential conflict arises between the best interests of particular patients and commercial or rationing prerogatives, doctors have a duty to explain the issues and dilemmas to their patients. Doctors shall state quite clearly what their intentions are and why they advocate particular patterns of diagnosis, treatment or resource use. Rationing of resources must be open to public scrutiny and points of conflict identified and presented in a rational, non-biased manner to the public.

50. Doctors who provide capital towards health services in the private sector are entitled to expect a reasonable return on investment. Where there may be a conflict of interests, the circumstances should be disclosed and open to scrutiny.

51. Like all professionals, doctors have the right to fair recompense for the use of their skills and experience. However, motives of profit must not be permitted to influence professional judgement on behalf of patients.

52. Doctors should insist that any contracts into which they enter, including those involving patients, be written in clear language such that all parties have a clear understanding of the intentions and rules.

53. Doctors who find themselves in a potentially controversial contractual or commercial situation should seek the advice of a suitable colleague or organisation.

CODE OF ETHICS OF THE CHILEAN MEDICAL ASSOCIATION

Chilean Medical Association

1983

• • •

Approved by the Honorable General Council in November 1983, the Code of Ethics of the Chilean Medical Association sets moral standards for the conduct of members of the association and "should only be used by and for physicians." Articles of particular note include: (1) article 25, which proscribes physician participation in torture; (2) article 26, which permits abortion only for therapeutic reasons and, along with articles 27–28, reflects the prevalence of Catholicism in Chile; (3) articles 27 and 28, which pertain to euthanasia and death with dignity; and (4) article 44, which provides for a patient or the patient's family to request a review board to investigate the clinical findings and recommendations of the attending physician.

Declaration of Principles

• • •

A respect for life and the human person is the basic foundation for the professional practice of medicine.

The ethical principles that govern the conduct of physicians oblige them to protect the human being from pain, suffering, and death without any discrimination.

Decorum, dignity, honesty, and moral integrity, as imperative norms in the life of a doctor, are attributes the medical community deems fundamental in its professional practice.

• • •

Title I

General Resolutions

• • •

ARTICLE 10. Doctor-patient confidentiality is both a right and an obligation of the profession. With respect to any patient this is imperative, even when the patient is no longer under a particular physician's care.

• • •

If a patient communicates to a physician the intent to commit a crime, such communication is not protected by the right and duty of doctor–patient confidentiality, and the physician must reveal any information necessary for the prevention of a crime or to protect any person(s) in danger.

. . .

Title II

On the Duties of the Doctor toward Patients

ARTICLE 13. The physician must attend to the needs of any person requiring his or her services and, in the absence of another colleague able to care for the patient, may not deny such attention.

ARTICLE 14. Physicians may not, under any circumstances, directly or indirectly reveal facts, data, or information that they have learned or that have been revealed to them in the course of their professional work, except by judicial order, or by freely expressed authorization by a patient who is of legal age and of sound mind.

Doctor-patient confidentiality is an objective right of the patient that the physician must absolutely respect as a natural right, based neither on promise nor on pact. Doctor-patient confidentiality includes the patient's name.

ARTICLE 15. In cases where it may be therapeutically necessary to have recourse to treatments involving known risk or serious disfiguring of the patient, the physician may not act without the express and informed consent of the patient or responsible family members when the patient is a minor or otherwise unable to make such decisions.

In emergency situations or in the absence of responsible family members and without the possibility of communication with them, or in the event that there be no next of kin, the physician may proceed without the above-mentioned authorization and without prejudice, after attempting to obtain the concurring opinion of another colleague in the treatment.

ARTICLE 16. No physician may participate or advise in any transaction involving the transplantation of organs if said transaction involves monetary gain.

. . .

ARTICLE 22. Scientific biomedical research on human beings is necessary; however, it is acceptable only when it does not involve serious health risks. It should always be carried out under direct medical supervision.

Its design and development should follow a strict protocol and be subject to scientific and ethical review. The patient or subject of the research must be informed of both potential risks and benefits, must give consent, and must reserve the right to abstain from any part of or withdraw from the study at any time.

. . .

ARTICLE 25. A physician shall not support or participate in the practice of torture or the infliction of any other cruel, inhumane, or degrading procedures, regardless of the offense(s) of which the victim of such procedures is accused or guilty, and regardless of the beliefs or motivation of the accused or guilty victim of such procedures, including armed conflict or civil war.

A physician must not provide any rationale, instrument, substance, or knowledge expertise that would facilitate the practice of torture or other forms of cruel, inhumane, or degrading treatment, or for the purpose of diminishing the victim's capacity to resist such treatment.

A physician must not be present before, during, or after any procedure in which torture or other forms of cruel, inhumane, or degrading treatment are used as a threat.

ARTICLE 26. A physician must respect human life from the moment of conception. Abortion may be performed only under the following circumstances:

a) it is performed for therapeutic reasons;
b) the decision is approved in writing by two physicians chosen for their competence;
c) the procedure is carried out by a specialist in the field.

If a physician considers that it is against his or her convictions to perform an abortion, he or she must withdraw, permitting the patient to continue medical care with another qualified physician.

ARTICLE 27. A physician must not under any circumstances deliberately end the life of a patient. No authority may order or permit a physician to do so. Furthermore, no patient or person responsible for making decisions for the patient may request this of a physician.

ARTICLE 28. Every person has the right to die with dignity. Thus, diagnostic and therapeutic procedures must be proportionate to the results that can be hoped for from such procedures.

A physician must relieve a patient's pain and suffering even though this may involve the risk of shortening the patient's life.

In the event of an imminent and inevitable death, were routine life support interrupted, a physician may in good faith make the decision to withhold any treatment that would prolong a precarious and painful condition. In a case where the patient is proven to be brain dead, the physician is authorized to withhold any and all types of treatment.

. . .

Title III

On Physicians' Relationship with Colleagues

. . .

ARTICLE 44. Any and all physicians must consult with one or more colleagues whenever the making of a diagnosis, the type of illness, or treatment requires such collaboration.

A patient or patient's family, with the knowledge of the attending physician, may ask that a Review Board be arranged if they deem it necessary.

It is a moral duty of the attending physician to accept the collaboration of colleagues convened on the Review Board, who shall examine the patient in the presence of the attending physician and one after the other, except in special cases. The findings of the Board shall be discussed among the attending and collaborating physicians before the Chief Physician makes them known to the patient or to the patient's family.

. . .

CODE OF MEDICAL ETHICS, BRAZIL

Federal Council of Medicine

1988

. . .

Brazil's Federal Council of Medicine approved the current Code of Medical Ethics in January 1988, rescinding the 1965 Code of Medical Ethics and the 1984 Brazilian Code of Medical Deontology. The preamble states that the code "contains the ethical standards governing physicians"; that "organizations delivering medical services are subject to the standards in this code"; and, interestingly, that "those who violate this code are subject to disciplinary action as stated by law." Other interesting features of the code include: (1) statements regarding occupational health and the natural environment (articles 12, 13); (2) the right of physicians to strike (article 24); and (3) the requirement that protocols for medical research be submitted to an independent committee for approval and monitoring (article 127).

Chapter I

Basic Principles

. . .

ART. 6 – The physician shall have utmost respect for human life, always acting in the interest of the patient. He/she will never use his/her knowledge to inflict physical or moral suffering, to end the life of an individual, or to allow cover-ups against his dignity and integrity.

ART. 7 – The physician shall practice his/her profession with ample autonomy and is not forced to provide professional services to an individual against his/her will, except in the absence of another physician, in emergency cases, or when his refusal could cause irreversible damage to the patient.

ART. 8 – The physician may not, under any circumstance or pretext, renounce his professional freedom and shall disallow any restriction or imposition that could harm the efficacy and appropriateness of his/her work.

. . .

ART. 11 – The physician shall keep information, obtained during the practice of his profession, confidential. The same applies to his/her work with businesses, except in cases when such information damages or poses a risk to the health of an employee, or the community.

ART. 12 – The physician shall promote an appropriate working environment for the individual, and the elimination, or control, of risks inherent in his/her work.

ART. 13 – The physician shall inform competent authorities of any forms of pollution and deterioration of the environment, that pose a risk to health and life.

ART. 14 – The physician shall promote the improvement of health conditions and medical service standards, and take part in responsibilities in relation to public health, health education, and health legislation.

. . .

Chapter II

Rights of the Physician

The physician has the right to:

ART. 20 – Practice Medicine without being discriminated against in terms of religion, race, sex, nationality, color, sexual choice, social status, political opinion, or for any other reason.

ART. 21 – Recommend adequate procedures to the patient, observing regularly accepted practice and respecting legal standards in force in the country.

. . .

ART. 24 – Suspend his/her activities, individually or collectively, when the public or private institution for which he/she works, does not offer minimal conditions for the practice of his/her profession, or does not pay accordingly, except in conditions of urgency and emergency. This decision shall be communicated immediately to the Regional Council of Medicine.

. . .

ART. 27 – When employed, dedicate the time and professional experience recommended for the performance of his/her duties, to the patient, avoiding excessive workloads or consultations that could harm the patient.

ART. 28 – Refuse to perform medical practices, although allowed by law, that are contrary to his/her conscience.

Chapter III

Professional Responsibility

The physician is forbidden:

. . .

ART. 40 – Not to inform the individual about working conditions that could pose a risk to his/her health. These facts must be communicated to those in charge, the authorities, and the Regional Council of Medicine.

ART. 41 – Not to inform the patient about social, environmental, or professional implications of his/her illness.

ART. 42 – To practice or recommend medical procedures, not necessary or forbidden by local law.

ART. 43 – Not to abide by specific legislation on organ or tissue transplants, sterilization, artificial insemination, and abortion.

. . .

Chapter IV

Human Rights

The physician is forbidden:

ART. 46 – To perform any medical procedure without previous explanation and consent of the patient or his/her legal representative, except in cases of imminent threat to life.

ART. 47 – To discriminate against a human being in any way or under any pretext.

ART. 48 – To exercise his/her authority in such a way that it limits the right of the patient to decide freely for him/herself or on his/her well-being.

ART. 49 – To participate in the practice of torture, or any other degrading procedures, that are inhuman or cruel; to be an accomplice in these kinds of practices, and not to denounce them when they come to his/her knowledge.

ART. 50 – To provide means, instruments, substances, or knowledge that facilitate the practice of torture or other kinds of degrading, inhuman, and cruel procedures, in relation to the individual.

ART. 51 – To force-feed any person on a hunger strike, who is considered capable, physically and mentally, of making perfect judgement of possible complications from this attitude. In these cases, the physician shall inform the individual of possible complications from prolonged lack of nutrition and treat him/her if there is imminent danger to life.

ART. 52 – To use any process that might change the personality or conscience of an individual, to decrease his/her physical or mental resistance during a police investigation or of any other kind.

ART. 53 – Not to respect the interest and integrity of an individual, by treating him/her in any institution where the person is being kept against his/her will.

Any procedures damaging the personality or physical or mental health of an individual, while under the care of a physician, shall compel the physician in charge to denounce this fact to the competent authorities and to the Regional Council of Medicine.

ART. 54 – To provide means, instruments, substances, knowledge, or to participate in any way, in the execution of a death penalty.

ART. 55 – To use the profession to corrupt customs or to commit or favor crime.

Chapter V

Relation with Patients and Family Members

The physician is forbidden:

ART. 56 – To disregard the right of the patient to decide freely about the performance of diagnostic or therapeutic practices, except in cases of imminent loss of life.

ART. 57 – Not to use all available diagnostic and treatment means within his/her reach in favor of the patient.

ART. 58 – Not to treat a patient, looking for his/her professional care, in an emergency, when there are no other physicians or medical services available.

ART. 59 – Not to inform the patient of the diagnosis, prognosis, risks and objectives of treatment, except when direct communication may be harmful to the patient. In this case, communication shall take place with the legal representative of the patient.

ART. 60 – To exaggerate the seriousness of a diagnosis or prognosis, to complicate treatment, or to exceed the number of visits, consultations, or any other medical procedures.

ART. 61 – To abandon a patient under his/her care.

§1 – Under circumstances, that in his/her view are harmful to the doctor–patient relationship or that interfere with full professional performance, a physician has the right to renounce treatment, as long as this fact is previously communicated to the patient or his/her legal representative, with the assurance of continuity of care and supplying all necessary information to the substituting physician.

§2 – Except in cases of just cause, communicated to the patient or his/her family members, the physician may not abandon the patient for having a chronic or incurable disease. The physician shall continue to treat him/her, even if only to alleviate physical or psychological suffering.

ART. 62 – To prescribe treatment or other procedures without examining the patient directly, except in emergency cases or the impossibility of performing such an examination. In this case, the examination shall be performed as soon as possible.

ART. 63 – Not to respect the modesty of any individual in his/her professional care.

ART. 64 – To oppose the realization of a medical inquiry requested by the patient or his legal representative.

ART. 65 – To take advantage of the doctor–patient relationship to obtain physical, emotional, financial, or political advantages.

ART. 66 – To use, in any case, means to shorten the life of a patient, even if requested to do so, by the patient or his legal representative.

ART. 67 – Not to respect the right of the patient to decide freely on a contraceptive or conceptive method. The physician shall always explain indication, reliability, and reversibility, as well as the risk of each method.

ART. 68 – To practice artificial insemination, without total consent by the participants, with the procedure duly explained.

ART. 69 – Not to maintain medical records for each patient.

ART. 70 – To deny the patient access to his/her medical records, clinical or similar records, as well as not to provide explanations necessary for their understanding, except when this incurs risks for the patient or third parties.

ART. 71 – Not to provide a medical opinion to the patient, upon referral or transfer for the continuity of care, or upon release, if requested to do so.

. . .

Chapter IX

Medical Confidentiality

The physician is forbidden:

ART. 102 – To reveal the fact that he is aware of information received during the practice of his/her profession, except for just cause, legal duty, or express authorization by the patient.

This is maintained:

a) Even if the fact is public knowledge or if the patient is deceased.
b) When testifying. In this instance, the physician shall present him/herself and declare his/her constraint.

ART. 103 – To reveal a professional secret relating to a minor, including to his/her parents or legal representatives, as long as the minor is capable of resolving his/her problem by his/her own means, except when the lack of revelation could imply damage to the patient.

ART. 104 – To make reference to identifiable clinical cases, exhibit patients or their photographs in professional announcements or during medical programs on radio, television or movies, as well as in articles, interviews or newspaper reports, magazines or other publications not specific to Medicine.

ART. 105 – To reveal confidential information obtained during the medical exam of workers, including upon demand by directors of businesses or institutions, except if silence poses a risk to the health of workers or the community.

ART. 106 – To provide insurance companies with any information about the circumstances of the death of his/her patient, beyond that contained in the death certificate, except by express authorization of the legal representative or heir.

ART. 107 – Not to inform his/her assistants and not to promote the respect of professional secrecy, as required by law.

ART. 108 – To facilitate the handling and knowledge of medical records, forms, and other kinds of medical observations, subject to professional secrecy, by persons not obligated by this commitment.

ART. 109 – Not to maintain professional secrecy when recovering professional fees by judicial or extra-judicial means.

. . .

Chapter XII

Medical Research

The physician is forbidden:

ART. 122 – To participate in any type of experiment with human beings with warlike, political, racial, or eugenic reasons.

ART. 123 – To perform research on an individual, without his/her express consent in writing, after having had the nature and consequence of research duly explained.

If the patient is not in condition to give his/her consent, research shall only be performed, in his/her own benefit, after express authorization by his/her legal representative.

ART. 124 – To use any type of experimental treatment, not approved for use in the country, without due authorization by competent authorities and without the consent of the patient or his legal representative, duly informed of the situation and possible consequences.

ART. 125 – To promote medical research in the community without knowledge by the community and with a purpose not directed at public health, in consideration of local characteristics.

ART. 126 – To obtain personal advantages or have any commercial interest or to renounce his/her professional independence in relation to medical research financing entities in which he/she participates.

ART. 127 – To perform medical research on individuals without having submitted the protocol for approval and monitoring of a commission not subject to any entity related to the researcher.

ART. 128 – To perform medical research on volunteers, healthy or not, who have a direct or indirect relation of dependency or subordination with the researcher.

ART. 129 – To perform or participate in medical research in which there is a need to suspend or to stop using recognized treatment, thereby harming the patient.

ART. 130 – To perform experiments with new clinical or surgical treatment on incurable or terminal patients, without reasonable hope for positive effects, imposing additional suffering.

. . .

EUROPEAN CODE OF MEDICAL ETHICS

Conférence Internationale des Ordres et des
Organismes d'Attributions Similaies

1987

. . .

Drafted in January 1987 by the Conférence Internationale des Ordres et des Organismes d'Attributions Similaires, this European Code of Medical Ethics represents one effort to articulate medical ethics guidelines for the European Community. The code represents a guide for the countries involved, each of which must decide whether further action at a national level is warranted. The twelve participating countries and their representative bodies include: Belgium, Conseil National de l'Ordre des Médecins Belges; Denmark, Danish Medical Association and National Board of Health; Spain, Consejo General de Colegios Oficiales de Medicos; France, Conseil National de l'Ordre des Médecins Français; Luxembourg, Collège Médical; Ireland, Medical Council; Italy, Federazione Nazionale degli Ordini dei Medici; The Netherlands, Koninklijke Nederlandsche Maatschappij tot Bevordering der Geneeskunst; Portugal, Ordem dos Medicos; Germany, Bundesärztekammer; United Kingdom, General Medical Council; and observer for Sweden, Association Médicale Suédoise.

This guide is intended to influence the professional conduct of doctors, in whatever branch of practice, in their contacts with patients, with society and between themselves. The guide also refers to the privileged position of doctors, upon which good medical practice depends. The Conference has recommended to its constituent regulatory bodies in each member state of the European Communities that they take such measures as may be necessary to ensure that their national requirements relating to the duties and privileges of doctors vis-à-vis their patients and society and in their professional relationships conform with the principles set out in this guide, and that there is provision within their legal systems for the effective enforcement of these principles.

ARTICLE 1

The doctor's vocation is to safeguard man's physical and mental health and relieve his suffering, while respecting human life and dignity with no discrimination on the grounds of age, race, religion, nationality, social status, political opinions or any other, whether in peace time or in war time.

Undertakings by the Doctor

ARTICLE 2

A doctor engaging in medical practice undertakes to give priority to the medical interests of the patient. The doctor may use his professional knowledge only to improve or maintain the health of those who place their trust in him; in no circumstances may he act to their detriment.

ARTICLE 3

A doctor engaging in medical practice must refrain from imposing on a patient his personal philosophical, moral or political opinions.

Enlightened Consent

ARTICLE 4

Except in an emergency, a doctor will explain to the patient the effects and the expected consequences of treatment. He will obtain the patient's consent, particularly when his proposed medical interventions present a serious risk.

The doctor may not substitute his own definition of the quality of life for that of his patient.

Moral and Technical Independence

ARTICLE 5

Both when given advice and when giving treatment, a doctor must make best use of his complete professional freedom and the technical and moral circumstances which permit him to act in complete independence.

The patient should be informed if these conditions are not met.

ARTICLE 6

When a doctor is working for a private or public authority or when he is acting on behalf of a third party, be it an individual or institution, he must also inform the patient of this.

Professional Confidentiality

ARTICLE 7

The doctor is necessarily the patient's confidant. He must guarantee to him complete confidentiality of all the information which he may have acquired and of the investigations which he may have undertaken in the course of his contacts with him.

The death of a patient does not absolve a doctor from the rule of professional secrecy.

ARTICLE 8

A doctor must respect the privacy of his patients and take all necessary steps to prevent the disclosure of anything which he may have learned in the course of his professional practice.

Where national law provides for exceptions to the principles of confidentiality, the doctor should be able to consult the Medical Council or equivalent professional authority.

ARTICLE 9

Doctors may not collaborate in the establishment of electronic medical data banks which could imperil or diminish the right of the patient to the safely protected confidentiality of his privacy. A nominated doctor should be responsible for ethical supervision and control of each computerised medical data bank.

Medical data banks must have no links with other data banks.

Standards of Medical Care

ARTICLE 10

The doctor must have access to all the resources of medical knowledge in order to utilise them as necessary for the benefit of his patient.

ARTICLE 11

He should not lay claim to a competence which he does not possess.

ARTICLE 12

He must call upon a more experienced colleague in any case which requires an examination or method of treatment beyond his own competence.

Care of the Terminally Ill

ARTICLE 13

While the practice of medicine must in all circumstances constantly respect the life, the moral autonomy and the free choice of the patient, the doctor may, in the case of an incurable and terminal illness, alleviate the physical and mental suffering of the patient by restricting his intervention to such treatment as is appropriate to preserve, so far as possible, the quality of a life which is drawing to its close.

It is essential to assist the dying patient right to the end and to take such action as will permit the patient to retain his dignity.

Removal of Organs

ARTICLE 14

In a case where it is impossible to reverse the terminal processes leading to the cessation of a patient's vital functions, doctors will establish that death has occurred, taking account of the most recent scientific data.

At least two doctors, acting individually, should take meticulous steps to verify that this situation has occurred, and record their findings in writing.

They should be independent of the team which is to carry out the transplantation and must, in all respects, give priority to the care of the dying patient.

ARTICLE 15

Doctors removing an organ for transplantation may give particular treatment designed to maintain the condition of that organ.

ARTICLE 16

Doctors removing organs for transplantation and those carrying out transplantations should take all practicable steps to ensure that the donor had not expressed opposition or left instructions to this effect either in writing or with his family.

Reproduction

ARTICLE 17

The doctor will furnish the patient, on request, with all relevant information on the subjects of reproduction and contraception.

ARTICLE 18

It is ethical for a doctor, by reason of his own beliefs, to refuse to intervene in the processes of reproduction or termination of pregnancy, and to suggest to the patients concerned that they consult other doctors.

Experimentation on Humans

ARTICLE 19

Progress in the field of medicine is based on research which must finally lead to experiments which have a direct bearing on humans.

ARTICLE 20

Details of all proposed experimentation involving patients must first be submitted to an ethical committee which is independent of the research team for opinions and advice.

ARTICLE 21

The free and informed consent of any person who is to be involved in a research project must be obtained after he has first been sufficiently informed of the aims, methods and expected benefits as well as the risks and potential problems, and of his right not to take part in experiments (or other research) and to withdraw from participation at any time.

Torture and Inhuman Treatment

ARTICLE 22

A doctor must never attend, take part in or carry out acts of torture or other kinds of cruel, inhuman or degrading treatment whatever the crime, accusation against, beliefs or motives of the victim or of those who commit these deeds, whatever the situation, including cases of civil or armed conflict.

ARTICLE 23

A doctor must never use his knowledge, his competence or his skills for the purpose of facilitating the use of torture or any other cruel, inhuman or degrading procedure for the purpose of weakening the resistance of a victim of these methods.

The Doctor and Society

ARTICLE 24

In order to accomplish his humanitarian duties, every doctor has the right to legal protection of his professional independence and his standing in society, in times of peace as in times of war.

ARTICLE 25

It is the duty of a doctor, whether acting alone or in conjunction with other doctors, to draw the attention of society to any deficiencies in the quality of health care or in the professional independence of doctors.

ARTICLE 26

Doctors must be involved in the development and the implementation of all collective measures designed to improve the prevention, diagnosis and treatment of disease. In particular, they must provide a medical contribution to the organisation of rescue services, particularly in the event of public disaster.

ARTICLE 27

They must participate, so far as their competence and available facilities permit, in constant improvement of the quality of care through research and continual refinement of methods of treatment, in accordance with advances in medical knowledge.

Relationships with Professional Colleagues

ARTICLE 28

The rules of professional etiquette were introduced in the interest of patients. They were designed to prevent patients becoming the victims of dishonest manoeuvres between doctors. The latter may, on the other hand, legitimately rely on their colleagues to adhere to the standards of conduct to which the profession as a whole subscribes.

ARTICLE 29

A doctor has a duty to inform the competent professional regulatory authorities of any lapses of which he may be aware on the part of his colleagues from the rules of medical ethics and good professional practice.

Publication of Findings

ARTICLE 30

It is the duty of a doctor to publish, initially in professional journals, any discoveries that he may have made or conclusions that he may have drawn from his scientific studies relevant to diagnosis or treatment. He must submit his findings in the appropriate form for review by his colleagues before releasing them to the lay public.

ARTICLE 31

Any exploitation or advertisement of a medical success to the profit of an individual or of a group or of an institution is contrary to medical ethics.

Continuity of Care

ARTICLE 32

A doctor, whatever his specialty, is obliged by his humanitarian duty to give emergency treatment to any patient in immediate danger, unless he is satisfied that other doctors will provide this care and are capable of doing so.

ARTICLE 33

The doctor who agrees to give care to a patient undertakes to ensure continuity of care when necessary with the help of assistants, locums or colleagues.

Freedom of Choice

ARTICLE 34

Freedom of choice constitutes a fundamental principle of the patient–doctor relationship. The doctor must respect, and make sure that others respect, the patient's freedom of choice of doctors.

The doctor, for his part, may refuse to treat a particular patient, unless the patient is in immediate danger.

Withdrawal of Services

ARTICLE 35

When a doctor decides to participate in an organised, collective withdrawal of services, he is not absolved of his ethical responsibilities vis-à-vis his patients to whom he must guarantee emergency services and such care as is required by those currently being treated.

Fees

ARTICLE 36

In fixing his fees, the doctor will take account, in the absence of any contract or of individual or collective agreement, of the importance of the service which has been given, any special circumstances in a particular case, his own competence and the financial situation of the patient.

CODE OF ETHICS FOR DOCTORS

Norwegian Medical Association

AMENDED 1992, 2000

• • •

Adopted in 1961 and most recently amended in 2000, the Norwegian Medical Association's Code of Ethics for Doctors is interesting in its freedom from the governmental intrusions that characterize U.S. codes. Other provisions of interest include the right to withhold information from patients (I, §3) and the admonition that physicians should take care of their own health (II, §3). Excerpts from the Norwegian code follow.

Adopted by the Representative Body in 1961 and subsequently amended, most recently in 2000.

<http://www.legeforeningen.no/index.db2?id=297>

I. General Provisions

§ 1. A doctor shall protect human health. A doctor shall cure, alleviate and console. A doctor shall help the ill to regain their health and the healthy to preserve theirs. A doctor shall base his practice on respect for fundamental human rights, and on truth and justice in relation to patients and to society.

§ 2. A doctor shall safeguard the interests and integrity of the individual patient. The patient shall be treated with compassion, care and respect. Cooperation with the patient should be based on mutual trust and where possible on informed consent.

§ 3. A patient is entitled to information on his or her condition and treatment and normally to access to the information in the patient's case sheet. The patient shall be informed to the extent he or she wishes. Information which may be thought to be particularly difficult to bear, shall be given with care.

§ 4. A doctor shall maintain confidentiality and exercise discretion in respect of information he or she obtains in his or her medical capacity. The ethical obligation to maintain professional secrecy and discretion may extend further than the statutory obligation. The giving of information must be grounded in the patient's implicit or explicit consent or in a statute.

§ 5. A doctor must when a patient's life is ending show respect for the patient's right of self-determination. Active euthanasia, i.e. measures intended to hasten a patient's death, must not be engaged in. A doctor must not help a patient to commit suicide. To terminate or to refrain from initiating treatment which is of no avail is not considered active euthanasia.

§ 6. When a patient is in urgent need of medical assistance, this shall be provided as soon as possible. The obligation to provide immediate assistance ceases to apply if the doctor has ascertained that another doctor is providing assistance.

A doctor can refuse to treat a patient provided the patient has reasonable access to treatment by another doctor.

§ 7. A doctor must not exploit a patient sexually, financially, religiously or in any other way. A patient's consent does not absolve the doctor of responsibility. A doctor must not enter into sexual relations with a person whose doctor he or she is.

§ 8. A doctor shall in his or her practice have due regard for his or her patient's financial circumstances and not charge unreasonable fees.

§ 9. In examinations and treatment a doctor shall only employ methods indicated by sound medical practice. Methods which expose the patient to unnecessary risk shall not be employed. If a doctor does not possess the skill a method calls for, he or she shall ensure that the patient receives other competent treatment.

A doctor must not use or recommend methods which lack foundations in scientific research or sufficient medical experience. A doctor must not allow him- or herself to be pressed into using medical methods which he or she regards as professionally incorrect.

When new methods are being tried out, regard for the patient on whom they are being tried shall be the primary concern.

§ 10. A doctor shall maintain and constantly seek to renew his or her knowledge.

A doctor should according to his or her competence contribute to the development and mediation of medical knowledge.

§ 11. A doctor should according to his or her ability contribute to objective information to the public and the authorities on medical matters. A doctor who pronounces on medical matters to the media should ensure that he or she will be able to check the form in which the pronouncements are made public.

§ 12. A doctor shall in his or her practice have due regard for the national economy. Unnecessary or excessively costly methods must not be employed.

A doctor must contribute to the distribution of medical resources in accordance with generally accepted ethical norms. A doctor must in no way seek to provide individual patients or groups with unjustified advantages, whether financial, in respect of priorities, or otherwise. A doctor must give notice of insufficient resources in his or her area of responsibility.

II. Rules Governing the Relations of Doctors with Their Colleagues and Collaborators

§ 1. A doctor must show respect for colleagues and collaborators, and assist, advise and guide them.

§ 2. A doctor who sees signs of professional or ethical failings in a colleague or collaborator should first take the matter up directly with the person concerned. The approach should be tactful, especially towards students or doctors in training.

If this does not have the desired effect, the doctor should take the matter up with the person's administrative superior, bodies of the Norwegian Medical Association, or the competent health authority.

A doctor who sees signs of illness or abuse of intoxicants in a colleague or collaborator should offer his/her assistance.

§ 3. A doctor should take care of his own health and seek help if it fails.

§ 4. A doctor should take care not to criticise colleagues and collaborators in the presence of patients and their relatives, but must always keep the patient's interests in view.

§ 5. Public and other debates between colleagues on medical questions and health policy issues must be conducted in an objective manner.

§ 6. The referring and referring back of patients between colleagues must be based on professional medical criteria and the patient's need for continuous health services.

§ 7. Doctors must communicate with one another openly and trustfully. Exchanges of information between doctors concerning patients must take place sufficiently quickly and cover what is professionally necessary.

§ 8. Practice with regard to referrals must not be governed by personal financial interests.

III. Advertisements and Other Information Concerning Medical Services

§ 1. Advertisements and other information concerning medical services may only state:

– the location, opening hours, and administration of the business,

– the type of practice, and the speciality (cf. § 2 below) and title (cf. § 3 below) of the practitioner,

– the diagnostic and therapeutic methods used, and

– the fees charged.

The information must reflect generally medically accepted and/or scientifically documented diagnosis of indications and/or methods. The information must contain nothing incorrect or misleading to the public.

Advertisements or other information may make no mention of possible or expected results of specific services, or of the quality of the services. No formulations may be used which could give the public the impression that by failing to avail oneself of the services advertised, one is placing one's own or other persons' somatic, mental or social health at risk.

The overall presentation of the advertisement or other information concerning medical services must accord with the intentions indicated in the above.

Commercial advertisements of medical services must state the name of a or the medically responsible doctor. That doctor is considered responsible for compliance with the provisions in this Chapter.

§ 2. A doctor who is not an approved specialist may only advertise general practice. An approved specialist may advertise his or her specialty on its own or together with "general practice". A specialty in a particular disease may only be advertised with the permission of the Council.

§ 3. A doctor may only use such titles and designations as his or her education and position entitle him to. He or she may not use titles and designations which may give an erroneous impression of his or her qualifications and work.

§ 4. A doctor may not advertise medicines or medical consumer goods. Mention in professional medical contexts in articles, lectures and the like, not made for gain, is not regarded as advertising.

IV. Rules Governing the Issuing by Doctors of Medical Certificates and Other Certified Documents

§ 1. A medical certificate is a declaration by a doctor concerning a person's state of health. Medical certificates comprise such documents as completed forms for the use of the National Insurance authorities, certificates for various purposes, and statements of expert opinion.

§ 2. A doctor shall not issue a medical certificate if he/she is in doubt as to his/her competence. If a doctor does not find objective grounds for issuing a certificate, a certificate shall not be issued.

§ 3. A doctor shall base his/her certificates on the necessary information and on examinations that are sufficiently extensive for the purpose.

§ 4. A medical certificate shall convey sufficient information for its purpose and be objective and neutral in its wording. Relevant information must not be withheld or distorted. A certificate shall not contain more information than necessary for its purpose. When medical documents intended for other purposes are attached to medical certificates, special care must be taken to observe professional secrecy.

§ 5. A medical certificate must clearly show to whom it is addressed, its purpose, the doctor's relation to the person concerned, and what the doctor's knowledge concerning the person is based on. Written certificates must be drawn up as separate documents and dated and signed.

§ 6. The person to whom a medical certificate relates is generally entitled to be informed of the contents of the certificate.

Regulations of the Council for Medical Ethics and the Divisional Medical Ethics Committees

Adopted by the Representative Body in 1997.

§ 1. The Council for Medical Ethics and the Divisional medical ethics committees are the Norwegian Medical Association's special bodies for dealing with ethical questions.

§ 2. The Council for Medical Ethics is the Association's highest competent body in matters concerning medical ethics. The Council's decisions are binding on members of the Association, and decisions in individual cases can not be reviewed by other bodies.

§ 3. The Council's main task is to advise members of the Association, its central bodies, and society on questions of medical ethics. The Council reports on matters of principle relating to questions of medical ethics, and deals with complaints against doctors on the basis of the Code of Ethics for Doctors.

The Council does not deal with matters relating to professional aspects of medical work or normally with cases undergoing public legal or administrative treatment.

§ 4. The Council consists of a chairperson, a deputy chairperson, and three other members, and is elected by the Representative Body for terms of four calendar years. Two deputy members are also elected, to step in in the event of lasting absence. The Central Board nominates persons for membership of the Council. The chairperson and deputy chairperson are elected separately. Members of the Central Board can not be members of the Council.

One of the Medical Association's lawyers serves as secretary to the Council.

§ 5. Each Division of the Norwegian Medical Association shall have a medical ethics committee of four members, and a deputy member who shall step in in the event of lasting absence, cf. §11 of the Bylaws of the Medical Association. The committees shall concern themselves with questions of medical ethics in cooperation with the Council, and deal with complaints at divisional level.

§ 6. Matters may be brought before the Council and the committees by individuals, organizations, or Medical Association bodies. The Council and the committees may also themselves bring matters up.

If a complaint appears to be due to a doctor's health problem, an offer of assistance should be made as mentioned in §12 of the Medical Association's Bylaws.

§ 7. The Council and the committees shall always consider first whether or not a matter falls within their scope, and can in that connection consider whether to send it from the committee to the Council or vice versa. Matters which raise important questions of principle are dealt with by the Council.

Cases of doubt as to which Divisional committee ought to handle a case are decided by the Council.

Decisions by medical ethics committees can be appealed to the Council within four weeks after receipt of notification of the decision.

The Council and the committees shall keep minutes of their proceedings. Committees shall send copies of all their minutes to the Council. The Council shall send a copy of its minutes to the committee concerned.

§ 8. When a matter has been brought before the Council or a committee, the person or persons concerned shall be entitled to comment. They can demand to present a verbal account of the matter at a meeting. If the case concerns a complaint, the complainant is entitled to comment on the reply given by the person complained against.

Members of the Medical Association are obliged to testify before the Council or a medical ethics committee. If no testimony has been received within the time limit, the matter can be decided on the basis of the information available.

Any person is entitled to assistance by a lawyer and/or a colleague in matters brought before the Council or a medical ethics committee.

§ 9. Parties in cases before the Council or a committee may submit reasoned requests that members whom they consider disqualified shall withdraw during the handling of the case. A Council or committee member may also request permission to step down if he/she believes that he/she is disqualified. Such questions are decided by the Council or by the committee concerned.

§ 10. For a decision by the Council or by a committee to be valid, it must be adopted with at least three votes in favour.

§ 11. A decision by the Council or a committee shall be made known to the persons concerned as soon as possible. The Council can decide to publish a decision, formulated so as to ensure anonymity, in the Journal of the Norwegian Medical Association.

§ 12. If the Council or a committee is of the opinion that a doctor has contravened the Code of Ethics, it can express its disapproval or reprimand the doctor. It may require that the doctor apologise for and/or discontinue the matter complained of.

If the Council finds that a doctor has committed such a serious contravention of the Code of Ethics for Doctors that he/she should be expelled from the Medical Association, the case and the expulsion proposal shall be sent to the Central Board. The expulsion can also be proposed of a doctor who refuses to comply with a Council decision.

FINAL REPORT CONCERNING BRAIN DEATH AND ORGAN TRANSPLANTATION

Japan Medical Association

1988

• • •

Traditional religious and cultural values surrounding death and dying inform the Japanese public's reluctance to accept brain-based criteria for determining death and the subsequent harvesting of organs for transplantation. Generally, the medical profession has been more amenable to the use of brain criteria for determining death. In 1988, the Bioethics Council of the Japan Medical Association issued its Final Report Concerning Brain Death and Organ Transplantation. The report recognizes the legitimacy of brain criteria for determining death, in addition to the traditional cardiac criteria. However, it also includes a clause that emphasizes the need to consider the wishes of the patient and/or the patient's family and to obtain their consent when using brain criteria to determine death. This compromise position permits the introduction of brain criteria for death while not offending those individuals who oppose it.

1. Definition of Death

   In addition to cardiac death heretofore, death of the brain (irreversible loss of brain function) can be considered as the state of death of the individual human being.

2. Brain Death Determination Criteria

   With the criteria of the Research Group of the Ministry of Health (Kazuo Takeuchi, Group Leader) as minimum required criteria, fundamental particulars should be determined by the ethics committees of university hospitals, etc., and determination should be carried out with certainty and circumspection according to these criteria in such a manner that no doubt remains.

3. Respecting the Wishes of the Patient Himself and His Family

   It is considered appropriate under present circumstances to carry out the determination of death resulting from brain death upon giving serious consideration to the wishes of the patient himself and his family and obtaining their consent.

4. Justifiability of the Determination of Death Resulting from Brain Death

   Together with being generally recognized by the Japan Medical Association and others, it is considered that the determination of death as a result of brain death is socially and legally justifiable when the consent on the part of the patient has been obtained and determination has been carried out by physicians in a reliable manner according to appropriate methods.

5. Time of Death as a Result of the Determination of Brain Death

   In regard to the time of a death as a result of a determination of brain death, it can be considered to be (1) the time when determination of brain death was first made or (2) the time of confirmation of brain death six or more hours subsequent to that. The time of death indicated on the death certificate can be either (1) or (2) above; however, as a precaution in case of disputes over inheritance after death, the other of the two should be recorded in the records of the patient's treatment.

6. Organ Transplantation

   The transplantation of organs is to be carried out in accordance with the guidelines established by the Japan Transplantation Association once the organ donor, organ recipient and the families involved have received thorough explanations and their consent given through their own free will has been obtained.

SUMMARY OF THE REPORT ON INFORMATION FROM DOCTORS AND CONSENT OF PATIENTS

Japan Medical Association

1991

• • •

In 1951, the Japan Medical Association (JMA) issued a Physician's Code of Ethics, which is of historic interest for its emphasis on the Confucian concept of jin, "loving kindness," in the practice of medicine. Medicine is considered a jin-jyutsu, "humanitarian art." Traditionally, in Japanese medical practice, the combination of jin with the concept of shinrai-kankei, "fiduciary relationship," which is a positive value between people, correlated with a tendency for patients to trust and adhere to professional advice without question and a predilection toward medical paternalism. Since the 1960s, a gradual trend has emerged in Japan toward reassessing the nature of the patient–physician relationship. Exposure to contemporary Western bioethics and greater recognition of patients' rights is reflected in a movement among Japanese medical professionals to redefine the formerly paternalistic fiduciary relationship in light of a new emphasis on shared information and decision making with their patients. Although the JMA has never technically rescinded its 1951 code, the code has been superseded in practice by more recent documents from the JMA Bioethics Council that reflect the trend away from medical paternalism. One such document is the 1991 Summary of the Report on Information from Doctors and Consent of Patients, which follows.

1. The Definition of Informed Consent

   In strict terms, informed consent refers to the system of determining of the selection of medical procedures, which is carried out once the physician, as obliged, provides the patient with thorough explanations regarding feasible procedures within the course of medical treatment activities.

   Informed consent is a concept which originated in U.S.A. as the principal statement of the rights of a patient and came to incorporate a specific content as a result of courtroom judicial precedents and so forth in connection with mishaps during medical treatment.

   It would seem necessary in the case of Japan, however, to examine its content independently and thereupon, with the opportunity offered by the informed consent, proceed with the structuring of a new relationship between physician and patient in the context of medical treatment.

2. The Relationship between the Physician's Explanation and Patient's Consent

   As a general rule, the patient's consent is obtained on the occasion of direct or indirect invasions of the patient's body; carrying out such invasions without consent could, legally speaking, entail the possible occurrence of problems of the criminal infliction of bodily harm or those of civil justice involving injury compensation.

Thus, the consent of the patient is premised on explanations by the physician; the physician must provide thorough explanations to the patient necessary to allow the patient to make judgments or selections.

3. The Current Meaning of Informed Consent

In Japan up to the present, there has been a tendency on the part of the patient to leave everything up to the physician. However, more and more we are seeing an increase in the comprehension of patients relating to medical treatments, changes in the structure of present-day illnesses, together with subdivision and specialization taking place in treatment methods, resulting in an increased emphasis on the frank and open interaction between physician and patient. There has also been a deeper concern for the problem of informed consent.

At this point, instead of simply adopting the American style of informed consent intact, it is more reasonable that we should embrace one which is relevant to our own society, one which sufficiently takes into account the sentiments of the people, the history of medical treatment, cultural background, the character of the nation and so forth.

4. Specific Content of Informed Consent and Its Configuration

THE PHYSICIAN'S EXPLANATION AND THE PATIENT'S CONSENT

The physician's explanations to the patient must be expressed in words which are easily understood, allowing effortless comprehension by the patient, with the minimum use of specialized terminology.

The patient's consent indicates that the patient has comprehended, is satisfied with and consents to the procedures which the physician proposes to take.

5. The Physician's Obligation to Explain and Its Limits

Explanations within the limits indicated below can be considered necessary under normal circumstances:

1. The disease name and its present condition>
2. Proposed treatment methods for the disease
3. The degree of risk involved in such treatment methods (the presence and extent of risk)
4. Other possible choices of treatment methods and their relative advantages and disadvantages.
5. Prognosis, that is, future assumptions relating to the patient's illness

Emergencies or cases in which the patient does not have the capacity to make judgments him or herself regarding consent after having been given explanations can be cited as exceptions to the general rule.

Cases in which the patient does not have the capacity to make judgments regarding consent after having been given explanations require that explanations be provided to the most appropriate next of kin and the patient's consent received by proxy. However, since the procedures in question are directed specifically to the patient, the inclinations of the patient should be taken into consideration when it is recognized that the patient does have judgmental capacity, though it may be impaired.

6. Informed Consent in Routine Diagnoses and Treatment

(1) Notification of Cancer

The following should be given thorough consideration as prior conditions upon the notification of cancer:

1. The purpose of notification must be explicit.
2. The family of the patient must be receptive.
3. Physician or others in the practice of medicine must have a satisfactory relationship with the family of the patient.
4. Mental care and support of the patient must be possible subsequent to notification.

(2) Living Wills

When a patient in terminal treatment has prepared a living will in advance and there is no hope of recovery, it is considered reasonable to respect the wishes of the patient not to engage in life-prolonging procedures, when such have been clearly stated.

(3) Others

If there is a necessity for blood transfusions in a patient who refuses such for religious reasons, the patient should be persuaded and then consent for transfusions obtained. However, if the patient persistently refuses, the will of the patient should be respected even though the outcome of not doing so would be disadvantageous to the patient. In such cases, it is considered that the physician does not assume any legal liability.

When the patient is a child, transfusions given contrary to the will of the parent can be considered permissible, even though the parent, as a follower of a religion, has refused such, since the child and the child's parents are fundamentally separate beings.

7. Informed Consent in Medical and Treatment Education

It cannot be denied that concern regarding informed consent among young physicians is lacking. It is of extreme importance that instruction regarding informed consent be promoted in the future both prior to graduation and thereafter through continuing education.

OATH OF SOVIET PHYSICIANS

1971

• • •

On 26 March 1971, the Presidium of the Supreme Soviet approved the text of the oath and ordered that all physicians and graduating medical students take the oath, sign a copy of it, and abide by it. The ruling went into effect on June 1, 1971. Distinctive features of this oath are: (1) dedication to preventive medicine; (2) commitment to the principles of communist morality; and (3) responsibility to the people and the Soviet government. The Soviet oath should be compared to the 1988 Regulations on Criteria for Medical Ethics and Their Implementation, issued by the Ministry of Health, People's Republic of China, and included in this section.

Having received the high title of physician and beginning a career in the healing arts, I solemnly swear:

to dedicate all my knowledge and all my strength to the care and improvement of human health, to treatment and prevention of disease, and to work conscientiously wherever the interests of the society will require it;

to be always ready to administer medical aid, to treat the patient with care and interest, and to keep professional secrets;

to constantly improve my medical knowledge and diagnostic and therapeutic skill, and to further medical science and the practice of medicine by my own work;

to turn, if the interests of my patients will require it, to my professional colleagues for advice and consultation, and to never refuse myself to give advice or help;

to keep and to develop the beneficial traditions of medicine in my country, to conduct all my actions according to the principles of the Communistic morale, to always keep in mind the high calling of the Soviet physician, and the high responsibility I have to my people and to the Soviet government.

I swear to be faithful to this Oath all my life long.

SOLEMN OATH OF A PHYSICIAN OF RUSSIA

1992

• • •

Approved by the Minister of Health and the Minister of Higher Education of the Russian Federation, this oath, which replaces the preceding Oath of Soviet Physicians, was first published in 1992. It is interesting to note the similarities between the new Russian oath and the Hippocratic Oath, indicating a conscious return to the Hippocratic tradition. While the Soviet oath bound physicians to the principles of communist morality and explicitly recognized their duty to the people and the Soviet state, the new oath focuses on the well-being of the individual patient.

In the presence of my Teachers and colleagues in the great science of doctoring, accepting with deep gratitude the rights of a physician granted to me

I SOLEMNLY PROMISE:

- to regard him who has taught me the art of doctoring as equal to my parents and to help him in his affairs and if he is in need;
- to impart any precepts, oral instruction, and all other learning to my pupils who are bound by the obligation of medical law but to no one else;
- I will conduct my life and my art purely and chastely, being charitable and not causing people harm;
- I will never deny medical assistance to anyone and will render it with equal diligence and patience to a patient of any means, nationality, religion, and conviction;
- no matter what house I may enter, I will go there for the benefit of the patient, remaining free of all intentional injustice and mischief, especially sexual relations;
- to prescribe dietetic measures and medical treatment for the patient's benefit according to my abilities and judgment, refraining from causing them any harm or injustice;
- I will never use my knowledge and skill to the detriment of anyone's health, even my enemy's;
- I will never give anyone a fatal drug if asked nor show ways to carry out such intentions;
- whatever I may see and hear during treatment or outside of treatment concerning a person's life, which should not be divulged, I will keep to myself, regarding such matters as secret;

• I promise to continue my study of the art of doctoring and do everything in my power to promote its advancement, reporting all my discoveries to the scientific world;

• I promise not to engage in the manufacture or sale of secret remedies;

• I promise to be just to my fellow doctors and not to insult their persons; however, if it is required for the benefit of a patient, I will speak the truth openly and impartially;

• in important cases I promise to seek the advice of doctors who are more versed and experienced than I; when I myself am summoned for consultation, I will acknowledge their merit and efforts according to my conscience.

If I fulfill this Oath without violating it, let me be given happiness in my life and art. If I transgress it and give a false Oath, let the opposite be my lot.

REGULATIONS ON CRITERIA FOR MEDICAL ETHICS AND THEIR IMPLEMENTATION

Ministry of Health, People's Republic of China

1988

• • •

The following regulations on medical ethics for healthcare providers were issued in December 1988 by the Ministry of Health of the People's Republic of China. The mention of socialist values in Article 1 may be compared to the statement regarding principles of communist morality found in the 1971 Soviet oath, which appears earlier in this section. It is notable, however, that these regulations do not mention responsibility to the State as did the Soviet oath. Also of note are the strong emphasis on education in medical ethics and the explicit application of the criteria to all healthcare workers.

Article 1. The purpose of the criteria is to strengthen the development of a society based on socialist values, to improve the quality of professional ethics of health-care workers and to promote health services.

Article 2. Medical ethics, which is also called professional ethics of health-care workers, guides the value system the health-care workers should have, covering all aspects from doctor–patient relationships to doctor–doctor relationships. The criteria for medical ethics form the code of conduct for health-care workers in their medical practice.

Article 3. The criteria for medical ethics include the following:

1. Heal the wounded, rescue the dying, and practice socialist humanitarianism. Keep the interests of the patient in your mind and try every means possible to relieve patient suffering.

2. Show respect to the patient's dignity and rights and treat all patients alike, whatever their nationality, race, sex, occupation, social position and economic status is.

3. Services should be provided in a civil, dignified, amiable, sympathetic, kind-hearted and courteous way.

4. Be honest in performing medical practice and conscious in observing medical discipline and law. Do not seek personal benefits through medical practice.

5. Keep the secrets related to the patient's illness and practice protective health-care service. In no case is one allowed to reveal the patient's health secret or compromise privacy.

6. Learn from other doctors and work together in cooperation. Handle professional relations between colleagues correctly.

7. Be rigorous in learning and practicing medicine and work hard to improve knowledge, ability, skills and service.

Article 4. Education in medical ethics is mandated for the implementation of these regulations and for supporting medical-ethical attitudes. Therefore, good control and assessment of medical ethics has to be introduced.

Article 5. Education on medical ethics and the promotion of medical ethics must be a part of managing and evaluating hospitals. Good and poor performance of working groups have to be judged and assessed according to these standards.

Article 6. Education in medical ethics should be conducted positively and unremittingly through linking theories with practice aiming to achieve actual and concrete results. It should be the rule to educate new health-care workers in medical ethics before they start their service; in no case are they allowed to practice before they get such an education.

Article 7. Every hospital should work out rules and regulations for the evaluation of medical ethics and should have a particular department to carry out the evaluation, regularly and irregularly. The results of the evaluation should be kept in record files.

Article 8. The evaluation of medical ethics should include self-evaluation, social evaluation, department evaluation and higher-level evaluation. Social evaluation is of particular importance and the opinions of the patients and public should be considered and health service should be offered under the surveillance of the masses.

Article 9. The result of the evaluation should be considered as an important standard in employment, promotion, payment and the hiring of health-care workers.

Article 10. Practice the rewarding of the best and the punishment of the worst. Those who observe medical ethics criteria should be rewarded and those who fail to observe criteria of medical ethics should be criticized and punished accordingly.

Article 11. These criteria are suitable for all health-care workers, including doctors, nurses, technicians and health-care administrators at all levels in all hospitals and clinics.

Article 12. Provincial health-care offices may work out detailed rules for the implementation of these criteria.

Article 13. These criteria become valid on the date they are issued.

ETHICAL AND RELIGIOUS DIRECTIVES FOR CATHOLIC HEALTH FACILITIES

United States Conference of Catholic Bishops

1971, REVISED 1975; 2001

• • •

The Catholic Church has published directives on medical ethics in several parts of the world, principally, though not exclusively, for use in its hospitals. These directives are considered binding not only on institutions but also on individuals: The medical staff, patients, and employees, regardless of their religion, are frequently expected to abide by such a code.

In the United States, a set of Ethical and Religious Directives for Catholic Hospitals was published in 1949 and revised in 1954. The directives printed here were originally approved as the national code by the U.S. Conference of Catholic Bishops and the United States Catholic Conference in 1971 and were revised in 1975 and again in 2001. Most distinctive are the directives on abortion, hysterectomy, sterilization, and artificial insemination.

<http://www.nccbuscc.org/bishops/directives.htm>

Preamble

Health care in the United States is marked by extraordinary change. Not only is there continuing change in clinical practice due to technological advances, but the health care system in the United States is being challenged by both institutional and social factors as well. At the same time,

there are a number of developments within the Catholic Church affecting the ecclesial mission of health care. Among these are significant changes in religious orders and congregations, the increased involvement of lay men and women, a heightened awareness of the Church's social role in the world, and developments in moral theology since the Second Vatican Council. A contemporary understanding of the Catholic health care ministry must take into account the new challenges presented by transitions both in the Church and in American society.

Throughout the centuries, with the aid of other sciences, a body of moral principles has emerged that expresses the Church's teaching on medical and moral matters and has proven to be pertinent and applicable to the ever-changing circumstances of health care and its delivery. In response to today's challenges, these same moral principles of Catholic teaching provide the rationale and direction for this revision of the *Ethical and Religious Directives for Catholic Health Care Services.*

These Directives presuppose our statement *Health and Health Care* published in 1981.[1] There we presented the theological principles that guide the Church's vision of health care, called for all Catholics to share in the healing mission of the Church, expressed our full commitment to the health care ministry, and offered encouragement to all those who are involved in it. Now, with American health care facing even more dramatic changes, we reaffirm the Church's commitment to health care ministry and the distinctive Catholic identity of the Church's institutional health care services.[2] The purpose of these *Ethical and Religious Directives* then is twofold: first, to reaffirm the ethical standards of behavior in health care that flow from the Church's teaching about the dignity of the human person; second, to provide authoritative guidance on certain moral issues that face Catholic health care today.

The *Ethical and Religious Directives* are concerned primarily with institutionally based Catholic health care services. They address the sponsors, trustees, administrators, chaplains, physicians, health care personnel, and patients or residents of these institutions and services. Since they express the Church's moral teaching, these Directives also will be helpful to Catholic professionals engaged in health care services in other settings. The moral teachings that we profess here flow principally from the natural law, understood in the light of the revelation Christ has entrusted to his Church. From this source the Church has derived its understanding of the nature of the human person, of human acts, and of the goals that shape human activity.

The Directives have been refined through an extensive process of consultation with bishops, theologians, sponsors, administrators, physicians, and other health care providers. While providing standards and guidance, the Directives do not cover in detail all of the complex issues that confront Catholic health care today. Moreover, the Directives will be reviewed periodically by the United States Conference of Catholic Bishops (formerly the National Conference of Catholic Bishops), in the light of authoritative church teaching, in order to address new insights from theological and medical research or new requirements of public policy.

The Directives begin with a general introduction that presents a theological basis for the Catholic health care ministry. Each of the six parts that follow is divided into two sections. The first section is in expository form; it serves as an introduction and provides the context in which concrete issues can be discussed from the perspective of the Catholic faith. The second section is in prescriptive form; the directives promote and protect the truths of the Catholic faith as those truths are brought to bear on concrete issues in health care.

General Introduction

The Church has always sought to embody our Savior's concern for the sick. The gospel accounts of Jesus' ministry draw special attention to his acts of healing: he cleansed a man with leprosy (Mt 8:1–4; Mk 1:40–42); he gave sight to two people who were blind (Mt 20:29–34; Mk 10:46–52); he enabled one who was mute to speak (Lk 11:14); he cured a woman who was hemorrhaging (Mt 9:20–22; Mk 5:25–34); and he brought a young girl back to life (Mt 9:18, 23–25; Mk 5:35–42). Indeed, the Gospels are replete with examples of how the Lord cured every kind of ailment and disease (Mt 9:35). In the account of Matthew, Jesus' mission fulfilled the prophecy of Isaiah: "He took away our infirmities and bore our diseases" (Mt 8:17; cf. Is 53:4).

Jesus' healing mission went further than caring only for physical affliction. He touched people at the deepest level of their existence; he sought their physical, mental, and spiritual healing (Jn 6:35, 11:25–27). He "came so that they might have life and have it more abundantly" (Jn 10:10).

The mystery of Christ casts light on every facet of Catholic health care: to see Christian love as the animating principle of health care; to see healing and compassion as a continuation of Christ's mission; to see suffering as a participation in the redemptive power of Christ's passion, death, and resurrection; and to see death, transformed by the resurrection, as an opportunity for a final act of communion with Christ.

For the Christian, our encounter with suffering and death can take on a positive and distinctive meaning through the redemptive power of Jesus' suffering and death. As St. Paul says, we are "always carrying about in the body the dying of Jesus, so that the life of Jesus may also be manifested in our body" (2 Cor 4:10). This truth does not lessen the pain and fear, but gives confidence and grace for bearing suffering rather than being overwhelmed by it. Catholic health care ministry bears witness to the truth that, for those who are in Christ, suffering and death are the birth pangs of the new creation. "God himself will always be with them [as their God]. He will wipe every tear from their eyes, and there shall be no more death or mourning, wailing or pain, [for] the old order has passed away" (Rev 21:3–4).

In faithful imitation of Jesus Christ, the Church has served the sick, suffering, and dying in various ways throughout history. The zealous service of individuals and communities has provided shelter for the traveler; infirmaries for the sick; and homes for children, adults, and the elderly.[3] In the United States, the many religious communities as well as dioceses that sponsor and staff this country's Catholic health care institutions and services have established an effective Catholic presence in health care. Modeling their efforts on the gospel parable of the Good Samaritan, these communities of women and men have exemplified authentic neighborliness to those in need (Lk 10:25–37). The Church seeks to ensure that the service offered in the past will be continued into the future.

While many religious communities continue their commitment to the health care ministry, lay Catholics increasingly have stepped forward to collaborate in this ministry. Inspired by the example of Christ and mandated by the Second Vatican Council, lay faithful are invited to a broader and more intense field of ministries than in the past.[4] By virtue of their Baptism, lay faithful are called to participate actively in the Church's life and mission.[5] Their participation and leadership in the health care ministry, through new forms of sponsorship and governance of institutional Catholic health care, are essential for the Church to continue her ministry of healing and compassion. They are joined in the Church's health care mission by many men and women who are not Catholic.

Catholic health care expresses the healing ministry of Christ in a specific way within the local church. Here the diocesan bishop exercises responsibilities that are rooted in his office as pastor, teacher, and priest. As the center of unity in the diocese and coordinator of ministries in the local church, the diocesan bishop fosters the mission of Catholic health care in a way that promotes collaboration among health care leaders, providers, medical professionals, theologians, and other specialists. As pastor, the diocesan bishop is in a unique position to encourage the faithful to greater responsibility in the healing ministry of the Church. As teacher, the diocesan bishop ensures the moral and religious identity of the health care ministry in whatever setting it is carried out in the diocese. As priest, the diocesan bishop oversees the sacramental care of the sick. These responsibilities will require that Catholic health care providers and the diocesan bishop engage in ongoing communication on ethical and pastoral matters that require his attention.

In a time of new medical discoveries, rapid technological developments, and social change, what is new can either be an opportunity for genuine advancement in human culture, or it can lead to policies and actions that are contrary to the true dignity and vocation of the human person. In consultation with medical professionals, church leaders review these developments, judge them according to the principles of right reason and the ultimate standard of revealed truth, and offer authoritative teaching and guidance about the moral and pastoral responsibilities entailed by the Christian faith.[6] While the Church cannot furnish a ready answer to every moral dilemma, there are many questions about which she provides normative guidance and direction. In the absence of a determination by the magisterium, but never contrary to church teaching, the guidance of approved authors can offer appropriate guidance for ethical decision making.

Created in God's image and likeness, the human family shares in the dominion that Christ manifested in his healing ministry. This sharing involves a stewardship over all material creation (Gn 1:26) that should neither abuse nor squander nature's resources. Through science the human race comes to understand God's wonderful work; and through technology it must conserve, protect, and perfect nature in harmony with God's purposes. Health care professionals pursue a special vocation to share in carrying forth God's life-giving and healing work.

The dialogue between medical science and Christian faith has for its primary purpose the common good of all human persons. It presupposes that science and faith do not contradict each other. Both are grounded in respect for truth and freedom. As new knowledge and new technologies expand, each person must form a correct conscience based on the moral norms for proper health care.

Part One

THE SOCIAL RESPONSIBILITY OF CATHOLIC HEALTH CARE SERVICES

INTRODUCTION

Their embrace of Christ's healing mission has led institutionally based Catholic health care services in the United States to become an integral part of the nation's health care system. Today, this complex health care system confronts a range of economic, technological, social, and moral challenges. The response of Catholic health care institutions and services to these challenges is guided by normative principles that inform the Church's healing ministry.

First, Catholic health care ministry is rooted in a commitment to promote and defend human dignity; this is the foundation of its concern to respect the sacredness of every human life from the moment of conception until death. The first right of the human person, the right to life, entails a right to the means for the proper development of life, such as adequate health care.[7]

Second, the biblical mandate to care for the poor requires us to express this in concrete action at all levels of Catholic health care. This mandate prompts us to work to ensure that our country's health care delivery system provides adequate health care for the poor. In Catholic institutions, particular attention should be given to the health care needs of the poor, the uninsured, and the underinsured.[8]

Third, Catholic health care ministry seeks to contribute to the common good. The common good is realized when economic, political, and social conditions ensure protection for the fundamental rights of all individuals and enable all to fulfill their common purpose and reach their common goals.[9]

Fourth, Catholic health care ministry exercises responsible stewardship of available health care resources. A just health care system will be concerned both with promoting equity of care—to assure that the right of each person to basic health care is respected—and with promoting the good health of all in the community. The responsible stewardship of health care resources can be accomplished best in dialogue with people from all levels of society, in accordance with the principle of subsidiarity and with respect for the moral principles that guide institutions and persons.

Fifth, within a pluralistic society, Catholic health care services will encounter requests for medical procedures contrary to the moral teachings of the Church. Catholic health care does not offend the rights of individual conscience by refusing to provide or permit medical procedures that are judged morally wrong by the teaching authority of the Church.

DIRECTIVES

1. A Catholic institutional health care service is a community that provides health care to those in need of it. This service must be animated by the Gospel of Jesus Christ and guided by the moral tradition of the Church.

2. Catholic health care should be marked by a spirit of mutual respect among care-givers that disposes them to deal with those it serves and their families with the compassion of Christ, sensitive to their vulnerability at a time of special need.

3. In accord with its mission, Catholic health care should distinguish itself by service to and advocacy for those people whose social condition puts them at the margins of our society and makes them particularly vulnerable to discrimination: the poor; the uninsured and the underinsured; children and the unborn; single parents; the elderly; those with incurable diseases and chemical dependencies; racial minorities; immigrants and refugees. In particular, the person with mental or physical disabilities, regardless of the cause or severity, must be treated as a unique person of incomparable worth, with the same right to life and to adequate health care as all other persons.

4. A Catholic health care institution, especially a teaching hospital, will promote medical research consistent with its mission of providing health care and with concern for the responsible stewardship of health care resources. Such medical research must adhere to Catholic moral principles.

5. Catholic health care services must adopt these Directives as policy, require adherence to them within the institution as a condition for medical privileges and employment, and provide appropriate instruction regarding the Directives for administration, medical and nursing staff, and other personnel.

6. A Catholic health care organization should be a responsible steward of the health care resources available to it. Collaboration with other health care providers, in ways that do not compromise Catholic social and moral teaching, can be an effective means of such stewardship.[10]

7. A Catholic health care institution must treat its employees respectfully and justly. This responsibility includes: equal employment opportunities for anyone qualified for the task, irrespective of a person's race, sex, age, national origin, or disability; a workplace that promotes employee participation; a work environment that ensures employee safety and well-being; just compensation and benefits; and recognition of the rights of employees to organize and bargain collectively without prejudice to the common good.

8. Catholic health care institutions have a unique relationship to both the Church and the wider community they serve. Because of the ecclesial nature of this relationship, the relevant requirements of canon law will be observed with regard to the foundation of a new Catholic health care institution; the substantial revision of the mission of an institution; and the sale, sponsorship transfer, or closure of an existing institution.

9. Employees of a Catholic health care institution must respect and uphold the religious mission of the institution and adhere to these Directives. They should maintain professional standards and promote the institution's commitment to human dignity and the common good.

Part Two

THE PASTORAL AND SPIRITUAL RESPONSIBILITY OF CATHOLIC HEALTH CARE

INTRODUCTION

The dignity of human life flows from creation in the image of God (Gn 1:26), from redemption by Jesus Christ (Eph 1:10; 1 Tm 2:4–6), and from our common destiny to share a life with God beyond all corruption (1 Cor 15:42–57). Catholic health care has the responsibility to treat those in need in a way that respects the human dignity and eternal destiny of all. The words of Christ have provided inspiration for Catholic health care: "I was ill and you cared for me" (Mt 25:36). The care provided assists those in need to experience their own dignity and value, especially when these are obscured by the burdens of illness or the anxiety of imminent death.

Since a Catholic health care institution is a community of healing and compassion, the care offered is not limited to the treatment of a disease or bodily ailment but embraces the physical, psychological, social, and spiritual dimensions of the human person. The medical expertise offered through Catholic health care is combined with other forms of care to promote health and relieve human suffering. For this reason, Catholic health care extends to the spiritual nature of the person. "Without health of the spirit, high technology focused strictly on the body offers limited hope for healing the whole person."[11] Directed to spiritual needs that are often appreciated more deeply during times of illness, pastoral care is an integral part of Catholic health care. Pastoral care encompasses the full range of spiritual services, including a listening presence; help in dealing with powerlessness, pain, and alienation; and assistance in recognizing and responding to God's will with greater joy and peace. It should be acknowledged, of course, that technological advances in medicine have reduced the length of hospital stays dramatically. It follows, therefore, that the pastoral care of patients, especially administration of the sacraments, will be provided more often than not at the parish level, both before and after one's hospitalization. For this reason, it is essential that there be very cordial and cooperative relationships between the personnel of pastoral care departments and the local clergy and ministers of care.

Priests, deacons, religious, and laity exercise diverse but complementary roles in this pastoral care. Since many areas of pastoral care call upon the creative response of these pastoral care-givers to the particular needs of patients or residents, the following directives address only a limited number of specific pastoral activities.

DIRECTIVES

10. A Catholic health care organization should provide pastoral care to minister to the religious and spiritual needs of all those it serves. Pastoral care personnel—clergy, religious, and lay alike—should have appropriate professional preparation, including an understanding of these Directives.

11. Pastoral care personnel should work in close collaboration with local parishes and community clergy. Appropriate pastoral services and/or referrals should be available to all in keeping with their religious beliefs or affiliation.

12. For Catholic patients or residents, provision for the sacraments is an especially important part of Catholic health care ministry. Every effort should be made to have priests assigned to hospitals and health care institutions to celebrate the Eucharist and provide the sacraments to patients and staff.

13. Particular care should be taken to provide and to publicize opportunities for patients or residents to receive the sacrament of Penance.

14. Properly prepared lay Catholics can be appointed to serve as extraordinary ministers of Holy Communion, in accordance with canon law and the policies of the local diocese. They should assist pastoral care personnel—clergy, religious, and laity—by providing supportive visits, advising patients regarding the availability of priests for the sacrament of Penance, and distributing Holy Communion to the faithful who request it.

15. Responsive to a patient's desires and condition, all involved in pastoral care should facilitate the availability of priests to provide the sacrament of Anointing of the Sick, recognizing that through this sacrament Christ provides grace and support to those who are seriously ill or weakened by advanced age. Normally, the sacrament is celebrated when the sick person is fully conscious. It may be conferred upon the sick who have lost consciousness or the use of reason, if there is reason to believe that they would have asked for the sacrament while in control of their faculties.

16. All Catholics who are capable of receiving Communion should receive Viaticum when they are in danger of death, while still in full possession of their faculties.[12]

17. Except in cases of emergency (i.e., danger of death), any request for Baptism made by adults or for infants should be referred to the chaplain of the institution. Newly born infants in danger of death, including those miscarried, should be baptized if this is possible.[13] In case of emergency, if a priest or a deacon is not available, anyone can validly baptize.[14] In the case of emergency Baptism, the chaplain or the director of pastoral care is to be notified.

18. When a Catholic who has been baptized but not yet confirmed is in danger of death, any priest may confirm the person.[15]

19. A record of the conferral of Baptism or Confirmation should be sent to the parish in which the institution is located and posted in its Baptism/ Confirmation registers.

20. Catholic discipline generally reserves the reception of the sacraments to Catholics. In accord with canon 844, §3, Catholic ministers may administer the sacraments of Eucharist, Penance, and Anointing of the Sick to members of the oriental churches that do not have full communion with the Catholic Church, or of other churches that in the judgment of the Holy See are in the same condition as the oriental churches, if such persons ask for the sacraments on their own and are properly disposed.

With regard to other Christians not in full communion with the Catholic Church, when the danger of death or other grave necessity is present, the four conditions of canon 844, §4, also must be present, namely, they cannot approach a minister of their own community; they ask for the sacraments on their own; they manifest Catholic faith in these sacraments; and they are properly disposed. The diocesan bishop has the responsibility to oversee this pastoral practice.

21. The appointment of priests and deacons to the pastoral care staff of a Catholic institution must have the explicit approval or confirmation of the local bishop in collaboration with the administration of the institution. The appointment of the director of the pastoral care staff should be made in consultation with the diocesan bishop.

22. For the sake of appropriate ecumenical and interfaith relations, a diocesan policy should be developed with regard to the appointment of non-Catholic members to the pastoral care staff of a Catholic health care institution. The director of pastoral care at a Catholic institution should be a Catholic; any exception to this norm should be approved by the diocesan bishop.

Part Three

THE PROFESSIONAL-PATIENT RELATIONSHIP

INTRODUCTION

A person in need of health care and the professional health care provider who accepts that person as a patient enter into a relationship that requires, among other things, mutual respect, trust, honesty, and appropriate confidentiality. The resulting free exchange of information must avoid manipulation, intimidation, or condescension. Such a relationship enables the patient to disclose personal information needed for effective care and permits the health care provider to use his or her professional competence most effectively to maintain or restore the patient's health. Neither the health care professional nor the patient acts independently of the other; both participate in the healing process.

Today, a patient often receives health care from a team of providers, especially in the setting of the modern acute-care hospital. But the resulting multiplication of relationships does not alter the personal character of the interaction between health care providers and the patient. The relationship of the person seeking health care and the professionals providing that care is an important part of the foundation on which diagnosis and care are provided. Diagnosis and care, therefore, entail a series of decisions with ethical as well as medical dimensions. The health care professional has the knowledge and experience to pursue the goals of healing, the maintenance of health, and the compassionate care of the dying, taking into account the patient's convictions and spiritual needs, and the moral responsibilities of all concerned. The person in need of health care depends on the skill of the health care provider to assist in preserving life and promoting health of body, mind, and spirit. The patient, in turn, has a responsibility to use these physical and mental resources in the service of moral and spiritual goals to the best of his or her ability.

When the health care professional and the patient use institutional Catholic health care, they also accept its public commitment to the Church's understanding of and witness to the dignity of the human person. The Church's moral teaching on health care nurtures a truly interpersonal professional-patient relationship. This professional–patient relationship is never separated, then, from the Catholic identity of the health care institution. The faith that inspires Catholic health care guides medical decisions in ways that fully respect the dignity of the person and the relationship with the health care professional.

DIRECTIVES

23. The inherent dignity of the human person must be respected and protected regardless of the nature of the person's health problem or social status. The respect for human dignity extends to all persons who are served by Catholic health care.

24. In compliance with federal law, a Catholic health care institution will make available to patients information about their rights, under the laws of their state, to make an advance directive for their medical treatment. The institution, however, will not honor an advance directive that is contrary to Catholic teaching. If the advance directive conflicts with Catholic teaching, an explanation should be provided as to why the directive cannot be honored.

25. Each person may identify in advance a representative to make health care decisions as his or her surrogate in the event that the person loses the capacity to make health care decisions. Decisions by the designated surrogate should be faithful to Catholic moral principles and to the person's intentions and values, or if the person's intentions are unknown, to the person's best interests. In the event that an advance directive is not executed, those who are in a position to know best the patient's wishes—usually family members and loved ones—should participate in the treatment decisions for the person who has lost the capacity to make health care decisions.

26. The free and informed consent of the person or the person's surrogate is required for medical treatments and procedures, except in an emergency situation when consent cannot be obtained and there is no indication that the patient would refuse consent to the treatment.

27. Free and informed consent requires that the person or the person's surrogate receive all reasonable information about the essential nature of the proposed treatment and its benefits; its risks, side-effects, consequences, and cost; and any reasonable and morally legitimate alternatives, including no treatment at all.

28. Each person or the person's surrogate should have access to medical and moral information and counseling so as to be able to form his or her conscience. The free and informed health care decision of the person or the person's surrogate is to be followed so long as it does not contradict Catholic principles.

29. All persons served by Catholic health care have the right and duty to protect and preserve their bodily and functional integrity.[16] The functional integrity of the person may be sacrificed to maintain the health or life of the person when no other morally permissible means is available.[17]

30. The transplantation of organs from living donors is morally permissible when such a donation will not sacrifice or seriously impair any essential bodily function and the anticipated benefit to the recipient

is proportionate to the harm done to the donor. Furthermore, the freedom of the prospective donor must be respected, and economic advantages should not accrue to the donor.

31. No one should be the subject of medical or genetic experimentation, even if it is therapeutic, unless the person or surrogate first has given free and informed consent. In instances of nontherapeutic experimentation, the surrogate can give this consent only if the experiment entails no significant risk to the person's well-being. Moreover, the greater the person's incompetency and vulnerability, the greater the reasons must be to perform any medical experimentation, especially nontherapeutic.

32. While every person is obliged to use ordinary means to preserve his or her health, no person should be obliged to submit to a health care procedure that the person has judged, with a free and informed conscience, not to provide a reasonable hope of benefit without imposing excessive risks and burdens on the patient or excessive expense to family or community.[18]

33. The well-being of the whole person must be taken into account in deciding about any therapeutic intervention or use of technology. Therapeutic procedures that are likely to cause harm or undesirable side-effects can be justified only by a proportionate benefit to the patient.

34. Health care providers are to respect each person's privacy and confidentiality regarding information related to the person's diagnosis, treatment, and care.

35. Health care professionals should be educated to recognize the symptoms of abuse and violence and are obliged to report cases of abuse to the proper authorities in accordance with local statutes.

36. Compassionate and understanding care should be given to a person who is the victim of sexual assault. Health care providers should cooperate with law enforcement officials and offer the person psychological and spiritual support as well as accurate medical information. A female who has been raped should be able to defend herself against a potential conception from the sexual assault. If, after appropriate testing, there is no evidence that conception has occurred already, she may be treated with medications that would prevent ovulation, sperm capacitation, or fertilization. It is not permissible, however, to initiate or to recommend treatments that have as their purpose or direct effect the removal, destruction, or interference with the implantation of a fertilized ovum.[19]

37. An ethics committee or some alternate form of ethical consultation should be available to assist by advising on particular ethical situations, by offering educational opportunities, and by reviewing and recommending policies. To these ends, there should be appropriate standards for medical ethical consultation within a particular diocese that will respect the diocesan bishop's pastoral responsibility as well as assist members of ethics committees to be familiar with Catholic medical ethics and, in particular, these Directives.

Part Four

ISSUES IN CARE FOR THE BEGINNING OF LIFE

INTRODUCTION

The Church's commitment to human dignity inspires an abiding concern for the sanctity of human life from its very beginning, and with the dignity of marriage and of the marriage act by which human life is transmitted. The Church cannot approve medical practices that undermine the biological, psychological, and moral bonds on which the strength of marriage and the family depends.

Catholic health care ministry witnesses to the sanctity of life "from the moment of conception until death."[20] The Church's defense of life encompasses the unborn and the care of women and their children during and after pregnancy. The Church's commitment to life is seen in its willingness to collaborate with others to alleviate the causes of the high infant mortality rate and to provide adequate health care to mothers and their children before and after birth.

The Church has the deepest respect for the family, for the marriage covenant, and for the love that binds a married couple together. This includes respect for the marriage act by which husband and wife express their love and cooperate with God in the creation of a new human being. The Second Vatican Council affirms:

> This love is an eminently human one.... It involves the good of the whole person.... The actions within marriage by which the couple are united intimately and chastely are noble and worthy ones. Expressed in a manner which is truly human, these actions signify and promote that mutual self-giving by which spouses enrich each other with a joyful and a thankful will.[21]

> Marriage and conjugal love are by their nature ordained toward the begetting and educating of children. Children are really the supreme gift of marriage and contribute very substantially to the welfare of their parents.... Parents should regard as their proper mission the task of transmitting human life and educating those to whom it has been

transmitted.... They are thereby cooperators with the love of God the Creator, and are, so to speak, the interpreters of that love.[22]

For legitimate reasons of responsible parenthood, married couples may limit the number of their children by natural means. The Church cannot approve contraceptive interventions that "either in anticipation of the marital act, or in its accomplishment or in the development of its natural consequences, have the purpose, whether as an end or a means, to render procreation impossible."[23] Such interventions violate "the inseparable connection, willed by God…between the two meanings of the conjugal act: the unitive and procreative meaning."[24]

With the advance of the biological and medical sciences, society has at its disposal new technologies for responding to the problem of infertility. While we rejoice in the potential for good inherent in many of these technologies, we cannot assume that what is technically possible is always morally right. Reproductive technologies that substitute for the marriage act are not consistent with human dignity. Just as the marriage act is joined naturally to procreation, so procreation is joined naturally to the marriage act. As Pope John XXIII observed:

> The transmission of human life is entrusted by nature to a personal and conscious act and as such is subject to all the holy laws of God: the immutable and inviolable laws which must be recognized and observed. For this reason, one cannot use means and follow methods which could be licit in the transmission of the life of plants and animals.[25]

Because the moral law is rooted in the whole of human nature, human persons, through intelligent reflection on their own spiritual destiny, can discover and cooperate in the plan of the Creator.[26]

Directives

38. When the marital act of sexual intercourse is not able to attain its procreative purpose, assistance that does not separate the unitive and procreative ends of the act, and does not substitute for the marital act itself, may be used to help married couples conceive.[27]

39. Those techniques of assisted conception that respect the unitive and procreative meanings of sexual intercourse and do not involve the destruction of human embryos, or their deliberate generation in such numbers that it is clearly envisaged that all cannot implant and some are simply being used to maximize the chances of others implanting, may be used as therapies for infertility.

40. Heterologous fertilization (that is, any technique used to achieve conception by the use of gametes coming from at least one donor other than the spouses) is prohibited because it is contrary to the covenant of marriage, the unity of the spouses, and the dignity proper to parents and the child.[28]

41. Homologous artificial fertilization (that is, any technique used to achieve conception using the gametes of the two spouses joined in marriage) is prohibited when it separates procreation from the marital act in its unitive significance (e.g., any technique used to achieve extra-corporeal conception).[29]

42. Because of the dignity of the child and of marriage, and because of the uniqueness of the mother–child relationship, participation in contracts or arrangements for surrogate motherhood is not permitted. Moreover, the commercialization of such surrogacy denigrates the dignity of women, especially the poor.[30]

43. A Catholic health care institution that provides treatment for infertility should offer not only technical assistance to infertile couples but also should help couples pursue other solutions (e.g., counseling, adoption).

44. A Catholic health care institution should provide prenatal, obstetric, and postnatal services for mothers and their children in a manner consonant with its mission.

45. Abortion (that is, the directly intended termination of pregnancy before viability or the directly intended destruction of a viable fetus) is never permitted. Every procedure whose sole immediate effect is the termination of pregnancy before viability is an abortion, which, in its moral context, includes the interval between conception and implantation of the embryo. Catholic health care institutions are not to provide abortion services, even based upon the principle of material cooperation. In this context, Catholic health care institutions need to be concerned about the danger of scandal in any association with abortion providers.

46. Catholic health care providers should be ready to offer compassionate physical, psychological, moral, and spiritual care to those persons who have suffered from the trauma of abortion.

47. Operations, treatments, and medications that have as their direct purpose the cure of a proportionately serious pathological condition of a pregnant woman are permitted when they cannot be safely postponed until the unborn child is viable, even if they will result in the death of the unborn child.

48. In case of extrauterine pregnancy, no intervention is morally licit which constitutes a direct abortion.[31]

49. For a proportionate reason, labor may be induced after the fetus is viable.

50. Prenatal diagnosis is permitted when the procedure does not threaten the life or physical integrity of the unborn child or the mother and does not subject them to disproportionate risks; when the diagnosis can provide information to guide preventative care for the mother or pre- or postnatal care for the child; and when the parents, or at least the mother, give free and informed consent. Prenatal diagnosis is not permitted when undertaken with the intention of aborting an unborn child with a serious defect.[32]

51. Nontherapeutic experiments on a living embryo or fetus are not permitted, even with the consent of the parents. Therapeutic experiments are permitted for a proportionate reason with the free and informed consent of the parents or, if the father cannot be contacted, at least of the mother. Medical research that will not harm the life or physical integrity of an unborn child is permitted with parental consent.[33]

52. Catholic health institutions may not promote or condone contraceptive practices but should provide, for married couples and the medical staff who counsel them, instruction both about the Church's teaching on responsible parenthood and in methods of natural family planning.

53. Direct sterilization of either men or women, whether permanent or temporary, is not permitted in a Catholic health care institution. Procedures that induce sterility are permitted when their direct effect is the cure or alleviation of a present and serious pathology and a simpler treatment is not available.[34]

54. Genetic counseling may be provided in order to promote responsible parenthood and to prepare for the proper treatment and care of children with genetic defects, in accordance with Catholic moral teaching and the intrinsic rights and obligations of married couples regarding the transmission of life.

Part Five

ISSUES IN CARE FOR THE DYING

INTRODUCTION

Christ's redemption and saving grace embrace the whole person, especially in his or her illness, suffering, and death.[35] The Catholic health care ministry faces the reality of death with the confidence of faith. In the face of death—for many, a time when hope seems lost—the Church witnesses to her belief that God has created each person for eternal life.[36]

Above all, as a witness to its faith, a Catholic health care institution will be a community of respect, love, and support to patients or residents and their families as they face the reality of death. What is hardest to face is the process of dying itself, especially the dependency, the helplessness, and the pain that so often accompany terminal illness. One of the primary purposes of medicine in caring for the dying is the relief of pain and the suffering caused by it. Effective management of pain in all its forms is critical in the appropriate care of the dying.

The truth that life is a precious gift from God has profound implications for the question of stewardship over human life. We are not the owners of our lives and, hence, do not have absolute power over life. We have a duty to preserve our life and to use it for the glory of God, but the duty to preserve life is not absolute, for we may reject life-prolonging procedures that are insufficiently beneficial or excessively burdensome. Suicide and euthanasia are never morally acceptable options.

The task of medicine is to care even when it cannot cure. Physicians and their patients must evaluate the use of the technology at their disposal. Reflection on the innate dignity of human life in all its dimensions and on the purpose of medical care is indispensable for formulating a true moral judgment about the use of technology to maintain life. The use of life-sustaining technology is judged in light of the Christian meaning of life, suffering, and death. Only in this way are two extremes avoided: on the one hand, an insistence on useless or burdensome technology even when a patient may legitimately wish to forgo it and, on the other hand, the withdrawal of technology with the intention of causing death.[37]

Some state Catholic conferences, individual bishops, and the USCCB Committee on Pro-Life Activities (formerly an NCCB committee) have addressed the moral issues concerning medically assisted hydration and nutrition. The bishops are guided by the Church's teaching forbidding euthanasia, which is "an action or an omission which of itself or by intention causes death, in order that all suffering may in this way be eliminated."[38] These statements agree that hydration and nutrition are not morally obligatory either when they bring no comfort to a person who is imminently dying or when they cannot be assimilated by a person's body. The USCCB Committee on Pro-Life Activities' report, in addition, points out the necessary distinctions between questions already resolved by the magisterium and those requiring further reflection, as, for example, the morality of withdrawing medically assisted hydration and nutrition from a person who is in the condition that is recognized by physicians as the "persistent vegetative state" (PVS).[39]

DIRECTIVES

55. Catholic health care institutions offering care to persons in danger of death from illness, accident, advanced age, or similar condition should provide them with appropriate opportunities to prepare for death. Persons in danger of death should be provided with whatever information is necessary to help them understand their condition and have the opportunity to discuss their condition with their family members and care providers. They should also be offered the appropriate medical information that would make it possible to address the morally legitimate choices available to them. They should be provided the spiritual support as well as the opportunity to receive the sacraments in order to prepare well for death.

56. A person has a moral obligation to use ordinary or proportionate means of preserving his or her life. Proportionate means are those that in the judgment of the patient offer a reasonable hope of benefit and do not entail an excessive burden or impose excessive expense on the family or the community.[40]

57. A person may forgo extraordinary or disproportionate means of preserving life. Disproportionate means are those that in the patient's judgment do not offer a reasonable hope of benefit or entail an excessive burden, or impose excessive expense on the family or the community.[41]

58. There should be a presumption in favor of providing nutrition and hydration to all patients, including patients who require medically assisted nutrition and hydration, as long as this is of sufficient benefit to outweigh the burdens involved to the patient.

59. The free and informed judgment made by a competent adult patient concerning the use or withdrawal of life-sustaining procedures should always be respected and normally complied with, unless it is contrary to Catholic moral teaching.

60. Euthanasia is an action or omission that of itself or by intention causes death in order to alleviate suffering. Catholic health care institutions may never condone or participate in euthanasia or assisted suicide in any way. Dying patients who request euthanasia should receive loving care, psychological and spiritual support, and appropriate remedies for pain and other symptoms so that they can live with dignity until the time of natural death.[42]

61. Patients should be kept as free of pain as possible so that they may die comfortably and with dignity, and in the place where they wish to die. Since a person has the right to prepare for his or her death while fully conscious, he or she should not be deprived of consciousness without a compelling reason. Medicines capable of alleviating or suppressing pain may be given to a dying person, even if this therapy may indirectly shorten the person's life so long as the intent is not to hasten death. Patients experiencing suffering that cannot be alleviated should be helped to appreciate the Christian understanding of redemptive suffering.

62. The determination of death should be made by the physician or competent medical authority in accordance with responsible and commonly accepted scientific criteria.

63. Catholic health care institutions should encourage and provide the means whereby those who wish to do so may arrange for the donation of their organs and bodily tissue, for ethically legitimate purposes, so that they may be used for donation and research after death.

64. Such organs should not be removed until it has been medically determined that the patient has died. In order to prevent any conflict of interest, the physician who determines death should not be a member of the transplant team.

65. use of tissue or organs from an infant may be permitted after death has been determined and with the informed consent of the parents or guardians.

66. Catholic health care institutions should not make use of human tissue obtained by direct abortions even for research and therapeutic purposes.[43]

Part Six

FORMING NEW PARTNERSHIPS WITH HEALTH CARE ORGANIZATIONS AND PROVIDERS

INTRODUCTION

Until recently, most health care providers enjoyed a degree of independence from one another. In ever-increasing ways, Catholic health care providers have become involved with other health care organizations and providers. For instance, many Catholic health care systems and institutions share in the joint purchase of technology and services with other local facilities or physicians' groups. Another phenomenon is the growing number of Catholic health care systems and institutions joining or co-sponsoring integrated delivery networks or managed care organizations in order to contract with insurers and other health care payers. In some instances, Catholic health care systems sponsor a health care plan or health maintenance organization. In many dioceses, new partnerships will result in a decrease in the number of health care providers, at times leaving the Catholic institution as the sole provider of health care services. At whatever level, new partnerships forge a variety of interwoven relationships: between the various institutional partners, between health care providers and the community, between physicians and health care services, and between health care services and payers.

On the one hand, new partnerships can be viewed as opportunities for Catholic health care institutions and services to witness to their religious and ethical commitments and so influence the healing profession. For example, new partnerships can help to implement the Church's social teaching. New partnerships can be opportunities to realign the local delivery system in order to provide a continuum of health care to the community; they can witness to a responsible stewardship of limited health care resources; and they can be opportunities to provide to poor and vulnerable persons a more equitable access to basic care.

On the other hand, new partnerships can pose serious challenges to the viability of the identity of Catholic health care institutions and services, and their ability to implement these Directives in a consistent way, especially when partnerships are formed with those who do not share Catholic moral principles. The risk of scandal cannot be underestimated when partnerships are not built upon common values and moral principles. Partnership opportunities for some Catholic health care providers may even threaten the continued existence of other Catholic institutions and services, particularly when partnerships are driven by financial considerations alone. Because of the potential dangers involved in the new partnerships that are emerging, an increased collaboration among Catholic-sponsored health care institutions is essential and should be sought before other forms of partnerships.

The significant challenges that new partnerships may pose, however, do not necessarily preclude their possibility on moral grounds. The potential dangers require that new partnerships undergo systematic and objective moral analysis, which takes into account the various factors that often pressure institutions and services into new partnerships that can diminish the autonomy and ministry of the Catholic partner. The following directives are offered to assist institutionally based Catholic health care services in this process of analysis. To this end, the United States Conference of Catholic Bishops has established the Ad Hoc Committee on Health Care Issues and the Church as a resource for bishops and health care leaders.

This new edition of the *Ethical and Religious Directives* omits the appendix concerning cooperation, which was contained in the 1995 edition. Experience has shown that the brief articulation of the principles of cooperation that was presented there did not sufficiently forestall certain possible misinterpretations and in practice gave rise to problems in concrete applications of the principles. Reliable theological experts should be consulted in interpreting and applying the principles governing cooperation, with the proviso that, as a rule, Catholic partners should avoid entering into partnerships that would involve them in cooperation with the wrongdoing of other providers.

DIRECTIVES

67. Decisions that may lead to serious consequences for the identity or reputation of Catholic health care services, or entail the high risk of scandal, should be made in consultation with the diocesan bishop or his health care liaison.

68. Any partnership that will affect the mission or religious and ethical identity of Catholic health care institutional services must respect church teaching and discipline. Diocesan bishops and other church authorities should be involved as such partnerships are developed, and the diocesan bishop should give the appropriate authorization before they are completed. The diocesan bishop's approval is required for partnerships sponsored by institutions subject to his governing authority; for partnerships sponsored by religious institutes of pontifical right, his *nihil obstat* should be obtained.

69. If a Catholic health care organization is considering entering into an arrangement with another organization that may be involved in activities judged morally wrong by the Church, participation in such activities, must be limited to what is in accord with the moral principles governing cooperation.

70. Catholic health care organizations are not permitted to engage in immediate material cooperation in actions that are intrinsically immoral, such as abortion, euthanasia, assisted suicide, and direct sterilization.[44]

71. The possibility of scandal must be considered when applying the principles governing cooperation.[45] Cooperation, which in all other respects is morally licit, may need to be refused because of the scandal that might be caused. Scandal can sometimes be avoided by an appropriate explanation of what is in fact being done at the health care facility under Catholic auspices. The diocesan bishop has final responsibility for assessing and addressing issues of scandal, considering not only the circumstances in his local diocese but also the regional and national implications of his decision.[46]

72. The Catholic partner in an arrangement has the responsibility periodically to assess whether the binding agreement is being observed and implemented in a way that is consistent with Catholic teaching.

Conclusion

Sickness speaks to us of our limitations and human frailty. It can take the form of infirmity resulting from the simple passing of years or injury from the exuberance of youthful energy. It can be temporary or chronic, debilitating, and even terminal. Yet the follower of Jesus faces illness and the consequences of the human condition aware that our Lord always shows compassion toward the infirm.

Jesus not only taught his disciples to be compassionate, but he also told them who should be the special object of their compassion. The parable of the feast with its humble guests was preceded by the instruction: "When you hold a banquet, invite the poor, the crippled, the lame, the blind" (Lk 14:13). These were people whom Jesus healed and loved.

Catholic health care is a response to the challenge of Jesus to go and do likewise. Catholic health care services rejoice in the challenge to be Christ's healing compassion in the world and see their ministry not only as an effort to restore and preserve health but also as a spiritual service and a sign of that final healing that will one day bring about the new creation that is the ultimate fruit of Jesus' ministry and God's love for us.

Notes

1. National Conference of Catholic Bishops, *Health and Health Care: A Pastoral Letter of the American Catholic Bishops* (Washington, D.C.: United States Catholic Conference, 1981).

2. Health care services under Catholic auspices are carried out in a variety of institutional settings (e.g., hospitals, clinics, out-patient facilities, urgent care centers, hospices, nursing homes, and parishes). Depending on the context, these Directives will employ the terms "institution" and/or "services" in order to encompass the variety of settings in which Catholic health care is provided.

3. *Health and Health Care,* p. 5.

4. Second Vatican Ecumenical Council, *Decree on the Apostolate of the Laity (Apostolicam Actuositatem)* (1965), no. 1.

5. Pope John Paul II, Post-Synodal Apostolic Exhortation, *On the Vocation and the Mission of the Lay Faithful in the Church and in the World (Christifideles Laici)* (Washington, D.C.: United States Catholic Conference, 1988), no. 29.

6. As examples, see Congregation for the Doctrine of the Faith, *Declaration on Procured Abortion* (1974); Congregation for the Doctrine of the Faith,

Declaration on Euthanasia (1980); Congregation for the Doctrine of the Faith, *Instruction on Respect for Human Life in its Origin and on the Dignity of Procreation: Replies to Certain Questions of the Day (Donum Vitae)* (Washington, D.C.: United States Catholic Conference, 1987).

7. Pope John XXIII, Encyclical Letter, *Peace on Earth (Pacem in Terris)* (Washington, D.C.: United States Catholic Conference, 1963), no. 11; *Health and Health Care,* pp. 5, 17–18; *Catechism of the Catholic Church,* 2nd ed. (Washington, D.C.: United States Catholic Conference, 2000), no. 2211.

8. Pope John Paul II, *On Social Concern, Encyclical Letter on the Occasion of the Twentieth Anniversary of "Populorum Progressio" (Sollicitudo Rei Socialis)* (Washington, D.C.: United States Catholic Conference, 1988), no. 43.

9. National Conference of Catholic Bishops, *Economic Justice for All: Pastoral Letter on Catholic Social Teaching and the U.S. Economy* (Washington, D.C.: United States Catholic Conference, 1986), no. 80.

10. The duty of responsible stewardship demands responsible collaboration. But in collaborative efforts, Catholic institutionally based health care services must be attentive to occasions when the policies and practices of other institutions are not compatible with the Church's authoritative moral teaching. At such times, Catholic health care institutions should determine whether or to what degree collaboration would be morally permissible. To make that judgment, the governing boards of Catholic institutions should adhere to the moral principles on cooperation. See Part Six.

11. *Health and Health Care,* p. 12.

12. Cf. *Code of Canon Law,* cc. 921–923.

13. Cf. ibid., c. 867, § 2, and c. 871.

14. To confer Baptism in an emergency, one must have the proper intention (to do what the Church intends by Baptism) and pour water on the head of the person to be baptized, meanwhile pronouncing the words: "I baptize you in the name of the Father, and of the Son, and of the Holy Spirit."

15. Cf. c. 883, 3.

16. For example, while the donation of a kidney represents loss of biological integrity, such a donation does not compromise functional integrity since human beings are capable of functioning with only one kidney.

17. Cf. directive 53.

18. *Declaration on Euthanasia,* Part IV; cf. also directives 56–57.

19. It is recommended that a sexually assaulted woman be advised of the ethical restrictions that prevent

Catholic hospitals from using abortifacient procedures; cf. Pennsylvania Catholic Conference, "Guidelines for Catholic Hospitals Treating Victims of Sexual Assault," *Origins* 22 (1993): 810.

20. Pope John Paul II, "Address of October 29, 1983, to the 35th General Assembly of the World Medical Association," *Acta Apostolicae Sedis* 76 (1984): 390.

21. Second Vatican Ecumenical Council, "Pastoral Constitution on the Church in the Modern World" (*Gaudium et Spes*) (1965), no. 49.

22. Ibid., no. 50.

23. Pope Paul VI, Encyclical Letter, *On the Regulation of Birth (Humanae Vitae)* (Washington, D.C.: United States Catholic Conference, 1968), no. 14.

24. Ibid., no. 12.

25. Pope John XXIII, Encyclical Letter, *Mater et Magistra* (1961), no. 193, quoted in Congregation for the Doctrine of the Faith, *Donum Vitae,* no. 4.

26. Pope John Paul II, Encyclical Letter, *The Splendor of Truth (Veritatis Splendor)* (Washington, D.C.: United States Catholic Conference, 1993), no. 50.

27. "Homologous artificial insemination within marriage cannot be admitted except for those cases in which the technical means is not a substitute for the conjugal act but serves to facilitate and to help so that the act attains its natural purpose" (*Donum Vitae,* Part II, B, no. 6; cf. also Part I, nos. 1, 6).

28. Ibid., Part II, A, no. 2.

29. "Artificial insemination as a substitute for the conjugal act is prohibited by reason of the voluntarily achieved dissociation of the two meanings of the conjugal act. Masturbation, through which the sperm is normally obtained, is another sign of this dissociation: even when it is done for the purpose of procreation, the act remains deprived of its unitive meaning: 'It lacks the sexual relationship called for by the moral order, namely, the relationship which realizes "the full sense of mutual self-giving and human procreation in the context of true love"'" (*Donum Vitae,* Part II, B, no. 6).

30. Ibid., Part II, A, no. 3.

31. Cf. directive 45.

32. *Donum Vitae,* Part I, no. 2.

33. Cf. ibid., no. 4.

34. Cf. Congregation for the Doctrine of the Faith, "Responses on Uterine Isolation and Related Matters," July 31, 1993, *Origins* 24 (1994): 211–212.

35. Pope John Paul II, Apostolic Letter, *On the Christian Meaning of Human Suffering (Salvifici Doloris)* (Washington, D.C.: United States Catholic Conference, 1984), nos. 25–27.

36. National Conference of Catholic Bishops, *Order of Christian Funerals* (Collegeville, Minn.: The Liturgical Press, 1989), no. 1.

37. *Declaration on Euthanasia.*

38. Ibid., Part II, p. 4.

39. Committee for Pro-Life Activities, National Conference of Catholic Bishops, *Nutrition and Hydration: Moral and Pastoral Reflections* (Washington, D.C.: United States Catholic Conference, 1992). On the importance of consulting authoritative teaching in the formation of conscience and in taking moral decisions, see *Veritatis Splendor,* nos. 63–64.

40. *Declaration on Euthanasia,* Part IV.

41. Ibid.

42. Cf. ibid.

43. *Donum Vitae,* Part I, no. 4.

44. While there are many acts of varying moral gravity that can be identified as intrinsically evil, in the context of contemporary health care the most pressing concerns are currently abortion, euthanasia, assisted suicide, and direct sterilization. See Pope John Paul II's *Ad Limina* Address to the bishops of Texas, Oklahoma, and Arkansas (Region X), in *Origins* 28 (1998): 283. See also "Reply of the Sacred Congregation for the Doctrine of the Faith on Sterilization in Catholic Hospitals" (*Quaecumque Sterilizatio*), March 13, 1975, *Origins* 10 (1976): 33–35: "Any cooperation institutionally approved or tolerated in actions which are in themselves, that is, by their nature and condition, directed to a contraceptive end…is absolutely forbidden. For the official approbation of direct sterilization and, a *fortiori,* its management and execution in accord with hospital regulations, is a matter which, in the objective order, is by its very nature (or intrinsically) evil." This directive supersedes the "Commentary on the Reply of the Sacred Congregation for the Doctrine of the Faith on Sterilization in Catholic Hospitals" published by the National Conference of Catholic Bishops on September 15, 1977 in *Origins* 11 (1977): 399–400.

45. See *Catechism of the Catholic Church*: "Scandal is an attitude or behavior which leads another to do evil" (no. 2284); "Anyone who uses the power at his disposal in such a way that it leads others to do wrong becomes guilty of scandal and responsible for the evil that he has directly or indirectly encouraged" (no. 2287).

46. See "The Pastoral Role of the Diocesan Bishop in Catholic Health Care Ministry," *Origins* 26 (1997): 703.

HEALTH ETHICS GUIDE

Catholic Health Association of Canada

2000

• • •

The full introduction to the "Health Ethics Guide" includes a summary of the basic principles that shape Catholic medical ethics. This 2000 "Health Guide" replaces the 1991 "Health Care Ethics Guide."

<http://www.chac.ca/publications/ethics.html>

• • •

The Catholic Health Organization

The ministry of Catholic organizations is one of the visible expressions of the ministry of Christ. As creatures of body and spirit, we need visible, tangible human institutions to assist us to live as a believing community bearing witness to the Good News as expressed in the Catholic faith. Catholic organizations fulfil this important role by being present to people at the critical points where life can be fostered, where people are born and die, where they learn and are taught, where they are cured and healed, and where they are assisted when in trouble. Catholics see this concrete involvement as a sacramental presence, an encounter with Christ.

Catholic health organizations have a distinct spiritual vision and culture that directs them to attend to the needs of the poor and vulnerable with compassion and dignity. It is that vision which defines the quality of their relationship with those in need of care.

Our distinctive vocation in Christian health care is not so much to heal better or more efficiently than anyone else; it is to bring comfort to people by giving them an experience that will strengthen their confidence in life. The ultimate goal of our care is to give those who are ill, through our care, a reason to hope. (Joseph Cardinal Bernadin, "What Makes a Hospital Catholic—A Response," *America*, Vol. 174, no. 15 (May 4, 1996), 9.)

Among the tangible signs that should identify Catholic organizations are the following: Catholic sponsorship and management; quality care; proper stewardship of resources for the community served; a culture that supports Christian ethical values and spiritual beliefs; recognition by the bishop of the diocese as an integral part of the apostolate; promotion of spiritual/religious care; mission and values integration; just working conditions; the availability of the sacraments, and the prominence of various Christian symbols.

The work of Catholic health organizations is a particular expression of the healing ministry of Christ. The physical, emotional and spiritual healing experienced by those cared for within these organizations is a sign of the presence and compassion of Christ the healer. Such organizations offer a privileged opportunity to provide the best possible care in a manner and atmosphere fully inspired by the gospel.

The basic orientation of Catholic health organizations and their personnel is respect for the dignity of every person and concern for the total well-being of persons receiving care. These organizations affirm the importance of family, friends and the community in the promotion of health. They also strive to provide for their personnel a milieu that is conducive to personal fulfillment.

As part of the history of health care institutions in Canada, religiously-based organizations have earned their rightful place in our country through their pioneering efforts, often undertaken in very demanding circumstances. Such centres continue to make a distinctive contribution to health care in Canada.

Ethical Reflection and Decision-Making

To witness to the teachings and values of Jesus Christ requires sound moral reflection and judgement. This is especially true in our technological world where there is an ever-increasing danger of reducing persons to objects. Judgements of what is right or wrong are ethical or moral decisions. Especially when rights, duties, or values appear to conflict, ethical reflection and discernment can assist everyone concerned.

The quality of ethical decisions depends not merely on abstract reasoning, but also on the lived faith, prudence and virtue of the decision-maker. The Catholic moral tradition is the fruit of an on-going dialogue between our understanding of human nature and our experience of God as revealed in Jesus Christ. It develops through prayer, study, reflection and the recognition of the Holy Spirit at work through various sources. Such sources include health and social service providers, the experience of the Christian community, moral theologians, ethicists, pastoral care workers, the local bishop, church teachings, and especially Sacred Scripture. No source of knowledge pertinent to the issue at hand should be neglected in the making of moral decisions.

The Catholic moral tradition presents a number of theological foundations that guide ethical reflection. These include a belief in the presence of God in human experience;

the conviction that all of creation is to be regarded as a gift of God's love; an awareness that we have a responsibility to work to eliminate sickness and suffering; an acknowledgement that, at times, there can be growth through suffering; and the recognition that the moral dimension of human existence requires that we act from an informed conscience.

The local bishop has the responsibility to provide leadership and to collaborate with the mission of Catholic organizations. In fulfilling his role as the primary teacher and pastor of the community, with the assistance of specialists in different disciplines, he has the task to ensure that the teaching of the church is reflected faithfully in the context of rapidly developing medical advances and of the increasing complexity of the human sciences. In order to truly respect dignity, promote justice and foster trust, the church must itself witness to these values.

Since the Christian moral tradition is a living tradition, our formulations of it are necessarily the product of a grasp of reality that is constantly being refined, of historically conditioned attitudes, and of limited philosophical concepts and language. At any given time in history, a particular formulation is only more or less adequate. Continued faithfulness to this living tradition presupposes growth in understanding of moral principles and their implications. It is also important to remember that Catholic teaching maintains a hierarchy of truths and values. This means that specific teachings have varying degrees of importance concerning one's faith and moral life.

The tradition is not always clear or unanimous concerning all moral issues. In such cases, it is the teaching of the Catholic Church that obligations are not to be imposed unless they are certain. Thus, in moral questions debated by moral theologians in the church, Catholic tradition upholds a person's liberty to follow those opinions that seem to be consistent with the wishes of the person receiving care and with the best standards of good care.

Christian Moral Values

Christian ethical reasoning is based upon a world view contained in the gospel as interpreted by the church. This world view gives rise to values and principles that direct ethical decision-making and that enable us to respond to the call to respect dignity, promote justice and foster trust.

Two fundamental values underlie the discussion of values in this guide.

I. DIGNITY OF EVERY HUMAN PERSON – All persons possess an intrinsic dignity and worth that is independent of what any other person thinks or says about them. (*Pastoral*

Constitution of the Church in the Modern World, Vatican Council II: Constitutions, Decrees, Declarations, Austin Flannery (ed.), New York, American Press, 1996, nos. 27, 29.) The basis for this dignity, in the Judeo-Christian tradition, is the belief that every human being is made in the image of God.

2. THE INTERCONNECTEDNESS OF EVERY HUMAN BEING — Human persons are social beings and cannot live or develop their potential outside of human relationships and community. (Ibid., nos. 12, 25.) This fundamental value affirms the interconnectedness of every human being with all persons, with all of creation, and with God. From these two fundamental values flow a number of related values.

3. STEWARDSHIP AND CREATIVITY – The scriptures present a view of creation as both gift and responsibility. We share a responsibility to respect, protect and care for all of creation and for ourselves. We are to use our own free and intelligent creativity to fashion a better world while respecting its true nature, appreciating its benefits and accepting its limitations.

4. RESPECT FOR HUMAN LIFE – Human life is sacred and inviolable in all of its phases and in every situation. (*Pontificia Academia Pro Vita, Final Declaration, 5th General Assembly* (February 24–27) 1999, no. 1.) Human life is a gift of God's love and the basis for all other human goods. Nevertheless, human bodily life is not an absolute good but is subordinated to the good of the whole person.

5. THE COMMON GOOD – Every individual has a duty to share in promoting the well-being of the community as well as a right to benefit from being a member of the community. Respect for human freedom necessitates that society seeks to enable men and women to assume responsibility for their own lives, and to encourage them to cooperate with each other in pursuit of the common good—the building of a just and compassionate social order in which true human growth for all persons is encouraged. By extension, the common good includes environmental concerns that have a direct relationship to the good of individuals and of society.

6. CHARITY OR SOLIDARITY – Charity is the Christian virtue urging us to respond to the needs of others. Solidarity (which includes empathy and compassion for others) is a contemporary way to express our interconnectedness to all human beings and our obligation to respond with love to their needs. This response is even more explicitly articulated in church teaching which exhorts individuals, organizations

and those who develop public policy to a preferential option for the poor and marginalized.

Christian Moral Principles

1. **TOTALITY AND INTEGRITY** – All our physical and psychological functions are to be developed, used, and cared for to protect our human dignity. Therefore, no human function can ever be sacrificed except for the saving or better functioning of the whole person. Basic human capacities may not be sacrificed if more harm than good would result to that person.

2. **DOUBLE EFFECT** – When an action may have both beneficial and harmful consequences, such as pain relief treatment for a terminally ill person—treatment that might shorten life—the action may be pursued if the following conditions are fulfilled: (i) the directly intended object of the act must not be intrinsically evil, i.e. contrary to one's fundamental commitment to God, neighbour or oneself; (ii) the intention of the agent must be to achieve the beneficial effects and to avoid the harmful effects as far as possible (i.e. the harmful effects should not be wanted, but only allowed); (iii) the foreseen beneficial effects are not achieved by means of the foreseen harmful effects; rather, the beneficial effects are inextricably and unavoidably linked to the harmful effects; (iv) the foreseen beneficial effects must be equal to or greater than the foreseen harmful effects.

3. **LEGITIMATE COOPERATION** – This principle applies to situations where an action involves more than one person, and sometimes when the persons have different intentions. It is unethical to cooperate formally with an immoral act, i.e. directly to intend the evil act itself. But sometimes it may be an ethical duty to cooperate materially with an immoral act, i.e. one does not intend the evil effects, but only the good effects, when only in this way can a greater harm be prevented. Two provisions must be considered, namely, (1) the cooperation is not immediate and, (2) the degree of cooperation and the danger of scandal is taken into account. (Refer to Appendix II, "The Principle of Legitimate Cooperation")

4. **SUBSIDIARITY** – According to this principle, decisions should be taken as close to the grass roots as possible. As applied to health needs, the principle suggests that the first responsibility for meeting these needs resides with the free and competent individual. Individuals, however, are not self-sufficient. They can achieve health and obtain health care only with the help of the community. The responsibility of fulfilling those needs that the individual cannot achieve alone must be assumed by larger or more complex groups, e.g. community organizations and different levels of government. (Refer to John Paul II, *Centesimus Annus*, no. 12)

5. **FREE AND INFORMED DECISION-MAKING** – The person receiving care is the primary decision-maker. No service or treatment is to be provided without his or her free and informed consent. For those not capable of making an informed decision, a proxy shall act for the person in accordance with their personal care directives. If an advance health care directive is inapplicable or unavailable, a proxy shall act for the person in accordance with their known needs, values and wishes. In emergency situations where the person receiving care is not capable of making an informed decision and a proxy is unavailable, the care provider may act in the proxy's stead.

6. **CONFIDENTIALITY** – Respect for the dignity of persons insists that persons receiving care be treated with trust, honesty and confidentiality. This includes privacy of personal information and freedom from unnecessary intrusions by others.

In this introductory section of the guide, we have highlighted the values and ethical principles of the Christian tradition that direct our efforts to enter into relationships that respect dignity, promote justice and foster truth. In the remainder of the guide we apply these values and ethical principles to seven key areas related to care in the fields of health and social services.

The Communal Nature of Care

INTRODUCTORY COMMENTS

Health and social service organizations operate in societies that are organized into complex networks of social groups, from the smallest family to local, national, international and global systems. These different social structures are contemporary expressions of the basic and diverse social needs of all persons. The interconnectedness of all human beings is a fundamental value.

While each person is unique, no one could exist for long or fulfil their potential apart from the human community. The community gives people opportunities to provide and obtain resources such as food, clothing, shelter and culture that are required to live a truly human life. Through sharing and communicating with others in community persons grow in knowledge and love. They achieve human fulfill- ment by serving others, since each one receives from and contributes in some way to the individual personal develop- ment of others. Indeed, every society in a certain sense is "personal," so that the person is the beginning, the subject and the aim of every social institution. (*Pastoral Constitution of the Church in the Modern Work, Vatican Council II: Constitutions, Decrees, Declarations,* Austin Flannery (ed.), New York, American Press, 1996, no. 25.)

The individual and social needs of people always must be kept in balance within a social order "founded on truth, built on justice, and animated by love.… Every social group must take account of the needs and legitimate aspirations of other groups, and even of the general welfare of the entire human family." (Ibid., no. 26.) This is achieved through cooperative activity and through social structures that seek to guarantee equity and to overcome domination of one group by another. Through such an approach, individuals and groups contribute to the well-being of others and receive from others what is needed to meet their own particu- lar needs.

Christian tradition uses the images of the human body and of the family to emphasize that human beings function often as organs of the greater civil society, united by com- mon ends and using common means. Every person shares responsibility for our society and society has a responsibility for each of its members. As Christians, we also live in society as members of a community of faith. The faith life of the Christian community is shaped by our baptismal call to share God's life and to work for the common good of all peoples. The fundamental law of this community is such that love of self, love of neighbour and love of God should not be separated.

Health care and social support are two of the responsi- bilities and benefits of society. *It is therefore necessary that (governments) give wholehearted and careful attention to the social as well as to the economic progress of the citizens, and to the development […] of such essential services as […] housing, public health, education […]* (John XXIII, *Pacem in Terris,* April 11, 1963, no. 63.)

Catholic health and social service organizations func- tion in civil society with a particular identity and mission. The specific way in which this mission is carried out distinguishes the service of Catholic care providers. This service is designated as "ministry" because it is motivated by the gospel and is part of an enduring faith tradition. Such an understanding of ministry challenges any system which might treat a person merely as a case, number or statistic. All those who are engaged in this ministry seek to create a community of compassion. They are dedicated to the care of persons in need, especially the most vulnerable, to the promotion of health in all its dimensions, and to forming healing relationships.

In society at large, Catholic health and social service organizations are a voice expressing a vision of life based on the moral and religious values of the Roman Catholic tradition. The care provided by these organizations is one expression within the local church of the healing ministry of Jesus Christ.

The Dignity of the Human Person

INTRODUCTORY COMMENTS

A fundamental value underlying ethics in health care and social services is respect for the dignity of each human person. This value aspires to protect the multiple interests of the person—from bodily to psychological to spiritual to cultural integrity. This respect for the dignity of each human person has been acknowledged and enshrined in the United Nations' *Universal Declaration of Human Rights.*

Human dignity is based on the physiological, psycho- logical, social and spiritual uniqueness of being a person. Persons are created with intelligence and free will, with a moral consciousness and a potential for self-fulfillment. They possess the radical capacity to know, to love, to choose freely and to determine the direction of their lives. Each person is irreplaceable, with an intrinsic value and purpose in life. All persons are equal in dignity and, therefore, are to be treated with equal respect.

Our Christian faith holds that all persons are created in the image and likeness of God, and are called to know, love and be in communion with God, with all other persons and creation for all eternity. We believe that God became human in Jesus Christ, enabling all human beings to share the dignity of being daughters or sons of God, sisters or brothers of Jesus Christ.

Respect is due to every person. In light of gospel values, differences of age, sex, race, religion, social and cultural background, health status, sexual orientation, intelligence, economic status, employment, or other qualitative distinc- tions do not take away from the dignity shared by all persons, whether or not they are aware of their dignity.

Human Reproduction

INTRODUCTORY COMMENTS

Human sexuality is a personal aspect of our identity that gives beauty, pleasure, power and mystery to our lives.

Because we are created in the image and likeness of God, human sexuality is good in all its dimensions: physical, psychological, spiritual and social.

Human sexuality has an interpersonal purpose. It is rooted in our basic human need to love and be loved, to live and grow through human relationships, to preserve and perpetuate society. The wonders of sexuality and birth are best shared in the family setting, and should be supported by instruction in both the parish and school.

Human sexuality is meant to nurture and sustain a woman's and a man's free gift of themselves in a permanent, loving and fruitful commitment of marriage. For Christians, this covenant of human love is a symbol of that faithful love existing between Christ and the church.

The love between a woman and a man is experienced in a unique way and completed through the marital act of sexual intercourse. This act can deepen the union of love, enabling the couple to share with God in the creation of human life. Men and women are called to be responsible stewards of God's gifts, always treating each other with loving respect. The unitive and procreative aspects of sexual intercourse are not to be separated.

Responsible parenthood requires that decisions about having children be made in a prayerful and discerning manner, considering what is most loving and life-giving and what is best for the overall welfare of the family.

Christianity looks upon the beginnings of human life with particular wonder and reverence. Catholic health care providers, therefore, are to surround obstetrical and perinatal care with an atmosphere respectful of human life, mindful of the parents' special circumstances and needs.

Organ and Tissue Donation and Transplantation

INTRODUCTORY COMMENTS

Human beings live and grow in mutual dependence with other members of the human community. Advances in medicine have made organ, blood and other tissue transplants a way to improve health and to give new life to countless people. Organ and tissue donation is an expression of respect for the dignity of persons, solidarity with other members of the human community, and charity in response to the needs and suffering of others.

From a Christian perspective, as members of the human community, we are co-creators and stewards of God's creation. We are to use our gifts to benefit ourselves, other

individuals and the common good. In honouring the sacredness of every human life, Christians are encouraged to be generous in their response to God's call to love through the self-giving that comes from volunteering to be an organ donor. (John Paul II, *Evangelium Vitae,* no. 86.)

In applying its ethical principles to the issue of organ and tissue donation and transplantation, the church teaches that transplanting organs and tissues from a dead person to a living person, and transplanting organs and tissues from a living person to another, are ethically acceptable, provided that the following criteria are met: there is a serious need on the part of the recipient that cannot usually be fulfilled in any other way; the functional integrity of the living donor as a human person is not impaired; the risk taken by the living donor as an act of charity is proportionate to the good resulting for the recipient; the donor's and the recipient's consent are free and informed.

Many Catholic health care organizations provide a crucial link in the donation and transplantation of organs and tissues. They have a responsibility to provide this service with respect. Health care professionals are ideally suited for promoting organ donation and for educating the public about the subject.

Schools, parishes and community organizations should highlight the merits of organ and tissue donation and transplantation. Such activities would help to bring this issue into peoples' homes and encourage them to express their wishes to family and care providers.

Care of the Dying Person

INTRODUCTORY COMMENTS

Because of the inherent dignity and value of the person, all human beings are to be respected at every stage of life.

Sickness, suffering and dying are an inevitable part of human experience. Although the harshness of these realities can be eased by medical and psychological advances, nonetheless, they are a reminder of the limits of human existence and they lead human beings to ask more profound questions about the meaning of life and the mystery of death.

Dying can be a time of deeper self-awareness and not merely an inevitable process to which persons must passively submit. It can be a time in which persons freely and consciously affirm the meaning of their lives. It can also be an occasion of profound reconciliation with family and friends. In the time between the diagnosis of a terminal illness and death many losses occur which affect both the dying person and family members. These losses may be physical, psychological, social, or spiritual in nature. Grief is an important dimension of the dying process. Spiritual and religious care, therefore, is an essential element of care for those who are dying.

As Christians, what may seem meaningless takes on new meaning when we walk with Jesus Christ in faith through his life, death and resurrection. Death is the end of life on earth and the beginning of an eternal life with God. This conviction has moved Christians throughout history to regard death with awe and profound respect. When suffering and sickness do occur, they can have a positive meaning in a person's life. They do not represent a punishment or curse. On the contrary, accepted as a means of drawing closer to Christ, they can be an aid to spiritual growth.

Advances in science and technology are dramatically improving our ability to cure illness, ease suffering and prolong life. Concerted efforts must be taken to alleviate sickness and suffering.

These advances also raise new ethical questions concerning end-of-life care, particularly around life-sustaining treatment. There are occasions when prolonging life by artificial means places onerous burdens on dying persons and their families. In the face of such issues, it is necessary to maintain a balance between two important obligations. We are obliged not to intentionally kill someone; assisted suicide and euthanasia are not acceptable options. At the same time, we are not obliged to use life-sustaining procedures which would impose burdens out of proportion with the benefits to be gained from such procedures.

Catholic health and social service organizations, along with local parish communities, should surround dying persons and their families with all the care resources available.

Research on Human Subjects

INTRODUCTORY COMMENTS

Research in the human sciences provides significant benefits for the human community. New knowledge and understanding in health care, the social sciences and technology help alleviate human suffering, improve treatments for illnesses and enhance health status. The findings of research involving human subjects can offer creative solutions and hope for research subjects, particular groups and society as a whole. The participation of individuals in research studies, as investigators or as subjects, is an affirmation of solidarity with others. The way research is carried out must always

respect the dignity and integrity of the persons involved and serve the common good.

Our Christian faith gives us an increased awareness of solidarity with others and challenges us to exercise leadership through participation in research. As co-creators with God, we are to use our gifts of intelligence and freedom to improve our bodies and to develop health care and social services that will benefit humankind, including medical technologies, methodologies and basic sciences.

Catholic health and social service organizations, as well as educational institutions engaged in research involving human subjects, have a responsibility to communicate and foster a respectful ethical attitude toward such research.

Governance and Administration

INTRODUCTORY COMMENTS

Catholic health and social service organizations are communities of service, united through collaborative activities and inspired by Roman Catholic moral principles for the purpose of providing an optimum level of care for those who are sick or in need, and promoting a healthy society. At the same time, they are occupational communities providing for personnel a means of personal and professional fulfillment and a means of earning a living.

To meet these obligations, the organization is called upon to act as a moral community by addressing the ethical dimension of decisions related to governance and administration, and by striving for effective communication and consultation with all members of the organization.

As a community of service that receives funds from the public to carry out its mission, the organization acts to meet obligations that correspond to its several roles:

- as an agency commissioned to provide services to the public;
- as a human community of service expressing solidarity with those in need of care;
- as a Christian community acting as a careful steward of God's gifts;
- as a church community committed to a preferential option for those who are poor and marginalized.

Work is a dimension of a person's creativity; it provides a community and a sense of meaning and purpose. As a community of work, the organization seeks to create an atmosphere within which work is viewed as more than an economic function. The personnel, in turn, are expected to carry out the mission of the organization. In their life and work personnel are guided by personal values that go beyond their role as employees. Personnel should be treated accordingly.

THE OATH OF A MUSLIM PHYSICIAN

Islamic Medical Association of North America

1977

. . .

Adopted in 1977 by the Islamic Medical Association of North America, the Oath of a Muslim Physician is a composite drawn from the historical and contemporary writings of Muslim physicians.

Praise be to Allah (God), the Teacher, the Unique, Majesty of the heavens, the Exalted, the Glorious, Glory be to Him, the Eternal Being Who created the Universe and all the creatures within, and the only Being Who containeth the infinity and the eternity. We serve no other god besides Thee and regard idolatry as an abominable injustice.

Give us the strength to be truthful, honest, modest, merciful and objective.

Give us the fortitude to admit our mistakes, to amend our ways and to forgive the wrongs of others.

Give us the wisdom to comfort and counsel all towards peace and harmony.

Give us the understanding that ours is a profession sacred that deals with your most precious gifts of life and intellect.

Therefore, make us worthy of this favoured station with honor, dignity and piety so that we may devote our lives in serving mankind, poor or rich, literate or illiterate, Muslim or non-Muslim, black or white with patience and tolerance with virtue and reverance, with knowledge and vigilance, with Thy love in our hearts and compassion for Thy servants, Thy most precious creation.

Hereby we take this oath in Thy name, the Creator of all the Heavens and the earth and follow Thy counsel as Thou hast revealed to Prophet Mohammad (pbuh).

"Whoever killeth a human being, not in lieu of another human being nor because of mischief on earth, it is as if he hath killed all mankind. And if he saveth a human life, he hath saved the life of all mankind." (Qur'an v/35)

ISLAMIC CODE OF MEDICAL ETHICS KUWAIT DOCUMENT

Islamic Organization for Medical Sciences

1981

. . .

The First International Conference on Islamic Medicine, held in Kuwait in January 1981, endorsed this Islamic Code of Medical Ethics with the hope that every Muslim doctor would "find in it the guiding light to maintain his professional behaviour within the boundaries of Islamic teachings." As do other Muslim medical ethics texts, the code draws on passages from the Qur'an and demonstrates an explicitly religious tone, more so even than most contemporary Judaeo-Christian medical ethics directives. The code includes an oath for physicians.

<http://www.islamset.com/ethics/code/cont2.html>

The Oath of the Doctor

I swear by God...The Great

To regard God in carrying out my profession

To protect human life in all stages and under all circumstances, doing my utmost to rescue it from death, malady, pain and anxiety...

To keep people's dignity, cover their privacies and lock up their secrets...

To be, all the way, an instrument of God's mercy, extending my medical care to near and far, virtuous and sinner and friend and enemy...

To strive in the pursuit of knowledge and harnessing it for the benefit but not the harm of Mankind...

To revere my teacher, teach my junior, and be brother to members of the Medical Profession joined in piety and charity...

To live my Faith in private and in public, avoiding whatever blemishes me in the eyes of God, His apostle and my fellow Faithful.

And may God be witness to this Oath.

. . .

Definition of Medical Profession

- "THERAPEUSIS" is a noble Profession. God honoured it by making it the miracle of Jesus son of Mary. Abraham enumerating his Lord's gifts upon him included "and if I fall ill He cures me."

- Like all aspects of knowledge, medical knowledge is part of the knowledge of God "who taught man what man never knew." The study of Medicine entails the revealing of God's signs in His creation. 'And in yourselves…do you not see?' The practice of Medicine brings God's mercy unto His subjects. Medical practice is therefore an act of worship and charity on top of being a career to make a living.

- But God's mercy is as accessible to all people including good and evil, virtuous and vicious and friend and foe—as are the rays of His sun, the comfort of His breeze, the coolness of His water and the bounty of His provision. And upon this basis must the medical profession operate, along the single track of God's mercy, never adversive and never punitive, never taking justice as its goal but mercy, under whatever situations and circumstances.

- In this respect the medical profession is unique. It shall never yield to social pressures motivated by enmity or feud be it personal, political or military. Enlightened statesmanship will do good by preserving the integrity of the medical profession and protecting its position beyond enmity or hostility.

- The provision of medical practice is a religious dictate upon the community, 'Fardh Kifaya,' that can be satisfied on behalf of the community by some citizens taking up medicine. It is the duty of the state to ensure the needs of the nation to doctors in the various needed specialities. In Islam, this is a duty that the ruler owes the nation.

- Need may arise to import from afar such medical expertise that is not locally available. It is the duty of the State to satisfy this need.

- It also behoves the State to recruit suitable candidates from the nation's youth to be trained as doctors. An ensuing duty therefore is to establish relevant schools, faculties, clinics, hospitals and institutions that are adequately equipped and manned to fulfill that purpose.

- "Medicine" is a religious necessity for society. In religious terms, whatever is necessary to satisfy that "necessity" automatically acquires the status of a "necessity." Exceptions shall therefore be made from certain general rules of jurisprudence for the sake of making medical education possible. One such example is the intimate inspection of the human body whether alive or dead, without in any way compromising the respect befitting the human body in life and death, and always in a climate of piety and awareness of the presence of God.

- The preservation of man's life should embrace also the utmost regard to his dignity, feelings, tenderness and the privacy of his sentiments and body parts. A patient is entitled to full attention, care and feeling of security while with his doctor. The doctor's privilege of being exempted from some general rules is only coupled with more responsibility and duty that he should carry out in conscientiousness and excellence in observing God, "excellence that entails that you worship God as if you see Him. For even though you don't see Him, He sees you."

. . .

Characters of the Physician

- The physician should be amongst those who believe in God, fulfill His rights, are aware of His greatness, obedient to His orders, refraining from His prohibitions, and observing Him in secret and in public.

- The physician should be endowed with wisdom and graceful admonition. He should be cheering not dispiriting, smiling and not frowning, loving and not hateful, tolerant and not edgy. He should never succumb to a grudge or fall short of clemency. He should be an instrument of God's justice, forgiveness and not punishment, coverage and not exposure.

- He should be so tranquil as never to be rash even when he is right…chaste of words even when joking…tame of voice and not noisy or loud, neat and trim and not shabby or unkempt…conducive of trust and inspiring of respect…well mannered in his dealings with the poor or rich, modest or great…in perfect control of his composure…and never compromising his dignity, however modest and forebearing.

- The physician should firmly know that "life" is God's…awarded only by Him…and that "Death" is the conclusion of one life and the beginning of another. Death is a solid truth…and it is the end of all but God. In his profession the Physician is a soldier for "Life" only…defending and preserving it as best as it can be, to the best of his ability.

- The Physician should offer the good example by caring for his own health. It is not befitting for him that his "do's" and "don'ts" are not observed primarily by himself. He should not turn his back on the lessons of medical progress, because he will never convince his patients unless they see the evidence of his own conviction…God addresses us in the Qoran by saying "and make not your own hands throw you into destruction." The Prophet says "your body has a right on you"…and the known dictum is "no harm or harming in Islam."

• • •

• The role of Physician is that of a catalyst through whom God, the Creator, works to preserve life and health. He is merely an instrument of God in alleviating people's illness. For being so designated the Physician should be grateful and forever seeking God's help. He should be modest, free from arrogance and pride and never fall into boasting or hint at self glorification through speech, writing or direct or subtle advertisement.

• The Physician should strive to keep abreast of scientific progress and innovation. His zeal or complacency and knowledge or ignorance, directly bear on the health and well-being of his patients. Responsibility for others should limit his freedom to expend his time. As the poor and needy have a recognized right in the money of the capable, so the patients own a share of the Doctor's time spent in study and in following the progress of medicine.

• The Physician should also know that the pursuit of knowledge has a double indication in Islam. Apart from the applied therapeutic aspect, pursuit of knowledge is in itself worship, according to the Qoranic guidance: "And say…My Lord…advance me in knowledge." and: "Among His worshippers…the learned fear Him most"…and: "God will raise up the ranks of those of you who believed and those who have been given knowledge."

Doctor-Doctor Relationship

• • •

• Physicians are jointly responsible for the health care of the Nation…and complement one another through the variety of their medical specialization be they preventive or therapeutic, in the private sector or in State employment…all abiding by the ethics and rules of their profession.

• • •

Doctor-Patient Relationship

• For the sake of the patient the Doctor was…and not the other way round. Health is the goal and medical care is the means…the "patient" is master and the "Doctor" is at his service. As the Prophet

says "The strongest should follow the pace of the weakest…for he is the one to be considered in deciding the pace of travel." Rules, schedules, time-tables and services should be so manipulated as to revolve around the patient and comply with his welfare and comfort as the top and overriding priority…other considerations coming next.

• • •

• The sphere of a Doctor's charity, nicety, tolerance and patience should be large enough to encompass the patient's relatives, friends and those who care for or worry about him…but without of course compromising the dictates of "Professional Secrecy".

• Health is a basic human necessity and is not a matter of luxury. It follows that the Medical Profession is unique in that the client is not denied the service even if he cannot afford the fee. Medical legislature should ensure medical help to all needy of it, by issuing and executing the necessary laws and regulations.

• • •

Professional Secrecy

Keeping other persons' secrets is decreed on all the Faithful…the more so if these were Doctors, for people willfully disclose their secrets and feelings to their doctors, confident of the time old heritage of Professional Secrecy, that the medical profession embraced since the dawn of history. The Prophet (peace be upon Him) described the three signs of the hypocrite as: "He lies when he speaks, he breaks his promise and he betrays when confided in." The Doctor shall put the seal of confidentiality on all information acquired by him through sight, hearing or deduction. Islamic spirit also requires that the items of the Law should stress the right of the patient to protect his secrets that he confides to his Doctor. A breach thereof would be detrimental to the practice of medicine, beside precluding several categories of patients from seeking medical help.

Doctor's Role During War

• Since the earliest battles of Islam it was decreed that the wounded is protected by his wound and the captive by his captivity. The faithful are praised in the Qoran as: "they offer food—dear as it is—to the needy, orphan or captive, (saying) we feed you for the sake of God without seeking any reward or gratitude from you." The Prophet (peace be upon Him) said to his companions: "I entrust the captives to your charity"…and they did…even giving them priority over themselves in the best of the food they shared. It is of interest to note that this was thirteen centuries prior to the Geneva Convention and the Red Cross.

• • •

- The Medical Profession shall not permit its technical, scientific or other resources to be utilized in any sort of harm or destruction or infliction upon man of physical, psychological, moral or other damage…regardless of all political or military considerations.

• • •

Responsibility and Liability

- The Practice of Medicine is lawful only to persons suitably educated, trained and qualified, fulfilling the criteria spelt out in the Law. A clear guidance is the Prophet's tradition: "*Who-so-ever treats people without knowledge of medicine, becomes liable*".
- With the availability of medical specialization, problem cases shall be referred to the relevant specialist. "*Each one is better suited to cope with what he was meant for*".
- In managing a medical case the Doctor shall do what he can to the best of his ability. If he does, without negligence, taking the measures and precautions expected from his equals then he is not to blame or punish even of the results were not satisfactory.
- The Doctor is the patient's agent on his body. The acceptance by the patient of a Doctor to treat him is considered an acceptance of any line of treatment the Doctor prescribes.
- If treatment entails surgical interference the initial acceptance referred to should be documented in writing, for the sake of protecting the Doctor against possible eventualities. If the patient declines or refuses the Doctor's prescribed plan of treatment, this refusal should also be documented by writing, witnesses, or patient's signature as the situation warrants or permits.
- When fear is the obstacle preventing the patient from consent, the Doctor may help his patient with a medicine such as a tranquilliser to free his patient from fear but without abolishing or suppressing his consciousness, so that the patient is able to make his choice in calmness and tranquillity. By far the best method to achieve this is the poise of the Doctor himself and his

personality, kindness, patience and the proper use of the spoken word.

- In situations where urgent and immediate surgical or other interference is necessary to save life, the Doctor should go ahead according to the Islamic rule' 'necessities override prohibitions'. His position shall be safe and secure whatever the result achieved, on condition that he has followed established medical methodology in a correct way. The "bad" inherent in not saving the patient outweighs the presumptive 'good' in leaving him to his self-destructive decision. The Islamic rule proclaims that "warding off" the 'bad' takes priority over bringing about the 'good'.

The Prophetic guidance is "Help your brother when he is right and when he is wrong". When concurring with helping a brother if right but surprised at helping him when wrong, the Prophet answered his companions: "Forbid him from being wrong…for this is the help he is in need of".

The Sanctity of Human Life

- "On that account we decreed for the Children of Israel that whoever kills a human soul for other than manslaughter or corruption in the land, it shall be as if he killed all mankind, and who-so-ever saves the life of one, it shall be as if he saved the life of all mankind." 5–32
- Human Life is sacred…and should not be willfully taken except upon the indications specified in Islamic Jurisprudence, all of which are outside the domain of the Medical Profession.
- A Doctor shall not take away life even when motivated by mercy. This is prohibited because this is not one of the legitimate indications for killing. Direct guidance in this respect is given by the Prophet's tradition: "In old times there was a man with an ailment that taxed his endurance. He cut his wrist with a knife and bled to death. God was displeased and said 'My subject hastened his end…I deny him paradise.'"

• • •

- The sanctity of human Life covers all its stages including intrauterine life of the embryo and fetus. This shall not be compromised by the Doctor save for the absolute medical necessity recognised by Islamic Jurisprudence.

• • •

- In his defence of Life, however, the Doctor is well advised to realize his limit and not transgress it. If it is scientifically certain that life cannot be restored, then it is futile to diligently keep on the vegetative state of the patient by heroic means of animation or preserve him by deep-freezing or other artificial methods. It is the process of life that the Doctor aims to maintain and not the process of dying. In any case, the Doctor shall not take a positive measure to terminate the patient's life.

- To declare a person dead is a grave responsibility that ultimately rests with the Doctor. He shall appreciate the seriousness of his verdict and pass it in all honesty and only when sure of it. He may dispel any trace of doubt by seeking counsel and resorting to modern scientific gear.

- The Doctor shall do his best that what remains of the life of an incurable patient will be spent under good care, moral support and freedom from pain and misery.

- The Doctor shall comply with the patient's right to know his illness. The Doctor's particular way of answering should however be tailored to the particular patient in question. It is the Doctor's duty to thoroughly study the psychological acumen of his patient. He shall never fall short of suitable vocabulary if the situation warrants the deletion of frightening nomenclature or coinage of new names, expressions or descriptions.

- In all cases the Doctor should have the ability to bolster his patient's faith and endow him with tranquility and peace of mind.

Doctor and Society

. . .

- The Medical Profession shall take it as duty to combat such health-destructive habits as smoking, uncleanliness, etc.

. . .

The combat and prevention of environmental pollution falls under this category.

The Doctor and Biomedical Advances

<http://www.islamset.com/ethics/code/cont2.html>

There is no censorship in Islam on scientific research, be it academic to reveal the signs of God in His creation, or applied aiming at the solution of a particular problem.

Freedom of scientific research shall not entail the subjugation of Man, telling him, harming him or subjecting him to definite or probable harm, with holding his therapeutic needs, defrauding him or exploiting his material need.

Freedom of scientific research shall not entail cruelty to animals, or their torture. Suitable protocols should be laid upon for the uncruel handling of experimental animals during experimentation.

The methodology of scientific research and the applications resultant thereof, shall not entail the commission of sin prohibited by Islam such as fornication, confounding of genealogy, deformity or tampering with the essence of the human personality, its freedom and eligibility to bear responsibility.

The Medical Profession has the right- and owes the duty of effective participation in the formulation and issuing of religious verdict concerning the lawfulness or otherwise of the unprecedented outcomes of current and future advances in biological science. The verdict should be reached in togetherness between Muslim specialists in jurisprudence and Muslim specialists in biosciences. Single-sided opinions have always suffered from lack of comprehension of technical or legal aspects.

The guiding rule in unprecedented matters falling under no extant text or law, is the Islamic dictum: "Wherever welfare is found, there exists the statute of God".

The individual patient is the collective responsibility of society, that has to ensure his health needs by any means inflicting no harm on others. This comprises the donation of body fluids or organs such as blood transfusion to the bleeding or a kidney transplant to the patient with bilateral irreparable renal damage. This is another 'Fardh Kifaya', a duty that donors fulfil on behalf of society. Apart from the technical procedure, the onus of public education falls on the medical Profession, which should also draw the procedural, organizational and technical regulations and the policy of priorities.

Organ donation shall never be the outcome of compulsion, family embarrassment, social or other pressure, or exploitation of financial need.

Donation shall not entail the exposure of the donor to harm.

The Medical Profession bears the greatest portion of responsibility for laying down the laws, rules and regulations organizing organ donation during life or after death by a statement in the donor's will or the consent of his family; as well as the establishment of tissue and organ banks for tissues amenable to storage. Cooperation with similar banks abroad is to be established on the basis of reciprocal aid.

On Medical Education

In planning the making of a Doctor, a principal goal is to make him a living example of all that God loves, free from all that God hates, well saturated with the love of God, of people and of knowledge.

The Medical Teacher owes his students the provision of the good example, adequate teaching, sound guidance and continual care in and out of classes and before and after graduation.

Medical Education picks from all trees without refractoriness or prejudice. Yet it has to be protected and purified from every positive activity towards atheism or infidelity.

Medical Education is neither passive nor authoritarian. It aims at sparking mental activity, fostering observation, analysis and reasoning, development of independent thought and the evolvement of fresh questions. The Qoran blamed those who said: " As such we have found our fathers and we will follow on their footsteps" an attitude which is only conductive to stagnation and arrest of progress.

"Faith" is remedial, a healer, a conqueror of stress and a procurer of cure. The training of the Doctor should prepare him to bolster "Faith" and avail the patient of its unlimited blessings.

Medical school curricula should include the teaching of matters of jurisprudence and worship pertaining to or influenced by various health aspects and problems.

Medical School curricula should familiarise the student with the medical and other scientific heritage of the era of Islamic civilization, the factors underlying the rise of Muslim civilization, those that lead to its eclipse, and the way(s) to its revival.

Medical school curricula should emphasize that medicine is worship both as an approach to belief by contemplation on the signs of God, as well as from the applied aspect by helping Man in distress.

Medical school curricula should comprise the teaching and study of this "Islamic Code of Medical Ethics".

SECTION III.

ETHICAL DIRECTIVES
FOR OTHER HEALTH-CARE PROFESSIONS

• • •

Code for Nurses, International Council of Nurses [1973, reaffirmed 1989; revised 2002]

Code for Nurses with Interpretive Statements, American Nurses' Association [1950, revised 1976, 1985, 2001]

Code of Ethics for Nursing, Canadian Nurses Association [1985, revised 1991]

Code of Ethics, American Chiropractic Association [1994–1995]

Principles of Ethics and Code of Professional Conduct with Advisory Opinions, American Dental Association [revised to June 2002]

Code of Ethics for the Profession of Dietetics, American Dietetic Association [1987, revised 1999]

Code of Ethics, American Association of Pastoral Counselors [last amended 1994]

Guidelines for the Chaplain's Role in Bioethics, College of Chaplains, American Protestant Health Association [1992]

Code of Ethics, American Pharmacists Association [1969, amended 1975, revised 1981, 1994]

Statement of Professional Standards: Codes of Ethics for Pharmacists, Fédération Internationale Pharmaceutique [1988, revised 1997]

Code of Ethics and Guide for Professional Conduct, American Physical Therapy Association [1981, last amended 1991]

Occupational Therapy Code of Ethics, American Occupational Therapy Association [1988, revised 2000]

Code of Ethics of the Physician Assistant Profession, American Academy of Physician Assistants [1983, amended 1985, reaffirmed 1990]

Ethical Principles of Psychologists and Code of Conduct, American Psychological Association [1992]

Code of Ethics, National Association of Social Workers [1979, revised 1990, 1996, 1999]

Code of Ethics, American College of Healthcare Executives [amended 1990]

Ethical Conduct for Health Care Institutions, American Hospital Association [1992]

This section demonstrates the great number and diversity of ethical directives for healthcare professionals other than physicians. The section opens with several codes of ethics for nurses, followed by ethics directives for other professional groups from chiropractors and dentists to social workers and hospital administrators.

Most of the documents in this section represent professional organizations in the United States.

CODE FOR NURSES

International Council of Nurses

1973, REAFFIRMED 1989, REVISED 2000

• • •

The International Council of Nurses first adopted an international code of ethics for nurses in 1953 and revised it in 1965. In 1973, the council adopted a new code, which was reaffirmed in 1989, and revised in 2000. The text of the International Code for Nurses follows.

<http://www.icn.ch/icncode.pdf>

Preamble

Nurses have four fundamental responsibilities: to promote health, to prevent illness, to restore health and to alleviate suffering. The need for nursing is universal.

Inherent in nursing is respect for human rights, including the right to life, to dignity and to be treated with respect. Nursing care is unrestricted by considerations of age, colour, creed, culture, disability or illness, gender, nationality, politics, race or social status.

Nurses render health services to the individual, the family and the community and co-ordinate their services with those of related groups.

THE CODE

The *ICN Code of Ethics for Nurses* has four principal elements that outline the standards of ethical conduct.

Elements of the Code

I. Nurses and people

The nurse's primary professional responsibility is to people requiring nursing care.

In providing care, the nurse promotes an environment in which the human rights, values, customs and spiritual beliefs of the individual, family and community are respected.

The nurse ensures that the individual receives sufficient information on which to base consent for care and related treatment.

The nurse holds in confidence personal information and uses judgement in sharing this information.

The nurse shares with society the responsibility for initiating and supporting action to meet the health and social needs of the public, in particular those of vulnerable populations.

The nurse also shares responsibility to sustain and protect the natural environment from depletion, pollution, degradation and destruction.

2. Nurses and practice

The nurse carries personal responsibility and accountability for nursing practice, and for maintaining competence by continual learning.

The nurse maintains a standard of personal health such that the ability to provide care is not compromised.

The nurse uses judgement regarding individual competence when accepting and delegating responsibility.

The nurse at all times maintains standards of personal conduct which reflect well on the profession and enhance public confidence.

The nurse, in providing care, ensures that use of technology and scientific advances are compatible with the safety, dignity and rights of people.

3. Nurses and the profession

The nurse assumes the major role in determining and implementing acceptable standards of clinical nursing practice, management, research and education.

The nurse is active in developing a core of research-based professional knowledge.

The nurse, acting through the professional organisation, participates in creating and maintaining equitable social and economic working conditions in nursing.

4. Nurses and co-workers

The nurse sustains a co-operative relationship with co-workers in nursing and other fields.

The nurse takes appropriate action to safeguard individuals when their care is endangered by a co-worker or any other person.

Suggestions for use of the ICN Code of Ethics for Nurses

The *ICN Code of Ethics for Nurses* is a guide for action based on social values and needs. It will have meaning only as a living document if applied to the realities of nursing and health care in a changing society.

To achieve its purpose the *Code* must be understood, internalised and used by nurses in all aspects of their work. It must be available to students and nurses throughout their study and work lives.

Applying the Elements of the ICN Code of Ethics for Nurses

The four elements of the *ICN Code of Ethics for Nurses*: nurses and people, nurses and practice, nurses and co-workers, and nurses and the profession, give a framework for the standards of conduct. The following chart will assist nurses to translate the standards into action. Nurses and nursing students can therefore:

- Study the standards under each element of the *Code*.
- Reflect on what each standard means to you. Think about how you can apply ethics in your nursing domain: practice, education, research or management.
- Discuss the *Code* with co-workers and others.
- Use a specific example from experience to identify ethical dilemmas and standards of conduct as outlined in the *Code*. Identify how you would resolve the dilemma.
- Work in groups to clarify ethical decision making and reach a consensus on standards of ethical conduct.
- Collaborate with your national nurses' association, co-workers, and others in the continuous application of ethical standards in nursing practice, education, management and research.

CODE FOR NURSES WITH INTERPRETIVE STATEMENTS

American Nurses' Association

1950, REVISED 1976, 1985, 2001

• • •

The 1985 Code for Nurses is a revised version of the code adopted by the American Nurses' Association (ANA) in 1950. The eleven-point code and the accompanying interpretive statements provide a framework for ethical decision making that includes several noteworthy aspects: (1) It identifies the values and beliefs that undergird the ethical standards; (2) it encompasses a breadth of social and professional concerns; (3) it manifests an awareness of the ethical implications of shifting professional roles and of the complexity of modern health care; and (4) it goes beyond prescriptive statements regarding personal and professional conduct by advocating a sense of accountability to the client.

Although the text of the code remains essentially unchanged from the 1976 revision, both the organization and the text of the interpretive statements have been modified somewhat. Among the changes: (1) The discussion of human dignity following point 1 is expanded and includes specific statements that "the nurse does not act deliberately to terminate the life of any person," but that nurses may provide symptomatic intervention to dying clients "even when the interventions entail substantial risks of hastening death"; and (2) a statement under point 11 in the 1976 code, that "quality health care is mandated as a right to all citizens," has been deleted. The 2001 ANA Code for Nurses and the text of selected interpretive statements are at <http://www.nursingworld. org/ethics/code/ethicscode150.htm>.

CODE OF ETHICS FOR NURSING

Canadian Nurses Association

1985, REVISED 1991

• • •

The introductory sections of the Canadian Nurses Association (CNA) code suggest a sophisticated view of the role of codes. For example, the code "provides clear direction for avoiding ethical violations," that is, "the neglect of moral obligation," but it cannot resolve "ethical dilemmas," in which there are "ethical reasons both for and against a particular course of action." The code also cannot relieve the "ethical distress" that occurs "when nurses experience the imposition of practices that provoke feelings of guilt, concern or distaste." The CNA code is unique in its explicit organization around values, which "express broad ideals of nursing"; obligations, which are "moral norms that have their basis in nursing values"; and limitations, which "describe exceptional circumstances in which a value or obligation cannot be applied."

Preamble

Nursing practice can be defined generally as a "dynamic, caring, helping relationship in which the nurse assists the client to achieve and maintain optimal health." Nurses in clinical practice, education, administration and research share the common goal of maintaining competent care and improving nursing practice. "Nurses direct their energies toward the promotion, maintenance and restoration of health, the prevention of illness, the alleviation of suffering and the ensuring of a peaceful death when life can no longer be sustained."

The nurse, by entering the profession, is committed to moral norms of conduct and assumes a professional commitment to health and the well-being of clients. As citizens, nurses continue to be bound by the moral and legal norms shared by all other participants in society. As individuals, nurses have a right to choose to live by their own values (their personal ethics) as long as those values do not compromise care of their clients.

· · ·

Ethical Problems

Situations often arise that present ethical problems for nurses in their practice. These situations tend to fall into three categories:

(a) Ethical violations involve the neglect of moral obligation; for example, a nurse who neglects to provide competent care to a client because of personal inconvenience has ethically failed the client.

(b) Ethical dilemmas arise where ethical reasons both for and against a particular course of action are present and one option must be selected. For example, a client who is likely to refuse some appropriate form of health care presents the nurse with an ethical dilemma. In this case, substantial moral reasons may be offered on behalf of several opposing options.

(c) Ethical distress occurs when nurses experience the imposition of practices that provoke feelings of guilt, concern or distaste. Such feelings may occur when nurses are ethically obliged to provide particular types of care despite their personal disagreement or discomfort with the course of treatment prescribed. For example, a nurse may think that continuing to tube feed an irreversibly unresponsive person is contrary to that client's well-being, but nonetheless is required to do so because that view is not shared by other caregivers.

This Code provides clear direction for avoiding ethical violations. When a course of action is mandated by the Code, and there exists no opposing ethical principle, ethical conduct requires that course of action.

This Code cannot serve the same function for all ethical dilemmas or for ethical distress. There is room within the profession of nursing for conscientious disagreement among nurses. The resolution of any dilemma often depends upon the specific circumstances of the case in question, and no particular resolution may be definitive of good nursing practice. Resolution may also depend upon the relative weight of the opposing principles, a matter about which reasonable people may disagree.

The Code cannot relieve ethical distress but it may serve as a guide for nurses to weigh and consider their responsibilities in the particular situation. Inevitably, nurses must reconcile their actions with their consciences in caring for clients.

The Code tries to provide guidance for those nurses who face ethical problems. Proper consideration of the Code should lead to better decision-making when ethical problems are encountered.

It should be noted that many problems or situations seen as ethical in nature are problems of miscommunication, failure of trust or management dilemmas in disguise. There is, therefore, a distinct need to clarify whether the problem is an ethical one or one of another sort.

Elements of the Code

This Code contains different elements designed to help the nurse in its interpretation. The values and obligations are presented by topic and not in order of importance. There is intentional variation in the normative terminology used in the Code (the nurse should or must) to indicate differences in the moral force of the statements; the term should indicates a moral preference, while must indicates an obligation. A number of distinctions between ethics and morals may be found in the literature. Since no distinction has been uniformly adopted by writers on ethics, these terms are used interchangeably in this Code.

- Values express broad ideals of nursing. They establish correct directions for nursing. In the absence of a conflict of ethics, the fact that a particular action promotes a value of nursing may be decisive in some specific instances. Nursing behaviour can always be appraised in terms of values: How closely did the behaviour approach the value? How widely did it deviate from the value? The values expressed in this Code must be adhered to by all nurses in their practice. Because they are so broad, however, values may not give specific guidance in difficult instances.

- Obligations are moral norms that have their basis in nursing values. However, obligations provide more specific direction for conduct than do values; obligations spell out what a value requires under particular circumstances.

- Limitations describe exceptional circumstances in which a value or obligation cannot be applied.

Limitations have been included separately to emphasize that, in the ordinary run of events, the values and obligations will be decisive.

It is also important to emphasize that even when a value or obligation must be limited, it nonetheless carries moral weight. For example, a nurse who is compelled to testify in a court of law on confidential matters is still subject to the values and obligations of confidentiality. While the requirement to testify is a justified limitation upon confidentiality, in other respects confidentiality must be observed. The nurse must only reveal that confidential information that is pertinent to the case at hand, and such revelation must take place within the appropriate context. The general obligation to preserve the client's confidences remains despite particular limiting circumstances.

Rights and Responsibilities

Clients possess both legal and moral rights. These serve as one foundation for the responsibilities of nurses. However, for several reasons this Code emphasizes the obligations of nurses, rather than the rights of clients. Because the rights of clients do not depend upon professional acceptance of those rights, it would be presumptuous for a profession to claim to define the rights of clients. Emphasizing the rights of clients may also seem unduly legalistic and restrictive, ignoring the fact that sometimes ethics require nurses to go beyond the letter of the law. (For one example, see Value II, Obligation 3.) Finally, because it is sometimes beyond the power of a nurse to secure the rights of a client—an achievement that requires the cooperative and scrupulous efforts of all members of the health care team—it is better for a professional code of nursing to emphasize the responsibilities of nurses rather than to detail the entitlements of clients.

Nurses, too, possess legal and moral rights, as persons and as professionals. It is beyond the scope of this Code to address the personal rights of nurses. However, to the extent that conditions of employment have an impact on the establishment of ethical nursing, this Code must deal with that issue.

The satisfaction of some ethical responsibilities requires action taken by the nursing profession as a whole. The fourth section of the Code contains values and obligations concerned with those collective responsibilities of nursing; this section is particularly addressed to professional associations. Ethical reflection must be ongoing and its facilitation is a continuing responsibility of the Canadian Nurses Association.

. . .

Clients

VALUE I: RESPECT FOR NEEDS AND VALUES OF CLIENTS

Value

A nurse treats clients with respect for their individual needs and values.

Obligations

1. The client's perceived best interests must be a prime concern of the nurse.

2. Factors such as the client's race, religion or absence thereof, ethnic origin, social or marital status, sex or sexual orientation, age, or health status must not be permitted to compromise the nurse's commitment to that client's care.

3. The expectations and normal life patterns of clients are acknowledged. Individualized programs of nursing care are designed to accommodate the psychological, social, cultural and spiritual needs of clients, as well as their biological needs.

4. The nurse does more than respond to the requests of clients; the nurse accepts an affirmative obligation within the context of health care to aid clients in their expression of needs and values, including their right to live at risk.

5. Recognizing the client's membership in a family and a community, the nurse, with the client's consent, should attempt to facilitate the participation of significant others in the care of the client.

VALUE II: RESPECT FOR CLIENT CHOICE

Value

Based upon respect for clients and regard for their right to control their own care, nursing care reflects respect for the right of choice held by clients.

Obligations

1. The competent client's consent is an essential precondition to the provision of health care. Nurses bear the primary responsibility to inform clients about the nursing care available to them.

2. Consent may be signified in many different ways. Verbal permission and knowledgeable cooperation are the usual forms by which clients consent to

nursing care. In each case, however, a valid consent represents the free choice of the competent client to undergo that care.

3. Consent, properly understood, is the process by which a client becomes an active participant in care. All clients should be aided in becoming active participants in their care to the maximum extent that circumstances permit. Professional ethics may require of the nurse actions that exceed the legal requirements of consent. For example, although a child may be legally incompetent to consent, nurses should nevertheless attempt to inform and involve the child.

4. Force, coercion and manipulative tactics must not be employed in the obtaining of consent.

5. Illness or other factors may compromise the client's capacity for self-direction. Nurses have a continuing obligation to value autonomy in such clients; for example, by creatively providing clients with opportunities for choices within their capabilities, the nurse helps them to maintain or regain some degree of autonomy.

6. Whenever information is provided to a client, this must be done in a truthful, understandable and sensitive way. The nurse must proceed with an awareness of the individual client's needs, interests and values.

7. Nurses have a responsibility to assess the understanding of clients about their care and to provide information and explanation when in possession of the knowledge required to respond accurately. When the client's questions require information beyond that known to the nurse, the client must be informed of that fact and assisted to obtain the information from a health care practitioner who is in possession of the required facts.

VALUE III: CONFIDENTIALITY

Value

The nurse holds confidential all information about a client learned in the health care setting.

Obligations

1. The rights of persons to control the amount of personal information revealed applies with special force in the health care setting. It is, broadly speaking, up to clients to determine who shall be told of their condition, and in what detail.

2. In describing professional confidentiality to a client, its boundaries should be revealed:

(a) Competent care requires that other members of a team of health personnel have access to or be provided with the relevant details of a client's condition.

(b) In addition, discussions of the client's care may be required for the purpose of teaching or quality assurance. In this case, special care must be taken to protect the client's anonymity.

Whenever possible, the client should be informed of these necessities at the onset of care.

3. An affirmative duty exists to institute and maintain practices that protect client confidentiality—for example, by limiting access to records or by choosing the most secure method of communicating client information.

4. Nurses have a responsibility to intervene if other participants in the health care delivery system fail to respect the confidentiality of client information.

Limitations

The nurse is not morally obligated to maintain confidentiality when the failure to disclose information will place the client or third parties in danger. Generally, legal requirements or privileges to disclose are morally justified by these same criteria. In facing such a situation, the first concern of the nurse must be the safety of the client or the third party.

Even when the nurse is confronted with the necessity to disclose, confidentiality should be preserved to the maximum possible extent. Both the amount of information disclosed and the number of people to whom disclosure is made should be restricted to the minimum necessary to prevent the feared harm.

VALUE IV: DIGNITY OF CLIENTS

Value

The nurse is guided by consideration for the dignity of clients.

Obligations

1. Nursing care must be done with consideration for the personal modesty of clients.

2. A nurse's conduct at all times should acknowledge the client as a person. For example, discussion of care in the presence of the client should actively involve or include that client.

3. Nurses have a responsibility to intervene when other participants in the health delivery system fail to respect any aspect of client dignity.

4. As ways of dealing with death and the dying process change, nursing is challenged to find new ways to preserve human values, autonomy and dignity. In assisting the dying client, measures must be taken to afford the client as much comfort, dignity and freedom from anxiety and pain as possible. Special consideration must be given to the need of the client's family or significant others to cope with their loss.

VALUE V: COMPETENT NURSING CARE

Value

The nurse provides competent care to clients.

Obligations

1. Nurses should engage in continuing education and in the upgrading of knowledge and skills relevant to their area of practice, that is, clinical practice, education, research or administration.

2. In seeking or accepting employment, nurses must accurately state their area of competence as well as limitations.

3. Nurses assigned to work outside an area of present competence must seek to do what, under the circumstances, is in the best interests of their clients. The nurse manager on duty, or others, must be informed of the situation at the earliest possible moment so that protective measures can be instituted. As a temporary measure, the safety and welfare of clients may be better served by the best efforts of the nurse under the circumstances than by no nursing care at all. Nurse managers are obligated to support nurses who are placed in such difficult situations and to make every effort to remedy the problem.

4. When called upon outside an employment setting to provide emergency care, nurses fulfil their obligations by providing the best care that circumstances, experience and education permit.

Limitations

A nurse is not ethically obliged to provide requested care when compliance would involve a violation of her or his moral beliefs. When that request falls within recognized forms of health care, however, the client must be referred to a health care practitioner who is willing to provide the service. Nurses who have or are likely to encounter such situations are morally obligated to seek to arrange conditions of employment so that the care of clients will not be jeopardized.

Nursing Roles and Relationships

VALUE VI: NURSING PRACTICE, EDUCATION, RESEARCH AND ADMINISTRATION

Value

The nurse maintains trust in nurses and nursing.

Obligations

1. Nurses accepting professional employment must ascertain to the best of their ability that conditions will permit the provision of care consistent with the values and obligations of the Code. Prospective employers should be informed of the provisions of the Code so that realistic and ethical expectations may be established at the beginning of the nurse–employer relationship.

2. Nurse managers, educators and peers are morally obligated to provide timely and accurate feedback to nurses, nurse managers, students of nursing and nurse educators. Objective performance appraisal is essential to the growth of nurses and is required by a concern for present and future clients.

3. Nurse managers bear special ethical responsibilities that flow from a concern for present and future clients. The nurse manager must seek to ensure that the competencies of personnel are used efficiently. Working within available resources, the nurse manager must seek to ensure the welfare of clients. When competent care is threatened due to inadequate resources or for some other reason, the nurse manager must act to minimize the present danger and to prevent future harm.

4. Student–teacher and student-client encounters are essential elements of nursing education. These encounters must be conducted in accordance with ethical nursing practices. The nurse educator is obligated to treat students of nursing with respect and honesty and to provide fair guidance in developing nursing competence. The nurse educator should ensure that students of nursing are acquainted with and comply with the provisions of the Code. Student–client encounters must be conducted with client consent and require special attention to the dignity of the client.

5. Research is necessary to the development of the profession of nursing. Nurses should be acquainted with advances in research, so that established results may be incorporated into clinical practice, education and administration. The individual nurse's competencies may also be used to promote, to

engage in or to assist health care research designed to enhance the health and welfare of clients.

The conduct of research must conform to ethical practice. The self-direction of clients takes on added importance in this context. Further direction is provided in the Canadian Nurses Association publication Ethical Guidelines for Nursing Research Involving Human Subjects.

VALUE VII: COOPERATION IN HEALTH CARE

Value

The nurse recognizes the contribution and expertise of colleagues from nursing and other disciplines as essential to excellent health care.

Obligations

1. The nurse functions as a member of the health care team.
2. The nurse should participate in the assessment, planning, implementation and evaluation of comprehensive programs of care for individual clients and client groups. The scope of a nurse's responsibility should be based upon education and experience, as well as legal considerations of licensure or registration.
3. The nurse accepts responsibility to work with colleagues and other health care professionals, with nursing interest groups and through professional nurses' associations to secure excellent care for clients.

VALUE VIII: PROTECTING CLIENTS FROM INCOMPETENCE

Value

The nurse takes steps to ensure that the client receives competent and ethical care.

Obligations

1. The first consideration of the nurse who suspects incompetence or unethical conduct must be the welfare of present clients or potential harm to future clients. Subject to that principle, the following must be considered:
   (a) The nurse is obliged to ascertain the facts of the situation before deciding upon the appropriate course of action.

   (b) Relationships in the health care team should not be disrupted unnecessarily. If a situation can be resolved without peril to present or future clients by direct discussion with the colleague suspected of providing incompetent or unethical care, that discussion should be done.
   (c) Institutional mechanisms for reporting incidents or risks of incompetent or unethical care must be followed.
   (d) The nurse must report any reportable offence stipulated in provincial or territorial professional nursing legislation.
   (e) It is unethical for a nurse to participate in efforts to deceive or mislead clients about the cause of alleged harm or injury resulting from unethical or incompetent conduct.
2. Guidance on activities that may be delegated by nurses to assistants and other health care workers is found in legislation and policy statements. When functions are delegated, the nurse should be satisfied about the competence of those who will be fulfilling these functions. The nurse has a duty to provide continuing supervision in such a case.
3. The nurse who attempts to protect clients or colleagues threatened by incompetent or unethical conduct may be placed in a difficult position. Colleagues and professional associations are morally obliged to support nurses who fulfil their ethical obligations under the Code.

VALUE IX: CONDITIONS OF EMPLOYMENT

Value

Conditions of employment should contribute in a positive way to client care and the professional satisfaction of nurses.

Obligations

1. Nurses accepting professional employment must ascertain, to the best of their ability, that employment conditions will permit provision of care consistent with the values and obligations of the Code.
2. Nurse managers must seek to ensure that the agencies where they are employed comply with all pertinent provincial or territorial legislation.
3. Nurse managers must seek to ensure the welfare of clients and nurses. When competent care is threatened due to inadequate resources or for some other reason, the nurse manager should act to minimize the present danger and to prevent future harm.

4. Nurse managers must seek to foster environments and conditions of employment that promote excellent care for clients and a good worklife for nurses.

5. Structures should exist in the work environment that provide nurses with means of recourse if conditions that promote a good worklife are absent.

VALUE X: JOB ACTION

Value

Job action by nurses is directed toward securing conditions of employment that enable safe and appropriate care for clients and contribute to the professional satisfaction of nurses.

Obligations

1. In the final analysis, the improvement of conditions of nursing employment is often to the advantage of clients. Over the short term, however, there is a danger that action directed toward this goal could work to the detriment of clients. In view of their ethical responsibility to current as well as future clients, nurses must respect the following principles:

   (a) The safety of clients is the first concern in planning and implementing any job action.

   (b) Individuals and groups of nurses participating in job actions share the ethical commitment to the safety of clients. However, their responsibilities may lead them to express this commitment in different but equally appropriate ways.

   (c) Clients whose safety requires ongoing or emergency nursing care are entitled to have those needs satisfied throughout the duration of any job action. Individuals and groups of nurses participating in job actions have a duty through coordination and communication to take steps to ensure the safety of clients.

   (d) Members of the public are entitled to know of the steps taken to ensure the safety of clients.

Nursing Ethics and Society

VALUE XI: ADVOCACY OF THE INTERESTS OF CLIENTS, THE COMMUNITY AND SOCIETY

Value

The nurse advocates the interests of clients.

Obligations

1. Advocating the interests of individual clients and groups of clients includes helping them to gain access to good health care. For example, by providing information to clients privately or publicly, the nurse enables them to satisfy their rights to health care.

2. When speaking in a public forum or in court, the nurse owes the public the same duties of accurate and relevant information as are owed to clients within the employment setting.

VALUE XII: REPRESENTING NURSING VALUES AND ETHICS

Value

The nurse represents the values and ethics of nursing before colleagues and others.

Obligations

1. Nurses serving on committees concerned with health care or research should see their role as including the vigorous representation of nursing's professional ethics.

2. Many public issues include health as a major component. Involvement in public activities may give the nurse the opportunity to further the objectives of nursing as well as to fulfil the duties of a citizen.

The Nursing Profession

VALUE XIII: RESPONSIBILITIES OF PROFESSIONAL NURSES' ASSOCIATIONS

Value

Professional nurses' organizations are responsible for clarifying, securing and sustaining ethical nursing conduct. The fulfillment of these tasks requires that professional nurses' organizations remain responsive to the rights, needs and legitimate interests of clients and nurses.

Obligations

1. Sustained communication and cooperation between the Canadian Nurses Association, provincial or territorial associations and other organizations of

nurses are essential steps toward securing ethical nursing conduct.

2. Activities of professional nurses' associations must at all times reflect a prime concern for excellent client care.

3. Professional nurses's associations should represent nursing interests and perspectives before nonnursing bodies, including legislatures, employers, the professional organizations of other health disciplines and the public communication media.

4. Professional nurses' associations should provide and encourage organizational structures that facilitate ethical nursing conduct.

   (a) Education in the ethical aspects of nursing should be available to nurses throughout their careers. Nurses' associations should actively support or develop structures to enhance sensitivity to, and application of, norms of ethical nursing conduct. Associations should also promote the development and dissemination of knowledge about ethical decision-making through nursing research.

   (b) Changing circumstances call for ongoing review of this Code. Supplementation of the Code may be necessary to address special situations. Professional associations should consider the ethics of nursing on a regular and continuing basis and be prepared to provide assistance to those concerned with its implementation.

CODE OF ETHICS

American Chiropractic Association

1994–1995

• • •

The current, 1994–1995 American Chiropractic Association (ACA) code differs significantly from an earlier, 1973 version. The current code rests on a single fundamental principle, "The greatest good for the patient," whereas the 1973 code also cited the Golden Rule—do unto others as you would have them do unto you—as a fundamental principle. In addition, the structure and language of the current code is much more modern than that of the 1973 code, which strongly resembled the American Medical Association Code of Medical Ethics of 1847 (see Section II) in the wording and ordering of its articles and subsections.

The 1994–1995 code is divided into four sections. Although the final section on "Administrative Procedures" is not printed below, it is noteworthy that two-thirds of the code is devoted to that section, which discusses the reporting and reviewing of alleged ethics violations.

Preamble

This Code of Ethics is based upon the fundamental principle that the ultimate end and object of the chiropractor's professional services and effort should be:

"The greatest good for the patient."

• • •

A. Responsibility to the Patient

A(1)   Doctors of chiropractic should hold themselves ready at all times to respond to the call of those needing their professional services, although they are free to accept or reject a particular patient except in an emergency.

A(2)   Doctors of chiropractic should attend their patients as often as they consider necessary to ensure the well-being of their patients.

A(3)   Having once undertaken to serve a patient, doctors of chiropractic should not neglect the patient. Doctors of chiropractic should take reasonable steps to protect their patients prior to withdrawing their professional services; such steps shall include: due notice to them allowing a reasonable time for obtaining professional services of others and delivering to their patients all papers and documents in compliance with A(5) of this Code of Ethics.

A(4)   Doctors of chiropractic should be honest and endeavor to practice with the highest degree of professional competency and honesty in the proper care of their patients.

A(5)   Doctors of chiropractic should comply with a patient's authorization to provide records, or copies of such records, to those whom the patient designates as authorized to inspect or receive all or part of such records. A reasonable charge may be made for the cost of duplicating records.

A(6)   Subject to the foregoing Section A(5), doctors of chiropractic should preserve and protect the patient's confidences and records, except as the patient directs or consents or the law requires otherwise. They should not discuss a patient's history, symptoms, diagnosis, or treatment with any third party until they have received the written consent of the patient or the patient's personal representative. They should not exploit the trust and dependency of their patients.

A(7)   Doctors of chiropractic owe loyalty, compassion and respect to their patients. Their clinical judgment and practice should be objective and exercised solely for the patient's benefit.

A(8)   Doctors of chiropractic should recognize and respect the right of every person to free choice of chiropractors or other health care providers and to the right to change such choice at will.

A(9)   Doctors of chiropractic are entitled to receive proper and reasonable compensation for their professional services commensurate with the value of the services they have rendered taking into consideration their experience, time required, reputation and the nature of the condition involved. Doctors of chiropractic should terminate a professional relationship when it becomes reasonably clear that the patient is not benefiting from it. Doctors of chiropractic should support and participate in proper activities designed to enable access to necessary chiropractic care on the part of persons unable to pay such reasonable fees.

A(10)   Doctors of chiropractic should maintain the highest standards of professional and personal conduct, and should refrain from all illegal conduct.

A(11)   Doctors of chiropractic should be ready to consult and seek the talents of other health care professionals when such consultation would benefit their patients or when their patients express a desire for such consultation.

A(12)   Doctors of chiropractic should employ their best good faith efforts that the patient possesses enough information to enable an intelligent choice in regard to proposed chiropractic treatment. The patient should make his or her own determination on such treatment.

A(13)   Doctors of chiropractic should utilize only those laboratory and X-ray procedures, and such devices or nutritional products that are in the best interest of the patient and

not in conflict with state statute or administrative rulings.

B. Responsibility to the Public

B(1)   Doctors of chiropractic should act as members of a learned profession dedicated to the promotion of health, the prevention of illness and the alleviation of suffering.

B(2)   Doctors of chiropractic should observe and comply with all laws, decisions and regulations of state governmental agencies and cooperate with the pertinent activities and policies of associations legally authorized to regulate or assist in the regulation of the chiropractic profession.

B(3)   Doctors of chiropractic should comport themselves as responsible citizens in the public affairs of their local community, state and nation in order to improve law, administrative procedures and public policies that pertain to chiropractic and the system of health care delivery. Doctors of chiropractic should stand ready to take the initiative in the proposal and development of measures to benefit the general public health and well-being, and should cooperate in the administration and enforcement of such measures and programs to the extent consistent with law.

B(4)   Doctors of chiropractic may advertise but should exercise utmost care that such advertising is relevant to health awareness, is accurate, truthful, not misleading or false or deceptive, and scrupulously accurate in representing the chiropractor's professional status and area of special competence. Communications to the public should not appeal primarily to an individual's anxiety or create unjustified expectations of results. Doctors of chiropractic should conform to all applicable state laws, regulations and judicial decisions in connection with professional advertising.

B(5)   Doctors of chiropractic should continually strive to improve their skill and competency by keeping abreast of current developments contained in the health and scientific literature, and by participating in continuing chiropractic educational programs and utilizing other appropriate means.

B(6)   Doctors of chiropractic may testify either as experts or when their patients are involved in court cases, workers' compensation proceedings or in other similar administrative proceedings in personal injury or related cases.

B(7)   The chiropractic profession should address itself to improvements in licensing procedures consistent with the development of the profession and of relevant advances in science.

B(8)   Doctors of chiropractic who are public officers should not engage in activities which are, or may be reasonably perceived to be in conflict with their official duties.

B(9)   Doctors of chiropractic should protect the public and reputation of the chiropractic profession by bringing to the attention of the appropriate public or private organization the actions of chiropractors who engage in deception, fraud or dishonesty, or otherwise engage in conduct inconsistent with this Code of Ethics or relevant provisions of applicable law or regulations within their states.

C. Responsibility to the Profession

C(1)   Doctors of chiropractic should assist in maintaining the integrity, competency and highest standards of the chiropractic profession.

C(2)   Doctors of chiropractic should by their behavior, avoid even the appearance of professional impropriety and should recognize that their public behavior may have an impact on the ability of the profession to serve the public. Doctors of chiropractic should promote public confidence in the chiropractic profession.

C(3)   As teachers, doctors of chiropractic should recognize their obligation to help others acquire knowledge and skill in the practice of the profession. They should maintain high standards of scholarship, education, training and objectivity in the accurate and full dissemination of information and ideas.

C(4)   Doctors of chiropractic should attempt to promote and maintain cordial relationships with other members of the chiropractic profession and other professions in an effort to promote information advantageous to the public's health and well-being.

. . .

PRINCIPLES OF ETHICS AND CODE OF PROFESSIONAL CONDUCT WITH ADVISORY OPINIONS

American Dental Association

REVISED TO JUNE 2002

• • •

Although most of the topics addressed in the 1994 American Dental Association code are the same as those found twenty years ago in the 1974 version, the organization and details of the code have been modified. The twenty-two sections of the 1974 code have been reduced to five main principles (which have been preserved in the latest 2002 version), and many of the remaining original sections now appear as subsections, which constitute the "code of professional conduct." The subsections are denoted as "advisory opinions." Some notable changes in content include the specification that dentists cannot ethically deny treatment to individuals who are HIV seropositive; addition of the obligation to safeguard the confidentiality of patient records; and removal of the former prohibition on advertising.

<http://www.ada.org/prof/prac/law/code/index.html>

I. Introduction

The dental profession holds a special position of trust within society. As a consequence, society affords the profession certain privileges that are not available to members of the public-at-large. In return, the profession makes a commitment to society that its members will adhere to high ethical standards of conduct. These standards are embodied in the *ADA Principles of Ethics and Code of Professional Conduct* (*ADA Code*). The *ADA Code* is, in effect, a written expression of the obligations arising from the implied contract between the dental profession and society.

Members of the ADA voluntarily agree to abide by the *ADA Code* as a condition of membership in the Association.

They recognize that continued public trust in the dental profession is based on the commitment of individual dentists to high ethical standards of conduct.

The *ADA Code* has three main components: The Principles of Ethics, the Code of Professional Conduct and the Advisory Opinions.

The Principles of Ethics are the aspirational goals of the profession. They provide guidance and offer justification for the *Code of Professional Conduct* and the *Advisory Opinions.* There are five fundamental principles that form the foundation of the *ADA Code*: patient autonomy, nonmaleficence, beneficence, justice and veracity. Principles can overlap each other as well as compete with each other for priority. More than one principle can justify a given element of the *Code of Professional Conduct.* Principles may at times need to be balanced against each other, but, otherwise, they are the profession's firm guideposts.

The *Code of Professional Conduct* is an expression of specific types of conduct that are either required or prohibited. The *Code of Professional Conduct* is a product of the ADA's legislative system. All elements of the *Code of Professional Conduct* result from resolutions that are adopted by the ADA's House of Delegates. The *Code of Professional Conduct* is binding on members of the ADA, and violations may result in disciplinary action.

The Advisory Opinions are interpretations that apply the *Code of Professional Conduct* to specific fact situations. They are adopted by the ADA's Council on Ethics, Bylaws and Judicial Affairs to provide guidance to the membership on how the Council might interpret the *Code of Professional Conduct* in a disciplinary proceeding.

The *ADA Code* is an evolving document and by its very nature cannot be a complete articulation of all ethical obligations. The *ADA Code* is the result of an on-going dialogue between the dental profession and society, and as such, is subject to continuous review.

Although ethics and the law are closely related, they are not the same. Ethical obligations may—and often do—exceed legal duties. In resolving any ethical problem not explicitly covered by the *ADA Code,* dentists should consider the ethical principles, the patient's needs and interests, and any applicable laws.

II. Preamble

The American Dental Association calls upon dentists to follow high ethical standards which have the benefit of the patient as their primary goal. Recognition of this goal, and of the education and training of a dentist, has resulted in society affording to the profession the privilege and obligation of self-government.

The Association believes that dentists should possess not only knowledge, skill and technical competence but also those traits of character that foster adherence to ethical principles. Qualities of compassion, kindness, integrity, fairness and charity complement the ethical practice of dentistry and help to define the true professional.

The ethical dentist strives to do that which is right and good. The *ADA Code* is an instrument to help the dentist in this quest.

III. Principles, Code of Professional Conduct And Advisory Opinions

The *Code of Professional Conduct* is organized into five sections. Each section falls under the Principle of Ethics that predominately applies to it. Advisory Opinions follow the section of the Code that they interpret.

Section I–Principle: Patient Autonomy

("Self-governance"). The dentist has a duty to respect the patient's rights to self-determination and confidentiality.

This principle expresses the concept that professionals have a duty to treat the patient according to the patient's desires, within the bounds of accepted treatment, and to protect the patient's confidentiality. Under this principle, the dentist's primary obligations include involving patients in treatment decisions in a meaningful way, with due consideration being given to the patient's needs, desires and abilities, and safeguarding the patient's privacy.

Code of Professional Conduct

I.A. PATIENT INVOLVEMENT

The dentist should inform the patient of the proposed treatment, and any reasonable alternatives, in a manner that allows the patient to become involved in treatment decisions.

I.B. PATIENT RECORDS

Dentists are obliged to safeguard the confidentiality of patient records. Dentists shall maintain patient records in a manner consistent with the protection of the welfare of the patient. Upon request of a patient or another dental practitioner, dentists shall provide any information that will be beneficial for the future treatment of that patient.

Advisory Opinions

I.B.I.COPIES OF RECORDS. A dentist has the ethical obligation on request of either the patient or the patient's new dentist to furnish, either gratuitously or for nominal cost, such dental records or copies or summaries of them, including dental X-rays or copies of them, as will be beneficial for the future treatment of that patient. This obligation exists whether or not the patient's account is paid in full.

I.B.2. CONFIDENTIALITY OF PATIENT RECORDS. The dominant theme in Code Section l-B is the protection of the confidentiality of a patient's records. The statement in this section that relevant information in the records should be released to another dental practitioner assumes that the dentist requesting the information is the patient's present dentist. The former dentist should be free to provide the present dentist with relevant information from the patient's records. This may often be required for the protection of both the patient and the present dentist. There may be circumstances where the former dentist has an ethical obligation to inform the present dentist of certain facts. Dentists should be aware, however, that the laws of the various jurisdictions in the United States are not uniform, and some confidentiality laws appear to prohibit the transfer of pertinent information, such as HIV seropositivity. Absent certain knowledge that the laws of the dentist's jurisdiction permit the forwarding of this information, a dentist should obtain the patient's written permission before forwarding health records which contain information of a sensitive nature, such as HIV seropositivity, chemical dependency or sexual preference. If it is necessary for a treating dentist to consult with another dentist or physician with respect to the patient, and the circumstances do not permit the patient to remain anonymous, the treating dentist should seek the permission of the patient prior to the release of data from the patient's records to the consulting practitioner. If the patient refuses, the treating dentist should then contemplate obtaining legal advice regarding the termination of the dentist/patient relationship.

Section 2–Principle: Nonmaleficence

Principle: Nonmaleficence

("Do no harm"). The dentist has a duty to refrain from harming the patient.

This principle expresses the concept that professionals have a duty to protect the patient from harm. Under this principle, the dentist's primary obligations include keeping knowledge and skills current, knowing one's own limitations and when to refer to a specialist or other professional, and knowing when and under what circumstances delegation of patient care to auxiliaries is appropriate.

Code of Professional Conduct

2.A. EDUCATION.

The privilege of dentists to be accorded professional status rests primarily in the knowledge, skill and experience with which they serve their patients and society. All dentists, therefore, have the obligation of keeping their knowledge and skill current.

2.B. CONSULTATION AND REFERRAL

Dentists shall be obliged to seek consultation, if possible, whenever the welfare of patients will be safeguarded or advanced by utilizing those who have special skills, knowledge, and experience. When patients visit or are referred to specialists or consulting dentists for consultation:

1. The specialists or consulting dentists upon completion of their care shall return the patient, unless the patient expressly reveals a different preference, to the referring dentist, or, if none, to the dentist of record for future care.

2. The specialists shall be obliged when there is no referring dentist and upon a completion of their treatment to inform patients when there is a need for further dental care.

Advisory Opinion

2.B.I. SECOND OPINIONS. A dentist who has a patient referred by a third party* for a "second opinion" regarding a diagnosis or treatment plan recommended by the patient's treating dentist should render the requested second opinion in accordance with this Code of Ethics. In the interest of the patient being afforded quality care, the dentist rendering the second opinion should not have a vested interest in the ensuing recommendation.

2.C. USE OF AUXILIARY PERSONNEL.

Dentists shall be obliged to protect the health of their patients by only assigning to qualified auxiliaries those duties which can be legally delegated. Dentists shall be further obliged to prescribe and supervise the patient care provided by all auxiliary personnel working under their direction.

2.D. PERSONAL IMPAIRMENT.

It is unethical for a dentist to practice while abusing controlled substances, alcohol or other chemical agents which impair the ability to practice. All dentists have an ethical obligation to urge chemically impaired colleagues to seek treatment. Dentists with first-hand knowledge that a colleague is practicing dentistry when so impaired have an ethical responsibility to report such evidence to the professional assistance committee of a dental society.

Advisory Opinion

2.D.1. ABILITY TO PRACTICE. A dentist who contracts any disease or becomes impaired in any way that might endanger patients or dental staff shall, with consultation and advice from a qualified physician or other authority, limit the activities of practice to those areas that do not endanger patients or dental staff. A dentist who has been advised to limit the activities of his or her practice should monitor the aforementioned disease or impairment and make additional limitations to the activities of the dentist's practice, as indicated.

2.E. POSTEXPOSURE, BLOODBORNE PATHOGENS

All dentists, regardless of their bloodborne pathogen status, have an ethical obligation to immediately inform any patient who may have been exposed to blood or other potentially infectious material in the dental office of the need for post exposure evaluation and follow-up and to immediately refer the patient to a qualified health care practitioner who can provide postexposure services. The dentist's ethical obligation in the event of an exposure incident extends to providing information concerning the dentist's own bloodborne pathogen status to the evaluating health care practitioner, if the dentist is the source individual, and to submitting to testing that will assist in the evaluation of the patient. If a staff member or other third person is the source individual, the dentist should encourage that person to cooperate as needed for the patient's evaluation.

2.F. PATIENT ABANDONMENT

Once a dentist has undertaken a course of treatment, the dentist should not discontinue that treatment without giving the patient adequate notice and the opportunity to obtain the services of another dentist. Care should be taken that the patient's oral health is not jeopardized in the process.

*A third party is any party to a dental prepayment contract that may collect premiums, assume financial risks, pay claims, and/or provide administrative services.

Section 3—Principle: Beneficence

Principle: Beneficence

("Do good"). The dentist has a duty to promote the patient's welfare.

This principle expresses the concept that professionals have a duty to act for the benefit of others. Under this principle, the dentist's primary obligation is service to the patient and the public-at-large. The most important aspect of this obligation is the competent and timely delivery of dental care within the bounds of clinical circumstances presented by the patient, with due consideration being given to the needs, desires and values of the patient. The same ethical considerations apply whether the dentist engages in fee-for-service, managed care or some other practice arrangement. Dentists may choose to enter into contracts governing the provision of care to a group of patients; however, contract obligations do not excuse dentists from their ethical duty to put the patient's welfare first.

Code of Professional Conduct

3.A. COMMUNITY SERVICE.

Since dentists have an obligation to use their skills, knowledge and experience for the improvement of the dental health of the public and are encouraged to be leaders in their community, dentists in such service shall conduct themselves in such a manner as to maintain or elevate the esteem of the profession.

3.B. GOVERNMENT OF A PROFESSION.

Every profession owes society the responsibility to regulate itself. Such regulation is achieved largely through the influence of the professional societies. All dentists, therefore, have the dual obligation of making themselves a part of a professional society and of observing its rules of ethics.

3.C. RESEARCH AND DEVELOPMENT.

Dentists have the obligation of making the results and benefits of their investigative efforts available to all when they are useful in safeguarding or promoting the health of the public.

3.D. PATENTS AND COPYRIGHTS.

Patents and copyrights may be secured by dentists provided that such patents and copyrights shall not be used to restrict research or practice.

3.E. ABUSE AND NEGLECT

Dentists shall be obliged to become familiar with the signs of abuse and neglect and to report suspected cases to the proper authorities, consistent with state laws.

3.E.1. REPORTING ABUSE AND NEGLECT

Advisory Opinion

3.E.1. REPORTING ABUSE AND NEGLECT The public and the profession are best served by dentists who are familiar with identifying the signs of abuse and neglect and knowledgeable about the appropriate intervention resources for all populations.

A dentist's ethical obligation to identify and report the signs of abuse and neglect is, at a minimum, to be consistent with a dentist's legal obligation in the jurisdiction where the dentist practices. Dentists, therefore, are ethically obliged to identify and report suspected cases of abuse and neglect to the same extent as they are legally obliged to do so in the jurisdiction where they practice. Dentists have a concurrent ethical obligation to respect an adult patient's right to self-determination and confidentiality and to promote the welfare of all patients. Care should be exercised to respect the wishes of an adult patient who asks that a suspected case of abuse and/or neglect not be reported, where such a report is not mandated by law. With the patient's permission, other possible solutions may be sought.

Dentists should be aware that jurisdictional laws vary in their definitions of abuse and neglect, in their reporting requirements and the extent to which immunity is granted to good faith reporters. The variances may raise potential legal and other risks that should be considered, while keeping in mind the duty to put the welfare of the patient first. Therefore a dentist's ethical obligation to identify and report suspected cases of abuse and neglect can vary from one jurisdiction to another.

Dentists are ethically obligated to keep current their knowledge of both identifying abuse and neglect and reporting it in the jurisdiction(s) where they practice.

Section 4—Principle: Justice

Principle: Justice

("Fairness"). The dentist has a duty to treat people fairly.

This principle expresses the concept that professionals have a duty to be fair in their dealings with patients, colleagues and society. Under this principle, the dentist's primary obligations include dealing with people justly and delivering dental care without prejudice. In its broadest sense, this principle expresses the concept that the dental profession should actively seek allies throughout society on specific activities that will help improve access to care for all.

Code of Professional Conduct

4.A. PATIENT SELECTION.

While dentists, in serving the public, may exercise reasonable discretion in selecting patients for their practices, dentists shall not refuse to accept patients into their practice or deny dental service to patients because of the patient's race, creed, color, sex or national origin.

Advisory Opinion

4.A.1. HIV POSITIVE PATIENTS. A dentist has the general obligation to provide care to those in need. A decision not to provide treatment to an individual because the individual has AIDS or is HIV seropositive, based solely on that fact, is unethical. Decisions with regard to the type of dental treatment provided or referrals made or suggested, in such instances should be made on the same basis as they are made with other patients, that is, whether the individual dentist believes he or she has need of another's skills, knowledge, equipment or experience and whether the dentist believes, after consultation with the patient's physician if appropriate, the patient's health status would be significantly compromised by the provision of dental treatment.

4.B. EMERGENCY SERVICE.

Dentists shall be obliged to make reasonable arrangements for the emergency care of their patients of record. Dentists shall be obliged when consulted in an emergency by patients not of record to make reasonable arrangements for emergency care. If treatment is provided, the dentist, upon completion of treatment, is obliged to return the patient to his or her regular dentist unless the patient expressly reveals a different preference.

4.C. JUSTIFIABLE CRITICISM.

Dentists shall be obliged to report to the appropriate reviewing agency as determined by the local component or constituent society instances of gross or continual faulty treatment by other dentists. Patients should be informed of their present oral health status without disparaging comment about prior services. Dentists issuing a public statement with respect to the profession shall have a reasonable basis to believe that the comments made are true.

Advisory Opinion

4.C.1. MEANING OF "JUSTIFIABLE." A dentist's duty to the public imposes a responsibility to report instances of gross or continual faulty treatment. However, the heading of this section is "Justifiable Criticism." Therefore, when informing a patient of the status of his or her oral health, the dentist should exercise care that the comments made are justifiable. For example, a difference of opinion as to preferred treatment should not be communicated to the patient in a manner which would imply mistreatment. There will necessarily be cases where it will be difficult to determine whether the comments made are justifiable. Therefore, this section is phrased to address the discretion of dentists and advises against disparaging statements against another dentist. However, it should be noted that, where comments are made which are obviously not supportable and therefore unjustified, such comments can be the basis for the institution of a disciplinary proceeding against the dentist making such statements.

4.D. EXPERT TESTIMONY.

Dentists may provide expert testimony when that testimony is essential to a just and fair disposition of a judicial or administrative action.

Advisory Opinion

4.D.I. CONTINGENT FEES.

It is unethical for a dentist to agree to a fee contingent upon the favorable outcome of the litigation in exchange for testifying as a dental expert.

4.E. REBATES AND SPLIT FEES.

Dentists shall not accept or tender "rebates" or "split fees."

Section 5—Principle: Veracity

Principle: Veracity

("Truthfulness"). The dentist has a duty to communicate truthfully.

This principle expresses the concept that professionals have a duty to be honest and trustworthy in their dealings with people. Under this principle, the dentist's primary obligations include respecting the position of trust inherent in the dentist-patient relationship, communicating truthfully and without deception, and maintaining intellectual integrity.

Code of Professional Conduct

5.A. REPRESENTATION OF CARE.

Dentists shall not represent the care being rendered to their patients in a false or misleading manner.

Advisory Opinions

5.A.I. DENTAL AMALGAM AND OTHER RESTORATIVE MATERIALS.

Based on available scientific data the ADA has determined that the removal of amalgam restorations from the non-allergic patient for the alleged purpose of removing toxic substances from the body, when such treatment is performed solely at the recommendation or suggestion of the dentist, is improper and unethical. The same principle of veracity applies to the dentist's recommendation concerning the removal of any dental restorative material.

5.A.2. UNSUBSTANTIATED REPRESENTATIONS.

A dentist who represents that dental treatment or diagnostic techniques recommended or performed by the dentist has the capacity to diagnose, cure or alleviate diseases, infections or other conditions, when such representations are not based upon accepted scientific knowledge or research, is acting unethically.

5.B. REPRESENTATION OF FEES.

Dentists shall not represent the fees being charged for providing care in a false or misleading manner.

Advisory Opinions

5.B.I. WAIVER OF COPAYMENT.

A dentist who accepts a third party* payment under a copayment plan as payment in full without disclosing to the third party* that the patient's payment portion will not be collected, is engaged in overbilling. The essence of this ethical impropriety is deception and misrepresentation; an overbilling dentist makes it appear to the third party* that the charge to the patient for services rendered is higher than it actually is.

5.B.2. OVERBILLING.

It is unethical for a dentist to increase a fee to a patient solely because the patient is covered under a dental benefits plan.

5.B.3. FEE DIFFERENTIAL.

Payments accepted by a dentist under a governmentally funded program, a component or constituent dental society sponsored access program, or a participating agreement entered into under a program of a third party* shall not be considered as evidence of overbilling in determining whether a charge to a patient, or to another third party* in behalf of a patient not covered under any of the aforecited programs constitutes overbilling under this section of the Code.

5.B.4. TREATMENT DATES.

A dentist who submits a claim form to a third party* reporting incorrect treatment dates for the purpose of assisting a patient in obtaining benefits under a dental plan, which benefits would otherwise be disallowed, is engaged in making an unethical, false or misleading representation to such third party.*

5.B.5. DENTAL PROCEDURES. A dentist who incorrectly describes on a third party* claim form a dental procedure in order to receive a greater payment or reimbursement or incorrectly makes a non-covered procedure appear to be a covered procedure on such a claim form is engaged in making an unethical, false or misleading representation to such third party.*

5.B.6. UNNECESSARY SERVICES. A dentist who recommends and performs unnecessary dental services or procedures is engaged in unethical conduct.

5.C. DISCLOSURE OF CONFLICT OF INTEREST.

A dentist who presents educational or scientific information in an article, seminar or other program shall disclose to the readers or participants any monetary or other special interest the dentist may have with a company whose products are promoted or endorsed in the presentation. Disclosure shall be made in any promotional material and in the presentation itself.

5.D. DEVICES AND THERAPEUTIC METHODS.

Except for formal investigative studies, dentists shall be obliged to prescribe, dispense, or promote only those devices, drugs and other agents whose complete formulae are available to the dental profession. Dentists shall have the further obligation of not holding out as exclusive any device, agent, method or technique if that representation would be false or misleading in any material respect.

Advisory Opinions

H5.D.I. REPORTING ADVERSE REACTIONS. A dentist who suspects the occurrence of an adverse reaction to a drug or dental device has an obligation to communicate that information to the broader medical and dental community, including, in the case of a serious adverse event, the Food and Drug Administration (FDA).

5.D.2 MARKETING OR SALE OF PRODUCTS OR PROCEDURES Dentists who, in the regular conduct of their practices, engage in or employ auxiliaries in the marketing or sale of products or procedures to their patients must take care not to exploit the trust inherent in the dentist-patient relationship for their own financial gain. Dentists should not induce their patients to purchase products or undergo procedures by misrepresenting the product's value, the necessity of the procedure or the dentist's professional expertise in recommending the product or procedure.

In the case of a health-related product, it is not enough for the dentist to rely on the manufacturer's or distributor's representations about the product's safety and efficacy. The dentist has an independent obligation to inquire into the truth and accuracy of such claims and verify that they are founded on accepted scientific knowledge or research.

Dentists should disclose to their patients all relevant information the patient needs to make an informed purchase decision, including whether the product is available elsewhere and whether there are any financial incentives for the dentist to recommend the product that would not be evident to the patient.

5.E. PROFESSIONAL ANNOUNCEMENT.

In order to properly serve the public, dentists should represent themselves in a manner that contributes to the esteem of the profession. Dentists should not misrepresent their training and competence in any way that would be false or misleading in any material respect.**

5.F. ADVERTISING.

Although any dentist may advertise, no dentist shall advertise or solicit patients in any form of communication in a manner that is false or misleading in any material respect.**

Advisory Opinions

5.F.I. ARTICLES AND NEWSLETTERS. If a dental health article, message or newsletter is published under a dentist's byline to the public without making truthful disclosure of the source and authorship or is designed to give rise to questionable expectations for the purpose of inducing the public to utilize the services of the sponsoring dentist, the dentist is engaged in making a false or misleading representation to the public in a material respect.

5.F.2. EXAMPLES OF "FALSE OR MISLEADING." The following examples are set forth to provide insight into the meaning of the term "false or misleading in a material respect." These examples are not meant to be all-inclusive. Rather, by restating the concept in alternative language and giving general examples, it is hoped that the membership will gain a better understanding of the term. With this in mind, statements shall be avoided which would: a) contain a material misrepresentation of fact, b) omit a fact necessary to make the statement considered as a whole not materially misleading, c) be intended or be likely to create an unjustified expectation about results the dentist can achieve, and d) contain a material, objective representation, whether express or implied, that the advertised services are superior in quality to those of other dentists, if that representation is not subject to reasonable substantiation.

Subjective statements about the quality of dental services can also raise ethical concerns. In particular, statements of opinion may be misleading if they are not honestly held, if they misrepresent the qualifications of the holder, or the basis of the opinion, or if the patient reasonably interprets them as implied statements of fact. Such statements will be evaluated on a case by case basis, considering how patients are likely to respond to the impression made by the advertisement as a whole. The fundamental issue is whether the advertisement, taken as a whole, is false or misleading in a material respect.

5.F.3. UNEARNED, NONHEALTH DEGREES. A dentist may use the title Doctor or Dentist, DDS, DMD or any additional earned, advanced academic degrees in health service areas in an announcement to the public. The announcement of an unearned academic degree may be misleading because of the likelihood that it will indicate to the public the attainment of specialty or diplomate status. For purposes of this advisory opinion, an unearned academic degree is one which is awarded by an educational institution not accredited by a generally recognized accrediting body or is an honorary degree.

The use of a nonhealth degree in an announcement to the public may be a representation which is misleading because the public is likely to assume that any degree announced is related to the qualifications of the dentist as a practitioner.

Some organizations grant dentists fellowship status as a token of membership in the organization or some other form of voluntary association. The use of such fellowships in advertising to the general public may be misleading because of the likelihood that it will indicate to the public attainment of education or skill in the field of dentistry.

Generally, unearned or nonhealth degrees and fellowships that designate association, rather than attainment, should be limited to scientific papers and curriculum vitae. In all instances, state law should be consulted. In any review by the council of the use of designations in advertising to the public, the council will apply the standard of whether the use of such is false or misleading in a material respect.

5.F.4. REFERRAL SERVICES. There are two basic types of referral services for dental care: not-for-profit and the commercial. The not-for-profit is commonly organized by dental societies or community services. It is open to all qualified practitioners in the area served. A fee is sometimes charged the practitioner to be listed with the service. A fee for such referral services is for the purpose of covering the expenses of the service and has no relation to the number of patients referred. In contrast, some commercial referral services restrict access to the referral service to a limited number of dentists in a particular geographic area. Prospective patients calling the service may be referred to a single subscribing dentist in the geographic area and the respective dentist billed for each patient referred. Commercial referral services often advertise to the public stressing that there is no charge for use of the service and the patient may not be informed of the referral fee paid by the dentist. There is a connotation to such advertisements that the referral that is being made is in the nature of a public service. A dentist is allowed to pay for any advertising permitted by the *Code,* but is generally not permitted to make payments to another person or entity for the referral of a patient for professional services. While the particular facts and circumstances relating to an individual commercial referral service will vary, the council believes that the aspects outlined above for commercial referral services violate the *Code* in that it constitutes advertising which is false or misleading in a material respect and violate the prohibitions in the *Code* against fee splitting.

5.F.5. INFECTIOUS DISEASE TEST RESULTS An advertisement or other communication intended to solicit patients which omits a material fact or facts necessary to put the information conveyed in the advertisement in a proper context can be misleading in a material respect. A dental practice should not seek to attract patients on the basis of partial truths which create a false impression.

For example, an advertisement to the public of HIV negative test results, without conveying additional information that will clarify the scientific significance of this fact contains a misleading omission. A dentist could satisfy his or her obligation under this advisory opinion to convey additional information by clearly stating in the advertisement or other communication: "This negative HIV test cannot guarantee that I am currently free of HIV."

5.G. NAME OF PRACTICE.

Since the name under which a dentist conducts his or her practice may be a factor in the selection process of the patient, the use of a trade name or an assumed name that is false or misleading in any material respect is unethical. Use of the name of a dentist no longer actively associated with the practice may be continued for a period not to exceed one year.**

Advisory Opinion

5.G.I. DENTIST LEAVING PRACTICE. Dentists leaving a practice who authorize continued use of their names should receive competent advice on the legal implications of this action. With permission of a departing dentist, his or her name may be used for more than one year, if, after the one year grace period has expired, prominent notice is provided to the public through such mediums as a sign at the office and a short statement on stationery and business cards that the departing dentist has retired from the practice.

5.H. ANNOUNCEMENT OF SPECIALIZATION AND LIMITATION OF PRACTICE.

This section and Section 5-I are designed to help the public make an informed selection between the practitioner who has completed an accredited program beyond the dental degree and a practitioner who has not completed such a program. The special areas of dental practice approved by the American Dental Association and the designation for ethical specialty announcement and limitation of practice are: dental public health, endodontics, oral and maxillofacial pathology, oral and maxillofacial radiology, oral and maxillofacial surgery, orthodontics and dentofacial orthopedics, pediatric dentistry, periodontics and prosthodontics. Dentists who choose to announce specialization should use "specialist in" or "practice limited to" and shall limit their practice exclusively to the announced special area(s) of dental practice, provided at the time of the announcement such dentists have met in each approved specialty for which they announce the existing educational requirements and standards set forth by the American Dental Association. Dentists who use their eligibility to announce as specialists to make the public believe that specialty services rendered in the dental office are being rendered by qualified specialists when such is not the case are engaged in unethical conduct. The burden of responsibility is on specialists to avoid any inference that general practitioners who are associated with specialists are qualified to announce themselves as specialists.

GENERAL STANDARDS.

The following are included within the standards of the American Dental Association for determining the education, experience and other appropriate requirements for announcing specialization and limitation of practice:

1. The special area(s) of dental practice and an appropriate certifying board must be approved by the American Dental Association.
2. Dentists who announce as specialists must have successfully completed an educational program accredited by the Commission on Dental Accreditation, two or more years in length, as specified by the Council on Dental Education and Licensure, or be diplomates of an American Dental Association recognized certifying board.

   The scope of the individual specialist's practice shall be governed by the educational standards for the specialty in which the specialist is announcing.

3. The practice carried on by dentists who announce as specialists shall be limited exclusively to the special area(s) of dental practices announced by the dentist.

STANDARDS FOR MULTIPLE-SPECIALTY ANNOUNCEMENTS.

Educational criteria for announcement by dentists in additional recognized specialty areas are the successful completion of an educational program accredited by the Commission on Dental Accreditation in each area for which the dentist wishes to announce. Dentists who completed their advanced education in programs listed by the Council on Dental Education and Licensure prior to the initiation of the accreditation process in 1967 and who are currently ethically announcing as specialists in a recognized area may announce in additional areas provided they are educationally qualified or are certified diplomates in each area for which they wish to announce. Documentation of successful completion of the educational program(s) must be submitted to the appropriate constituent society. The documentation must assure that the duration of the program(s) is a minimum of two years except for oral and maxillofacial surgery which must have been a minimum of three years in duration.**

Advisory Opinions

5.H.I. DUAL DEGREED DENTISTS. Nothing in Section 5-H shall be interpreted to prohibit a dual degreed dentist who practices medicine or osteopathy under a valid state license from announcing to the public as a dental specialist provided the dentist meets the educational, experience and other standards set forth in the *Code* for specialty announcement and further providing that the announcement is truthful and not materially misleading.

5.H.2. SPECIALIST ANNOUNCEMENT OF CREDENTIALS IN NON-SPECIALTY INTEREST AREAS. A dentist who is qualified to announce specialization under this section may not announce to the public that he or she is certified or a diplomate or otherwise similarly credentialed in an area of dentistry not recognized as a specialty area by the American Dental Association unless:

1. The organization granting the credential grants certification or diplomate status based on the following: a) the dentist's successful completion of a formal, full-time advanced education program (graduate or postgraduate level) of at least 12 months' duration; and b) the dentist's training and experience; and c) successful completion of an oral and written examination based on psychometric principles; and

2. The announcement includes the following language: [Name of announced area of dental practice] is not recognized as a specialty area by the American Dental Association.

Nothing in this advisory opinion affects the right of a properly qualified dentist to announce specialization in an ADA-recognized specialty area(s) as provided for under Section 5.H of this *Code* or the responsibility of such dentist to limit his or her practice exclusively to the special area(s) of dental practice announced. Specialists shall not announce their credentials in a manner that implies specialization in a non-specialty interest area.

See also: Report of the Council on Ethics, Bylaws and Judicial Affairs on Advisory Opinion 5.H.2. Specialist Announcement of Credentials in Non-Specialty Interest Areas

5.I. GENERAL PRACTITIONER ANNOUNCEMENT OF SERVICES.

General dentists who wish to announce the services available in their practices are permitted to announce the availability of those services so long as they avoid any communications that express or imply specialization. General dentists shall also state that the services are being provided by general dentists. No dentist shall announce available services in any way that would be false or misleading in any material respect.**

Advisory Opinions

5. I.I. GENERAL PRACTITIONER ANNOUNCEMENT OF CREDENTIALS IN NON-SPECIALTY INTEREST AREAS A general dentist may not announce to the public that he or she is certified or a diplomate or otherwise similarly credentialed in an area of dentistry not recognized as a specialty area by the American Dental Association unless:

1. The organization granting the credential grants certification or diplomate status based on the following: a) the dentist's successful completion of a formal, full-time advanced education program (graduate or postgraduate level) of at least 12 months duration; and b) the dentist's training and experience; and c) successful completion of an oral and written examination based on psychometric principles;

2. The dentist discloses that he or she is a general dentist; and

3. The announcement includes the following language: [Name of announced area of dental practice] is not recognized as a specialty area by the American Dental Association.

5.I.2. CREDENTIALS IN GENERAL DENTISTRY. General dentists may announce fellowships or other credentials earned in the area of general dentistry so long as they avoid any communications that express or imply specialization and the announcement includes the disclaimer that the dentist is a general dentist. The use of abbreviations to designate credentials shall be avoided when such use would lead the reasonable person to believe that the designation represents an academic degree, when such is not the case.

See also: Report of the ADA Council on Ethics, Bylaws and Judicial Affairs On Advisory Opinion 5.I.2. Credentials in General Dentistry

*A third party is any party to a dental prepayment contract that may collect premiums, assume financial risks, pay claims and/or provide administrative services.

**Advertising, solicitation of patients or business or other promotional activities by dentists or dental care delivery organizations shall not be considered unethical or improper, except for those promotional activities which are false or misleading in any material respect. Notwithstanding any *ADA Principles of Ethics and Code of Professional Conduct* or other standards of dentist conduct which may be differently worded, this shall be the sole standard for determining the ethical propriety of such promotional activities. Any provision of an ADA constituent or component society's code of ethics or other standard of dentist conduct relating to dentists' or dental care delivery organizations' advertising, solicitation, or other promotional activities which is worded differently from the above standard shall be deemed to be in conflict with the *ADA Principles of Ethics and Code of Professional Conduct.*

• • •

CODE OF ETHICS FOR THE PROFESSION OF DIETETICS

American Dietetic Association

1987, REVISED 1999

• • •

The current Code of Ethics for the Profession of Dietetics was adopted by the American Dietetic Association (ADA) in 1999. Whereas most professional codes apply only to members of the authoring organization, the ADA code applies both to members of the ADA and to nonmembers who are credentialed as "registered dieticians" (RDs) or "dietetic technicians, registered" (DTRs) by the Commission on Dietetic Registration, the ADA's credentialing agency. Certain provisions, however, apply only to one group or the other. The code is supplemented by a detailed Consideration of Ethics Issues which outlines how ethics cases will be handled.

<http://www.eatright.org/adacode.html>

Principles

1. The dietetics practitioner conducts himself/herself with honesty, integrity, and fairness.

2. The dietetics practitioner practices dietetics based on scientific principles and current information.

3. The dietetics practitioner presents substantiated information and interprets controversial information without personal bias, recognizing that legitimate differences of opinion exist.

4. The dietetics practitioner assumes responsibility and accountability for personal competence in practice, continually striving to increase professional knowledge and skills and to apply them in practice.

5. The dietetics practitioner recognizes and exercises professional judgment within the limits of his/her qualifications and collaborates with others, seeks counsel, or makes referrals as appropriate.

6. The dietetics practitioner provides sufficient information to enable clients and others to make their own informed decisions.

7. The dietetics practitioner protects confidential information and makes full disclosure about any limitations on his/her ability to guarantee full confidentiality.

8. The dietetics practitioner provides professional services with objectivity and with respect for the unique needs and values of individuals.

9. The dietetics practitioner provides professional services in a manner that is sensitive to cultural differences and does not discriminate against others on the basis of race, ethnicity, creed, religion, disability, sex, age, sexual orientation, or national origin.

10. The dietetics practitioner does not engage in sexual harassment in connection with professional practice.

11. The dietetics practitioner provides objective evaluations of performance for employees and coworkers, candidates for employment, students, professional association memberships, awards, or scholarships. The dietetics practitioner makes all reasonable effort to avoid bias in any kind of professional evaluation of others.

12. The dietetics practitioner is alert to situations that might cause a conflict of interest or have the appearance of a conflict. The dietetics practitioner provides full disclosure when a real or potential conflict of interest arises.

13. The dietetics practitioner who wishes to inform the public and colleagues of his/her services does so by using factual information. The dietetics practitioner does not advertise in a false or misleading manner.

14. The dietetics practitioner promotes or endorses products in a manner that is neither false nor misleading.

15. The dietetics practitioner permits the use of his/her name for the purpose of certifying that dietetics services have been rendered only if he/she has provided or supervised the provision of those services.

16. The dietetics practitioner accurately presents professional qualifications and credentials.

    a. The dietetics practitioner uses Commission on Dietetic Registration awarded credentials ("RD" or "Registered Dietitian"; "DTR" or "Dietetic Technician, Registered"; "CSP" or "Certified Specialist in Pediatric Nutrition"; "CSR" or "Certified Specialist in Renal Nutrition"; and "FADA" or "Fellow of The American Dietetic Association") only when the credential is current and authorized by the Commission on Dietetic Registration. The dietetics practitioner provides accurate information and complies with all requirements of the Commission on Dietetic Registration program in which he/she is seeking initial or continued credentials from the Commission on Dietetic Registration.

    b. The dietetics practitioner is subject to disciplinary action for aiding another person in violating any Commission on Dietetic Registration requirements or aiding another person in representing himself/herself as Commission on Dietetic Registration credentialed when he/she is not.

17. The dietetics practitioner withdraws from professional practice under the following circumstances:

    a. The dietetics practitioner has engaged in any substance abuse that could affect his/her practice;

    b. The dietetics practitioner has been adjudged by a court to be mentally incompetent;

    c. The dietetics practitioner has an emotional or mental disability that affects his/her practice in a manner that could harm the client or others.

18. The dietetics practitioner complies with all applicable laws and regulations concerning the profession and is subject to disciplinary action under the following circumstances:

    a. The dietetics practitioner has been convicted of a crime under the laws of the United States which is a felony or a misdemeanor, an essential element of which is dishonesty, and which is related to the practice of the profession.

b. The dietetics practitioner has been disciplined by a state, and at least one of the grounds for the discipline is the same or substantially equivalent to these principles.

c. The dietetics practitioner has committed an act of misfeasance or malfeasance which is directly related to the practice of the profession as determined by a court of competent jurisdiction, a licensing board, or an agency of a governmental body.

19. The dietetics practitioner supports and promotes high standards of professional practice. The dietetics practitioner accepts the obligation to protect clients, the public, and the profession by upholding the Code of Ethics for the Profession of Dietetics and by reporting alleged violations of the Code through the defined review process of The American Dietetic Association and its credentialing agency, the Commission on Dietetic Registration.

CODE OF ETHICS

American Association of Pastoral Counselors

LAST AMENDED 1994

• • •

Amended in 1994, the current Code of Ethics of the American Association of Pastoral Counselors contains many of the same elements as other professional codes, for example, statements pertaining to confidentiality, professional qualifications, and the welfare of the individuals they serve. In addition, the code contains aspects unique to the profession, such as avoiding the imposition of one's personal theology on clients and maintaining a responsible association with one's faith group.

Principle I – Prologue

As members of the American Association of Pastoral Counselors, we are committed to the various theologies, traditions, and values of our faith communities and to the dignity and worth of each individual. We are dedicated to advancing the welfare of those who seek our assistance and to the maintenance of high standards of professional conduct and competence. We are accountable for our ministry whatever its setting. This accountability is expressed in relationships to clients, colleagues, students, our faith communities, and through the acceptance and practice of the principles and procedures of this Code of Ethics.

In order to uphold our standards, as members of AAPC we covenant to accept the following foundational premises:

A. To maintain responsible association with the faith group in which we have ecclesiastical standing.

B. To avoid discriminating against or refusing employment, educational opportunity or professional assistance to anyone on the basis of race, gender, sexual orientation, religion, or national origin.

C. To remain abreast of new developments in the field through both educational activities and clinical experience. We agree at all levels of membership to continue post-graduate education and professional growth including supervision, consultation, and active participation in the meetings and affairs of the Association.

D. To seek out and engage in collegial relationships, recognizing that isolation can lead to a loss of perspective and judgement.

E. To manage our personal lives in a healthful fashion and to seek appropriate assistance for our own personal problems or conflicts.

F. To diagnose or provide treatment only for those problems or issues that are within the reasonable boundaries of our competence.

G. To establish and maintain appropriate professional relationship boundaries.

Principle II – Professional Practices

In all professional matters members of AAPC maintain practices that protect the public and advance the profession.

A. We use our knowledge and professional associations for the benefit of the people we serve and not to secure unfair personal advantage.

B. We clearly represent our level of membership and limit our practice to that level.

C. Fees and financial arrangements, as with all contractual matters, are always discussed without hesitation or equivocation at the onset and are established in a straight-forward, professional manner.

D. We are prepared to render service to individuals and communities in crisis without regard to financial remuneration when necessary.

E. We neither receive nor pay a commission for referral of a client.

F. We conduct our practice, agency, regional and Association fiscal affairs with due regard to recognized business and accounting procedures.

G. Upon the transfer of a pastoral counseling practice or the sale of real, personal, tangible or intangible property or assets used in such practice, the privacy and well being of the client shall be of primary concern.

1. Client names and records shall be excluded from the transfer or sale.

2. Any fees paid shall be for services rendered, consultation, equipment, real estate, and the name and logo of the counseling agency.

H. We are careful to represent facts truthfully to clients, referral sources, and third party payors regarding credentials and services rendered. We shall correct any misrepresentation of our professional qualifications or affiliations.

I. We do not malign colleagues or other professionals.

Principle III – Client Relationships

It is the responsibility of members of AAPC to maintain relationships with clients on a professional basis.

A. We do not abandon or neglect clients. If we are unable, or unwilling for appropriate reasons, to provide professional help or continue a professional relationship, every reasonable effort is made to arrange for continuation of treatment with another professional.

B. We make only realistic statements regarding the pastoral counseling process and its outcome.

C. We show sensitive regard for the moral, social, and religious standards of clients and communities. We avoid imposing our beliefs on others, although we may express them when appropriate in the pastoral counseling process.

D. Counseling relationships are continued only so long as it is reasonably clear that the clients are benefiting from the relationship.

E. We recognize the trust placed in and unique power of the therapeutic relationship. While acknowledging the complexity of some pastoral relationships, we avoid exploiting the trust and dependency of clients. We avoid those dual relationships with clients (e.g., business or close personal relationships) which could impair our professional judgement, compromise the integrity of the treatment, and/or use the relationship for our own gain.

F. We do not engage in harassment, abusive words or actions, or exploitative coercion of clients or former clients.

G. All forms of sexual behavior or harassment with clients are unethical, even when a client invites or consents to such behavior or involvement. Sexual behavior is defined as, but not limited to, all forms of overt and covert seductive speech, gestures, and behavior as well as physical contact of a sexual nature; harassment is defined as but not limited to, repeated comments, gestures or physical contacts of a sexual nature.

H. We recognize that the therapist/client relationship involves a power imbalance, the residual effects of which are operative following the termination of the therapy relationship. Therefore, all sexual behavior or harassment as defined in Principle III, G with former clients is unethical.

Principle IV – Confidentiality

As members of AAPC we respect the integrity and protect the welfare of all persons with whom we are working and have an obligation to safeguard information about them that has been obtained in the course of the counseling process.

A. All records kept on a client are stored or disposed of in a manner that assures security and confidentiality.

B. We treat all communications from clients with professional confidence.

C. Except in those situations where the identity of the client is necessary to the understanding of the case, we use only the first names of our clients when engaged in supervision or consultation. It is our responsibility to convey the importance of confidentiality to the supervisor/consultant; this is particularly important when the supervision is shared by other professionals, as in a supervisory group.

D. We do not disclose client confidences to anyone, except: as mandated by law; to prevent a clear and immediate danger to someone; in the course of a civil, criminal or disciplinary action arising from the counseling where the pastoral counselor is a defendant; for purposes of supervision or consultation; or by previously obtained written permission. In cases involving more than one person (as client) written permission must be obtained from all legally accountable persons who have been present during the counseling before any disclosure can be made.

E. We obtain informed written consent of clients before audio and/or video tape recording or permitting third party observation of their sessions.

F. We do not use these standards of confidentiality to avoid intervention when it is necessary, e.g., when there is evidence of abuse of minors, the elderly, the disabled, the physically or mentally incompetent.

G. When current or former clients are referred to in a publication, while teaching or in a public presentation, their identity is thoroughly disguised.

H. We as members of AAPC agree that as an express condition of our membership in the Association,

Association ethics communications, files, investigative reports, and related records are strictly confidential and waive their right to use same in a court of law to advance any claim against another member. Any member seeking such records for such purpose shall be subject to disciplinary action for attempting to violate the confidentiality requirements of the organization. This policy is intended to promote pastoral and confessional communications without legal consequences and to protect potential privacy and confidentiality interests of third parties.

Principle V – Supervisee, Student & Employee Relationships

As members of AAPC we have an ethical concern for the integrity and welfare of our supervisees, students and employees. These relationships are maintained on a professional and confidential basis. We recognize our influential position with regard to both current and former supervisees, students and employees, and avoid exploiting their trust and dependency. We make every effort to avoid dual relationships with such persons that could impair our judgement or increase the risk of personal and/or financial exploitation.

A. We do not engage in ongoing counseling relationships with current supervisees, students and employees.

B. We do not engage in sexual or other harassment of supervisees, students, employees, research subjects or colleagues.

C. All forms of sexual behavior, as defined in Principle III.G, with our supervisees, students, research subjects and employees (except in employee situations involving domestic partners) are unethical.

D. We advise our students, supervisees, and employees against offering or engaging in, or holding themselves out as competent to engage in, professional services beyond their training, level of experience and competence.

E. We do not harass or dismiss an employee who has acted in a reasonable, responsible and ethical manner to protect, or intervene on behalf of, a client or other member of the public or another employee.

Principle VI – Interprofessional Relationships

As members of AAPC we relate to and cooperate with other professional persons in our community and beyond. We are part of a network of health care professionals and are expected to develop and maintain interdisciplinary and interprofessional relationships.

A. We do not offer ongoing clinical services to persons currently receiving treatment from another professional without prior knowledge of and in consultation with the other professional, with the clients' informed consent. Soliciting such clients is unethical.

B. We exercise care and interprofessional courtesy when approached for services by persons who claim or appear to have inappropriately terminated treatment with another professional.

Principle VII – Advertising

Any advertising by or for a member of AAPC, including announcements, public statements and promotional activities, is undertaken with the purpose of helping the public make informed judgements and choices.

. . .

GUIDELINES FOR THE CHAPLAINS' ROLE IN BIOETHICS

College of Chaplains, American Protestant Health Association

1992

. . .

This document differs from codes of ethics in its focus on the role of chaplains in clinical settings, particularly within healthcare institutions. Certified chaplains are recognized to be essential members of the healthcare team; they help to identify and integrate the spiritual and moral perspectives of patients with those of other healthcare disciplines to form a holistic approach to bioethics.

<http://www.professionalchaplains.org/stage/index.html>

Introduction

Advances in medical science and technology, the evolution of integrated delivery systems, and the changing economics of health care present benefits and ethical dilemmas. Ethical conflicts can arise in the clinical setting and at the organizational level. The obligations of health care organizations include provision of a forum for ethical reflection, a deliberate process for ethics consultation, and persons trained in ethics consultation.

Health care ethics committees may serve three functions: (1) education, (2) consultation, and (3) review and recommendation of institutional policies and procedures. Health care organizations that have a formal health care ethics committee often include a certified Chaplain on that committee. As members of health care ethics committees, Chaplains play a crucial role in health care ethics reflection. Chaplains may be of assistance to health care ethics committees as they discuss the questions of philosophy, theology, spirituality, human values, and morals which are integral to ethical questions.

While some Chaplains have education and/or training in ethics, their roles as Chaplains differ from those of ethicists. Chaplains identify and clarify the patient's spiritual and moral perspectives as essential ingredients in the process of health care ethics reflection. Integration of these perspectives with those of other health care disciplines fosters a holistic approach to health care ethics.

These Guidelines provide primary principles for the effective inclusion of pastoral/spiritual care in the process of health care ethics reflection. While each health care institution has a particular context within which ethical reflection is done, these Guidelines are generally applicable to a variety of health care settings. The Guidelines emphasize pastoral/spiritual care's unique perspective as integral to the ethical reflection process of a health care organization.

Principle I

The health care organization includes a certified chaplain on its health care ethics committee.

INTERPRETATION – *A certified Chaplain can make unique contributions to a health care ethics committee. Certified Chaplains have theological education on at least the master's level or its equivalent that includes formal training in pastoral theology and clinical pastoral education.*

Guideline 1

Chaplains offer pastoral/spiritual care to health care ethics committee members and to medical and health care professionals involved in health care ethics discussion and consultation.

Guideline 2

Chaplains serve as resource persons to religious/faith group leaders and to the health care ethics committee concerning the

spiritual and value dimensions and values of illness and health even if patients or their families have no apparent religious affiliation.

Principle II

Chaplains develop a continuing education plan for themselves and their colleagues that addresses health care ethics theories and approaches related to the spiritual, religious, cultural, and philosophical values represented in persons served by their health care institutions, thus, contributing to the institution's education program.

INTERPRETATION – *Certified Chaplains commit to yearly continuing education for themselves in order to maintain certification and serve as resource persons in their organizations' educational programs in health care ethics.*

Guideline 1

The Chaplain seeks continuing education in health care ethics and ethics consultation in order to achieve a working knowledge of basic principles, ethical decision-making, current issues, and developing trends.

Guideline 2

Chaplains participate in and serve as resource persons to the organization's health care ethics education program to patients, staff, and community with the goal of providing a forum for discussion of various spiritual and religious perspectives on health care ethics issues.

Guideline 3

Chaplains are included in peer review as the multi-disciplinary team seeks to teach health care ethics theories, principles, and options that apply in specific situations.

Guideline 4

Chaplains contribute as resource persons and speakers in the organization's education programs for patients, health care professionals, and the community.

Guideline 5

Chaplains bring expertise in spiritual, theological, ethical, and moral values to the multi-disciplinary team in the clinical setting.

Guideline 6

Chaplains bring expertise in spiritual, theological, ethical, and moral values to the multi-disciplinary reflection and discourse on ethical issues, dilemmas, case studies, and retrospective reviews.

Principle III

Chaplains participate in the health care ethics consultation services of the facility or organization.

INTERPRETATION – *A health care ethics committee may provide the service of consultation to physicians, nurses, administration, patients, and families. Consultation does not take the place of or interfere with the patient-physician relationship. Consultation helps clarify ethical options through reflective discussion in the context of health care ethics principles and good medical practice.*

Guideline 1

The Chaplain's role is to maintain contact with the patient and/or the patient's decision-maker(s) during the ethics consultation process.

- The Chaplain may serve as a resource to the health care ethics consultation process, helping to interpret the process and facilitate the patient and the patient's decision-maker's understanding of and participation in the consultation process.

Guideline 2

The Chaplain may assist in facilitating group process.

- The Chaplain may facilitate and be a resource in supporting group process, i.e., consultative process, staff and patient decision-makers' concerns, etc.

Guideline 3

The Chaplain clarifies theological beliefs and values that influence decision-making.

- The Chaplain's function is to identify spiritual, moral, religious, cultural, and philosophical values which influence decisions.
- The Chaplain provides validation and recognition of the importance of personal beliefs, which will help individuals trust the consultation process.
- The Chaplain serves as an advocate for the spiritual values and religious beliefs held by the

patient, even when those values and beliefs are not those of the Chaplain.

- The Chaplain assures that the religious, cultural, and philosophic values of the patient are considered during discussion of appropriate medical treatment, even when those values and beliefs are other than those of the Chaplain.

Guideline 4

The Chaplain provides pastoral care to those involved in the health care ethics consultation process.

- Chaplains may provide continuing support to the patient, family, and staff during and following the consultation process.

Guideline 5

The Chaplain serves as liaison with the patient's own clergy.

- The Chaplain is the liaison with the religious community. The Chaplain develops programs and strategies to develop positive relationships with community clergy and other designated religious representatives who visit congregants and may be involved in the decision-making process.
- The Chaplain provides consultations, referrals, professional resources, and educational opportunities for community clergy.
- The Chaplain facilitates the pastoral ministry and the role of community clergy in the decision-making process for their congregants who are patients.

Principle IV

Chaplains assist the health care organization in its review and recommendation of policies that have health care ethics implications in the services provided by the organization.

INTERPRETATION – *Health care ethics committees are usually responsible for reviewing existing or proposed policies and procedures for the organization, medical staff, nursing staff, etc. As members of the health care ethics committee, Chaplains offer input from their discipline of pastoral/spiritual care.*

Guideline 1

Chaplains serve as resource persons for understanding and interpreting faith communities, religious traditions, and belief systems as they might relate to or be affected by proposed policies and procedures.

Guideline 2

Chaplains serve as resource person to staff who have spiritual and religious concerns which arise in the implementation of policies and procedures with ethical implications.

Principle V
Chaplains provide pastoral and spiritual care to those involved in the ethical reflection process.

INTERPRETATION – *The ministry of Chaplains includes a wide repertoire of services including pastoral presence, pastoral conversation, pastoral/spiritual care, and pastoral counseling. Experiencing such services, patients, families, health care staff, and employees feel affirmed, understood, and supported in their particular predicament and in their right to have a particular ethical perspective. Those involved in the process can be enabled to explore the relationships of the physical issues of health and illness, psychological dimensions of the situation, i.e., anxiety, fear, trust, etc., and the spiritual issues, i.e., meaning, hope, ultimate concern, and God's presence. Issues vary greatly from person to person depending upon the situation and belief system of the individual. Pastoral/spiritual care offers support for all involved and creates an atmosphere of sensitivity and trust in the context of health care ethics decision-making.*

Guideline 1

Chaplains offer religious resources and support from the patient's and family's faith system and community as appropriate.

Guideline 2

Chaplains facilitate the ministry of community clergy and faith group leaders for the purpose of offering support and the opportunity for patients and families to explore the values, beliefs, and meaning inherent in the patient's situation.

Principle VI
Chaplains provide specific evaluation of the process of ethical reflection from a spiritual perspective as well as from a clinical perspective.

INTERPRETATION – *Evaluation of the health care ethics reflection process utilized in a case consultation, policy review,*

or educational event is an important part of quality improvement. Each discipline, including pastoral/spiritual care, has its own perspective and responsibility to contribute to the evaluation process.

Guideline 1

Chaplains have the responsibility to be advocates for patients, families, and health care staff in behalf of their particular spiritual values. The role of the Chaplain is to help ensure that the health care ethics reflection process is as attentive, respectful, and inclusive of patients' values and wishes as possible.

Guideline 2

Pastoral intervention in the health care ethics process is evaluated regularly through peer review and input from a clinically trained and experienced ethicist. The health care organization provides opportunities and encouragement for Chaplains to attend and participate in regional and/or national health care ethics workshops, conferences, and other educational events.

Principle VII
Chaplains provide for alternate coverage of the chaplain's role in the health care ethics reflection process when it is appropriate for the chaplain designated to exclude her/himself.

INTERPRETATION – *The Chaplain charged with the responsibility to serve on the health care ethics committee or to participate in the consultation service may withdraw from participation so that objectivity and professionalism can be maintained in the process.*

Guideline 1

If the Chaplain does not have adequate knowledge about an issue, particularly a patient's or family's spiritual perspective, the Chaplain seeks consultation or makes an appropriate referral.

Guideline 2

If the Chaplain has a personal relationship with one or more of the significant parties involved in the case being reviewed, designating another certified Chaplain to participate in the ethics process maintains objective and professional integrity.

Guideline 3

Chaplains are familiar with the process for health care ethics consultation in their organizations. When patients with whom they have pastoral relationships are brought to the attention of the health care ethics service for consultation or for education purposes, other pastoral care staff persons or community clergy can be involved when and to the degree appropriate. In this process, confidentiality is maintained.

PRINCIPLE VIII

Chaplains in administrative and managerial roles assist in the identification and consideration of values in matters of the health care organization.

INTERPRETATION – *Organizational values and ethics reflect consistency at all levels and in all services of the health care organization. The certified Chaplain who is in an administrative position and/or works at a managerial level has knowledge and experience of health care ethics, organizational ethics, and spiritual values related to the organization.*

Guideline 1

Chaplains bring expertise in spiritual dimensions, theological considerations, ethical issues, and moral values to the administrative and managerial teams.

Guideline 2

Chaplains with managerial/administrative responsibilities serve as resource persons to the administrators, board members, owners, etc. concerning the exploration of the spiritual dimensions, theological considerations, ethical issues, and moral values of the health care organization.

Conclusion

Spiritual and religious dimensions of health care ethics issues and dilemmas must be considered and included in the process of health care ethics reflection. The Association of Professional Chaplains provides resources and a Bioethics Committee to assist members of the APC as well as other health care providers to facilitate, promote, enhance, and strengthen the role of Chaplains in this important endeavor.

Approved by the Board of Directors 10/2000

CODE OF ETHICS

American Pharmacists Association

1969, AMENDED 1975, REVISED 1981, 1994

• • •

The current code of the American Pharmacists Association (APhA) was approved in 1969, amended in 1975 and 1981, and last revised in 1994. Since the 1969 code, the Association has introduced gender-neutral language and removed the prohibition on advertising. The name of the organization was changed from American Pharmaceutical Association in 2003.

<http://www.aphanet.org/>

Preamble

Pharmacists are health professionals who assist individuals in making the best use of medications. This Code, prepared and supported by pharmacists, is intended to state publicly the principles that form the fundamental basis of the roles and responsibilities of pharmacists. These principles, based on moral obligations and virtues, are established to guide pharmacists in relationships with patients, health professionals, and society.

I. A pharmacist respects the covenantal relationship between the patient and pharmacist.

Considering the patient-pharmacist relationship as a covenant means that a pharmacist has moral obligations in response to the gift of trust received from society. In return for this gift, a pharmacist promises to help individuals achieve optimum benefit from their medications, to be committed to their welfare, and to maintain their trust.

II. A pharmacist promotes the good of every patient in a caring, compassionate, and confidential manner.

A pharmacist places concern for the well-being of the patient at the center of professional practice. In doing so, a pharmacist considers needs stated by the patient as well as those defined by health science. A pharmacist is dedicated to protecting the dignity of the patient. With a caring attitude and a compassionate spirit, a pharmacist focuses on serving the patient in a private and confidential manner.

III. A pharmacist respects the autonomy and dignity of each patient.

A pharmacist promotes the right of self-determination and recognizes individual self-worth by encouraging patients to participate in decisions about their health. A pharmacist communicates with patients in terms that are understandable. In all cases, a pharmacist respects personal and cultural differences among patients.

IV. A pharmacist acts with honesty and integrity in professional relationships.

A pharmacist has a duty to tell the truth and to act with conviction of conscience. A pharmacist avoids discriminatory practices, behavior or work conditions that impair professional judgment, and actions that compromise dedication to the best interests of patients.

V. A pharmacist maintains professional competence.

A pharmacist has a duty to maintain knowledge and abilities as new medications, devices, and technologies become available and as health information advances.

VI. A pharmacist respects the values and abilities of colleagues and other health professionals.

When appropriate, a pharmacist asks for the consultation of colleagues or other health professionals or refers the patient. A pharmacist acknowledges that colleagues and other health professionals may differ in the beliefs and values they apply to the care of the patient.

VII. A pharmacist serves individual, community, and societal needs.

The primary obligation of a pharmacist is to individual patients. However, the obligations of a pharmacist may at times extend beyond the individual to the community and society. In these situations, the pharmacist recognizes the responsibilities that accompany these obligations and acts accordingly.

VIII. A pharmacist seeks justice in the distribution of health resources.

When health resources are allocated, a pharmacist is fair and equitable, balancing the needs of patients and society.

* adopted by the membership of the American Pharmaceutical Association October 27, 1994.

STATEMENT OF PROFESSIONAL STANDARDS: CODE OF ETHICS FOR PHARMACISTS

Fédération Internationale Pharmaceutique

1988, REVISED 1997

• • •

In 1988, the Fédération Internationale Pharmaceutique adopted sixteen guidelines for ethical behavior by pharmacists. The guidelines, which are deliberately broad so that nations may adapt them in creating their own ethics codes, mention several topics of particular note: (1) the independence of the profession, extending to the refusal to dispense medications, including prescriptions, if it serves the patient's health; (2) the role of pharmacists as health educators; and (3) respect for the freedom of choice of patients. A more recent statement was adopted by the Council of the International Pharmaceutical Federation (FIP) at its Council meeting in Vancouver on 5th September 1997.

<http://www.fip.org/pdf/codeeth.pdf>

Introduction:

A profession is identified by the willingness of individual practitioners to comply with ethical and professional standards which exceed minimum legal requirements.

Pharmacists are health professionals who help people to maintain good health, to avoid ill health and, where appropriate, to acquire and make the best use of their medicines. The role of the pharmacist has changed significantly in the last twenty years. Whilst the fundamental ethical principles remain essentially the same, this Code of Ethics has been redrafted to reaffirm and state publicly the principles that form the basis of the roles and responsibilities of pharmacists. These principles, based on moral obligations and values, are established to enable national pharmaceutical organisations through their Codes of Ethics to guide pharmacists in their relationships with patients, other health professionals, and society generally.

Pharmacists seek to act with fairness and equity in the allocation of health resources available to them.

Principles:

In the practice of their profession:

1. **The pharmacist's prime responsibility is the good of the individual.**

   Obligations:

   –to be objective,

   –to put the good of the individual before personal or commercial interests (including financial interest),

   –to promote the individual's right of access to safe and effective treatment.

2. **The pharmacist shows the same dedication to all.**

   Obligations:

   –to show respect for life and human dignity,

   –to not discriminate between people,

   –to strive to treat and inform each individual according to personal circumstances.

3. **The pharmacist respects the individual's right to freedom of choice of treatment.**

   Obligation:

   –to ensure that where the pharmacist is involved in developing care and treatment plans, this is done in consultation with the individual.

4. **The pharmacist respects and safeguards the individual's right to confidentiality.**

   Obligation:

   –to not disseminate information, which identifies the individual, without informed consent or due cause.

5. **The pharmacist cooperates with colleagues and other professionals and respects their values and abilities.**

   Obligation:

   –to cooperate with colleagues, and other professionals and agencies in efforts to promote good health and treat and prevent ill health.

6. **The pharmacist acts with honesty and integrity in professional relationships.**

   Obligations:

   –to act with conviction of conscience,

   –to avoid practices, behaviour or work conditions that could impair professional judgement.

7. **The pharmacist serves the needs of the individual, the community and society.**

   Obligation:

   –to recognise the responsibilities associated with serving the needs of the individual on the one hand and society at large on the other.

8. **The pharmacist maintains and develops professional knowledge and skills.**

   Obligation:

   –to ensure competency in each pharmaceutical service provided, by continually updating knowledge and skills.

9. **The pharmacist ensures continuity of care in the event of labour disputes, pharmacy closure or conflict with personal moral beliefs.**

   Obligation:

   –to refer the patient to another pharmacist.

   –To ensure that when a pharmacy closes, the patients are informed of the pharmacy to which their records, if held, have been transferred.

CODE OF ETHICS AND GUIDE FOR PROFESSIONAL CONDUCT

American Physical Therapy Association

1981, LAST AMENDED 1991

• • •

The American Physical Therapy Association Code of Ethics articulates eleven ethical principles for the physical therapy profession, which are developed further in the Guide for Professional Conduct. The eleven principles are printed here.

<http://www.apta.org/PT_Practice/ethics_pt/code_ethics>

• • •

Preamble

This Code of Ethics of the American Physical Therapy Association sets forth principles for the ethical practice of physical therapy. All physical therapists are responsible for maintaining and promoting ethical practice. To this end, the physical therapist shall act in the best interest of the patient/client. This Code of Ethics shall be binding on all physical therapists.

Principle 1

A physical therapist shall respect the rights and dignity of all individuals and shall provide compassionate care.

Principle 2

A physical therapist shall act in a trustworthy manner towards patients/clients, and in all other aspects of physical therapy practice.

Principle 3

A physical therapist shall comply with laws and regulations governing physical therapy and shall strive to effect changes that benefit patients/clients.

Principle 4

A physical therapist shall exercise sound professional judgment.

Principle 5

A physical therapist shall achieve and maintain professional competence.

Principle 6

A physical therapist shall maintain and promote high standards for physical therapy practice, education and research.

Principle 7

A physical therapist shall seek only such remuneration as is deserved and reasonable for physical therapy services.

Principle 8

A physical therapist shall provide and make available accurate and relevant information to patients/clients about their care and to the public about physical therapy services.

Principle 9

A physical therapist shall protect the public and the profession from unethical, incompetent, and illegal acts.

Principle 10

A physical therapist shall endeavor to address the health needs of society.

Priniciple 11

A physical therapist shall respect the rights, knowledge, and skills of colleagues and other health care professionals.

OCCUPATIONAL THERAPY CODE OF ETHICS

American Occupational Therapy Association

1988, REVISED 2000

• • •

The Occupational Therapy Code of Ethics, revised in 2000, updates the 1988 Code. Although the code is enforceable only with respect to members of the association, it is interesting because it expressly applies to all "occupational therapy personnel," including therapists, assistants, and students.

http://www.aota.org/general/coe.asp

• • •

The American Occupational Therapy Association and its component members are committed to furthering people's ability to function fully within their total environment. To this end the occupational therapist renders service to clients in all stages of health and illness, to institutions, to other professionals and colleagues, to students, and to the general public. A more recent code was adopted in 2000. This document is heavily principle-based, with references to beneficence, nonmalificence, and justice, as well as fidelity and veracity.

Preamble

The American Occupational Therapy Association's Code of Ethics is a public statement of the common set of values and principles used to promote and maintain high standards of behavior in occupational therapy. The American Occupational Therapy Association and its members are committed to furthering the ability of individuals, groups, and systems to function within their total environment. To this end, occupational therapy personnel (including all staff and personnel who work and assist in providing occupational therapy services, (e.g., aides, orderlies, secretaries, technicians) have a responsibility to provide services to recipients in any stage of health and illness who are individuals, research participants, institutions and businesses, other professionals and colleagues, students, and to the general public.

The *Occupational Therapy Code of Ethics* is a set of principles that applies to occupational therapy personnel at all levels. These principles to which occupational therapists and occupational therapy assistants aspire are part of a lifelong effort to act in an ethical manner. The various roles of practitioner (occupational therapist and occupational therapy assistant), educator, fieldwork educator, clinical supervisor, manager, administrator, consultant, fieldwork coordinator, faculty program director, researcher/scholar, private practice owner, entrepreneur, and student are assumed.

Any action in violation of the spirit and purpose of this Code shall be considered unethical. To ensure compliance with the Code, the Commission on Standards and Ethics (SEC) establishes and maintains the enforcement procedures. Acceptance of membership in the American Occupational Therapy Association commits members to adherence to the Code of Ethics and its enforcement procedures. The Code of Ethics, Core Values and Attitudes of Occupational Therapy Practice (AOTA, 1993), and the Guidelines to the Occupational Therapy Code of Ethics (AOTA, 1998) are aspirational documents designed to be used together to guide occupational therapy personnel.

Principle I. Occupational therapy personnel shall demonstrate a concern for the well-being of the recipients of their services. (beneficence)

A. Occupational therapy personnel shall provide services in a fair and equitable manner. They shall recognize and appreciate the cultural components of economics, geography, race, ethnicity, religious and political factors, marital status, sexual orientation, and disability of all recipients of their services.

B. Occupational therapy practitioners shall strive to ensure that fees are fair and reasonable and commensurate with services performed. When occupational therapy practitioners set fees, they shall set fees considering institutional, local, state, and federal requirements, and with due regard for the service recipient's ability to pay.

C. Occupational therapy personnel shall make every effort to advocate for recipients to obtain needed services through available means.

Principle 2. Occupational therapy personnel shall take reasonable precautions to avoid imposing or inflicting harm upon the recipient of services or to his or her property. (nonmaleficence)

A. Occupational therapy personnel shall maintain relationships that do not exploit the recipient of services sexually, physically, emotionally, financially, socially, or in any other manner.

B. Occupational therapy practitioners shall avoid relationships or activities that interfere with professional judgment and objectivity.

Principle 3. Occupational therapy personnel shall respect the recipient and/or their surrogate(s) as well as the recipient's rights. (autonomy, privacy, confidentiality)

A. Occupational therapy practitioners shall collaborate with service recipients or their surrogate(s) in setting goals and priorities throughout the intervention process.

B. Occupational therapy practitioners shall fully inform the service recipients of the nature, risks, and potential outcomes of any interventions.

C. Occupational therapy practitioners shall obtain informed consent from participants involved in research activities and indicate that they have fully informed and advised the participants of potential risks and outcomes. Occupational therapy practitioners shall endeavor to ensure that the participant(s) comprehend these risks and outcomes.

D. Occupational therapy personnel shall respect the individual's right to refuse professional services or involvement in research or educational activities.

E. Occupational therapy personnel shall protect all privileged confidential forms of written, verbal, and electronic communication gained from educational, practice, research, and investigational activities unless otherwise mandated by local, state, or federal regulations.

Principle 4. Occupational therapy personnel shall achieve and continually maintain high standards of competence. (duties)

A. Occupational therapy practitioners shall hold the appropriate national and state credentials for the services they provide.

B. Occupational therapy practitioners shall use procedures that conform to the standards of practice and other appropriate AOTA documents relevant to practice.

C. Occupational therapy practitioners shall take responsibility for maintaining and documenting competence by participating in professional development and educational activities.

D. Occupational therapy practitioners shall critically examine and keep current with emerging knowledge relevant to their practice so they may perform their duties on the basis of accurate information.

E. Occupational therapy practitioners shall protect service recipients by ensuring that duties assumed by or assigned to other occupational therapy personnel match credentials, qualifications, experience, and scope of practice.

F. Occupational therapy practitioners shall provide appropriate supervision to individuals for whom the practitioners have supervisory responsibility in accordance with Association policies, local, state and federal laws, and institutional values.

G. Occupational therapy practitioners shall refer to or consult with other service providers whenever such a referral or consultation would be helpful to the care of the recipient of service. The referral or consultation process should be done in collaboration with the recipient of service.

Principle 5. Occupational therapy personnel shall comply with laws and Association policies guiding the profession of occupational therapy. (justice)

A. Occupational therapy personnel shall familiarize themselves with and seek to understand and abide by applicable Association policies; local, state, and federal laws; and institutional rules.

B. Occupational therapy practitioners shall remain abreast of revisions in those laws and Association policies that apply to the profession of occupational therapy and shall inform employers, employees, and colleagues of those changes.

C. Occupational therapy practitioners shall require those they supervise in occupational therapy-related activities to adhere to the Code of Ethics.

D. Occupational therapy practitioners shall take reasonable steps to ensure employers are aware of occupational therapy's ethical obligations, as set forth in this Code of Ethics, and of the implications of those obligations for occupational therapy practice, education, and research.

E. Occupational therapy practitioners shall record and report in an accurate and timely manner all information related to professional activities.

Principle 6. Occupational therapy personnel shall provide accurate information about occupational therapy services. (veracity)

A. Occupational therapy personnel shall accurately represent their credentials, qualifications, education, experience, training, and competence. This is of particular importance for those to whom occupational therapy personnel provide their services or with whom occupational therapy practitioners have a professional relationship.

B. Occupational therapy personnel shall disclose any professional, personal, financial, business, or volunteer affiliations that may pose a conflict of interest to those with whom they may establish a professional, contractual, or other working relationship.

C. Occupational therapy personnel shall refrain from using or participating in the use of any form of communication that contains false, fraudulent, deceptive, or unfair statements or claims.

D. Occupational therapy practitioners shall accept the responsibility for their professional actions which reduce the public's trust in occupational therapy services and those that perform those services.

Principle 7. Occupational therapy personnel shall treat colleagues and other professionals with fairness, discretion, and integrity. (fidelity)

A. Occupational therapy personnel shall preserve, respect, and safeguard confidential information about colleagues and staff, unless otherwise mandated by national, state, or local laws.

B. Occupational therapy practitioners shall accurately represent the qualifications, views, contributions, and findings of colleagues.

C. Occupational therapy personnel shall take adequate measures to discourage, prevent, expose, and correct any breaches of the Code of Ethics and report any breaches of the Code of Ethics to the appropriate authority.

D. Occupational therapy personnel shall familiarize themselves with established policies and procedures for handling concerns about this Code of Ethics, including familiarity with national, state, local, district, and territorial procedures for handling ethics complaints. These include policies and procedures created by the American Occupational Therapy Association, licensing and regulatory bodies, employers, agencies, certification boards, and other organizations who have jurisdiction over occupational therapy practice.

CODE OF ETHICS OF THE PHYSICIAN ASSISTANT PROFESSION

American Academy of Physician Assistants

1983, AMENDED 1985, REAFFIRMED 1990

• • •

The American Academy of Physician Assistants' (AAPA) current Code of Ethics was adopted in 1983, amended in 1985, and reaffirmed in 1990. In addition to standard features, the code explicitly recognizes that: (1) It is necessarily limited and does not preclude additional, equally imperative, obligations; (2) physician assistants should use their skills "to contribute to an improved community"; and (3) physician assistants "shall place service before material gain." The AAPA also has issued Guidelines for Professional Conduct, which interpret and elaborate upon the principles found in the code of ethics.

<http://www.aapa.org/images/GECINSERTATION.pdf>

The American Academy of Physician Assistants recognizes its responsibility to aid the profession in maintaining high standards in the provision of quality and accessible health care services. The following principles delineate the standards governing the conduct of physician assistants in their professional interactions with patients, colleagues, other health professionals and the general public. Realizing that no code can encompass all ethical responsibilities of the physician assistant, this enumeration of obligations in the Code of Ethics is not comprehensive and does not constitute a denial of the existence of other obligations, equally imperative, though not specifically mentioned.

Physician assistants shall be committed to providing competent medical care, assuming as their primary responsibility the health, safety, welfare and dignity of all humans.

Physician assistants shall extend to each patient the full measure of their ability as dedicated, empathetic health care providers and shall assume responsibility for the skillful and proficient transactions of their professional duties.

Physician assistants shall deliver needed health care services to health consumers without regard to sex, age, race, creed, socioeconomic and political status.

Physician assistants shall adhere to all state and federal laws governing informed consent concerning the patient's health care.

Physician assistants shall seek consultation with their supervising physician, other health providers, or qualified professionals having special skills, knowledge or experience whenever the welfare of the patient will be safeguarded or advanced by such consultation. Supervision should include ongoing communication between the physician and the physician assistant regarding the care of all patients.

Physician assistants shall take personal responsibility for being familiar with and adhering to all federal/state laws applicable to the practice of their profession.

Physician assistants shall provide only those services for which they are qualified via education and/or experience and by pertinent legal regulatory process.

Physician assistants shall not misrepresent in any manner, either directly or indirectly, their skills, training, professional credentials, identity, or services.

Physician assistants shall uphold the doctrine of confidentiality regarding privileged patient information, unless required to release such information by law or such information becomes necessary to protect the welfare of the patient or the community.

Physician assistants shall strive to maintain and increase the quality of individual health care service through individual study and continuing education.

Physician assistants shall have the duty to respect the law, to uphold the dignity of the physician assistant profession and to accept its ethical principles. The physician assistant shall not participate in or conceal any activity that will bring discredit or dishonor to the physician assistant profession and shall expose, without fear or favor, any illegal or unethical conduct in the medical profession.

Physician assistants, ever cognizant of the needs of the community, shall use the knowledge and experience acquired as professionals to contribute to an improved community.

Physician assistants shall place service before material gain and must carefully guard against conflicts of professional interest.

Physician assistants shall strive to maintain a spirit of cooperation with their professional organizations and the general public.

ETHICAL PRINCIPLES OF PSYCHOLOGISTS AND CODE OF CONDUCT

American Psychological Association

1992, REVISED 2002

• • •

A substantially revised version of the Ethical Principles of Psychologists and Code of Conduct was adopted by the American Psychological Association (APA) in 1992. The 1992 revision, which is still current, consists of an introduction, a preamble, six general principles, and specific ethical standards. The preamble and general principles represent "aspirational goals to guide psychologists toward the highest ideals of psychology," whereas the ethical standards establish "enforceable rules for conduct." The standards are noteworthy for the scope of the topics addressed, including sexual harassment, misuse of influence, and informed consent, that pertain to therapeutic and research relationships, as well as those that pertain to the care and use of animals in research.

The preamble, general principles, and excerpts from the ethical standards follow.

<http://www.apa.org/ethics/code2002.html>

• • •

Preamble

Psychologists are committed to increasing scientific and professional knowledge of behavior and people's understanding of themselves and others and to the use of such knowledge to improve the condition of individuals, organizations, and society. Psychologists respect and protect civil and human rights and the central importance of freedom of inquiry and expression in research, teaching, and publication. They strive to help the public in developing informed judgments and choices concerning human behavior. In doing so, they perform many roles, such as researcher, educator, diagnostician, therapist, supervisor, consultant, administrator, social interventionist, and expert witness. This Ethics Code provides a common set of principles and standards upon which psychologists build their professional and scientific work.

This Ethics Code is intended to provide specific standards to cover most situations encountered by psychologists.

It has as its goals the welfare and protection of the individuals and groups with whom psychologists work and the education of members, students, and the public regarding ethical standards of the discipline.

The development of a dynamic set of ethical standards for psychologists' work-related conduct requires a personal commitment and lifelong effort to act ethically; to encourage ethical behavior by students, supervisees, employees, and colleagues; and to consult with others concerning ethical problems.

GENERAL PRINCIPLES

This section consists of General Principles. General Principles, as opposed to Ethical Standards, are aspirational in nature. Their intent is to guide and inspire psychologists toward the very highest ethical ideals of the profession. General Principles, in contrast to Ethical Standards, do not represent obligations and should not form the basis for imposing sanctions. Relying upon General Principles for either of these reasons distorts both their meaning and purpose.

Principle A: Beneficence and Nonmaleficence

Psychologists strive to benefit those with whom they work and take care to do no harm. In their professional actions, psychologists seek to safeguard the welfare and rights of those with whom they interact professionally and other affected persons, and the welfare of animal subjects of research. When conflicts occur among psychologists' obligations or concerns, they attempt to resolve these conflicts in a responsible fashion that avoids or minimizes harm. Because psychologists' scientific and professional judgments and actions may affect the lives of others, they are alert to and guard against personal, financial, social, organizational, or political factors that might lead to misuse of their influence. Psychologists strive to be aware of the possible effect of their own physical and mental health on their ability to help those with whom they work.

Principle B: Fidelity and Responsibility

Psychologists establish relationships of trust with those with whom they work. They are aware of their professional and scientific responsibilities to society and to the specific communities in which they work. Psychologists uphold professional standards of conduct, clarify their professional roles and obligations, accept appropriate responsibility for their behavior, and seek to manage conflicts of interest that could lead to exploitation or harm. Psychologists consult with, refer to, or cooperate with other professionals and institutions to the extent needed to serve the best interests of those with whom they work. They are concerned about the ethical compliance of their colleagues' scientific and professional conduct. Psychologists strive to contribute a portion of their professional time for little or no compensation or personal advantage.

Principle C: Integrity

Psychologists seek to promote accuracy, honesty, and truthfulness in the science, teaching, and practice of psychology. In these activities psychologists do not steal, cheat, or engage in fraud, subterfuge, or intentional misrepresentation of fact. Psychologists strive to keep their promises and to avoid unwise or unclear commitments. In situations in which deception may be ethically justifiable to maximize benefits and minimize harm, psychologists have a serious obligation to consider the need for, the possible consequences of, and their responsibility to correct any resulting mistrust or other harmful effects that arise from the use of such techniques.

Principle D: Justice

Psychologists recognize that fairness and justice entitle all persons to access to and benefit from the contributions of psychology and to equal quality in the processes, procedures, and services being conducted by psychologists. Psychologists exercise reasonable judgment and take precautions to ensure that their potential biases, the boundaries of their competence, and the limitations of their expertise do not lead to or condone unjust practices.

Principle E: Respect for People's Rights and Dignity

Psychologists respect the dignity and worth of all people, and the rights of individuals to privacy, confidentiality, and self-determination. Psychologists are aware that special safeguards may be necessary to protect the rights and welfare of persons or communities whose vulnerabilities impair autonomous decision making. Psychologists are aware of and respect cultural, individual, and role differences, including those based on age, gender, gender identity, race, ethnicity, culture, national origin, religion, sexual orientation, disability, language, and socioeconomic status and consider these factors when working with members of such groups. Psychologists try to eliminate the effect on their work of biases based on those factors, and they do not knowingly participate in or condone activities of others based upon such prejudices.

ETHICAL STANDARDS

I. Resolving Ethical Issues

I.01 MISUSE OF PSYCHOLOGISTS' WORK

If psychologists learn of misuse or misrepresentation of their work, they take reasonable steps to correct or minimize the misuse or misrepresentation.

I.02 CONFLICTS BETWEEN ETHICS AND LAW, REGULATIONS, OR OTHER GOVERNING LEGAL AUTHORITY

If psychologists' ethical responsibilities conflict with law, regulations, or other governing legal authority, psychologists make known their commitment to the Ethics Code and take steps to resolve the conflict. If the conflict is unresolvable via such means, psychologists may adhere to the requirements of the law, regulations, or other governing legal authority.

I.03 CONFLICTS BETWEEN ETHICS AND ORGANIZATIONAL DEMANDS

If the demands of an organization with which psychologists are affiliated or for whom they are working conflict with this Ethics Code, psychologists clarify the nature of the conflict, make known their commitment to the Ethics Code, and to the extent feasible, resolve the conflict in a way that permits adherence to the Ethics Code.

I.04 INFORMAL RESOLUTION OF ETHICAL VIOLATIONS

When psychologists believe that there may have been an ethical violation by another psychologist, they attempt to resolve the issue by bringing it to the attention of that individual, if an informal resolution appears appropriate and the intervention does not violate any confidentiality rights that may be involved. (See also Standards 1.02, Conflicts Between Ethics and Law, Regulations, or Other Governing Legal Authority, and 1.03, Conflicts Between Ethics and Organizational Demands.)

I.05 REPORTING ETHICAL VIOLATIONS

If an apparent ethical violation has substantially harmed or is likely to substantially harm a person or organization and is not appropriate for informal resolution under Standard 1.04, Informal Resolution of Ethical Violations, or is not resolved properly in that fashion, psychologists take further action appropriate to the situation. Such action might include referral to state or national committees on professional ethics, to state licensing boards, or to the appropriate institutional authorities. This standard does not apply when an intervention would violate confidentiality rights or when psychologists have been retained to review the work of another psychologist whose professional conduct is in question. (See also Standard 1.02, Conflicts Between Ethics and Law, Regulations, or Other Governing Legal Authority.)

I.06 COOPERATING WITH ETHICS COMMITTEES

Psychologists cooperate in ethics investigations, proceedings, and resulting requirements of the APA or any affiliated state psychological association to which they belong. In doing so, they address any confidentiality issues. Failure to cooperate is itself an ethics violation. However, making a request for deferment of adjudication of an ethics complaint pending the outcome of litigation does not alone constitute noncooperation.

I.07 IMPROPER COMPLAINTS

Psychologists do not file or encourage the filing of ethics complaints that are made with reckless disregard for or willful ignorance of facts that would disprove the allegation.

I.08 UNFAIR DISCRIMINATION AGAINST COMPLAINANTS AND RESPONDENTS

Psychologists do not deny persons employment, advancement, admissions to academic or other programs, tenure, or promotion, based solely upon their having made or their being the subject of an ethics complaint. This does not preclude taking action based upon the outcome of such proceedings or considering other appropriate information.

2. Competence

2.01 BOUNDARIES OF COMPETENCE

(a) Psychologists provide services, teach, and conduct research with populations and in areas only within the boundaries of their competence, based on their education, training, supervised experience, consultation, study, or professional experience.

(b) Where scientific or professional knowledge in the discipline of psychology establishes that an understanding of factors associated with age, gender, gender identity, race, ethnicity, culture, national origin, religion, sexual orientation, disability, language, or socioeconomic status is essential for effective implementation of their services or research, psychologists have or obtain the training, experience, consultation, or supervision necessary to ensure the competence of their services, or they make appropriate referrals, except as provided in Standard 2.02, Providing Services in Emergencies.

(c) Psychologists planning to provide services, teach, or conduct research involving populations, areas, techniques, or technologies new to them undertake

relevant education, training, supervised experience, consultation, or study.

(d) When psychologists are asked to provide services to individuals for whom appropriate mental health services are not available and for which psychologists have not obtained the competence necessary, psychologists with closely related prior training or experience may provide such services in order to ensure that services are not denied if they make a reasonable effort to obtain the competence required by using relevant research, training, consultation, or study.

(e) In those emerging areas in which generally recognized standards for preparatory training do not yet exist, psychologists nevertheless take reasonable steps to ensure the competence of their work and to protect clients/patients, students, supervisees, research participants, organizational clients, and others from harm.

(f) When assuming forensic roles, psychologists are or become reasonably familiar with the judicial or administrative rules governing their roles.

2.02 PROVIDING SERVICES IN EMERGENCIES

In emergencies, when psychologists provide services to individuals for whom other mental health services are not available and for which psychologists have not obtained the necessary training, psychologists may provide such services in order to ensure that services are not denied. The services are discontinued as soon as the emergency has ended or appropriate services are available.

2.03 MAINTAINING COMPETENCE

Psychologists undertake ongoing efforts to develop and maintain their competence.

2.04 BASES FOR SCIENTIFIC AND PROFESSIONAL JUDGMENTS

Psychologists' work is based upon established scientific and professional knowledge of the discipline. (See also Standards 2.01e, Boundaries of Competence, and 10.01b, Informed Consent to Therapy.)

2.05 DELEGATION OF WORK TO OTHERS

Psychologists who delegate work to employees, supervisees, or research or teaching assistants or who use the services of others, such as interpreters, take reasonable steps to (1) avoid delegating such work to persons who have a multiple relationship with those being served that would likely lead to exploitation or loss of objectivity; (2) authorize only those responsibilities that such persons can be expected to perform competently on the basis of their education, training, or experience, either independently or with the level of supervision being provided; and (3) see that such persons perform these services competently. (See also Standards 2.02, Providing Services in Emergencies; 3.05, Multiple Relationships; 4.01, Maintaining Confidentiality; 9.01, Bases for Assessments; 9.02, Use of Assessments; 9.03, Informed Consent in Assessments; and 9.07, Assessment by Unqualified Persons.)

2.06 PERSONAL PROBLEMS AND CONFLICTS

(a) Psychologists refrain from initiating an activity when they know or should know that there is a substantial likelihood that their personal problems will prevent them from performing their work-related activities in a competent manner.

(b) When psychologists become aware of personal problems that may interfere with their performing work-related duties adequately, they take appropriate measures, such as obtaining professional consultation or assistance, and determine whether they should limit, suspend, or terminate their work-related duties. (See also Standard 10.10, Terminating Therapy.)

3. Human Relations

3.01 UNFAIR DISCRIMINATION

In their work-related activities, psychologists do not engage in unfair discrimination based on age, gender, gender identity, race, ethnicity, culture, national origin, religion, sexual orientation, disability, socioeconomic status, or any basis proscribed by law.

3.02 SEXUAL HARASSMENT

Psychologists do not engage in sexual harassment. Sexual harassment is sexual solicitation, physical advances, or verbal or nonverbal conduct that is sexual in nature, that occurs in connection with the psychologist's activities or roles as a psychologist, and that either (1) is unwelcome, is offensive, or creates a hostile workplace or educational environment, and the psychologist knows or is told this or (2) is sufficiently severe or intense to be abusive to a reasonable person in the context. Sexual harassment can consist of a single intense or severe act or of multiple persistent or pervasive acts. (See also Standard 1.08, Unfair Discrimination Against Complainants and Respondents.)

3.03 OTHER HARASSMENT

Psychologists do not knowingly engage in behavior that is harassing or demeaning to persons with whom they interact in their work based on factors such as those persons' age, gender, gender identity, race, ethnicity, culture, national origin, religion, sexual orientation, disability, language, or socioeconomic status.

3.04 AVOIDING HARM

Psychologists take reasonable steps to avoid harming their clients/patients, students, supervisees, research participants, organizational clients, and others with whom they work, and to minimize harm where it is foreseeable and unavoidable.

3.05 MULTIPLE RELATIONSHIPS

(a) A multiple relationship occurs when a psychologist is in a professional role with a person and (1) at the same time is in another role with the same person, (2) at the same time is in a relationship with a person closely associated with or related to the person with whom the psychologist has the professional relationship, or (3) promises to enter into another relationship in the future with the person or a person closely associated with or related to the person.

A psychologist refrains from entering into a multiple relationship if the multiple relationship could reasonably be expected to impair the psychologist's objectivity, competence, or effectiveness in performing his or her functions as a psychologist, or otherwise risks exploitation or harm to the person with whom the professional relationship exists.

Multiple relationships that would not reasonably be expected to cause impairment or risk exploitation or harm are not unethical.

(b) If a psychologist finds that, due to unforeseen factors, a potentially harmful multiple relationship has arisen, the psychologist takes reasonable steps to resolve it with due regard for the best interests of the affected person and maximal compliance with the Ethics Code.

(c) When psychologists are required by law, institutional policy, or extraordinary circumstances to serve in more than one role in judicial or administrative proceedings, at the outset they clarify role expectations and the extent of confidentiality and thereafter as changes occur. (See also Standards 3.04, Avoiding Harm, and 3.07, Third-Party Requests for Services.)

3.06 CONFLICT OF INTEREST

Psychologists refrain from taking on a professional role when personal, scientific, professional, legal, financial, or other interests or relationships could reasonably be expected to (1) impair their objectivity, competence, or effectiveness in performing their functions as psychologists or (2) expose the person or organization with whom the professional relationship exists to harm or exploitation.

3.07 THIRD-PARTY REQUESTS FOR SERVICES

When psychologists agree to provide services to a person or entity at the request of a third party, psychologists attempt to clarify at the outset of the service the nature of the relationship with all individuals or organizations involved. This clarification includes the role of the psychologist (e.g., therapist, consultant, diagnostician, or expert witness), an identification of who is the client, the probable uses of the services provided or the information obtained, and the fact that there may be limits to confidentiality. (See also Standards 3.05, Multiple Relationships, and 4.02, Discussing the Limits of Confidentiality.)

3.08 EXPLOITATIVE RELATIONSHIPS

Psychologists do not exploit persons over whom they have supervisory, evaluative, or other authority such as clients/patients, students, supervisees, research participants, and employees. (See also Standards 3.05, Multiple Relationships; 6.04, Fees and Financial Arrangements; 6.05, Barter With Clients/Patients; 7.07, Sexual Relationships With Students and Supervisees; 10.05, Sexual Intimacies With Current Therapy Clients/Patients; 10.06, Sexual Intimacies With Relatives or Significant Others of Current Therapy Clients/Patients; 10.07, Therapy With Former Sexual Partners; and 10.08, Sexual Intimacies With Former Therapy Clients/Patients.)

3.09 COOPERATION WITH OTHER PROFESSIONALS

When indicated and professionally appropriate, psychologists cooperate with other professionals in order to serve their clients/patients effectively and appropriately. (See also Standard 4.05, Disclosures.)

3.10 INFORMED CONSENT

(a) When psychologists conduct research or provide assessment, therapy, counseling, or consulting services in person or via electronic transmission or other forms of communication, they obtain the informed consent of the individual or individuals using language that is reasonably understandable to that person or persons except when conducting such activities without consent is mandated by law or governmental regulation or as otherwise provided in this Ethics Code. (See also Standards 8.02, Informed Consent to Research; 9.03, Informed Consent in Assessments; and 10.01, Informed Consent to Therapy.)

(b) For persons who are legally incapable of giving informed consent, psychologists nevertheless (1) provide an appropriate explanation, (2) seek the individual's assent, (3) consider such persons' preferences and best interests, and (4) obtain appropriate permission from a legally authorized person, if such substitute consent is permitted or required by law. When consent by a legally authorized person is not permitted or required by law, psychologists take reasonable steps to protect the individual's rights and welfare.

(c) When psychological services are court ordered or otherwise mandated, psychologists inform the individual of the nature of the anticipated services, including whether the services are court ordered or mandated and any limits of confidentiality, before proceeding.

(d) Psychologists appropriately document written or oral consent, permission, and assent. (See also Standards 8.02, Informed Consent to Research; 9.03, Informed Consent in Assessments; and 10.01, Informed Consent to Therapy.)

3.11 PSYCHOLOGICAL SERVICES DELIVERED TO OR THROUGH ORGANIZATIONS

(a) Psychologists delivering services to or through organizations provide information beforehand to clients and when appropriate those directly affected by the services about (1) the nature and objectives of the services, (2) the intended recipients, (3) which of the individuals are clients, (4) the relationship the psychologist will have with each person and the organization, (5) the probable uses of services provided and information obtained, (6) who will have access to the information, and (7) limits of confidentiality. As soon as feasible, they provide information about the results and conclusions of such services to appropriate persons.

(b) If psychologists will be precluded by law or by organizational roles from providing such information to particular individuals or groups, they so inform those individuals or groups at the outset of the service.

3.12 INTERRUPTION OF PSYCHOLOGICAL SERVICES

Unless otherwise covered by contract, psychologists make reasonable efforts to plan for facilitating services in the event that psychological services are interrupted by factors such as the psychologist's illness, death, unavailability, relocation, or retirement or by the client's/patient's relocation or financial limitations. (See also Standard 6.02c, Maintenance, Dissemination, and Disposal of Confidential Records of Professional and Scientific Work.)

4. Privacy and Confidentiality

4.01 MAINTAINING CONFIDENTIALITY

Psychologists have a primary obligation and take reasonable precautions to protect confidential information obtained through or stored in any medium, recognizing that the extent and limits of confidentiality may be regulated by law or established by institutional rules or professional or scientific relationship. (See also Standard 2.05, Delegation of Work to Others.)

4.02 DISCUSSING THE LIMITS OF CONFIDENTIALITY

(a) Psychologists discuss with persons (including, to the extent feasible, persons who are legally incapable of giving informed consent and their legal representatives) and organizations with whom they establish a scientific or professional relationship (1) the relevant limits of confidentiality and (2) the foreseeable uses of the information generated through their psychological activities. (See also Standard 3.10, Informed Consent.)

(b) Unless it is not feasible or is contraindicated, the discussion of confidentiality occurs at the outset of the relationship and thereafter as new circumstances may warrant.

(c) Psychologists who offer services, products, or information via electronic transmission inform clients/patients of the risks to privacy and limits of confidentiality.

4.03 RECORDING

Before recording the voices or images of individuals to whom they provide services, psychologists obtain permission from all such persons or their legal representatives. (See also Standards 8.03, Informed Consent for Recording Voices and Images in Research; 8.05, Dispensing With Informed Consent for Research; and 8.07, Deception in Research.)

4.04 MINIMIZING INTRUSIONS ON PRIVACY

(a) Psychologists include in written and oral reports and consultations, only information germane to the purpose for which the communication is made.

(b) Psychologists discuss confidential information obtained in their work only for appropriate scientific or professional purposes and only with persons clearly concerned with such matters.

4.05 DISCLOSURES

(a) Psychologists may disclose confidential information with the appropriate consent of the organizational client, the individual client/patient, or another legally authorized person on behalf of the client/patient unless prohibited by law.

(b) Psychologists disclose confidential information without the consent of the individual only as mandated by law, or where permitted by law for a valid purpose such as to (1) provide needed professional services; (2) obtain appropriate professional consultations; (3) protect the client/patient, psychologist, or others from harm; or (4) obtain payment for services from a client/patient, in which instance disclosure is limited to the minimum that is necessary to achieve the purpose. (See also Standard 6.04e, Fees and Financial Arrangements.)

4.06 CONSULTATIONS

When consulting with colleagues, (1) psychologists do not disclose confidential information that reasonably could lead to the identification of a client/patient, research participant, or other person or organization with whom they have a confidential relationship unless they have obtained the prior consent of the person or organization or the disclosure cannot be avoided, and (2) they disclose information only to the extent necessary to achieve the purposes of the consultation. (See also Standard 4.01, Maintaining Confidentiality.)

4.07 USE OF CONFIDENTIAL INFORMATION FOR DIDACTIC OR OTHER PURPOSES

Psychologists do not disclose in their writings, lectures, or other public media, confidential, personally identifiable information concerning their clients/patients, students, research participants, organizational clients, or other recipients of their services that they obtained during the course of their work, unless (1) they take reasonable steps to disguise the person or organization, (2) the person or organization has consented in writing, or (3) there is legal authorization for doing so.

5. Advertising and Other Public Statements

5.01 AVOIDANCE OF FALSE OR DECEPTIVE STATEMENTS

(a) Public statements include but are not limited to paid or unpaid advertising, product endorsements, grant applications, licensing applications, other credentialing applications, brochures, printed matter, directory listings, personal resumes or curricula vitae, or comments for use in media such as print or electronic transmission, statements in legal proceedings, lectures and public oral presentations, and published materials. Psychologists do not knowingly make public statements that are false, deceptive, or fraudulent concerning their research, practice, or other work activities or those of persons or organizations with which they are affiliated.

(b) Psychologists do not make false, deceptive, or fraudulent statements concerning (1) their training, experience, or competence; (2) their academic degrees; (3) their credentials; (4) their institutional or association affiliations; (5) their services; (6) the scientific or clinical basis for, or results or degree of success of, their services; (7) their fees; or (8) their publications or research findings.

(c) Psychologists claim degrees as credentials for their health services only if those degrees (1) were earned from a regionally accredited educational institution or (2) were the basis for psychology licensure by the state in which they practice.

5.02 STATEMENTS BY OTHERS

(a) Psychologists who engage others to create or place public statements that promote their professional practice, products, or activities retain professional responsibility for such statements.

(b) Psychologists do not compensate employees of press, radio, television, or other communication media in return for publicity in a news item. (See also Standard 1.01, Misuse of Psychologists' Work.)

(c) A paid advertisement relating to psychologists' activities must be identified or clearly recognizable as such.

5.03 DESCRIPTIONS OF WORKSHOPS AND NON-DEGREE-GRANTING EDUCATIONAL PROGRAMS

To the degree to which they exercise control, psychologists responsible for announcements, catalogs, brochures, or advertisements describing workshops, seminars, or other non-degree-granting educational programs ensure that they accurately describe the audience for which the program is intended, the educational objectives, the presenters, and the fees involved.

5.04 MEDIA PRESENTATIONS

When psychologists provide public advice or comment via print, Internet, or other electronic transmission, they take precautions to ensure that statements (1) are based on their professional knowledge, training, or experience in accord with appropriate psychological literature and practice; (2) are otherwise consistent with this Ethics Code; and (3) do not indicate that a professional relationship has been established with the recipient. (See also Standard 2.04, Bases for Scientific and Professional Judgments.)

5.05 TESTIMONIALS

Psychologists do not solicit testimonials from current therapy clients/patients or other persons who because of their particular circumstances are vulnerable to undue influence.

5.06 IN-PERSON SOLICITATION

Psychologists do not engage, directly or through agents, in uninvited in-person solicitation of business from actual or potential therapy clients/patients or other persons who because of their particular circumstances are vulnerable to undue influence. However, this prohibition does not preclude (1) attempting to implement appropriate collateral contacts for the purpose of benefiting an already engaged therapy client/patient or (2) providing disaster or community outreach services.

6. Record Keeping and Fees

6.01 DOCUMENTATION OF PROFESSIONAL AND SCIENTIFIC WORK AND MAINTENANCE OF RECORDS

Psychologists create, and to the extent the records are under their control, maintain, disseminate, store, retain, and dispose of records and data relating to their professional and scientific work in order to (1) facilitate provision of services later by them or by other professionals, (2) allow for replication of research design and analyses, (3) meet institutional requirements, (4) ensure accuracy of billing and payments, and (5) ensure compliance with law. (See also Standard 4.01, Maintaining Confidentiality.)

6.02 MAINTENANCE, DISSEMINATION, AND DISPOSAL OF CONFIDENTIAL RECORDS OF PROFESSIONAL AND SCIENTIFIC WORK

(a) Psychologists maintain confidentiality in creating, storing, accessing, transferring, and disposing of records under their control, whether these are written, automated, or in any other medium. (See also Standards 4.01, Maintaining Confidentiality, and 6.01, Documentation of Professional and Scientific Work and Maintenance of Records.)

(b) If confidential information concerning recipients of psychological services is entered into databases or systems of records available to persons whose access has not been consented to by the recipient, psychologists use coding or other techniques to avoid the inclusion of personal identifiers.

(c) Psychologists make plans in advance to facilitate the appropriate transfer and to protect the confidentiality of records and data in the event of psychologists' withdrawal from positions or practice. (See also Standards 3.12, Interruption of Psychological Services, and 10.09, Interruption of Therapy.)

6.03 WITHHOLDING RECORDS FOR NONPAYMENT

Psychologists may not withhold records under their control that are requested and needed for a client's/patient's emergency treatment solely because payment has not been received.

6.04 FEES AND FINANCIAL ARRANGEMENTS

(a) As early as is feasible in a professional or scientific relationship, psychologists and recipients of psychological services reach an agreement specifying compensation and billing arrangements.

(b) Psychologists' fee practices are consistent with law.

(c) Psychologists do not misrepresent their fees.

(d) If limitations to services can be anticipated because of limitations in financing, this is discussed with the recipient of services as early as is feasible. (See also Standards 10.09, Interruption of Therapy, and 10.10, Terminating Therapy.)

(e) If the recipient of services does not pay for services as agreed, and if psychologists intend to use collection agencies or legal measures to collect the fees, psychologists first inform the person that such measures will be taken and provide that person an opportunity to make prompt payment. (See also Standards 4.05, Disclosures; 6.03, Withholding Records for Nonpayment; and 10.01, Informed Consent to Therapy.)

6.05 BARTER WITH CLIENTS/PATIENTS

Barter is the acceptance of goods, services, or other nonmonetary remuneration from clients/patients in return for psychological services. Psychologists may barter only if (1) it is not clinically contraindicated, and (2) the resulting arrangement is not exploitative. (See also Standards 3.05, Multiple Relationships, and 6.04, Fees and Financial Arrangements.)

6.06 ACCURACY IN REPORTS TO PAYORS AND FUNDING SOURCES

In their reports to payors for services or sources of research funding, psychologists take reasonable steps to ensure the accurate reporting of the nature of the service provided or research conducted, the fees, charges, or payments, and where applicable, the identity of the provider, the findings, and the diagnosis. (See also Standards 4.01, Maintaining Confidentiality; 4.04, Minimizing Intrusions on Privacy; and 4.05, Disclosures.)

6.07 REFERRALS AND FEES

When psychologists pay, receive payment from, or divide fees with another professional, other than in an employer-employee relationship, the payment to each is based on the services provided (clinical, consultative, administrative, or other) and is not based on the referral itself. (See also Standard 3.09, Cooperation With Other Professionals.)

7. Education and Training

7.01 DESIGN OF EDUCATION AND TRAINING PROGRAMS

Psychologists responsible for education and training programs take reasonable steps to ensure that the programs are designed to provide the appropriate knowledge and proper experiences, and to meet the requirements for licensure, certification, or other goals for which claims are made by the program. (See also Standard 5.03, Descriptions of Workshops and Non-Degree-Granting Educational Programs.)

7.02 DESCRIPTIONS OF EDUCATION AND TRAINING PROGRAMS

Psychologists responsible for education and training programs take reasonable steps to ensure that there is a current and accurate description of the program content (including participation in required course- or program-related counseling, psychotherapy, experiential groups, consulting projects, or community service), training goals and objectives, stipends and benefits, and requirements that must be met for satisfactory completion of the program. This information must be made readily available to all interested parties.

7.03 ACCURACY IN TEACHING

(a) Psychologists take reasonable steps to ensure that course syllabi are accurate regarding the subject matter to be covered, bases for evaluating progress, and the nature of course experiences. This standard does not preclude an instructor from modifying course content or requirements when the instructor considers it pedagogically necessary or desirable, so long as students are made aware of these modifications in a manner that enables them to fulfill course requirements. (See also Standard 5.01, Avoidance of False or Deceptive Statements.)

(b) When engaged in teaching or training, psychologists present psychological information accurately. (See also Standard 2.03, Maintaining Competence.)

7.04 STUDENT DISCLOSURE OF PERSONAL INFORMATION

Psychologists do not require students or supervisees to disclose personal information in course- or program-related activities, either orally or in writing, regarding sexual history, history of abuse and neglect, psychological treatment, and relationships with parents, peers, and spouses or significant others except if (1) the program or training facility has clearly identified this requirement in its admissions and program materials or (2) the information is necessary to evaluate or obtain assistance for students whose personal problems could reasonably be judged to be preventing them from performing their training- or professionally related activities in a competent manner or posing a threat to the students or others.

7.05 MANDATORY INDIVIDUAL OR GROUP THERAPY

(a) When individual or group therapy is a program or course requirement, psychologists responsible for that program allow students in undergraduate and graduate programs the option of selecting such therapy from practitioners unaffiliated with the program. (See also Standard 7.02, Descriptions of Education and Training Programs.)

(b) Faculty who are or are likely to be responsible for evaluating students' academic performance do not themselves provide that therapy. (See also Standard 3.05, Multiple Relationships.)

7.06 ASSESSING STUDENT AND SUPERVISEE PERFORMANCE

(a) In academic and supervisory relationships, psychologists establish a timely and specific process for providing feedback to students and supervisees. Information regarding the process is provided to the student at the beginning of supervision.

(b) Psychologists evaluate students and supervisees on the basis of their actual performance on relevant and established program requirements.

7.07 SEXUAL RELATIONSHIPS WITH STUDENTS AND SUPERVISEES

Psychologists do not engage in sexual relationships with students or supervisees who are in their department, agency, or training center or over whom psychologists have or are likely to have evaluative authority. (See also Standard 3.05, Multiple Relationships.)

8. Research and Publication

8.01 INSTITUTIONAL APPROVAL

When institutional approval is required, psychologists provide accurate information about their research proposals and obtain approval prior to conducting the research. They conduct the research in accordance with the approved research protocol.

8.02 INFORMED CONSENT TO RESEARCH

(a) When obtaining informed consent as required in Standard 3.10, Informed Consent, psychologists inform participants about (1) the purpose of the research, expected duration, and procedures; (2) their right to decline to participate and to withdraw from the research once participation has begun; (3) the foreseeable consequences of declining or withdrawing; (4) reasonably foreseeable factors that may be expected to influence their willingness to participate such as potential risks, discomfort, or adverse effects; (5) any prospective research benefits; (6) limits of confidentiality; (7) incentives for participation; and (8) whom to contact for questions about the research and research participants' rights. They provide opportunity for the prospective participants to ask questions and receive answers. (See also Standards 8.03, Informed Consent for Recording Voices and Images in Research; 8.05, Dispensing With Informed Consent for Research; and 8.07, Deception in Research.)

(b) Psychologists conducting intervention research involving the use of experimental treatments clarify to participants at the outset of the research (1) the experimental nature of the treatment; (2) the services that will or will not be available to the control group(s) if appropriate; (3) the means by which assignment to treatment and control groups will be made; (4) available treatment alternatives if an individual does not wish to participate in the research or wishes to withdraw once a study has begun; and (5) compensation for or monetary costs of participating including, if appropriate, whether reimbursement from the participant or a third-party payor will be sought. (See also Standard 8.02a, Informed Consent to Research.)

8.03 INFORMED CONSENT FOR RECORDING VOICES AND IMAGES IN RESEARCH

Psychologists obtain informed consent from research participants prior to recording their voices or images for data collection unless (1) the research consists solely of naturalistic observations in public places, and it is not anticipated that the recording will be used in a manner that could cause personal identification or harm, or (2) the research design includes deception, and consent for the use of the recording is obtained during debriefing. (See also Standard 8.07, Deception in Research.)

8.04 CLIENT/PATIENT, STUDENT, AND SUBORDINATE RESEARCH PARTICIPANTS

(a) When psychologists conduct research with clients/ patients, students, or subordinates as participants, psychologists take steps to protect the prospective participants from adverse consequences of declining or withdrawing from participation.

(b) When research participation is a course requirement or an opportunity for extra credit, the prospective participant is given the choice of equitable alternative activities.

8.05 DISPENSING WITH INFORMED CONSENT FOR RESEARCH

Psychologists may dispense with informed consent only (1) where research would not reasonably be assumed to create distress or harm and involves (a) the study of normal educational practices, curricula, or classroom management methods conducted in educational settings; (b) only anonymous questionnaires, naturalistic observations, or archival research for which disclosure of responses would not place participants at risk of criminal or civil liability or damage their financial standing, employability, or reputation, and confidentiality is protected; or (c) the study of factors related to job or organization effectiveness conducted in organizational settings for which there is no risk to participants' employability, and confidentiality is protected or (2) where otherwise permitted by law or federal or institutional regulations.

8.06 OFFERING INDUCEMENTS FOR RESEARCH PARTICIPATION

(a) Psychologists make reasonable efforts to avoid offering excessive or inappropriate financial or other inducements for research participation when such inducements are likely to coerce participation.

(b) When offering professional services as an inducement for research participation, psychologists clarify the nature of the services, as well as the risks, obligations, and limitations. (See also Standard 6.05, Barter With Clients/Patients.)

8.07 DECEPTION IN RESEARCH

(a) Psychologists do not conduct a study involving deception unless they have determined that the use of deceptive techniques is justified by the study's significant prospective scientific, educational, or applied value and that effective nondeceptive alternative procedures are not feasible.

(b) Psychologists do not deceive prospective participants about research that is reasonably expected to cause physical pain or severe emotional distress.

(c) Psychologists explain any deception that is an integral feature of the design and conduct of an experiment to participants as early as is feasible,

preferably at the conclusion of their participation, but no later than at the conclusion of the data collection, and permit participants to withdraw their data. (See also Standard 8.08, Debriefing.)

8.08 DEBRIEFING

(a) Psychologists provide a prompt opportunity for participants to obtain appropriate information about the nature, results, and conclusions of the research, and they take reasonable steps to correct any misconceptions that participants may have of which the psychologists are aware.

(b) If scientific or humane values justify delaying or withholding this information, psychologists take reasonable measures to reduce the risk of harm.

(c) When psychologists become aware that research procedures have harmed a participant, they take reasonable steps to minimize the harm.

8.09 HUMANE CARE AND USE OF ANIMALS IN RESEARCH

(a) Psychologists acquire, care for, use, and dispose of animals in compliance with current federal, state, and local laws and regulations, and with professional standards.

(b) Psychologists trained in research methods and experienced in the care of laboratory animals supervise all procedures involving animals and are responsible for ensuring appropriate consideration of their comfort, health, and humane treatment.

(c) Psychologists ensure that all individuals under their supervision who are using animals have received instruction in research methods and in the care, maintenance, and handling of the species being used, to the extent appropriate to their role. (See also Standard 2.05, Delegation of Work to Others.)

(d) Psychologists make reasonable efforts to minimize the discomfort, infection, illness, and pain of animal subjects.

(e) Psychologists use a procedure subjecting animals to pain, stress, or privation only when an alternative procedure is unavailable and the goal is justified by its prospective scientific, educational, or applied value.

(f) Psychologists perform surgical procedures under appropriate anesthesia and follow techniques to avoid infection and minimize pain during and after surgery.

(g) When it is appropriate that an animal's life be terminated, psychologists proceed rapidly, with an effort to minimize pain and in accordance with accepted procedures.

8.10 REPORTING RESEARCH RESULTS

(a) Psychologists do not fabricate data. (See also Standard 5.01a, Avoidance of False or Deceptive Statements.)

(b) If psychologists discover significant errors in their published data, they take reasonable steps to correct such errors in a correction, retraction, erratum, or other appropriate publication means.

8.11 PLAGIARISM

Psychologists do not present portions of another's work or data as their own, even if the other work or data source is cited occasionally.

8.12 PUBLICATION CREDIT

(a) Psychologists take responsibility and credit, including authorship credit, only for work they have actually performed or to which they have substantially contributed. (See also Standard 8.12b, Publication Credit.)

(b) Principal authorship and other publication credits accurately reflect the relative scientific or professional contributions of the individuals involved, regardless of their relative status. Mere possession of an institutional position, such as department chair, does not justify authorship credit. Minor contributions to the research or to the writing for publications are acknowledged appropriately, such as in footnotes or in an introductory statement.

(c) Except under exceptional circumstances, a student is listed as principal author on any multiple-authored article that is substantially based on the student's doctoral dissertation. Faculty advisors discuss publication credit with students as early as feasible and throughout the research and publication process as appropriate. (See also Standard 8.12b, Publication Credit.)

8.13 DUPLICATE PUBLICATION OF DATA

Psychologists do not publish, as original data, data that have been previously published. This does not preclude republishing data when they are accompanied by proper acknowledgment.

8.14 SHARING RESEARCH DATA FOR VERIFICATION

(a) After research results are published, psychologists do not withhold the data on which their conclusions are based from other competent professionals who seek to verify the substantive claims through reanalysis and who intend to use such data only for that purpose, provided that the confidentiality of the participants can be protected and unless legal rights concerning proprietary data preclude their release.

This does not preclude psychologists from requiring that such individuals or groups be responsible for costs associated with the provision of such information.

(b) Psychologists who request data from other psychologists to verify the substantive claims through reanalysis may use shared data only for the declared purpose. Requesting psychologists obtain prior written agreement for all other uses of the data.

8.15 REVIEWERS

Psychologists who review material submitted for presentation, publication, grant, or research proposal review respect the confidentiality of and the proprietary rights in such information of those who submitted it.

9. Assessment

9.01 BASES FOR ASSESSMENTS

(a) Psychologists base the opinions contained in their recommendations, reports, and diagnostic or evaluative statements, including forensic testimony, on information and techniques sufficient to substantiate their findings. (See also Standard 2.04, Bases for Scientific and Professional Judgments.)

(b) Except as noted in 9.01c, psychologists provide opinions of the psychological characteristics of individuals only after they have conducted an examination of the individuals adequate to support their statements or conclusions. When, despite reasonable efforts, such an examination is not practical, psychologists document the efforts they made and the result of those efforts, clarify the probable impact of their limited information on the reliability and validity of their opinions, and appropriately limit the nature and extent of their conclusions or recommendations. (See also Standards 2.01, Boundaries of Competence, and 9.06, Interpreting Assessment Results.)

(c) When psychologists conduct a record review or provide consultation or supervision and an individual examination is not warranted or necessary for the opinion, psychologists explain this and the sources of information on which they based their conclusions and recommendations.

9.02 USE OF ASSESSMENTS

(a) Psychologists administer, adapt, score, interpret, or use assessment techniques, interviews, tests, or instruments in a manner and for purposes that are appropriate in light of the research on or evidence of the usefulness and proper application of the techniques.

(b) Psychologists use assessment instruments whose validity and reliability have been established for use with members of the population tested. When such validity or reliability has not been established, psychologists describe the strengths and limitations of test results and interpretation.

(c) Psychologists use assessment methods that are appropriate to an individual's language preference and competence, unless the use of an alternative language is relevant to the assessment issues.

9.03 INFORMED CONSENT IN ASSESSMENTS

(a) Psychologists obtain informed consent for assessments, evaluations, or diagnostic services, as described in Standard 3.10, Informed Consent, except when (1) testing is mandated by law or governmental regulations; (2) informed consent is implied because testing is conducted as a routine educational, institutional, or organizational activity (e.g., when participants voluntarily agree to assessment when applying for a job); or (3) one purpose of the testing is to evaluate decisional capacity. Informed consent includes an explanation of the nature and purpose of the assessment, fees, involvement of third parties, and limits of confidentiality and sufficient opportunity for the client/patient to ask questions and receive answers.

(b) Psychologists inform persons with questionable capacity to consent or for whom testing is mandated by law or governmental regulations about the nature and purpose of the proposed assessment services, using language that is reasonably understandable to the person being assessed.

(c) Psychologists using the services of an interpreter obtain informed consent from the client/patient to use that interpreter, ensure that confidentiality of test results and test security are maintained, and include in their recommendations, reports, and diagnostic or evaluative statements, including forensic testimony, discussion of any limitations on the data obtained. (See also Standards 2.05, Delegation of Work to Others; 4.01, Maintaining Confidentiality; 9.01, Bases for Assessments; 9.06, Interpreting Assessment Results; and 9.07, Assessment by Unqualified Persons.)

9.04 RELEASE OF TEST DATA

(a) The term *test data* refers to raw and scaled scores, client/patient responses to test questions or stimuli, and psychologists' notes and recordings concerning client/patient statements and behavior during an examination. Those portions of test materials that include client/patient responses are included in the definition of *test data*. Pursuant to a client/patient release, psychologists provide test data to the client/patient or other persons identified in the release. Psychologists may refrain from releasing test data to protect a client/patient or others from substantial harm or misuse or misrepresentation of the data or the test, recognizing that in many instances release of confidential information under these circumstances is regulated by law. (See also Standard 9.11, Maintaining Test Security.)

(b) In the absence of a client/patient release, psychologists provide test data only as required by law or court order.

9.05 TEST CONSTRUCTION

Psychologists who develop tests and other assessment techniques use appropriate psychometric procedures and current scientific or professional knowledge for test design, standardization, validation, reduction or elimination of bias, and recommendations for use.

9.06 INTERPRETING ASSESSMENT RESULTS

When interpreting assessment results, including automated interpretations, psychologists take into account the purpose of the assessment as well as the various test factors, test-taking abilities, and other characteristics of the person being assessed, such as situational, personal, linguistic, and cultural differences, that might affect psychologists' judgments or reduce the accuracy of their interpretations. They indicate any significant limitations of their interpretations. (See also Standards 2.01b and c, Boundaries of Competence, and 3.01, Unfair Discrimination.)

9.07 ASSESSMENT BY UNQUALIFIED PERSONS

Psychologists do not promote the use of psychological assessment techniques by unqualified persons, except when such use is conducted for training purposes with appropriate supervision. (See also Standard 2.05, Delegation of Work to Others.)

9.08 OBSOLETE TESTS AND OUTDATED TEST RESULTS

(a) Psychologists do not base their assessment or intervention decisions or recommendations on data or test results that are outdated for the current purpose.

(b) Psychologists do not base such decisions or recommendations on tests and measures that are obsolete and not useful for the current purpose.

9.09 TEST SCORING AND INTERPRETATION SERVICES

(a) Psychologists who offer assessment or scoring services to other professionals accurately describe the purpose, norms, validity, reliability, and applications of the procedures and any special qualifications applicable to their use.

(b) Psychologists select scoring and interpretation services (including automated services) on the basis of evidence of the validity of the program and procedures as well as on other appropriate considerations. (See also Standard 2.01b and c, Boundaries of Competence.)

(c) Psychologists retain responsibility for the appropriate application, interpretation, and use of assessment instruments, whether they score and interpret such tests themselves or use automated or other services.

9.10 EXPLAINING ASSESSMENT RESULTS

Regardless of whether the scoring and interpretation are done by psychologists, by employees or assistants, or by automated or other outside services, psychologists take reasonable steps to ensure that explanations of results are given to the individual or designated representative unless the nature of the relationship precludes provision of an explanation of results (such as in some organizational consulting, preemployment or security screenings, and forensic evaluations), and this fact has been clearly explained to the person being assessed in advance.

9.11. MAINTAINING TEST SECURITY

The term *test materials* refers to manuals, instruments, protocols, and test questions or stimuli and does not include *test data* as defined in Standard 9.04, Release of Test Data. Psychologists make reasonable efforts to maintain the integrity and security of test materials and other assessment techniques consistent with law and contractual obligations, and in a manner that permits adherence to this Ethics Code.

10. Therapy

10.01 INFORMED CONSENT TO THERAPY

(a) When obtaining informed consent to therapy as required in Standard 3.10, Informed Consent, psychologists inform clients/patients as early as is feasible in the therapeutic relationship about the nature and anticipated course of therapy, fees, involvement of third parties, and limits of confidentiality and provide sufficient opportunity for the client/patient to ask questions and receive answers. (See also Standards 4.02, Discussing the Limits of Confidentiality, and 6.04, Fees and Financial Arrangements.)

(b) When obtaining informed consent for treatment for which generally recognized techniques and procedures have not been established, psychologists

inform their clients/patients of the developing nature of the treatment, the potential risks involved, alternative treatments that may be available, and the voluntary nature of their participation. (See also Standards 2.01e, Boundaries of Competence, and 3.10, Informed Consent.)

(c) When the therapist is a trainee and the legal responsibility for the treatment provided resides with the supervisor, the client/patient, as part of the informed consent procedure, is informed that the therapist is in training and is being supervised and is given the name of the supervisor.

10.02 THERAPY INVOLVING COUPLES OR FAMILIES

(a) When psychologists agree to provide services to several persons who have a relationship (such as spouses, significant others, or parents and children), they take reasonable steps to clarify at the outset (1) which of the individuals are clients/patients and (2) the relationship the psychologist will have with each person. This clarification includes the psychologist's role and the probable uses of the services provided or the information obtained. (See also Standard 4.02, Discussing the Limits of Confidentiality.)

(b) If it becomes apparent that psychologists may be called on to perform potentially conflicting roles (such as family therapist and then witness for one party in divorce proceedings), psychologists take reasonable steps to clarify and modify, or withdraw from, roles appropriately. (See also Standard 3.05c, Multiple Relationships.)

10.03 GROUP THERAPY

When psychologists provide services to several persons in a group setting, they describe at the outset the roles and responsibilities of all parties and the limits of confidentiality.

10.04 PROVIDING THERAPY TO THOSE SERVED BY OTHERS

In deciding whether to offer or provide services to those already receiving mental health services elsewhere, psychologists carefully consider the treatment issues and the potential client's/patient's welfare. Psychologists discuss these issues with the client/patient or another legally authorized person on behalf of the client/patient in order to minimize the risk of confusion and conflict, consult with the other service providers when appropriate, and proceed with caution and sensitivity to the therapeutic issues.

10.05 SEXUAL INTIMACIES WITH CURRENT THERAPY CLIENTS/PATIENTS

Psychologists do not engage in sexual intimacies with current therapy clients/patients.

10.06 SEXUAL INTIMACIES WITH RELATIVES OR SIGNIFICANT OTHERS OF CURRENT THERAPY CLIENTS/PATIENTS

Psychologists do not engage in sexual intimacies with individuals they know to be close relatives, guardians, or significant others of current clients/patients. Psychologists do not terminate therapy to circumvent this standard.

10.07 THERAPY WITH FORMER SEXUAL PARTNERS

Psychologists do not accept as therapy clients/patients persons with whom they have engaged in sexual intimacies.

10.08 SEXUAL INTIMACIES WITH FORMER THERAPY CLIENTS/PATIENTS

(a) Psychologists do not engage in sexual intimacies with former clients/patients for at least two years after cessation or termination of therapy.

(b) Psychologists do not engage in sexual intimacies with former clients/patients even after a two-year interval except in the most unusual circumstances. Psychologists who engage in such activity after the two years following cessation or termination of therapy and of having no sexual contact with the former client/patient bear the burden of demonstrating that there has been no exploitation, in light of all relevant factors, including (1) the amount of time that has passed since therapy terminated; (2) the nature, duration, and intensity of the therapy; (3) the circumstances of termination; (4) the client's/patient's personal history; (5) the client's/patient's current mental status; (6) the likelihood of adverse impact on the client/patient; and (7) any statements or actions made by the therapist during the course of therapy suggesting or inviting the possibility of a posttermination sexual or romantic relationship with the client/patient. (See also Standard *3.05, Multiple Relationships.*)

10.09 INTERRUPTION OF THERAPY

When entering into employment or contractual relationships, psychologists make reasonable efforts to provide for orderly and appropriate resolution of responsibility for client/patient care in the event that the employment or contractual relationship ends, with paramount consideration given to the welfare of the client/patient. (See also Standard *3.12, Interruption of Psychological Services.*)

10.10 TERMINATING THERAPY

(a) Psychologists terminate therapy when it becomes reasonably clear that the client/patient no longer needs the service, is not likely to benefit, or is being harmed by continued service.

(b) Psychologists may terminate therapy when threatened or otherwise endangered by the client/patient or another person with whom the client/patient has a relationship.

(c) Except where precluded by the actions of clients/patients or third-party payors, prior to termination psychologists provide pretermination counseling and suggest alternative service providers as appropriate.

HISTORY AND EFFECTIVE DATE

This version of the APA Ethics Code was adopted by the American Psychological Association's Council of Representatives during its meeting, August 21, 2002, and is effective beginning June 1, 2003. Inquiries concerning the substance or interpretation of the APA Ethics Code should be addressed to the Director, Office of Ethics, American Psychological Association, 750 First Street, NE, Washington, DC 20002–4242. The Ethics Code and information regarding the Code can be found on the APA web site, <http://www.apa.org/ethics.> The standards in this Ethics Code will be used to adjudicate complaints brought concerning alleged conduct occurring on or after the effective date. Complaints regarding conduct occurring prior to the effective date will be adjudicated on the basis of the version of the Ethics Code that was in effect at the time the conduct occurred.

The APA has previously published its Ethics Code as follows:

American Psychological Association (1953). Ethical standards of psychologists. Washington, DC: Author.

American Psychological Association (1959). Ethical standards of psychologists. American Psychologist, 14, 279–282.

American Psychological Association (1963). Ethical standards of psychologists. American Psychologist, 18, 56–60.

American Psychological Association (1968). Ethical standards of psychologists. American Psychologist, 23, 357–361.

American Psychological Association (1977, March). Ethical standards of psychologists. APA Monitor, 22–23.

American Psychological Association (1979). Ethical standards of psychologists. Washington, DC: Author.

American Psychological Association (1981). Ethical principles of psychologists. American Psychologist, 36, 633–638.

American Psychological Association (1990). Ethical principles of psychologists (Amended June 2, 1989). American Psychologist, 45, 390–395.

American Psychological Association (1992). Ethical principles of psychologists and code of conduct. *American Psychologist, 47,* 1597–1611.

Request copies of the APA's Ethical Principles of Psychologists and Code of Conduct from the APA Order Department, 750 First Street, NE, Washington, DC 20002–4242, or phone (202) 336–5510.

CODE OF ETHICS

National Association of Social Workers

1979, REVISED 1990, 1996, 1999

• • •

The current Code of Ethics of the National Association of Social Workers (NASW) was adopted by the NASW Delegate Assembly in 1979 and revised in 1990, 1996 and 1999.

The Code is based primarily on certain core values such as service, justice, dignity, competence, integrity and the importance of human relationships.

Preamble

The primary mission of the social work profession is to enhance human well-being and help meet the basic human needs of all people, with particular attention to the needs and empowerment of people who are vulnerable, oppressed, and living in poverty. A historic and defining feature of social work is the profession's focus on individual well-being in a social context and the well-being of society. Fundamental to social work is attention to the environmental forces that create, contribute to, and address problems in living.

Social workers promote social justice and social change with and on behalf of clients. "Clients" is used inclusively to refer to individuals, families, groups, organizations, and communities. Social workers are sensitive to cultural and ethnic diversity and strive to end discrimination, oppression, poverty, and other forms of social injustice. These activities may be in the form of direct practice, community organizing, supervision, consultation, administration, advocacy, social and political action, policy development and implementation, education, and research and evaluation. Social workers seek to enhance the capacity of people to address their own needs. Social workers also seek to promote the responsiveness of organizations, communities, and other social institutions to individuals' needs and social problems.

The mission of the social work profession is rooted in a set of core values. These core values, embraced by social workers throughout the profession's history, are the foundation of social work's unique purpose and perspective:

• service
• social justice
• dignity and worth of the person
• importance of human relationships
• integrity
• competence.

This constellation of core values reflects what is unique to the social work profession. Core values, and the principles that flow from them, must be balanced within the context and complexity of the human experience.

Purpose of the NASW Code of Ethics

Professional ethics are at the core of social work. The profession has an obligation to articulate its basic values, ethical principles, and ethical standards. The *NASW Code of Ethics* sets forth these values, principles, and standards to guide social workers' conduct. The *Code* is relevant to all social workers and social work students, regardless of their professional functions, the settings in which they work, or the populations they serve.

The *NASW Code of Ethics* serves six purposes:

1. The *Code* identifies core values on which social work's mission is based.
2. The *Code* summarizes broad ethical principles that reflect the profession's core values and establishes a set of specific ethical standards that should be used to guide social work practice.
3. The *Code* is designed to help social workers identify relevant considerations when professional obligations conflict or ethical uncertainties arise.
4. The *Code* provides ethical standards to which the general public can hold the social work profession accountable.
5. The *Code* socializes practitioners new to the field to social work's mission, values, ethical principles, and ethical standards.
6. The *Code* articulates standards that the social work profession itself can use to assess whether social workers have engaged in unethical conduct. NASW has formal procedures to adjudicate ethics complaints filed against its members.* In subscribing to this *Code*, social workers are required to cooperate in its implementation, participate in NASW adjudication proceedings, and abide by any NASW disciplinary rulings or sanctions based on it.

*For information on NASW adjudication procedures, see *NASW Procedures for the Adjudication of Grievances*.

The *Code* offers a set of values, principles, and standards to guide decision making and conduct when ethical issues arise. It does not provide a set of rules that prescribe how social workers should act in all situations. Specific applications of the *Code* must take into account the context in which it is being considered and the possibility of conflicts among the *Code*'s values, principles, and standards. Ethical responsibilities flow from all human relationships, from the personal and familial to the social and professional.

Further, the *NASW Code of Ethics* does not specify which values, principles, and standards are most important and ought to outweigh others in instances when they conflict. Reasonable differences of opinion can and do exist among social workers with respect to the ways in which values, ethical principles, and ethical standards should be rank ordered when they conflict. Ethical decision making in a given situation must apply the informed judgment of the individual social worker and should also consider how the issues would be judged in a peer review process where the ethical standards of the profession would be applied.

Ethical decision making is a process. There are many instances in social work where simple answers are not available to resolve complex ethical issues. Social workers should take into consideration all the values, principles, and standards in this *Code* that are relevant to any situation in which ethical judgment is warranted. Social workers' decisions and actions should be consistent with the spirit as well as the letter of this *Code*.

In addition to this *Code*, there are many other sources of information about ethical thinking that may be useful. Social workers should consider ethical theory and principles generally, social work theory and research, laws, regulations, agency policies, and other relevant codes of ethics, recognizing that among codes of ethics social workers should consider the *NASW Code of Ethics* as their primary source. Social workers also should be aware of the impact on ethical decision making of their clients' and their own personal values and cultural and religious beliefs and practices. They should be aware of any conflicts between personal and professional values and deal with them responsibly. For additional guidance social workers should consult the relevant literature on professional ethics and ethical decision making and seek appropriate consultation when faced with ethical dilemmas. This may involve consultation with an agency-based or social work organization's ethics committee, a regulatory body, knowledgeable colleagues, supervisors, or legal counsel.

Instances may arise when social workers' ethical obligations conflict with agency policies or relevant laws or regulations. When such conflicts occur, social workers must make a responsible effort to resolve the conflict in a manner that is consistent with the values, principles, and standards expressed in this *Code*. If a reasonable resolution of the conflict does not appear possible, social workers should seek proper consultation before making a decision.

The *NASW Code of Ethics* is to be used by NASW and by individuals, agencies, organizations, and bodies (such as licensing and regulatory boards, professional liability insurance providers, courts of law, agency boards of directors, government agencies, and other professional groups) that choose to adopt it or use it as a frame of reference. Violation of standards in this *Code* does not automatically imply legal liability or violation of the law. Such determination can only be made in the context of legal and judicial proceedings. Alleged violations of the *Code* would be subject to a peer review process. Such processes are generally separate from legal or administrative procedures and insulated from legal review or proceedings to allow the profession to counsel and discipline its own members.

A code of ethics cannot guarantee ethical behavior. Moreover, a code of ethics cannot resolve all ethical issues or disputes or capture the richness and complexity involved in striving to make responsible choices within a moral community. Rather, a code of ethics sets forth values, ethical principles, and ethical standards to which professionals aspire and by which their actions can be judged. Social workers' ethical behavior should result from their personal commitment to engage in ethical practice. The *NASW Code of Ethics* reflects the commitment of all social workers to uphold the profession's values and to act ethically. Principles and standards must be applied by individuals of good character who discern moral questions and, in good faith, seek to make reliable ethical judgments.

Ethical Principles

The following broad ethical principles are based on social work's core values of service, social justice, dignity and worth of the person, importance of human relationships, integrity, and competence. These principles set forth ideals to which all social workers should aspire.

VALUE: *Service*

ETHICAL PRINCIPLE: *Social workers' primary goal is to help people in need and to address social problems.*

Social workers elevate service to others above self-interest. Social workers draw on their knowledge, values, and skills to help people in need and to address social problems. Social workers are encouraged to volunteer some portion of their professional skills with no expectation of significant financial return (pro bono service).

VALUE: *Social Justice*

ETHICAL PRINCIPLE: *Social workers challenge social injustice.*

Social workers pursue social change, particularly with and on behalf of vulnerable and oppressed individuals and groups of people. Social workers' social change efforts are focused primarily on issues of poverty, unemployment, discrimination, and other forms of social injustice. These activities seek to promote sensitivity to and knowledge about oppression and cultural and ethnic diversity. Social workers strive to ensure access to needed information, services, and resources; equality of opportunity; and meaningful participation in decision making for all people.

VALUE: *Dignity and Worth of the Person*

ETHICAL PRINCIPLE: *Social workers respect the inherent dignity and worth of the person.*

Social workers treat each person in a caring and respectful fashion, mindful of individual differences and cultural and ethnic diversity. Social workers promote clients' socially responsible self-determination. Social workers seek to enhance clients' capacity and opportunity to change and to address their own needs. Social workers are cognizant of their dual responsibility to clients and to the broader society. They seek to resolve conflicts between clients' interests and the broader society's interests in a socially responsible manner consistent with the values, ethical principles, and ethical standards of the profession.

VALUE: *Importance of Human Relationships*

ETHICAL PRINCIPLE: *Social workers recognize the central importance of human relationships.*

Social workers understand that relationships between and among people are an important vehicle for change. Social workers engage people as partners in the helping process. Social workers seek to strengthen relationships among people in a purposeful effort to promote, restore, maintain, and enhance the well-being of individuals, families, social groups, organizations, and communities.

VALUE: *Integrity*

ETHICAL PRINCIPLE: *Social workers behave in a trustworthy manner.*

Social workers are continually aware of the profession's mission, values, ethical principles, and ethical standards and

practice in a manner consistent with them. Social workers act honestly and responsibly and promote ethical practices on the part of the organizations with which they are affiliated.

VALUE: *Competence*

ETHICAL PRINCIPLE: *Social workers practice within their areas of competence and develop and enhance their professional expertise.*

Social workers continually strive to increase their professional knowledge and skills and to apply them in practice. Social workers should aspire to contribute to the knowledge base of the profession.

Ethical Standards

The following ethical standards are relevant to the professional activities of all social workers. These standards concern (1) social workers' ethical responsibilities to clients, (2) social workers' ethical responsibilities to colleagues, (3) social workers' ethical responsibilities in practice settings, (4) social workers' ethical responsibilities as professionals, (5) social workers' ethical responsibilities to the social work profession, and (6) social workers' ethical responsibilities to the broader society.

Some of the standards that follow are enforceable guidelines for professional conduct, and some are aspirational. The extent to which each standard is enforceable is a matter of professional judgment to be exercised by those responsible for reviewing alleged violations of ethical standards.

I. Social Workers' Ethical Responsibilities to Clients

1.01 COMMITMENT TO CLIENTS

Social workers' primary responsibility is to promote the well-being of clients. In general, clients' interests are primary. However, social workers' responsibility to the larger society or specific legal obligations may on limited occasions supersede the loyalty owed clients, and clients should be so advised. (Examples include when a social worker is required by law to report that a client has abused a child or has threatened to harm self or others.)

1.02 SELF-DETERMINATION

Social workers respect and promote the right of clients to self-determination and assist clients in their efforts to identify and clarify their goals. Social workers may limit clients' right to self-determination when, in the social workers' professional judgment, clients' actions or potential actions pose a serious, foreseeable, and imminent risk to themselves or others.

1.03 INFORMED CONSENT

(a) Social workers should provide services to clients only in the context of a professional relationship based, when appropriate, on valid informed consent. Social workers should use clear and understandable language to inform clients of the purpose of the services, risks related to the services, limits to services because of the requirements of a third-party payer, relevant costs, reasonable alternatives, clients' right to refuse or withdraw consent, and the time frame covered by the consent. Social workers should provide clients with an opportunity to ask questions.

(b) In instances when clients are not literate or have difficulty understanding the primary language used in the practice setting, social workers should take steps to ensure clients' comprehension. This may include providing clients with a detailed verbal explanation or arranging for a qualified interpreter or translator whenever possible.

(c) In instances when clients lack the capacity to provide informed consent, social workers should protect clients' interests by seeking permission from an appropriate third party, informing clients consistent with the clients' level of understanding. In such instances social workers should seek to ensure that the third party acts in a manner consistent with clients' wishes and interests. Social workers should take reasonable steps to enhance such clients' ability to give informed consent.

(d) In instances when clients are receiving services involuntarily, social workers should provide information about the nature and extent of services and about the extent of clients' right to refuse service.

(e) Social workers who provide services via electronic media (such as computer, telephone, radio, and television) should inform recipients of the limitations and risks associated with such services.

(f) Social workers should obtain clients' informed consent before audiotaping or videotaping clients or permitting observation of services to clients by a third party.

1.04 COMPETENCE

(a) Social workers should provide services and represent themselves as competent only within the boundaries of their education, training, license, certification, consultation received, supervised experience, or other relevant professional experience.

(b) Social workers should provide services in substantive areas or use intervention techniques or approaches that are new to them only after engaging in appropriate study, training, consultation, and supervision from people who are competent in those interventions or techniques.

(c) When generally recognized standards do not exist with respect to an emerging area of practice, social workers should exercise careful judgment and take responsible steps (including appropriate education, research, training, consultation, and supervision) to ensure the competence of their work and to protect clients from harm.

1.05 CULTURAL COMPETENCE AND SOCIAL DIVERSITY

(a) Social workers should understand culture and its function in human behavior and society, recognizing the strengths that exist in all cultures.

(b) Social workers should have a knowledge base of their clients' cultures and be able to demonstrate competence in the provision of services that are sensitive to clients' cultures and to differences among people and cultural groups.

(c) Social workers should obtain education about and seek to understand the nature of social diversity and oppression with respect to race, ethnicity, national origin, color, sex, sexual orientation, age, marital status, political belief, religion, and mental or physical disability.

1.06 CONFLICTS OF INTEREST

(a) Social workers should be alert to and avoid conflicts of interest that interfere with the exercise of professional discretion and impartial judgment. Social workers should inform clients when a real or potential conflict of interest arises and take reasonable steps to resolve the issue in a manner that makes the clients' interests primary and protects clients' interests to the greatest extent possible. In some cases, protecting clients' interests may require termination of the professional relationship with proper referral of the client.

(b) Social workers should not take unfair advantage of any professional relationship or exploit others to further their personal, religious, political, or business interests.

(c) Social workers should not engage in dual or multiple relationships with clients or former clients in which there is a risk of exploitation or potential harm to the client. In instances when dual or multiple relationships are unavoidable, social workers should take steps to protect clients and are responsible for setting clear, appropriate, and culturally sensitive boundaries. (Dual or multiple relationships occur when social workers relate to clients in more than one relationship, whether professional, social, or business. Dual or multiple relationships can occur simultaneously or consecutively.)

(d) When social workers provide services to two or more people who have a relationship with each other (for example, couples, family members), social workers should clarify with all parties which individuals will be considered clients and the nature of social workers' professional obligations to the various individuals who are receiving services. Social workers who anticipate a conflict of interest among the individuals receiving services or who anticipate having to perform in potentially conflicting roles (for example, when a social worker is asked to testify in a child custody dispute or divorce proceedings involving clients) should clarify their role with the parties involved and take appropriate action to minimize any conflict of interest.

1.07 PRIVACY AND CONFIDENTIALITY

(a) Social workers should respect clients' right to privacy. Social workers should not solicit private information from clients unless it is essential to providing services or conducting social work evaluation or research. Once private information is shared, standards of confidentiality apply.

(b) Social workers may disclose confidential information when appropriate with valid consent from a client or a person legally authorized to consent on behalf of a client.

(c) Social workers should protect the confidentiality of all information obtained in the course of professional service, except for compelling professional reasons. The general expectation that social workers will keep information confidential does not apply when disclosure is necessary to prevent serious, foreseeable, and imminent harm to a client or other identifiable person. In all instances, social workers should disclose the least amount of confidential information necessary to achieve the desired purpose; only information that is directly relevant to the purpose for which the disclosure is made should be revealed.

(d) Social workers should inform clients, to the extent possible, about the disclosure of confidential information and the potential consequences, when feasible before the disclosure is made. This applies whether social workers disclose confidential information on the basis of a legal requirement or client consent.

(e) Social workers should discuss with clients and other interested parties the nature of confidentiality and limitations of clients' right to confidentiality. Social workers should review with clients circumstances where confidential information may be requested and where disclosure of confidential information may be legally required. This discussion should occur as soon as possible in the social worker–client relationship and as needed throughout the course of the relationship.

(f) When social workers provide counseling services to families, couples, or groups, social workers should seek agreement among the parties involved concerning each individual's right to confidentiality and obligation to preserve the confidentiality of information shared by others. Social workers should inform participants in family, couples, or group counseling that social workers cannot guarantee that all participants will honor such agreements.

(g) Social workers should inform clients involved in family, couples, marital, or group counseling of the social worker's, employer's, and agency's policy concerning the social worker's disclosure of confidential information among the parties involved in the counseling.

(h) Social workers should not disclose confidential information to third-party payers unless clients have authorized such disclosure.

(i) Social workers should not discuss confidential information in any setting unless privacy can be ensured. Social workers should not discuss confidential information in public or semipublic areas such as hallways, waiting rooms, elevators, and restaurants.

(j) Social workers should protect the confidentiality of clients during legal proceedings to the extent permitted by law. When a court of law or other legally authorized body orders social workers to disclose confidential or privileged information without a client's consent and such disclosure could cause harm to the client, social workers should request that the court withdraw the order or limit the order as narrowly as possible or maintain the records under seal, unavailable for public inspection.

(k) Social workers should protect the confidentiality of clients when responding to requests from members of the media.

(l) Social workers should protect the confidentiality of clients' written and electronic records and other sensitive information. Social workers should take reasonable steps to ensure that clients' records are stored in a secure location and that clients' records are not available to others who are not authorized to have access.

(m) Social workers should take precautions to ensure and maintain the confidentiality of information transmitted to other parties through the use of computers, electronic mail, facsimile machines, telephones and telephone answering machines, and other electronic or computer technology. Disclosure of identifying information should be avoided whenever possible.

(n) Social workers should transfer or dispose of clients' records in a manner that protects clients' confidentiality and is consistent with state statutes governing records and social work licensure.

(o) Social workers should take reasonable precautions to protect client confidentiality in the event of the social worker's termination of practice, incapacitation, or death.

(p) Social workers should not disclose identifying information when discussing clients for teaching or training purposes unless the client has consented to disclosure of confidential information.

(q) Social workers should not disclose identifying information when discussing clients with consultants unless the client has consented to disclosure of confidential information or there is a compelling need for such disclosure.

(r) Social workers should protect the confidentiality of deceased clients consistent with the preceding standards.

I.08 ACCESS TO RECORDS

(a) Social workers should provide clients with reasonable access to records concerning the clients. Social workers who are concerned that clients' access to their records could cause serious misunderstanding or harm to the client should provide assistance in interpreting the records and consultation with the client regarding the records. Social workers should limit clients' access to their records, or portions of their records, only in exceptional circumstances when there is compelling evidence that such access would cause serious harm to the client. Both clients' requests and the rationale for withholding some or all of the record should be documented in clients' files.

(b) When providing clients with access to their records, social workers should take steps to protect the confidentiality of other individuals identified or discussed in such records.

I.09 SEXUAL RELATIONSHIPS

(a) Social workers should under no circumstances engage in sexual activities or sexual contact with current clients, whether such contact is consensual or forced.

(b) Social workers should not engage in sexual activities or sexual contact with clients' relatives or other individuals with whom clients maintain a close personal relationship when there is a risk of exploitation or potential harm to the client. Sexual activity or sexual contact with clients' relatives or

other individuals with whom clients maintain a personal relationship has the potential to be harmful to the client and may make it difficult for the social worker and client to maintain appropriate professional boundaries. Social workers—not their clients, their clients' relatives, or other individuals with whom the client maintains a personal relationship—assume the full burden for setting clear, appropriate, and culturally sensitive boundaries.

(c) Social workers should not engage in sexual activities or sexual contact with former clients because of the potential for harm to the client. If social workers engage in conduct contrary to this prohibition or claim that an exception to this prohibition is warranted because of extraordinary circumstances, it is social workers—not their clients—who assume the full burden of demonstrating that the former client has not been exploited, coerced, or manipulated, intentionally or unintentionally.

(d) Social workers should not provide clinical services to individuals with whom they have had a prior sexual relationship. Providing clinical services to a former sexual partner has the potential to be harmful to the individual and is likely to make it difficult for the social worker and individual to maintain appropriate professional boundaries.

I.10 PHYSICAL CONTACT

Social workers should not engage in physical contact with clients when there is a possibility of psychological harm to the client as a result of the contact (such as cradling or caressing clients). Social workers who engage in appropriate physical contact with clients are responsible for setting clear, appropriate, and culturally sensitive boundaries that govern such physical contact.

I.11 SEXUAL HARASSMENT

Social workers should not sexually harass clients. Sexual harassment includes sexual advances, sexual solicitation, requests for sexual favors, and other verbal or physical conduct of a sexual nature.

I.12 DEROGATORY LANGUAGE

Social workers should not use derogatory language in their written or verbal communications to or about clients. Social workers should use accurate and respectful language in all communications to and about clients.

I.13 PAYMENT FOR SERVICES

(a) When setting fees, social workers should ensure that the fees are fair, reasonable, and commensurate with the services performed. Consideration should be given to clients' ability to pay.

(b) Social workers should avoid accepting goods or services from clients as payment for professional services. Bartering arrangements, particularly involving services, create the potential for conflicts of interest, exploitation, and inappropriate boundaries in social workers' relationships with clients. Social workers should explore and may participate in bartering only in very limited circumstances when it can be demonstrated that such arrangements are an accepted practice among professionals in the local community, considered to be essential for the provision of services, negotiated without coercion, and entered into at the client's initiative and with the client's informed consent. Social workers who accept goods or services from clients as payment for professional services assume the full burden of demonstrating that this arrangement will not be detrimental to the client or the professional relationship.

(c) Social workers should not solicit a private fee or other remuneration for providing services to clients who are entitled to such available services through the social workers' employer or agency.

1.14 CLIENTS WHO LACK DECISION-MAKING CAPACITY

When social workers act on behalf of clients who lack the capacity to make informed decisions, social workers should take reasonable steps to safeguard the interests and rights of those clients.

1.15 INTERRUPTION OF SERVICES

Social workers should make reasonable efforts to ensure continuity of services in the event that services are interrupted by factors such as unavailability, relocation, illness, disability, or death.

1.16 TERMINATION OF SERVICES

(a) Social workers should terminate services to clients and professional relationships with them when such services and relationships are no longer required or no longer serve the clients' needs or interests.

(b) Social workers should take reasonable steps to avoid abandoning clients who are still in need of services. Social workers should withdraw services precipitously only under unusual circumstances, giving careful consideration to all factors in the situation and taking care to minimize possible adverse effects. Social workers should assist in making appropriate arrangements for continuation of services when necessary.

(c) Social workers in fee-for-service settings may terminate services to clients who are not paying an overdue balance if the financial contractual arrangements have been made clear to the client, if the

client does not pose an imminent danger to self or others, and if the clinical and other consequences of the current nonpayment have been addressed and discussed with the client.

(d) Social workers should not terminate services to pursue a social, financial, or sexual relationship with a client.

(e) Social workers who anticipate the termination or interruption of services to clients should notify clients promptly and seek the transfer, referral, or continuation of services in relation to the clients' needs and preferences.

(f) Social workers who are leaving an employment setting should inform clients of appropriate options for the continuation of services and of the benefits and risks of the options.

2. Social Workers' Ethical Responsibilities to Colleagues

2.01 RESPECT

(a) Social workers should treat colleagues with respect and should represent accurately and fairly the qualifications, views, and obligations of colleagues.

(b) Social workers should avoid unwarranted negative criticism of colleagues in communications with clients or with other professionals. Unwarranted negative criticism may include demeaning comments that refer to colleagues' level of competence or to individuals' attributes such as race, ethnicity, national origin, color, sex, sexual orientation, age, marital status, political belief, religion, and mental or physical disability.

(c) Social workers should cooperate with social work colleagues and with colleagues of other professions when such cooperation serves the well-being of clients.

2.02 CONFIDENTIALITY

Social workers should respect confidential information shared by colleagues in the course of their professional relationships and transactions. Social workers should ensure that such colleagues understand social workers' obligation to respect confidentiality and any exceptions related to it.

2.03 INTERDISCIPLINARY COLLABORATION

(a) Social workers who are members of an interdisciplinary team should participate in and contribute to decisions that affect the well-being of clients by drawing on the perspectives, values, and experiences of the social work profession. Professional and ethical obligations of the interdisciplinary team as a whole and of its individual members should be clearly established.

(b) Social workers for whom a team decision raises ethical concerns should attempt to resolve the disagreement through appropriate channels. If the disagreement cannot be resolved, social workers should pursue other avenues to address their concerns consistent with client well-being.

2.04 DISPUTES INVOLVING COLLEAGUES

(a) Social workers should not take advantage of a dispute between a colleague and an employer to obtain a position or otherwise advance the social workers' own interests.

(b) Social workers should not exploit clients in disputes with colleagues or engage clients in any inappropriate discussion of conflicts between social workers and their colleagues.

2.05 CONSULTATION

(a) Social workers should seek the advice and counsel of colleagues whenever such consultation is in the best interests of clients.

(b) Social workers should keep themselves informed about colleagues' areas of expertise and competencies. Social workers should seek consultation only from colleagues who have demonstrated knowledge, expertise, and competence related to the subject of the consultation.

(c) When consulting with colleagues about clients, social workers should disclose the least amount of information necessary to achieve the purposes of the consultation.

2.06 REFERRAL FOR SERVICES

(a) Social workers should refer clients to other professionals when the other professionals' specialized knowledge or expertise is needed to serve clients fully or when social workers believe that they are not being effective or making reasonable progress with clients and that additional service is required.

(b) Social workers who refer clients to other professionals should take appropriate steps to facilitate an orderly transfer of responsibility. Social workers who refer clients to other professionals should disclose, with clients' consent, all pertinent information to the new service providers.

(c) Social workers are prohibited from giving or receiving payment for a referral when no professional service is provided by the referring social worker.

2.07 SEXUAL RELATIONSHIPS

(a) Social workers who function as supervisors or educators should not engage in sexual activities or contact with supervisees, students, trainees, or other colleagues over whom they exercise professional authority.

(b) Social workers should avoid engaging in sexual relationships with colleagues when there is potential for a conflict of interest. Social workers who become involved in, or anticipate becoming involved in, a sexual relationship with a colleague have a duty to transfer professional responsibilities, when necessary, to avoid a conflict of interest.

2.08 SEXUAL HARASSMENT

Social workers should not sexually harass supervisees, students, trainees, or colleagues. Sexual harassment includes sexual advances, sexual solicitation, requests for sexual favors, and other verbal or physical conduct of a sexual nature.

2.09 IMPAIRMENT OF COLLEAGUES

(a) Social workers who have direct knowledge of a social work colleague's impairment that is due to personal problems, psychosocial distress, substance abuse, or mental health difficulties and that interferes with practice effectiveness should consult with that colleague when feasible and assist the colleague in taking remedial action.

(b) Social workers who believe that a social work colleague's impairment interferes with practice effectiveness and that the colleague has not taken adequate steps to address the impairment should take action through appropriate channels established by employers, agencies, NASW, licensing and regulatory bodies, and other professional organizations.

2.10 INCOMPETENCE OF COLLEAGUES

(a) Social workers who have direct knowledge of a social work colleague's incompetence should consult with that colleague when feasible and assist the colleague in taking remedial action.

(b) Social workers who believe that a social work colleague is incompetent and has not taken adequate steps to address the incompetence should take action through appropriate channels established by employers, agencies, NASW, licensing and regulatory bodies, and other professional organizations.

2.11 UNETHICAL CONDUCT OF COLLEAGUES

(a) Social workers should take adequate measures to discourage, prevent, expose, and correct the unethical conduct of colleagues.

(b) Social workers should be knowledgeable about established policies and procedures for handling concerns about colleagues' unethical behavior. Social workers should be familiar with national, state, and local procedures for handling ethics complaints. These include policies and procedures created by NASW, licensing and regulatory bodies, employers, agencies, and other professional organizations.

(c) Social workers who believe that a colleague has acted unethically should seek resolution by discussing their concerns with the colleague when feasible and when such discussion is likely to be productive.

(d) When necessary, social workers who believe that a colleague has acted unethically should take action through appropriate formal channels (such as contacting a state licensing board or regulatory body, an NASW committee on inquiry, or other professional ethics committees).

(e) Social workers should defend and assist colleagues who are unjustly charged with unethical conduct.

3. Social Workers' Ethical Responsibilities in Practice Settings

3.01 SUPERVISION AND CONSULTATION

(a) Social workers who provide supervision or consultation should have the necessary knowledge and skill to supervise or consult appropriately and should do so only within their areas of knowledge and competence.

(b) Social workers who provide supervision or consultation are responsible for setting clear, appropriate, and culturally sensitive boundaries.

(c) Social workers should not engage in any dual or multiple relationships with supervisees in which there is a risk of exploitation of or potential harm to the supervisee.

(d) Social workers who provide supervision should evaluate supervisees' performance in a manner that is fair and respectful.

3.02 EDUCATION AND TRAINING

(a) Social workers who function as educators, field instructors for students, or trainers should provide instruction only within their areas of knowledge and competence and should provide instruction based on the most current information and knowledge available in the profession.

(b) Social workers who function as educators or field instructors for students should evaluate students' performance in a manner that is fair and respectful.

(c) Social workers who function as educators or field instructors for students should take reasonable steps to ensure that clients are routinely informed when services are being provided by students.

(d) Social workers who function as educators or field instructors for students should not engage in any dual or multiple relationships with students in which there is a risk of exploitation or potential harm to the student. Social work educators and field instructors are responsible for setting clear, appropriate, and culturally sensitive boundaries.

3.03 PERFORMANCE EVALUATION

Social workers who have responsibility for evaluating the performance of others should fulfill such responsibility in a fair and considerate manner and on the basis of clearly stated criteria.

3.04 CLIENT RECORDS

(a) Social workers should take reasonable steps to ensure that documentation in records is accurate and reflects the services provided.

(b) Social workers should include sufficient and timely documentation in records to facilitate the delivery of services and to ensure continuity of services provided to clients in the future.

(c) Social workers' documentation should protect clients' privacy to the extent that is possible and appropriate and should include only information that is directly relevant to the delivery of services.

(d) Social workers should store records following the termination of services to ensure reasonable future access. Records should be maintained for the number of years required by state statutes or relevant contracts.

3.05 BILLING

Social workers should establish and maintain billing practices that accurately reflect the nature and extent of services provided and that identify who provided the service in the practice setting.

3.06 CLIENT TRANSFER

(a) When an individual who is receiving services from another agency or colleague contacts a social worker for services, the social worker should carefully consider the client's needs before agreeing to provide services. To minimize possible confusion and conflict, social workers should discuss with potential clients the nature of the clients' current relationship with other service providers and the implications, including possible benefits or risks, of entering into a relationship with a new service provider.

(b) If a new client has been served by another agency or colleague, social workers should discuss with the client whether consultation with the previous service provider is in the client's best interest.

3.07 ADMINISTRATION

(a) Social work administrators should advocate within and outside their agencies for adequate resources to meet clients' needs.

(b) Social workers should advocate for resource allocation procedures that are open and fair. When not all clients' needs can be met, an allocation procedure should be developed that is nondiscriminatory and based on appropriate and consistently applied principles.

(c) Social workers who are administrators should take reasonable steps to ensure that adequate agency or organizational resources are available to provide appropriate staff supervision.

(d) Social work administrators should take reasonable steps to ensure that the working environment for which they are responsible is consistent with and encourages compliance with the NASW Code of Ethics. Social work administrators should take reasonable steps to eliminate any conditions in their organizations that violate, interfere with, or discourage compliance with the *Code*.

3.08 CONTINUING EDUCATION AND STAFF DEVELOPMENT

Social work administrators and supervisors should take reasonable steps to provide or arrange for continuing education and staff development for all staff for whom they are responsible. Continuing education and staff development should address current knowledge and emerging developments related to social work practice and ethics.

3.09 COMMITMENTS TO EMPLOYERS

(a) Social workers generally should adhere to commitments made to employers and employing organizations.

(b) Social workers should work to improve employing agencies' policies and procedures and the efficiency and effectiveness of their services.

(c) Social workers should take reasonable steps to ensure that employers are aware of social workers' ethical obligations as set forth in the NASW Code of Ethics and of the implications of those obligations for social work practice.

(d) Social workers should not allow an employing organization's policies, procedures, regulations, or administrative orders to interfere with their ethical practice of social work. Social workers should take reasonable steps to ensure that their employing organizations' practices are consistent with the NASW Code of Ethics.

(e) Social workers should act to prevent and eliminate discrimination in the employing organization's work assignments and in its employment policies and practices.

(f) Social workers should accept employment or arrange student field placements only in organizations that exercise fair personnel practices.

(g) Social workers should be diligent stewards of the resources of their employing organizations, wisely conserving funds where appropriate and never misappropriating funds or using them for unintended purposes.

3.10 LABOR-MANAGEMENT DISPUTES

(a) Social workers may engage in organized action, including the formation of and participation in labor unions, to improve services to clients and working conditions.

(b) The actions of social workers who are involved in labor-management disputes, job actions, or labor strikes should be guided by the profession's values, ethical principles, and ethical standards. Reasonable differences of opinion exist among social workers concerning their primary obligation as professionals during an actual or threatened labor strike or job action. Social workers should carefully examine relevant issues and their possible impact on clients before deciding on a course of action.

4. Social Workers' Ethical Responsibilities as Professionals

4.01 COMPETENCE

(a) Social workers should accept responsibility or employment only on the basis of existing competence or the intention to acquire the necessary competence.

(b) Social workers should strive to become and remain proficient in professional practice and the performance of professional functions. Social workers should critically examine and keep current with emerging knowledge relevant to social work. Social workers should routinely review the professional literature and participate in continuing education relevant to social work practice and social work ethics.

(c) Social workers should base practice on recognized knowledge, including empirically based knowledge, relevant to social work and social work ethics.

4.02 DISCRIMINATION

Social workers should not practice, condone, facilitate, or collaborate with any form of discrimination on the basis of race, ethnicity, national origin, color, sex, sexual orientation, age, marital status, political belief, religion, or mental or physical disability.

4.03 PRIVATE CONDUCT

Social workers should not permit their private conduct to interfere with their ability to fulfill their professional responsibilities.

4.04 DISHONESTY, FRAUD, AND DECEPTION

Social workers should not participate in, condone, or be associated with dishonesty, fraud, or deception.

4.05 IMPAIRMENT

(a) Social workers should not allow their own personal problems, psychosocial distress, legal problems, substance abuse, or mental health difficulties to interfere with their professional judgment and performance or to jeopardize the best interests of people for whom they have a professional responsibility.

(b) Social workers whose personal problems, psychosocial distress, legal problems, substance abuse, or mental health difficulties interfere with their professional judgment and performance should immediately seek consultation and take appropriate remedial action by seeking professional help, making adjustments in workload, terminating practice, or taking any other steps necessary to protect clients and others.

4.06 MISREPRESENTATION

(a) Social workers should make clear distinctions between statements made and actions engaged in as a private individual and as a representative of the social work profession, a professional social work organization, or the social worker's employing agency.

(b) Social workers who speak on behalf of professional social work organizations should accurately represent the official and authorized positions of the organizations.

(c) Social workers should ensure that their representations to clients, agencies, and the public of professional qualifications, credentials, education, competence, affiliations, services provided, or results to be achieved are accurate. Social workers should claim only those relevant professional credentials they actually possess and take steps to correct any inaccuracies or misrepresentations of their credentials by others.

4.07 SOLICITATIONS

(a) Social workers should not engage in uninvited solicitation of potential clients who, because of their circumstances, are vulnerable to undue influence, manipulation, or coercion.

(b) Social workers should not engage in solicitation of testimonial endorsements (including solicitation of consent to use a client's prior statement as a testimonial endorsement) from current clients or from other people who, because of their particular circumstances, are vulnerable to undue influence.

4.08 ACKNOWLEDGING CREDIT

(a) Social workers should take responsibility and credit, including authorship credit, only for work they have actually performed and to which they have contributed.

(b) Social workers should honestly acknowledge the work of and the contributions made by others.

5. Social Workers' Ethical Responsibilities to the Social Work Profession

5.01 INTEGRITY OF THE PROFESSION

(a) Social workers should work toward the maintenance and promotion of high standards of practice.

(b) Social workers should uphold and advance the values, ethics, knowledge, and mission of the profession. Social workers should protect, enhance, and improve the integrity of the profession through appropriate study and research, active discussion, and responsible criticism of the profession.

(c) Social workers should contribute time and professional expertise to activities that promote respect for the value, integrity, and competence of the social work profession. These activities may include teaching, research, consultation, service, legislative testimony, presentations in the community, and participation in their professional organizations.

(d) Social workers should contribute to the knowledge base of social work and share with colleagues their knowledge related to practice, research, and ethics. Social workers should seek to con-tribute to the profession's literature and to share their knowledge at professional meetings and conferences.

(e) Social workers should act to prevent the unauthorized and unqualified practice of social work.

5.02 EVALUATION AND RESEARCH

(a) Social workers should monitor and evaluate policies, the implementation of programs, and practice interventions.

(b) Social workers should promote and facilitate evaluation and research to contribute to the development of knowledge.

(c) Social workers should critically examine and keep current with emerging knowledge relevant to social work and fully use evaluation and research evidence in their professional practice.

(d) Social workers engaged in evaluation or research should carefully consider possible consequences and should follow guidelines developed for the protection of evaluation and research participants. Appropriate institutional review boards should be consulted.

(e) Social workers engaged in evaluation or research should obtain voluntary and written informed consent from participants, when appropriate, without any implied or actual deprivation or penalty for refusal to participate; without undue inducement to participate; and with due regard for participants' well-being, privacy, and dignity. Informed consent should include information about the nature, extent, and duration of the participation requested and disclosure of the risks and benefits of participation in the research.

(f) When evaluation or research participants are incapable of giving informed consent, social workers should provide an appropriate explanation to the participants, obtain the participants' assent to the extent they are able, and obtain written consent from an appropriate proxy.

(g) Social workers should never design or conduct evaluation or research that does not use consent procedures, such as certain forms of naturalistic observation and archival research, unless rigorous and responsible review of the research has found it to be justified because of its prospective scientific, educational, or applied value and unless equally effective alternative procedures that do not involve waiver of consent are not feasible.

(h) Social workers should inform participants of their right to withdraw from evaluation and research at any time without penalty.

(i) Social workers should take appropriate steps to ensure that participants in evaluation and research have access to appropriate supportive services.

(j) Social workers engaged in evaluation or research should protect participants from unwarranted physical or mental distress, harm, danger, or deprivation.

(k) Social workers engaged in the evaluation of services should discuss collected information only for professional purposes and only with people professionally concerned with this information.

(l) Social workers engaged in evaluation or research should ensure the anonymity or confidentiality of participants and of the data obtained from them. Social workers should inform participants of any limits of confidentiality, the measures that will be taken to ensure confidentiality, and when any records containing research data will be destroyed.

(m) Social workers who report evaluation and research results should protect participants' confidentiality by omitting identifying information unless proper consent has been obtained authorizing disclosure.

(n) Social workers should report evaluation and research findings accurately. They should not fabricate or falsify results and should take steps to correct any errors later found in published data using standard publication methods.

(o) Social workers engaged in evaluation or research should be alert to and avoid conflicts of interest and dual relationships with participants, should inform participants when a real or potential conflict of interest arises, and should take steps to resolve the issue in a manner that makes participants' interests primary.

(p) Social workers should educate themselves, their students, and their colleagues about responsible research practices.

6. Social Workers' Ethical Responsibilities to the Broader Society

6.01 SOCIAL WELFARE

Social workers should promote the general welfare of society, from local to global levels, and the development of people, their communities, and their environments. Social workers should advocate for living conditions conducive to the fulfillment of basic human needs and should promote social, economic, political, and cultural values and institutions that are compatible with the realization of social justice.

6.02 PUBLIC PARTICIPATION

Social workers should facilitate informed participation by the public in shaping social policies and institutions.

6.03 PUBLIC EMERGENCIES

Social workers should provide appropriate professional services in public emergencies to the greatest extent possible.

6.04 SOCIAL AND POLITICAL ACTION

(a) Social workers should engage in social and political action that seeks to ensure that all people have equal access to the resources, employment, services, and opportunities they require to meet their basic human needs and to develop fully. Social workers should be aware of the impact of the political arena on practice and should advocate for changes in policy and legislation to improve social conditions in order to meet basic human needs and promote social justice.

(b) Social workers should act to expand choice and opportunity for all people, with special regard for vulnerable, disadvantaged, oppressed, and exploited people and groups.

(c) Social workers should promote conditions that encourage respect for cultural and social diversity within the United States and globally. Social workers should promote policies and practices that demonstrate respect for difference, support the expansion of cultural knowledge and resources, advocate for programs and institutions that demonstrate cultural competence, and promote policies that safeguard the rights of and confirm equity and social justice for all people.

(d) Social workers should act to prevent and eliminate domination of, exploitation of, and discrimination against any person, group, or class on the basis of race, ethnicity, national origin, color, sex, sexual orientation, age, marital status, political belief, religion, or mental or physical disability.

CODE OF ETHICS

American College of Healthcare Executives

AMENDED 1990

• • •

The American College of Healthcare Executives' Code of Ethics sets standards for the ethical behavior of health-care executives both in their professional relationships and in their personal behavior, particularly when it relates to their professional role and identity. Of particular note are statements about assuring "all people…reasonable access to healthcare services" and establishing "a resource allocation process that considers ethical ramifications," as well as a section addressing conflicts of interest and a section on responsibilities to community and society

<http://www.ache.org/ABT_ACHE/code.cfm>

• • •

Preface

The *Code of Ethics* is administered by the Ethics Committee, which is appointed by the Board of Governors upon nomination by the Chairman. It is composed of at least nine Diplomates or Fellows of the College, each of whom serves a three-year term on a staggered basis, with three members retiring each year. *The Ethics Committee shall:*

• Review and evaluate annually the *Code of Ethics,* and make any necessary recommendations for updating the Code.

• Review and recommend action to the Board of Governors on allegations brought forth regarding breaches of the *Code of Ethics.*

• Develop ethical policy statements to serve as guidelines of ethical conduct for healthcare executives and their professional relationships.

• Prepare an annual report of observations, accomplishments, and recommendations to the Board of Governors, and such other periodic reports as required.

The Ethics Committee invokes the *Code of Ethics* under authority of the ACHE *Bylaws,* Article II, Membership, Section 6, Resignation and Termination of Membership; Transfer to Inactive Status, subsection (b), as follows:

Membership may be terminated or rendered inactive by action of the Board of Governors as a result of violation of the *Code of Ethics;* nonconformity with the Bylaws or Regulations Governing Admission, Advancement, Recertification, and Reappointment; conviction of a felony; or conviction of a crime of moral turpitude or a crime relating to the healthcare management profession. No such termination of membership or imposition of inactive status shall be effected without affording a reasonable opportunity for the member to consider the charges and to appear in his or her own defense before the Board of Governors or its designated hearing committee, as outlined in the "Grievance Procedure," Appendix I of the College's *Code of Ethics.*

Preamble

The purpose of the *Code of Ethics* of the American College of Healthcare Executives is to serve as a guide to conduct for members. It contains standards of ethical behavior for healthcare executives in their professional relationships. These relationships include members of the healthcare executive's organization and other organizations. Also included are patients or others served, colleagues, the community and society as a whole. The *Code of Ethics* also incorporates standards of ethical behavior governing personal behavior, particularly when that conduct directly relates to the role and identity of the healthcare executive.

The fundamental objectives of the healthcare management profession are to enhance overall quality of life, dignity and well-being of every individual needing healthcare services; and to create a more equitable, accessible, effective and efficient healthcare system.

Healthcare executives have an obligation to act in ways that will merit the trust, confidence and respect of healthcare professionals and the general public. Therefore, healthcare executives should lead lives that embody an exemplary system of values and ethics.

In fulfilling their commitments and obligations to patients or others served, healthcare executives function as moral advocates. Since every management decision affects the health and well-being of both individuals and communities, healthcare executives must carefully evaluate the possible outcomes of their decisions. In organizations that deliver healthcare services, they must work to safeguard and foster the rights, interests and prerogatives of patients or others served. The role of moral advocate requires that healthcare executives speak out and take actions necessary to promote such rights, interests and prerogatives if they are threatened.

I. The Healthcare Executive's Responsibilities to the Profession of Healthcare Management

The healthcare executive shall:

A. Uphold the values, ethics and mission of the healthcare management profession;

B. Conduct all personal and professional activities with honesty, integrity, respect, fairness and good faith in a manner that will reflect well upon the profession;

C. Comply with all laws pertaining to healthcare management in the jurisdictions in which the healthcare executive is located, or conducts professional activities;

D. Maintain competence and proficiency in healthcare management by implementing a personal program of assessment and continuing professional education;

E. Avoid the exploitation of professional relationships for personal gain;

F. Use this Code to further the interests of the profession and not for selfish reasons;

G. Respect professional confidences;

H. Enhance the dignity and image of the healthcare management profession through positive public information programs; and

I. Refrain from participating in any activity that demeans the credibility and dignity of the healthcare management profession.

II. The Healthcare Executive's Responsibilities to Patients or Others Served, to the Organization, and to Employees

A. RESPONSIBILITIES TO PATIENTS OR OTHERS SERVED

The healthcare executive shall, within the scope of his or her authority:

1. Work to ensure the existence of a process to evaluate the quality of care or service rendered;

2. Avoid practicing or facilitating discrimination and institute safeguards to prevent discriminatory organizational practices;

3. Work to ensure the existence of a process that will advise patients or others served of the rights, opportunities, responsibilities, and risks regarding available healthcare services;

4. Work to provide a process that ensures the autonomy and self-determination of patients or others served; and

5. Work to ensure the existence of procedures that will safeguard the confidentiality and privacy of patients or others served.

B. RESPONSIBILITIES TO THE ORGANIZATION

The healthcare executive shall, within the scope of his or her authority:

1. Provide healthcare services consistent with available resources and work to ensure the existence of a resource allocation process that considers ethical ramifications;

2. Conduct both competitive and cooperative activities in ways that improve community healthcare services;

3. Lead the organization in the use and improvement of standards of management and sound business practices;

4. Respect the customs and practices of patients or others served, consistent with the organization's philosophy; and

5. Be truthful in all forms of professional and organizational communication, and avoid disseminating information that is false, misleading, or deceptive.

C. RESPONSIBILITIES TO EMPLOYEES

Healthcare executives have an ethical and professional obligation to employees of the organizations they manage that encompass but are not limited to:

1. Working to create a working environment conducive for underscoring employee ethical conduct and behavior;

2. Working to ensure that individuals may freely express ethical concerns and providing mechanisms for discussing and addressing such concerns;

3. Working to ensure a working environment that is free from harassment, sexual and other; coercion of any kind, especially to perform illegal or unethical acts; and discrimination on the basis of race, creed, color, sex, ethnic origin, age, or disability;

4. Working to ensure a working environment that is conducive to proper utilization of employees' skills and abilities;

5. Paying particular attention to the employee's work environment and job safety; and

6. Working to establish appropriate grievance and appeals mechanisms.

III. Conflicts of Interest

A conflict of interest may be only a matter of degree, but exists when the healthcare executive:

A. Acts to benefit directly or indirectly by using authority or inside information, or allows a friend, relative or associate to benefit from such authority or information.

B. Uses authority or information to make a decision to intentionally affect the organization in an adverse manner.

The healthcare executive shall:

A. Conduct all personal and professional relationships in such a way that all those affected are assured that management decisions are made in the best interests of the organization and the individuals served by it;

B. Disclose to the appropriate authority any direct or indirect financial or personal interests that pose potential or actual conflicts of interest;

C. Accept no gifts or benefits offered with the express or implied expectation of influencing a management decision; and

D. Inform the appropriate authority and other involved parties of potential or actual conflicts of interest related to appointments or elections to boards or committees inside or outside the healthcare executive's organization.

IV. The Healthcare Executive's Responsibilities to Community and Society

The healthcare executive shall:

A. Work to identify and meet the healthcare needs of the community;

B. Work to ensure that all people have reasonable access to healthcare services;

C. Participate in public dialogue on healthcare policy issues and advocate solutions that will improve health status and promote quality healthcare;

D. Consider the short-term and long-term impact of management decisions on both the community and on society; and

E. Provide prospective consumers with adequate and accurate information, enabling them to make enlightened judgments and decisions regarding services.

V. The Healthcare Executive's Responsibility to Report Violations of the Code

A member of the College who has reasonable grounds to believe that another member has violated this Code has a duty to communicate such facts to the Ethics Committee.

Appendix I

American College of Healthcare Executives Grievance Procedure

1. In order to be processed by the College, a complaint must be filed in writing to the Ethics Committee of the College within three years of the date of discovery of the alleged violation; and the Committee has the responsibility to look into incidents brought to its attention regardless of the informality of the information, provided the information can be documented or supported or may be a matter of public record. The three-year period within which a complaint must be filed shall temporarily cease to run during intervals when the accused member is in inactive status, or when the accused member resigns from the College.

2. The Committee chairman initially will determine whether the complaint falls within the purview of the Ethics Committee and whether immediate investigation is necessary. However, all letters of complaint that are filed with the Ethics Committee will appear on the agenda of the next committee meeting. The Ethics Committee shall have the final discretion to determine whether a complaint falls within the purview of the Ethics Committee.

3. If a grievance proceeding is initiated by the Ethics Committee:

   a. Specifics of the complaint will be sent to the respondent by certified mail. In such mailing, committee staff will inform the respondent that the grievance proceeding has been initiated, and that the respondent may respond directly to the Ethics Committee; the respondent also will be asked to cooperate with the Regent investigating the complaint.

b. The Ethics Committee shall refer the matter to the appropriate Regent who is deemed best able to investigate the alleged infraction. The Regent shall make inquiry into the matter, and in the process the respondent shall be given an opportunity to be heard.

c. Upon completion of the inquiry, the Regent shall present a complete report and recommended disposition of the matter in writing to the Ethics Committee. Absent unusual circumstances, the Regent is expected to complete his or her report and recommended disposition, and provide them to the Committee, within 60 days.

4. Upon the Committee's receipt of the Regent's report and recommended disposition, the Committee shall review them and make its written recommendation to the Board of Governors as to what action shall be taken and the reason or reasons therefor. A copy of the Committee's recommended decision along with the Regent's report and recommended disposition to the Board will be mailed to the respondent by certified mail. In such mailing, the respondent will be notified that within 30 days after his or her receipt of the Ethics Committee's recommended decision, the respondent may file a written appeal of the recommended decision with the Board of Governors.

5. Any written appeal submitted by the respondent must be received by the Board of Governors within 30 days after the recommended decision of the Ethics Committee is received by the respondent. The Board of Governors shall not take action on the Ethics Committee's recommended decision until the 30-day appeal period has elapsed. If no appeal to the Board of Governors is filed in a timely fashion, the Board shall review the recommended decision and determine action to be taken.

6. If an appeal to the Board of Governors is timely filed, the College Chairman shall appoint an ad hoc committee consisting of three Fellows to hear the matter. At least 30 days' notice of the formation of this committee, and of the hearing date, time and place, with an opportunity for representation, shall be mailed to the respondent. Reasonable requests for postponement shall be given consideration.

7. This ad hoc committee shall give the respondent adequate opportunity to present his or her case at the hearing, including the opportunity to submit a written statement and other documents deemed relevant by the respondent, and to be represented if so desired. Within a reasonable period of time following the hearing, the ad hoc committee shall write a detailed report with recommendations to the Board of Governors.

8. The Board of Governors shall decide what action to take after reviewing the report of the ad hoc committee. The Board shall provide the respondent with a copy of its decision. The decision of the Board of Governors shall be final. The Board of Governors shall have the authority to accept or reject any of the findings or recommended decisions of the Regent, the Ethics Committee or the ad hoc committee, and to order whatever level of discipline it feels is justified.

9. At each level of the grievance proceeding, the Board of Governors shall have the sole discretion to notify or contact the complainant relating to the grievance proceeding; provided, however, that the complainant shall be notified as to whether the complaint was reviewed by the Ethics Committee and whether the Ethics Committee or the Board of Governors has taken final action with respect to the complaint.

10. No individual shall serve on the ad hoc committee described above, or otherwise participate in these grievance proceedings on behalf of the College, if he or she is in direct economic competition with the respondent or otherwise has a financial conflict of interest in the matter, unless such conflict is disclosed to and waived in writing by the respondent.

11. All information obtained, reviewed, discussed and otherwise used or developed in a grievance proceeding that is not otherwise publicly known, publicly available, or part of the public domain is considered to be privileged and strictly confidential information of the College, and is not to be disclosed to anyone outside of the grievance proceeding except as determined by the Board of Governors or as required by law; provided, however, that an individual's membership status is not confidential and may be made available to the public upon request.

Appendix II

Ethics Committee Action

Once the grievance proceeding has been initiated, the Ethics Committee may take any of the following actions based upon its findings:

1. Determine the grievance complaint to be invalid.

2. Dismiss the grievance complaint.

3. Recommend censure.

4. Recommend transfer to inactive status for a specified minimum period of time.

5. Recommend expulsion.

Appendices I and II, entitled "American College of Healthcare Executives Grievance Procedure" and "Ethics Committee Action," respectively, are a material part of this Code of Ethics and are incorporated herein by reference.

ETHICAL CONDUCT FOR HEALTH CARE INSTITUTIONS

American Hospital Association

1992

• • •

In 1973, the American Hospital Association (AHA) developed its Guidelines on Ethical Conduct and Relationships for Health Care Institutions, the precursor to the present document, as a complement to the preceding code of ethics for health-care executives. This AHA code of ethics for health-care institutions, which addresses the major areas affecting their ethical conduct, is different because it is written for institutions, that is, their "mission, programs, and services," rather than for people.

Points of interest include (1) responsibility for "fair and effective use" of available resources and helping to resolve the problem of providing care to medically indigent individuals; (2) respect for the spiritual needs and cultural beliefs of patients and families; (3) accommodation, to the extent possible, of "the desire of employees and medical staff to embody religious and/or moral values in their professional activities"; and (4) sensitivity to "institutional decisions that employees might interpret as compromising their ability to provide high-quality health care."

Introduction

Health care institutions, by virtue of their roles as health care providers, employers, and community health resources, have special responsibilities for ethical conduct and ethical practices that go beyond meeting minimum legal and regulatory standards. Their broad range of patient care, education, public health, social service, and business functions is essential to the health and well being of their communities. These roles and functions demand that health care organizations conduct themselves in an ethical manner that emphasizes a basic community service orientation and justifies the public trust. The health care institution's mission and values should be embodied in all its programs, services, and activities.

Because health care organizations must frequently seek a balance among the interests and values of individuals, the institution, and society, they often face ethical dilemmas in meeting the needs of their patients and their communities. This advisory is intended to assist members of the American Hospital Association to better identify and understand the ethical aspects and implications of institutional policies and practices. It is offered with the understanding that each institution's leadership in making policy and decisions must take into account the needs and values of the institution, its physicians, other caregivers, and employees and those of individual patients, their families, and the community as a whole.

• • •

Community Role

- Health care institutions should be concerned with the overall health status of their communities while continuing to provide direct patient services. They should take a leadership role in enhancing public health and continuity of care in the community by communicating and working with other health care and social agencies to improve the availability and provision of health promotion, education, and patient care services.

- Health care institutions are responsible for fair and effective use of available health care delivery resources to promote access to comprehensive and affordable health care services of high quality. This responsibility extends beyond the resources of the given institution to include efforts to coordinate with other health care organizations and professionals and to share in community solutions for providing care for the medically indigent and others in need of specific health services.

- All health care institutions are responsible for meeting community service obligations which may include special initiatives for care for the poor and uninsured, provision of needed medical or social services, education, and various programs designed to meet the specific needs of their communities.

- Health care institutions, being dependent upon community confidence and support, are accountable to the public, and therefore their communications and disclosure of information and data related to the institution should be clear, accurate, and sufficiently complete to assure that it is not misleading. Such disclosure should be aimed primarily at better public understanding of health issues, the services available to prevent and treat illness, and patient rights and responsibilities relating to health care decisions.

- Advertising may be used to advance the health care organization's goals and objectives and should, in all cases, support the mission of the health care organization. Advertising may be used to educate the public, to report to the community, to increase awareness of available services, to increase support for the organization, and to recruit employees. Health care advertising should be truthful, fair, accurate, complete, and sensitive to the health care needs of the public. False or misleading statements, or statements that might lead the uninformed to draw false conclusions about the health care facility, its competitors, or other health care providers are unacceptable and unethical.

- As health care institutions operate in an increasingly challenging environment, they should consider the overall welfare of their communities and their own missions in determining their activities, service mixes, and business. Health care organizations should be particularly sensitive to potential conflicts of interests involving individuals or groups associated with the medical staff, governing board, or executive management. Examples of such conflicts include ownership or other financial interests in competing provider organizations or groups contracting with the health care institution.

Patient Care

- Health care institutions are responsible for providing each patient with care that is both appropriate and necessary for the patient's condition. Development and maintenance of organized programs for utilization review and quality improvement and of procedures to verify the credentials of physicians and other health professionals are basic to this obligation.
- Health care institutions in conjunction with attending physicians are responsible for assuring reasonable continuity of care and for informing patients of patient care alternatives when acute care is no longer needed.
- Health care institutions should ensure that the health care professionals and organizations with which they are formally or informally affiliated have appropriate credentials and/or accreditation and participate in organized programs to assess and assure continuous improvement in quality of care.
- Health care institutions should have policies and practices that assure that patient transfers are medically appropriate and legally permissible. Health care institutions should inform patients of the need for and alternatives to such transfers.
- Health care institutions should have policies and practices that support informed consent for diagnostic and therapeutic procedures and use of advance directives. Policies and practices must

respect and promote the patient's responsibility for decision making.

- Health care institutions are responsible for assuring confidentiality of patient-specific information. They are responsible for providing safeguards to prevent unauthorized release of information and establishing procedures for authorizing release of data.
- Health care institutions should assure that the psychological, social, spiritual, and physical needs and cultural beliefs and practices of patients and families are respected and should promote employee and medical staff sensitivity to the full range of such needs and practices. The religious and social beliefs and customs of patients should be accommodated whenever possible.
- Health care institutions should have specific mechanisms or procedures to resolve conflicting values and ethical dilemmas as well as complaints and disputes among patients their families, medical staff, employees, the institution, and the community.

Organizational Conduct

- The policies and practices of health care institutions should respect and support the professional ethical codes and responsibilities of their employees and medical staff members and be sensitive to institutional decisions that employees might interpret as compromising their ability to provide high-quality health care.
- Health care institutions should provide for fair and equitably-administered employee compensation, benefits, and other policies and practices.
- To the extent possible and consistent with the ethical commitments of the institution, health care institutions should accommodate the desires of employees and medical staff to embody religious and/or moral values in their professional activities.
- Health care institutions should have written policies on conflict of interest that apply to officers, governing board members, and medical staff, as well as others who may make or influence decisions for or on behalf of the institution, including contract employees. Particular attention should be given to potential conflicts related to referral sources, vendors, competing health care services, and investments. These policies should recognize that individuals in decision-making or administrative positions often have duality of interests that may not always present conflicts. But they should provide mechanisms for identifying and addressing dualities when they do exist.

• Health care institutions should communicate their mission, values, and priorities to their employees and volunteers, whose patient care and service activities are the most visible embodiment of the institution's ethical commitments and values.

SECTION IV.

ETHICAL DIRECTIVES
FOR HUMAN RESEARCH

• • •

German Guidelines on Human Experimentation [1931]

Nuremberg Code [1947]

Principles for Those in Research and Experimentation, World Medical Association [1954]

Article Seven, International Covenant on Civil and Political Rights, General Assembly of the United Nations [1958]

Declaration of Helsinki, World Medical Association [1964, revised 1975, 1983, 1989, 1996, 2000]

The Belmont Report: Ethical Principles and Guidelines for the Protection of Human Subjects of Research, National Commission for the Protection of Human Subjects of Biomedical and Behavioral Research [1979]

DHHS Regulations for the Protection of Human Subjects (45 CFR 46) [June 18, 1991]

Summary Report of the International Summit Conference on Bioethics [1987]

Recommendation No. R (90) 3 of the Committee of Ministers to Member States Concerning Medical Research on Human Beings, Council of Europe [1990]

International Ethical Guidelines for Biomedical Research Involving Human Subjects, Council for International Organizations of Medical Sciences (CIOMS) in collaboration with the World Health Organization [1993, revised 2000]

Directives pertaining to the ethics of research on human subjects generally fall into two categories: (1) national or international policies and/or laws and (2) policies of professional groups, e.g., medicine, nursing, epidemiology, and psychology. In addition, directives may pertain either to research in general or to specific types of research. For example, the U.S. Food and Drug Administration (FDA), the Recombinant DNA Advisory Committee of the National Institutes of Health, and the Medical Research Council of Canada all have guidelines governing gene therapy, investigational drugs, or reproductive technologies; and the Ethics Committee of the American Fertility Society has issued a comprehensive document, "Ethical Considerations of the New Reproductive Technologies."

Due to space limitations, research directives issued by professional associations and those pertaining to specific areas of research are not printed in this section; but a selection of such documents are listed in the bibliography to the Appendix. In addition, some of the professional codes included in other sections contain guidelines on research.

The documents in this section are organized chronologically except for the 1991 United States DHHS regulations, which follow The Belmont Report because of the two documents' interdependence.

GERMAN GUIDELINES ON HUMAN EXPERIMENTATION

1931

• • •

The following guidelines for therapeutic and scientific research on human subjects, which are thought to be the first of their kind, were published originally as a Circular of the Reich Minister of the Interior dated February 28, 1931. The guidelines remained in force until 1945, but were not included in the Reich legislation validated at the end of World War II. It is interesting to note the disjunction between the guidelines and the practice of the Nazi researchers.

1. In order that medical science may continue to advance, the initiation in appropriate cases of therapy involving new and as yet insufficiently tested means and procedures cannot be avoided. Similarly, scientific experimentation involving human subjects cannot be completely excluded as such, as this would hinder or even prevent progress in the diagnosis, treatment, and prevention of diseases.

   The freedom to be granted to the physician accordingly shall be weighed against his special duty to remain aware at all times of his major responsibility for the life and health of any person on whom he undertakes innovative therapy or performs an experiment.

2. For the purposes of these Guidelines, "innovative therapy" means interventions and treatment methods that involve humans and serve a therapeutic

purpose, in other words that are carried out in a particular, individual case in order to diagnose, treat, or prevent a disease or suffering or to eliminate a physical defect, although their effects and consequences cannot be sufficiently evaluated on the basis of existing experience.

3. For the purposes of these Guidelines, "scientific experimentation" means interventions and treatment methods that involve humans and are undertaken for research purposes without serving a therapeutic purpose in an individual case, and whose effects and consequences cannot be sufficiently evaluated on the basis of existing experience.

4. Any innovative therapy must be justified and performed in accordance with the principles of medical ethics and the rules of medical practice and theory.

   In all cases, the question of whether any adverse effects which may occur are proportionate to the anticipated benefits shall be examined and assessed.

   Innovative therapy may be carried out only it if has been tested in advance in animal trials (where these are possible).

5. Innovative therapy may be carried out only after the subject or his legal representative has unambiguously consented to the procedure in the light of relevant information provided in advance.

   Where consent is refused, innovative therapy may be initiated only if it constitutes an urgent procedure to preserve life or prevent serious damage to health and prior consent could not be obtained under the circumstances.

6. The question of whether to use innovative therapy must be examined with particular care where the subject is a child or a person under 18 years of age.

7. Exploitation of social hardship in order to undertake innovative therapy is incompatible with the principles of medical ethics.

8. Extreme caution shall be exercised in connection with innovative therapy involving live microorganisms, especially live pathogens. Such therapy shall be considered permissible only if the procedure can be assumed to be relatively safe and similar benefits are unlikely to be achieved under the circumstances by any other method.

9. In clinics, policlinics, hospitals, or other treatment and care establishments, innovative therapy may be carried out only by the physician in charge or by another physician acting in accordance with his express instructions and subject to his complete responsibility.

10. A report shall be made in respect of any innovative therapy, indicating the purpose of the procedure, the

justification for it, and the manner in which it is carried out. In particular, the report shall include a statement that the subject or, where appropriate, his legal representative has been provided in advance with relevant information and has given his consent.

Where therapy has been carried out without consent, under the conditions referred to in the second paragraph of Section 5, the statement shall give full details of these conditions.

11. The results of any innovative therapy may be published only in a manner whereby the patient's dignity and the dictates of humanity are fully respected.

12. Sections 4–11 of these Guidelines shall be applicable, *mutatis mutandis,* to scientific experimentation (cf. Section 3).

The following additional requirements shall apply to such experimentation:

(a) experimentation shall be prohibited in all cases where consent has not been given;

(b) experimentation involving human subjects shall be avoided if it can be replaced by animal studies. Experimentation involving human subjects may be carried out only after all data that can be collected by means of those biological methods (laboratory testing and animal studies) that are available to medical science for purposes of clarification and confirmation of the validity of the experiment have been obtained. Under these circumstances, motiveless and unplanned experimentation involving human subjects shall obviously be prohibited;

(c) experimentation involving children or young persons under 18 years of age shall be prohibited if it in any way endangers the child or young person;

(d) experimentation involving dying subjects is incompatible with the principles of medical ethics and shall therefore be prohibited.

13. While physicians and, more particularly, those in charge of hospital establishments may thus be expected to be guided by a strong sense of responsibility towards their patients, they should at the same time not be denied the satisfying responsibility (*verantwortungsfreudigkeit*) of seeking new ways to protect or treat patients or alleviate or remedy their suffering where they are convinced, in the light of their medical experience, that known methods are likely to fail.

14. Academic training courses should take every suitable opportunity to stress the physician's special duties when carrying out a new form of therapy or a scientific experiment as well as when publishing his results.

NUREMBERG CODE

1947

• • •

The Nuremberg Military Tribunal's decision in the case of the United States v. Karl Brandt et al. includes what is now called the Nuremberg Code, a ten-point statement delimiting permissible medical experimentation on human subjects. According to this statement, human experimentation is justified only if its results benefit society and it is carried out in accord with basic principles that "satisfy moral, ethical, and legal concepts."

1. The voluntary consent of the human subject is absolutely essential.

   This means that the person involved should have legal capacity to give consent; should be so situated as to be able to exercise free power of choice, without the intervention of any element of force, fraud, deceit, duress, over-reaching, or other ulterior form of constraint or coercion; and should have sufficient knowledge and comprehension of the elements of the subject matter involved as to enable him to make an understanding and enlightened decision. This latter element requires that before the acceptance of an affirmative decision by the experimental subject there should be made known to him the nature, duration, and purpose of the experiment; the method and means by which it is to be conducted; all inconveniences and hazards reasonably to be expected; and the effects upon his health or person which may possibly come from his participation in the experiment.

   The duty and responsibility for ascertaining the quality of the consent rests upon each individual who initiates, directs or engages in the experiment. It is a personal duty and responsibility which may not be delegated to another with impunity.

2. The experiment should be such as to yield fruitful results for the good of society, unprocurable by other methods or means of study, and not random and unnecessary in nature.

3. The experiment should be so designed and based on the results of animal experimentation and a knowledge of the natural history of the disease or other problem under study that the anticipated results will justify the performance of the experiment.

4. The experiment should be so conducted as to avoid all unnecessary physical and mental suffering and injury.

5. No experiment should be conducted where there is an a priori reason to believe that death or disabling injury will occur; except, perhaps, in those experiments where the experimental physicians also serve as subjects.

6. The degree of risk to be taken should never exceed that determined by the humanitarian importance of the problem to be solved by the experiment.

7. Proper preparations should be made and adequate facilities provided to protect the experimental subject against even remote possibilities of injury, disability, or death.

8. The experiment should be conducted only by scientifically qualified persons. The highest degree of skill and care should be required through all stages of the experiment of those who conduct or engage in the experiment.

9. During the course of the experiment the human subject should be at liberty to bring the experiment to an end if he has reached the physical or mental state where continuation of the experiment seems to him to be impossible.

10. During the course of the experiment the scientist in charge must be prepared to terminate the experiment at any stage, if he has probable cause to believe, in the exercise of the good faith, superior skill and careful judgment required of him that a continuation of the experiment is likely to result in injury, disability, or death to the experimental subject.

PRINCIPLES FOR THOSE IN RESEARCH AND EXPERIMENTATION

World Medical Association

1954

• • •

Formulated by the Committee on Medical Ethics and adopted by the Eighth General Assembly of the World Medical Association (WMA), this document is the first set of guidelines governing research issued by the WMA and is the historical predecessor of the Declaration of Helsinki.

1. Scientific and Moral Aspects of Experimentation

   The word experimentation applies not only to experimentation itself but also to the experimenter. An individual cannot and should not attempt any kind of experimentation. Scientific qualities are indisputable and must always be respected. Likewise, there must be strict adherence to the general rules of respect of the individual.

2. Prudence and Discretion in the Publication of the First Results of Experimentation

   This principle applies primarily to the medical press and we are proud to note that in the majority of cases this rule has been adhered to by the editors of our journals. Then there is the general press which does not in every instance have the same rules of prudence and discretion as the medical press. The World Medical Association draws attention to the detrimental effects of premature or unjustified statements. In the interest of the public, each national association should consider methods of avoiding this danger.

3. Experimentation on Healthy Subjects

   Every step must be taken in order to make sure that those who submit themselves to experimentation be fully informed. The paramount factor in experimentation on human beings is the responsibility of the research worker and not the willingness of the person submitting to the experiment.

4. Experimentation on Sick Subjects

   Here it may be that in the presence of individual and desperate cases one may attempt an operation or a treatment of a rather daring nature. Such exceptions will be rare and require the approval either of the person or his next of kin. In such a situation it is the doctor's conscience which will make the decision.

5. Necessity of Informing the Person Who Submits to Experimentation of the Nature of the Experimentation, the Reasons for the Experiment, and the Risks Involved

   It should be required that each person who submits to experimentation be informed of the nature of, the reason for, and the risk of the proposed experiment. If the patient is irresponsible, consent should be obtained from the individual who is legally responsible for the individual. In both instances, consent should be obtained in writing.

ARTICLE SEVEN, INTERNATIONAL COVENANT ON CIVIL AND POLITICAL RIGHTS

General Assembly of the United Nations

1958

• • •

Prepared by the Commission on Human Rights, the draft Covenant on Civil and Political Rights was first considered by the Third (Social,

Humanitarian, and Cultural) Committee of the General Assembly of the United Nations in 1954. Article Seven of the draft covenant was adopted in 1958. Discussion of the article focused primarily on the second sentence. Some members argued that emphasis on one type of cruel and inhuman treatment weakened the article. However, it was generally agreed that that sentence was directed against criminal experimentation, such as that conducted by Nazi physician-researchers, and should be retained. The difficulty lay in prohibiting criminal experimentation without hindering legitimate research.

The committee entertained many amendments. Two notable discussions involved the "free consent" requirement and the phrase "…involving risk, where such is not required by his state of physical or mental health," which appeared at the end of the second sentence in the original draft. The committee ultimately retained the "free consent" requirement as an important criterion for determining when experimentation amounted to "cruel, inhuman, or degrading treatment." The committee also deleted the final phrase on the grounds that the term "experimentation" did not cover medical treatment that was required in the interest of an individual's health, and inclusion of the phrase would confuse the meaning of the provision by implying that scientific or medical practices directed toward an individual's welfare came within the scope of the article.

ARTICLE 7.

No one shall be subjected to torture or to cruel, inhuman or degrading treatment or punishment. In particular, no one shall be subjected without his free consent to medical or scientific experimentation.

DECLARATION OF HELSINKI

World Medical Association

1964, REVISED 1975, 1983, 1989, 1996, 2000

• • •

The Declaration of Helsinki, which offers recommendations for conducting experiments using human subjects, was adopted in 1962 and revised by the 18th World Medical Assembly at Helsinki, Finland, in 1964. Subsequent revisions were approved in Tokyo (1975), Venice (1983), Hong Kong (1989), Somerset West, Republic of South Africa (1996), and Edinburgh (2000).

<http://www.wma.net/e/policy/17-c_e.html>

A. INTRODUCTION

1. The World Medical Association has developed the Declaration of Helsinki as a statement of ethical principles to provide guidance to physicians and other participants in medical research involving human subjects. Medical research involving human subjects includes research on identifiable human material or identifiable data.

2. It is the duty of the physician to promote and safeguard the health of the people. The physician's knowledge and conscience are dedicated to the fulfillment of this duty.

3. The Declaration of Geneva of the World Medical Association binds the physician with the words, "The health of my patient will be my first consideration," and the International Code of Medical Ethics declares that, "A physician shall act only in the patient's interest when providing medical care which might have the effect of weakening the physical and mental condition of the patient."

4. Medical progress is based on research which ultimately must rest in part on experimentation involving human subjects.

5. In medical research on human subjects, considerations related to the well-being of the human subject should take precedence over the interests of science and society.

6. The primary purpose of medical research involving human subjects is to improve prophylactic, diagnostic and therapeutic procedures and the understanding of the aetiology and pathogenesis of disease. Even the best proven prophylactic, diagnostic, and therapeutic methods must continuously be challenged through research for their effectiveness, efficiency, accessibility and quality.

7. In current medical practice and in medical research, most prophylactic, diagnostic and therapeutic procedures involve risks and burdens.

8. Medical research is subject to ethical standards that promote respect for all human beings and protect their health and rights. Some research populations are vulnerable and need special protection. The particular needs of the economically and medically disadvantaged must be recognized. Special attention is also required for those who cannot give or refuse consent for themselves, for those who may be subject to giving consent under duress, for those who will not benefit personally from the research and for those for whom the research is combined with care.

9. Research Investigators should be aware of the ethical, legal and regulatory requirements for research on human subjects in their own countries as well as applicable international requirements. No national ethical, legal or regulatory requirement should be allowed to reduce or eliminate any of the protections for human subjects set forth in this Declaration.

B. BASIC PRINCIPLES FOR ALL MEDICAL RESEARCH

10. It is the duty of the physician in medical research to protect the life, health, privacy, and dignity of the human subject.

11. Medical research involving human subjects must conform to generally accepted scientific principles, be based on a thorough knowledge of the scientific literature, other relevant sources of information, and on adequate laboratory and, where appropriate, animal experimentation.

12. Appropriate caution must be exercised in the conduct of research which may affect the environment, and the welfare of animals used for research must be respected.

13. The design and performance of each experimental procedure involving human subjects should be clearly formulated in an experimental protocol. This protocol should be submitted for consideration, comment, guidance, and where appropriate, approval to a specially appointed ethical review committee, which must be independent of the investigator, the sponsor or any other kind of undue influence. This independent committee should be in conformity with the laws and regulations of the country in which the research experiment is performed. The committee has the right to monitor ongoing trials. The researcher has the obligation to provide monitoring information to the committee, especially any serious adverse events. The researcher should also submit to the committee, for review, information regarding funding, sponsors, institutional affiliations, other potential conflicts of interest and incentives for subjects.

14. The research protocol should always contain a statement of the ethical considerations involved and should indicate that there is compliance with the principles enunciated in this Declaration.

15. Medical research involving human subjects should be conducted only by scientifically qualified persons and under the supervision of a clinically competent medical person. The responsibility for the human subject must always rest with a medically qualified person and never rest on the subject of the research, even though the subject has given consent.

16. Every medical research project involving human subjects should be preceded by careful assessment of predictable risks and burdens in comparison with foreseeable benefits to the subject or to others. This does not preclude the participation of healthy volunteers in medical research. The design of all studies should be publicly available.

17. Physicians should abstain from engaging in research projects involving human subjects unless they are confident that the risks involved have been adequately assessed and can be satisfactorily managed. Physicians should cease any investigation if the risks are found to outweigh the potential benefits or if there is conclusive proof of positive and beneficial results.

18. Medical research involving human subjects should only be conducted if the importance of the objective outweighs the inherent risks and burdens to the subject. This is especially important when the human subjects are healthy volunteers.

19. Medical research is only justified if there is a reasonable likelihood that the populations in which the research is carried out stand to benefit from the results of the research.

20. The subjects must be volunteers and informed participants in the research project.

21. The right of research subjects to safeguard their integrity must always be respected. Every precaution should be taken to respect the privacy of the subject, the confidentiality of the patient's information and to minimize the impact of the study on the subject's physical and mental integrity and on the personality of the subject.

22. In any research on human beings, each potential subject must be adequately informed of the aims, methods, sources of funding, any possible conflicts of interest, institutional affiliations of the researcher, the anticipated benefits and potential risks of the study and the discomfort it may entail. The subject should be informed of the right to abstain from participation in the study or to withdraw consent to participate at any time without reprisal. After ensuring that the subject has understood the information, the physician should then obtain the subject's freely-given informed consent, preferably in writing. If the consent cannot be obtained in writing, the non-written consent must be formally documented and witnessed.

23. When obtaining informed consent for the research project the physician should be particularly cautious if the subject is in a dependent relationship with the physician or may consent under duress. In that case the informed consent should be obtained by a well-informed physician who is not engaged in the investigation and who is completely independent of this relationship.

24. For a research subject who is legally incompetent, physically or mentally incapable of giving consent or is a legally incompetent minor, the investigator must obtain informed consent from the legally authorized representative in accordance with applicable law. These groups should not be

included in research unless the research is necessary to promote the health of the population represented and this research cannot instead be performed on legally competent persons.

25. When a subject deemed legally incompetent, such as a minor child, is able to give assent to decisions about participation in research, the investigator must obtain that assent in addition to the consent of the legally authorized representative.

26. Research on individuals from whom it is not possible to obtain consent, including proxy or advance consent, should be done only if the physical/mental condition that prevents obtaining informed consent is a necessary characteristic of the research population. The specific reasons for involving research subjects with a condition that renders them unable to give informed consent should be stated in the experimental protocol for consideration and approval of the review committee. The protocol should state that consent to remain in the research should be obtained as soon as possible from the individual or a legally authorized surrogate.

27. Both authors and publishers have ethical obligations. In publication of the results of research, the investigators are obliged to preserve the accuracy of the results. Negative as well as positive results should be published or otherwise publicly available. Sources of funding, institutional affiliations and any possible conflicts of interest should be declared in the publication. Reports of experimentation not in accordance with the principles laid down in this Declaration should not be accepted for publication.

C. ADDITIONAL PRINCIPLES FOR MEDICAL RESEARCH COMBINED WITH MEDICAL CARE

28. The physician may combine medical research with medical care, only to the extent that the research is justified by its potential prophylactic, diagnostic or therapeutic value. When medical research is combined with medical care, additional standards apply to protect the patients who are research subjects.

29. The benefits, risks, burdens and effectiveness of a new method should be tested against those of the best current prophylactic, diagnostic, and therapeutic methods. This does not exclude the use of placebo, or no treatment, in studies where no proven prophylactic, diagnostic or therapeutic method exists. See footnote

30. At the conclusion of the study, every patient entered into the study should be assured of access to the best proven prophylactic, diagnostic and therapeutic methods identified by the study.

31. The physician should fully inform the patient which aspects of the care are related to the research. The refusal of a patient to participate in a study must never interfere with the patient-physician relationship.

32. In the treatment of a patient, where proven prophylactic, diagnostic and therapeutic methods do not exist or have been ineffective, the physician, with informed consent from the patient, must be free to use unproven or new prophylactic, diagnostic and therapeutic measures, if in the physician's judgement it offers hope of saving life, re-establishing health or alleviating suffering. Where possible, these measures should be made the object of research, designed to evaluate their safety and efficacy. In all cases, new information should be recorded and, where appropriate, published. The other relevant guidelines of this Declaration should be followed.

Footnote: Note of Clarification on Paragraph 29 of the WMA Declaration of Helsinki

The WMA hereby reaffirms its position that extreme care must be taken in making use of a placebo-controlled trial and that in general this methodology should only be used in the absence of existing proven therapy. However, a placebo-controlled trial may be ethically acceptable, even if proven therapy is available, under the following circumstances:

— Where for compelling and scientifically sound methodological reasons its use is necessary to determine the efficacy or safety of a prophylactic, diagnostic or therapeutic method; or

— Where a prophylactic, diagnostic or therapeutic method is being investigated for a minor condition and the patients who receive placebo will not be subject to any additional risk of serious or irreversible harm.

All other provisions of the Declaration of Helsinki must be adhered to, especially the need for appropriate ethical and scientific review.

The Declaration of Helsinki (Document 17.C) is an official policy document of the World Medical Association, the global representative body for physicians. It was first adopted in 1964 (Helsinki, Finland) and revised in 1975 (Tokyo, Japan), 1983 (Venice, Italy), 1989 (Hong Kong), 1996 (Somerset-West, South Africa) and 2000 (Edinburgh, Scotland). Note of clarification on Paragraph 29 added by the WMA General Assembly, Washington 2002.

THE BELMONT REPORT: ETHICAL PRINCIPLES AND GUIDELINES FOR THE PROTECTION OF HUMAN SUBJECTS OF RESEARCH

National Commission for the Protection of Human Subjects of Biomedical and Behavioral Research

1979

• • •

The National Commission for the Protection of Human Subjects of Biomedical and Behavioral Research was created when the National Research Act (P.L. 93–348) became law on July 12, 1974. One of its mandates was to identify the basic ethical principles that should underlie research involving human subjects and to develop guidelines to ensure that such research is conducted in accordance with those principles. Since the first set of federal guidelines for human experimentation applicable to all programs under the auspices of what was then the Department of Health, Education, and Welfare (DHEW) was enacted in 1971, the National Commission's task, in part, was to identify and articulate the theoretical principles upon which those already existing guidelines were based.

After nearly four years of deliberation, the commission published its findings as the Belmont Report, which is printed below. The current, 1991 revision of the 1971 federal guidelines for human experimentation are also included in this section of the Appendix. Federal regulations require that every U.S. research institution that receives federal funds for research involving human subjects adopt a statement of principles to govern the protection of human subjects of research, and virtually all such institutions have endorsed the Belmont principles. Many research institutions outside of the United States also endorse the Belmont principles; however, the majority of foreign institutions cite the Declaration of Helsinki as their core ethical standard.

Scientific research has produced substantial social benefits. It has also posed some troubling ethical questions. Public attention was drawn to these questions by reported abuses of human subjects in biomedical experiments, especially during the Second World War. During the Nuremberg War Crime Trials, the Nuremberg code was drafted as a set of standards for judging physicians and scientists who had conducted biomedical experiments on concentration camp prisoners. This code became the prototype of many later codes intended to assure that research involving human subjects would be carried out in an ethical manner.

The codes consist of rules, some general, others specific, that guide the investigators or the reviewers of research in their work. Such rules often are inadequate to cover complex situations; at times they come into conflict, and they are frequently difficult to interpret or apply. Broader ethical principles will provide a basis on which specific rules may be formulated, criticized and interpreted.

Three principles, or general prescriptive judgments, that are relevant to research involving human subjects are identified in this statement. Other principles may also be relevant. These three are comprehensive, however, and are stated at a level of generalization that should assist scientists, subjects, reviewers and interested citizens to understand the ethical issues inherent in research involving human subjects. These principles cannot always be applied so as to resolve beyond dispute particular ethical problems. The objective is to provide an analytical framework that will guide the resolution of ethical problems arising from research involving human subjects.

This statement consists of a distinction between research and practice, a discussion of the three basic ethical principles, and remarks about the application of these principles.

A. Boundaries Between Practice and Research

It is important to distinguish between biomedical and behavioral research, on the one hand, and the practice of accepted therapy on the other, in order to know what activities ought to undergo review for the protection of human subjects of research. The distinction between research and practice is blurred partly because both often occur together (as in research designed to evaluate a therapy) and partly because notable departures from standard practice are often called "experimental" when the terms "experimental" and "research" are not carefully defined.

For the most part, the term "practice" refers to interventions that are designed solely to enhance the well-being of an individual patient or client and that have a reasonable expectation of success. The purpose of medical or behavioral practice is to provide diagnosis, preventive treatment or therapy to particular individuals. By contrast, the term "research" designates an activity designed to test an hypothesis, permit conclusions to be drawn, and thereby to develop or contribute to generalizable knowledge (expressed, for example, in theories, principles, and statements of relationships). Research is usually described in a formal protocol that sets forth an objective and a set of procedures designed to reach that objective.

When a clinician departs in a significant way from standard or accepted practice, the innovation does not, in and of itself, constitute research. The fact that a procedure is "experimental," in the sense of new, untested or different, does not automatically place it in the category of research.

Radically new procedures of this description should, however, be made the object of formal research at an early stage in order to determine whether they are safe and effective. Thus, it is the responsibility of medical practice committees, for example, to insist that a major innovation be incorporated into a formal research project.

Research and practice may be carried on together when research is designed to evaluate the safety and efficacy of a therapy. This need not cause any confusion regarding whether or not the activity requires review; the general rule is that if there is any element of research in an activity, that activity should undergo review for the protection of human subjects.

B. Basic Ethical Principles

The expression "basic ethical principles" refers to those general judgments that serve as a basic justification for the many particular ethical prescriptions and evaluations of human actions. Three basic principles, among those generally accepted in our cultural tradition, are particularly relevant to the ethics of research involving human subjects: the principles of respect for persons, beneficence and justice.

1. Respect for Persons. — Respect for persons incorporates at least two ethical convictions: first, that individuals should be treated as autonomous agents, and second, that persons with diminished autonomy are entitled to protection. The principle of respect for persons thus divides into two separate moral requirements: the requirement to acknowledge autonomy and the requirement to protect those with diminished autonomy.

An autonomous person is an individual capable of deliberation about personal goals and of acting under the direction of such deliberation. To respect autonomy is to give weight to autonomous persons' considered opinions and choices while refraining from obstructing their actions unless they are clearly detrimental to others. To show lack of respect for an autonomous agent is to repudiate that person's considered judgments, to deny an individual the freedom to act on those considered judgments, or to withhold information necessary to make a considered judgment, when there are no compelling reasons to do so.

However, not every human being is capable of self-determination. The capacity for self-determination matures during an individual's life, and some individuals lose this capacity wholly or in part because of illness, mental disability, or circumstances that severely restrict liberty. Respect for the immature and the incapacitated may require protecting them as they mature or while they are incapacitated.

Some persons are in need of extensive protection, even to the point of excluding them from activities which may harm them; other persons require little protection beyond making sure they undertake activities freely and with awareness of possible adverse consequences. The extent of protection afforded should depend upon the risk of harm and the likelihood of benefit. The judgment that any individual lacks autonomy should be periodically reevaluated and will vary in different situations.

In most cases of research involving human subjects, respect for persons demands that subjects enter into the research voluntarily and with adequate information. In some situations, however, application of the principle is not obvious. The involvement of prisoners as subjects of research provides an instructive example. On the one hand, it would seem that the principle of respect for persons requires that prisoners not be deprived of the opportunity to volunteer for research. On the other hand, under prison conditions they may be subtly coerced or unduly influenced to engage in research activities for which they would not otherwise volunteer. Respect for persons would then dictate that prisoners be protected. Whether to allow prisoners to "volunteer" or to "protect" them presents a dilemma. Respecting persons, in most hard cases, is often a matter of balancing competing claims urged by the principle of respect itself.

2. Beneficence. — Persons are treated in an ethical manner not only by respecting their decisions and protecting them from harm, but also by making efforts to secure their well-being. Such treatment falls under the principle of beneficence. The term "beneficence" is often understood to cover acts of kindness or charity that go beyond strict obligation. In this document, beneficence is understood in a stronger sense, as an obligation. Two general rules have been formulated as complementary expressions of beneficent actions in this sense: (1) do not harm and (2) maximize possible benefits and minimize possible harms.

The Hippocratic maxim "do no harm" has long been a fundamental principle of medical ethics. Claude Bernard extended it to the realm of research, saying that one should not injure one person regardless of the benefits that might come to others. However, even avoiding harm requires learning what is harmful; and, in the process of obtaining this information, persons may be exposed to risk of harm. Further, the Hippocratic Oath requires physicians to benefit their patients "according to their best judgment." Learning what will in fact benefit may require exposing persons to risk. The problem posed by these imperatives is to decide when it is justifiable to seek certain benefits despite the risks involved, and when the benefits should be foregone because of the risks.

The obligations of beneficence affect both individual investigators and society at large, because they extend both to particular research projects and to the entire enterprise of research. In the case of particular projects, investigators and members of their institutions are obliged to give forethought to the maximization of benefits and the reduction of risk that might occur from the research investigation. In the case of scientific research in general, members of the larger society are obliged to recognize the longer term benefits and risks that may result from the improvement of knowledge and from the development of novel medical, psychotherapeutic, and social procedures.

The principle of beneficence often occupies a well-defined justifying role in many areas of research involving human subjects. An example is found in research involving children. Effective ways of treating childhood diseases and fostering healthy development are benefits that serve to justify research involving children—even when individual research subjects are not direct beneficiaries. Research also makes it possible to avoid the harm that may result from the application of previously accepted routine practices that on closer investigation turn out to be dangerous. But the role of the principle of beneficence is not always so unambiguous. A difficult ethical problem remains, for example, about research that presents more than minimal risk without immediate prospect of direct benefit to the children involved. Some have argued that such research is inadmissible, while others have pointed out that this limit would rule out much research promising great benefit to children in the future. Here again, as with all hard cases, the different claims covered by the principle of beneficence may come into conflict and force difficult choices.

3. Justice. — Who ought to receive the benefits of research and bear its burdens? This is a question of justice, in the sense of "fairness in distribution" or "what is deserved." An injustice occurs when some benefit to which a person is entitled is denied without good reason or when some burden is imposed unduly. Another way of conceiving the principle of justice is that equals ought to be treated equally. However, this statement requires explication. Who is equal and who is unequal? What considerations justify departure from equal distribution? Almost all commentators allow that distinctions based on experience, age, deprivation, competence, merit and position do sometimes constitute criteria justifying differential treatment for certain purposes. It is necessary, then, to explain in what respects people should be treated equally. There are several widely accepted formulations of just ways to distribute burdens and benefits. Each formulation mentions some relevant property on the basis of which burdens and benefits should be distributed. These formulations are (1) to each person an equal share, (2) to each person according to individual need, (3) to each person

according to individual effort, (4) to each person according to societal contribution, and (5) to each person according to merit.

Questions of justice have long been associated with social practices such as punishment, taxation and political representation. Until recently these questions have not generally been associated with scientific research. However, they are foreshadowed even in the earliest reflections on the ethics of research involving human subjects. For example, during the 19th and early 20th centuries the burdens of serving as research subjects fell largely upon poor ward patients, while the benefits of improved medical care flowed primarily to private patients. Subsequently, the exploitation of unwilling prisoners as research subjects in Nazi concentration camps was condemned as a particularly flagrant injustice. In this country, in the 1940's, the Tuskegee syphilis study used disadvantaged, rural black men to study the untreated course of a disease that is by no means confined to that population. These subjects were deprived of demonstrably effective treatment in order not to interrupt the project, long after such treatment became generally available.

Against this historical background, it can be seen how conceptions of justice are relevant to research involving human subjects. For example, the selection of research subjects needs to be scrutinized in order to determine whether some classes (e.g., welfare patients, particularly racial and ethnic minorities, or persons confined to institutions) are being systematically selected simply because of their easy availability, their compromised position, or their manipulability, rather than for reasons directly related to the problem being studied. Finally, whenever research supported by public funds leads to the development of therapeutic devices and procedures, justice demands both that these not provide advantages only to those who can afford them and that such research should not unduly involve persons from groups unlikely to be among the beneficiaries of subsequent applications of the research.

C. Applications

Applications of the general principles to the conduct of research leads to consideration of the following requirements: informed consent, risk/benefit assessment, and the selection of subjects of research.

1. Informed Consent. — Respect for persons requires that subjects, to the degree that they are capable, be given the opportunity to choose what shall or shall not happen to them. This opportunity is provided when adequate standards for informed consent are satisfied.

While the importance of informed consent is unquestioned, controversy prevails over the nature and possibility of an informed consent. Nonetheless, there is widespread agreement that the consent process can be analyzed as containing three elements: information, comprehension and voluntariness.

Information. Most codes of research establish specific items for disclosure intended to assure that subjects are given sufficient information. These items generally include: the research procedure, their purposes, risks and anticipated benefits, alternative procedures (where therapy is involved), and a statement offering the subject the opportunity to ask questions and to withdraw at any time from the research. Additional items have been proposed, including how subjects are selected, the person responsible for the research, etc.

However, a simple listing of items does not answer the question of what the standard should be for judging how much and what sort of information should be provided. One standard frequently invoked in medical practice, namely the information commonly provided by practitioners in the field or in the locale, is inadequate since research takes place precisely when a common understanding does not exist. Another standard, currently popular in malpractice law, requires the practitioner to reveal the information that reasonable persons would wish to know in order to make a decision regarding their care. This, too, seems insufficient since the research subject, being in essence a volunteer, may wish to know considerably more about risks gratuitously undertaken than do patients who deliver themselves into the hand of a clinician for needed care. It may be that a standard of "the reasonable volunteer" should be proposed: the extent and nature of information should be such that persons, knowing that the procedure is neither necessary for their care nor perhaps fully understood, can decide whether they wish to participate in the furthering of knowledge. Even when some direct benefit to them is anticipated, the subjects should understand clearly the range of risk and the voluntary nature of participation.

A special problem of consent arises where informing subjects of some pertinent aspect of the research is likely to impair the validity of the research. In many cases, it is sufficient to indicate to subjects that they are being invited to participate in research of which some features will not be revealed until the research is concluded. In all cases of research involving incomplete disclosure, such research is justified only if it is clear that (1) incomplete disclosure is truly necessary to accomplish the goals of the research, (2) there are no undisclosed risks to subjects that are more than minimal, and (3) there is an adequate plan for debriefing subjects, when appropriate, and for dissemination of research results to them. Information about risks should never be withheld for the purpose of eliciting the cooperation of subjects, and truthful answers should always be given to direct questions about the research. Care should be taken to distinguish cases in which disclosure would destroy or invalidate the research from cases in which disclosure would simply inconvenience the investigator.

Comprehension. The manner and context in which information is conveyed is as important as the information itself. For example, presenting information in a disorganized and rapid fashion, allowing too little time for consideration or curtailing opportunities for questioning, all may adversely affect a subject's ability to make an informed choice.

Because the subject's ability to understand is a function of intelligence, rationality, maturity and language, it is necessary to adapt the presentation of the information to the subject's capacities. Investigators are responsible for ascertaining that the subject has comprehended the information. While there is always an obligation to ascertain that the information about risk to subjects is complete and adequately comprehended, when the risks are more serious, that obligation increases. On occasion, it may be suitable to give some oral or written tests of comprehension.

Special provision may need to be made when comprehension is severely limited—for example, by conditions of immaturity or mental disability. Each class of subjects that one might consider as incompetent (e.g., infants and young children, mentally disabled patients, the terminally ill and the comatose) should be considered on its own terms. Even for these persons, however, respect requires giving them the opportunity to choose to the extent they are able, whether or not to participate in research. The objections of these subjects to involvement should be honored, unless the research entails providing them a therapy unavailable elsewhere. Respect for persons also requires seeking the permission of other parties in order to protect the subjects from harm. Such persons are thus respected both by acknowledging their own wishes and by the use of third parties to protect them from harm.

The third parties chosen should be those who are most likely to understand the incompetent subject's situation and to act in that person's best interest. The person authorized to act on behalf of the subject should be given an opportunity to observe the research as it proceeds in order to be able to withdraw the subject from the research, if such action appears in the subject's best interest.

Voluntariness. An agreement to participate in research constitutes a valid consent only if voluntarily given. This element of informed consent requires conditions free of coercion and undue influence. Coercion occurs when an overt threat of harm is intentionally presented by one person to another in order to obtain compliance. Undue influence, by contrast, occurs through an offer of an excessive, unwarranted, inappropriate or improper reward or other overture in order to obtain compliance. Also, inducements that would ordinarily be acceptable may become undue influences if the subject is especially vulnerable.

Unjustifiable pressures usually occur when persons in positions of authority or commanding influence—especially where possible sanctions are involved—urge a course of action for a subject. A continuum of such influencing factors exists, however, and it is impossible to state precisely where justifiable persuasion ends and undue influence begins. But undue influence would include actions such as manipulating a person's choice through the controlling influence of a close relative and threatening to withdraw health services to which an individual would otherwise be entitled.

2. Assessment of Risks and Benefits. — The assessment of risks and benefits requires a careful arrayal of relevant data, including, in some cases, alternative ways of obtaining the benefits sought in the research. Thus, the assessment presents both an opportunity and a responsibility to gather systematic and comprehensive information about proposed research. For the investigator, it is a means to examine whether the proposed research is properly designed. For a review committee, it is a method for determining whether the risks that will be presented to subjects are justified. For prospective subjects, the assessment will assist the determination whether or not to participate.

The Nature and Scope of Risks and Benefits. The requirement that research be justified on the basis of a favorable risk/benefit assessment bears a close relation to the principle of beneficence, just as the moral requirement that informed consent be obtained is derived primarily from the principle of respect for persons. The term "risk" refers to a possibility that harm may occur. However, when expressions such as "small risk" or "high risk" are used, they usually refer (often ambiguously) both to the chance (probability) of experiencing a harm and the severity (magnitude) of the envisioned harm.

The term "benefit" is used in the research context to refer to something of positive value related to health or welfare. Unlike "risk," "benefit" is not a term that expresses probabilities. Risk is properly contrasted to probability of benefits, and benefits are properly contrasted with harms rather than risks of harm. Accordingly, so-called risk benefit assessments are concerned with the probabilities and magnitudes of possible harms and anticipated benefits. Many kinds of possible harms and benefits need to be taken into account. There are, for example, risks of psychological harm, physical harm, legal harm, social harm and economic harm

and the corresponding benefits. While the most likely types of harms to research subjects are those of psychological or physical pain or injury, other possible kinds should not be overlooked.

Risks and benefits of research may affect the individual subjects, the families of the individual subjects, and society at large (or special groups of subjects in society). Previous codes and Federal regulations have required that risks to subjects be outweighed by the sum of both the anticipated benefit to the subject, if any, and the anticipated benefit to society in the form of knowledge to be gained from the research. In balancing these different elements, the risks and benefits affecting the immediate research subject will normally carry special weight. On the other hand, interests other than those of the subject may on some occasions be sufficient by themselves to justify the risks involved in the research, so long as the subjects' rights have been protected. Beneficence thus requires that we protect against risk of harm to subjects and also that we be concerned about the loss of the substantial benefits that might be gained from research.

The Systematic Assessment of Risks and Benefits. It is commonly said that benefits and risks must be "balanced" and shown to be "in a favorable ratio." The metaphorical character of these terms draws attention to the difficulty of making precise judgments. Only on rare occasions will quantitative techniques be available for the scrutiny of research protocols. However, the idea of systematic, nonarbitrary analysis of risks and benefits should be emulated insofar as possible. This ideal requires those making decisions about the justifiability of research to be thorough in the accumulation and assessment of information about all aspects of the research, and to consider alternatives systematically. This procedure renders the assessment of research more rigorous and precise, while making communication between review board members and investigators less subject to misinterpretation, misinformation and conflicting judgments. Thus, there should first be a determination of the validity of the presuppositions of the research; then the nature, probability and magnitude of risk should be distinguished with as much clarity as possible. The method of ascertaining risks should be explicit, especially where there is no alternative to the use of such vague categories as small or slight risk. It should also be determined whether an investigator's estimates of the probability of harm or benefits are reasonable, as judged by known facts or other available studies.

Finally, assessment of the justifiability of research should reflect at least the following considerations: (i) Brutal or inhumane treatment of human subjects is never morally justified. (ii) Risks should be reduced to those necessary to achieve the research objective. It should be determined whether it is in fact necessary to use human subjects at all. Risk can perhaps never be entirely eliminated, but it can often be reduced by careful attention to alternative procedures. (iii) When research involves significant risk of serious impairment, review committees should be extraordinarily insistent on the justification of the risk (looking usually to the likelihood of benefit to the subject—or, in some rare cases, to the manifest voluntariness of the participation). (iv) When vulnerable populations are involved in research, the appropriateness of involving them should itself be demonstrated. A number of variables go into such judgments, including the nature and degree of risk, the condition of the particular population involved, and the nature and level of the anticipated benefits. (v) Relevant risks and benefits must be thoroughly arrayed in documents and procedures used in the informed consent process.

3. Selection of Subjects. — Just as the principle of respect for persons finds expression in the requirements for consent, and the principle of beneficence in risk benefit assessment, the principle of justice gives rise to moral requirements that there be fair procedures and outcomes in the selection of research subjects.

Justice is relevant to the selection of subjects of research at two levels: the social and the individual. Individual justice in the selection of subjects would require that researchers exhibit fairness: thus, they should not offer potentially beneficial research only to some patients who are in their favor or select only "undesirable" persons for risky research. Social justice requires that distinction be drawn between classes of subjects that ought, and ought not, to participate in any particular kind of research, based on the ability of members of that class to bear burdens and on the appropriateness of placing further burdens on already burdened persons. Thus, it can be considered a matter of social justice that there is an order of preference in the selection of classes of subjects (e.g., adults before children) and that some classes of potential subjects (e.g., the institutionalized mentally infirm or prisoners) may be involved as research subjects, if at all, only on certain conditions.

Injustice may appear in the selection of subjects, even if individual subjects are selected fairly by investigators and treated fairly in the course of research. Thus injustice arises from social, racial, sexual and cultural biases institutionalized in society. Thus, even if individual researchers are treating their research subjects fairly, and even if IRBs are taking care to assure that subjects are selected fairly within a particular institution, unjust social patterns may nevertheless appear in the overall distribution of the burdens and benefits of research. Although individual institutions or investigators may not be able to resolve a problem that is pervasive in their social setting, they can consider distributive justice in selecting research subjects.

Some populations, especially institutionalized ones, are already burdened in many ways by their infirmities and environments. When research is proposed that involves risks and does not include a therapeutic component, other less burdened classes of persons should be called upon first to accept these risks of research, except where the research is directly related to the specific conditions of the class involved. Also, even though public funds for research may often flow in the same directions as public funds for health care, it seems unfair that populations dependent on public health care constitute a pool of preferred research subjects if more advantaged populations are likely to be the recipients of the benefits.

One special instance of injustice results from the involvement of vulnerable subjects. Certain groups, such as racial minorities, the economically disadvantaged, the very sick, and the institutionalized may continually be sought as research subjects, owing to their ready availability in settings where research is conducted. Given their dependent status and their frequently compromised capacity for free consent, they should be protected against the danger of being involved in research solely for administrative convenience, or because they are easy to manipulate as a result of their illness or socioeconomic condition.

DHHS REGULATIONS FOR THE PROTECTION OF HUMAN SUBJECTS (45 CFR 46)

JUNE 18, 1991

• • •

Between 1953 and 1971 various agencies within the U.S. Department of Health, Education, and Welfare (DHEW), now the Department of Health and Human Services (DHHS), issued their own guidelines on human experimentation. Finally, in 1971, the first set of federal guidelines for human experimentation applicable to all DHEW programs was established. Those guidelines were revised slightly and officially published (May 30, 1974) as part of the Code of Federal Regulations (Title 45, Subtitle A, Part 46).

In 1981, the regulations underwent a major revision in light of various reports by the National Commission for the Protection of Human Subjects of Biomedical and Behavioral Research, which also issued the Belmont Report (see preceding document). The regulations were expanded to include guidelines for research involving fetuses, pregnant women, and human in vitro fertilization (Subpart B); children (Subpart C); and prisoners (Subpart D).

In June 1991, a revised Federal Policy for the Protection of Human Subjects (Subpart A) was adopted as "the Common Rule" by fifteen federal departments and agencies and the Office of Science and Technology Policy. Subparts B, C, and D remain directly applicable only to DHHS-supported human subjects research. The regulations were most recently revised November 13, 2001.

Subpart A–Federal Policy for the Protection of Human Subjects

(Basic DHHS Policy for Protection of Human Research Subjects)

. . .

<http://ohrp.osophs.dhhs.gov/humansubjects/guidance/45cfr46.htm>

§46.101 To what does this policy apply?

(a) Except as provided in paragraph (b) of this section, this policy applies to all research involving human subjects conducted, supported or otherwise subject to regulation by any Federal Department or Agency which takes appropriate administrative action to make the policy applicable to such research. This includes research conducted by Federal civilian employees or military personnel, except that each Department or Agency head may adopt such procedural modifications as may be appropriate from an administrative standpoint. It also includes research conducted, supported, or otherwise subject to regulation by the Federal Government outside the United States.

(1) Research that is conducted or supported by a Federal Department or Agency, whether or not it is regulated as defined in §46.102(e), must comply with all sections of this policy.

(2) Research that is neither conducted nor supported by a Federal Department or Agency but is subject to regulation as defined in §46.102(e) must be reviewed and approved, in compliance with §46.101, §46.102, and §46.107 through §46.117 of this policy, by an Institutional Review Board (IRB) that operates in accordance with the pertinent requirements of this policy.

(b) Unless otherwise required by Department or Agency heads, research activities in which the only involvement of human subjects will be in one or more of the following categories are exempt from this policy:1

(1) Research conducted in established or commonly accepted educational settings, involving normal educational practices, such as (i) research on regular and special education instructional strategies, or (ii) research on the effectiveness of or the comparison among instructional techniques, curricula, or classroom management methods.

(2) Research involving the use of educational tests (cognitive, diagnostic, aptitude, achievement), survey procedures, interview procedures or observation of public behavior, unless: (i) information obtained is recorded in such a manner that human subjects can be identified, directly or through identifiers linked to the subjects; and (ii) any disclosure of the human subjects' responses outside the research could reasonably place the subjects at risk of criminal or civil liability or be damaging to the subjects' financial standing, employability, or reputation.

(3) Research involving the use of educational tests (cognitive, diagnostic, aptitude, achievement), survey procedures, interview procedures, or observation of public behavior that is not exempt under paragraph (b)(2) of this section, if:

(i) the human subjects are elected or appointed public officials or candidates for public office; or (ii) Federal statute(s) require(s) without exception that the confidentiality of the personally identifiable information will be maintained throughout the research and thereafter.

(4) Research involving the collection or study of existing data, documents, records, pathological specimens, or diagnostic specimens, if these sources are publicly available or if the information is recorded by the investigator in such a manner that subjects cannot be identified, directly or through identifiers linked to the subjects.

(5) Research and demonstration projects which are conducted by or subject to the approval of Department or Agency heads, and which are designed to study, evaluate, or otherwise examine:

(i) Public benefit or service programs; (ii) procedures for obtaining benefits or services under those programs; (iii) possible changes in or alternatives to those programs or procedures; or (iv) possible changes in methods or levels of payment for benefits or services under those programs.

(6) Taste and food quality evaluation and consumer acceptance studies, (i) if wholesome foods

without additives are consumed or (ii) if a food is consumed that contains a food ingredient at or below the level and for a use found to be safe, or agricultural chemical or environmental contaminant at or below the level found to be safe, by the Food and Drug Administration or approved by the Environmental Protection Agency or the Food Safety and Inspection Service of the U.S. Department of Agriculture.

(c) Department or Agency heads retain final judgment as to whether a particular activity is covered by this policy.

(d) Department or Agency heads may require that specific research activities or classes of research activities conducted, supported, or otherwise subject to regulation by the Department or Agency but not otherwise covered by this policy, comply with some or all of the requirements of this policy.

(e) Compliance with this policy requires compliance with pertinent Federal laws or regulations which provide additional protections for human subjects.

(f) This policy does not affect any State or local laws or regulations which may otherwise be applicable and which provide additional protections for human subjects.

(g) This policy does not affect any foreign laws or regulations which may otherwise be applicable and which provide additional protections to human subjects of research.

(h) When research covered by this policy takes place in foreign countries, procedures normally followed in the foreign countries to protect human subjects may differ from those set forth in this policy. [An example is a foreign institution which complies with guidelines consistent with the World Medical Assembly Declaration (Declaration of Helsinki amended 1989) issued either by sovereign states or by an organization whose function for the protection of human research subjects is internationally recognized.] In these circumstances, if a Department or Agency head determines that the procedures prescribed by the institution afford protections that are at least equivalent to those provided in this policy, the Department or Agency head may approve the substitution of the foreign procedures in lieu of the procedural requirements provided in this policy. Except when otherwise required by statute, Executive Order, or the Department or Agency head, notices of these actions as they occur will be published in the Federal Register or will be otherwise published as provided in Department or Agency procedures.

(i) Unless otherwise required by law, Department or Agency heads may waive the applicability of some or all of the provisions of this policy to specific

research activities or classes or research activities otherwise covered by this policy. Except when otherwise required by statute or Executive Order, the Department or Agency head shall forward advance notices of these actions to the Office for Protection from Research Risks, National Institutes of Health, Department of Health and Human Services (DHHS), and shall also publish them in the Federal Register or in such other manner as provided in Department or Agency procedures.[1]

[1] Institutions with DHHS-approved assurances on file will abide by provisions of Title 45 CFR Part 46 Subparts A-D. Some of the other departments and agencies have incorporated all provisions of Title 45 CFR Part 46 into their policies and procedures as well. However, the exemptions at 45 CFR 46.101(b) do not apply to research involving prisoners, fetuses, pregnant women, or human in vitro fertilization, Subparts B and C. The exemption at 45 CFR 46.101(b)(2), for research involving survey or interview procedures or observation of public behavior, does not apply to research with children, Subpart D, except for research involving observations of public behavior when the investigator(s) do not participate in the activities being observed.

§46.102 Definitions.

(a) *Department or Agency* head means the head of any Federal Department or Agency and any other officer or employee of any Department or Agency to whom authority has been delegated.

(b) *Institution* means any public or private entity or Agency (including Federal, State, and other agencies).

(c) *Legally authorized representative* means an individual or judicial or other body authorized under applicable law to consent on behalf of a prospective subject to the subject's participation in the procedure(s) involved in the research.

(d) *Research* means a systematic investigation, including research development, testing and evaluation, designed to develop or contribute to generalizable knowledge. Activities which meet this definition constitute research for purposes of this policy, whether or not they are conducted or supported under a program which is considered research for other purposes. For example, some demonstration and service programs may include research activities.

(e) *Research subject to regulation,* and similar terms are intended to encompass those research activities for which a Federal Department or Agency has specific responsibility for regulating as a research activity, (for example, Investigational New Drug requirements administered by the Food and Drug

Administration). It does not include research activities which are incidentally regulated by a Federal Department or Agency solely as part of the Department's or Agency's broader responsibility to regulate certain types of activities whether research or non-research in nature (for example, Wage and Hour requirements administered by the Department of Labor).

(f) *Human subject* means a living individual about whom an investigator (whether professional or student) conducting research obtains

(1) data through intervention or interaction with the individual, or

(2) identifiable private information.

Intervention includes both physical procedures by which data are gathered (for example, venipuncture) and manipulations of the subject or the subject's environment that are performed for research purposes. *Interaction* includes communication or inter-personal contact between investigator and subject. *Private information* includes information about behavior that occurs in a context in which an individual can reasonably expect that no observation or recording is taking place, and information which has been provided for specific purposes by an individual and which the individual can reasonably expect will not be made public (for example, a medical record). Private information must be individually identifiable (i.e., the identity of the subject is or may readily be ascertained by the investigator or associated with the information) in order for obtaining the information to constitute research involving human subjects.

(g) *IRB* means an Institutional Review Board established in accord with and for the purposes expressed in this policy.

(h) *IRB approval* means the determination of the IRB that the research has been reviewed and may be conducted at an institution within the constraints set forth by the IRB and by other institutional and Federal requirements.

(i) *Minimal risk* means that the probability and magnitude of harm or discomfort anticipated in the research are not greater in and of themselves than those ordinarily encountered in daily life or during the performance of routine physical or psychological examinations or tests.

(j) *Certification* means the official notification by the institution to the supporting Department or Agency, in accordance with the requirements of this policy, that a research project or activity involving human subjects has been reviewed and approved by an IRB in accordance with an approved assurance.

§46.103 Assuring compliance with this policy—research conducted or supported by any Federal Department or Agency.

(a) Each institution engaged in research which is covered by this policy and which is conducted or supported by a Federal Department or Agency shall provide written assurance satisfactory to the Department or Agency head that it will comply with the requirements set forth in this policy. In lieu of requiring submission of an assurance, individual Department or Agency heads shall accept the existence of a current assurance, appropriate for the research in question, on file with the Office for Protection from Research Risks, National Institutes Health, DHHS, and approved for Federal-wide use by that office. When the existence of an DHHS-approved assurance is accepted in lieu of requiring submission of an assurance, reports (except certification) required by this policy to be made to Department and Agency heads shall also be made to the Office for Protection from Research Risks, National Institutes of Health, DHHS.

(b) Departments and agencies will conduct or support research covered by this policy only if the institution has an assurance approved as provided in this section, and only if the institution has certified to the Department or Agency head that the research has been reviewed and approved by an IRB provided for in the assurance, and will be subject to continuing review by the IRB. Assurances applicable to federally supported or conducted research shall at a minimum include:

(1) A statement of principles governing the institution in the discharge of its responsibilities for protecting the rights and welfare of human subjects of research conducted at or sponsored by the institution, regardless of whether the research is subject to Federal regulation. This may include an appropriate existing code, declaration, or statement of ethical principles, or a statement formulated by the institution itself. This requirement does not preempt provisions of this policy applicable to Department- or Agency-supported or regulated research and need not be applicable to any research exempted or waived under §46.101 (b) or (i).

(2) Designation of one or more IRBs established in accordance with the requirements of this policy, and for which provisions are made for meeting space and sufficient staff to support the IRB's review and recordkeeping duties.

(3) A list of IRB members identified by name; earned degrees; representative capacity; indications of experience such as board certifications,

licenses, etc., sufficient to describe each member's chief anticipated contributions to IRB deliberations; and any employment or other relationship between each member and the institution; for example: full-time employee, part-time employee, member of governing panel or board, stockholder, paid or unpaid consultant. Changes in IRB membership shall be reported to the Department or Agency head, unless in accord with §46.103(a) of this policy, the existence of a DHHS-approved assurance is accepted. In this case, change in IRB membership shall be reported to the Office for Protection from Research Risks, National Institutes of Health, DHHS.

(4) Written procedures which the IRB will follow (i) for conducting its initial and continuing review of research and for reporting its findings and actions to the investigator and the institution; (ii) for determining which projects require review more often than annually and which projects need verification from sources other than the investigators that no material changes have occurred since previous IRB review; and (iii) for ensuring prompt reporting to the IRB of proposed changes in a research activity, and for ensuring that such changes in approved research, during the period for which IRB approval has already been given, may not be initiated without IRB review and approval except when necessary to eliminate apparent immediate hazards to the subject.

(5) Written procedures for ensuring prompt reporting to the IRB, appropriate institutional officials, and the Department or Agency head of (i) any unanticipated problems involving risks to subjects or others or any serious or continuing noncompliance with this policy or the requirements or determinations of the IRB; and (ii) any suspension or termination of IRB approval.

(c) The assurance shall be executed by an individual authorized to act for the institution and to assume on behalf of the institution the obligations imposed by this policy and shall be filed in such form and manner as the Department or Agency head prescribes.

(d) The Department or Agency head will evaluate all assurances submitted in accordance with this policy through such officers and employees of the Department or Agency and such experts or consultants engaged for this purpose as the Department or Agency head determines to be appropriate. The Department or Agency head's evaluation will take into consideration the adequacy of the proposed IRB in light of the anticipated scope of the institution's research activities and the types of subject populations likely to be involved, the appropriateness of the proposed initial and continuing review procedures in light of the probable risks, and the size and complexity of the institution.

(e) On the basis of this evaluation, the Department or Agency head may approve or disapprove the assurance, or enter into negotiations to develop an approvable one. The Department or Agency head may limit the period during which any particular approved assurance or class of approved assurances shall remain effective or otherwise condition or restrict approval.

(f) Certification is required when the research is supported by a Federal Department or Agency and not otherwise exempted or waived under §46.101 (b) or (i). An institution with an approved assurance shall certify that each application or proposal for research covered by the assurance and by §46.103 of this policy has been reviewed and approved by the IRB. Such certification must be submitted with the application or proposal or by such later date as may be prescribed by the Department or Agency to which the application or proposal is submitted. Under no condition shall research covered by §46.103 of the policy be supported prior to receipt of the certification that the research has been reviewed and approved by the IRB. Institutions without an approved assurance covering the research shall certify within 30 days after receipt of a request for such a certification from the Department or Agency, that the application or proposal has been approved by the IRB. If the certification is not submitted within these time limits, the application or proposal may be returned to the institution.

(Approved by the Office of Management and Budget under Control Number 9999–0020.)

§§46.104–46.106 [Reserved]

§46.107 IRB membership.

(a) Each IRB shall have at least five members, with varying backgrounds to promote complete and adequate review of research activities commonly conducted by the institution. The IRB shall be sufficiently qualified through the experience and expertise of its members, and the diversity of the members, including consideration of race, gender, and cultural backgrounds and sensitivity to such issues as community attitudes, to promote respect for its advice and counsel in safeguarding the rights and welfare of human subjects. In addition to possessing the professional competence necessary to review specific research activities, the IRB shall be able to ascertain the acceptability of proposed research in terms of institutional commitments and regulations, applicable law, and standards of professional conduct and practice. The IRB shall therefore include persons knowledgeable in these areas. If an IRB regularly reviews research that involves a vulnerable category of subjects, such as children, prisoners, pregnant women, or handicapped or mentally disabled persons, consideration shall be given to the inclusion of one or more individuals who are knowledgeable about and experienced in working with these subjects.

(b) Every nondiscriminatory effort will be made to ensure that no IRB consists entirely of men or entirely of women, including the institution's consideration of qualified persons of both sexes, so long as no selection is made to the IRB on the basis of gender. No IRB may consist entirely of members of one profession.

(c) Each IRB shall include at least one member whose primary concerns are in scientific areas and at least one member whose primary concerns are in nonscientific areas.

(d) Each IRB shall include at least one member who is not otherwise affiliated with the institution and who is not part of the immediate family of a person who is affiliated with the institution.

(e) No IRB may have a member participate in the IRB's initial or continuing review of any project in which the member has a conflicting interest, except to provide information requested by the IRB.

(f) An IRB may, in its discretion, invite individuals with competence in special areas to assist in the review of issues which require expertise beyond or in addition to that available on the IRB. These individuals may not vote with the IRB.

§46.108 IRB functions and operations.

In order to fulfill the requirements of this policy each IRB shall:

(a) Follow written procedures in the same detail as described in §46.103(b)(4) and to the extent required by §46.103(b)(5).

(b) Except when an expedited review procedure is used (see §46.110), review proposed research at convened meetings at which a majority of the members of the IRB are present, including at least one member whose primary concerns are in nonscientific areas. In order for the research to be approved, it shall receive the approval of a majority of those members present at the meeting

§46.109 IRB review of research.

(a) An IRB shall review and have authority to approve, require modifications in (to secure approval), or disapprove all research activities covered by this policy.

(b) An IRB shall require that information given to subjects as part of informed consent is in accordance with §46.116. The IRB may require that information, in addition to that specifically mentioned in §46.116, be given to the subjects when in the IRB's judgment the information would meaningfully add to the protection of the rights and welfare of subjects.

(c) An IRB shall require documentation of informed consent or may waive documentation in accordance with §46.117.

(d) An IRB shall notify investigators and the institution in writing of its decision to approve or disapprove the proposed research activity, or of modifications required to secure IRB approval of the research activity. If the IRB decides to disapprove a research activity, it shall include in its written notification a statement of the reasons for its decision and give the investigator an opportunity to respond in person or in writing.

(e) An IRB shall conduct continuing review of research covered by this policy at intervals appropriate to the degree of risk, but not less than once per year, and shall have authority to observe or have a third party observe the consent process and the research.

(Approved by the Office of Management and Budget under Control Number 9999–0020.)

§46.110 Expedited review procedures for certain kinds of research involving no more than minimal risk, and for minor changes in approved research.

(a) The Secretary, HHS, has established, and published as a Notice in the Federal Register, a list of categories of research that may be reviewed by the IRB through an expedited review procedure. The list will be amended, as appropriate, after consultation with other departments and agencies, through periodic republication by the Secretary, HHS, in the Federal Register. A copy of the list is available from the Office for Protection from Research Risks, National Institutes of Health, DHHS, Bethesda, Maryland 20892.

(b) An IRB may use the expedited review procedure to review either or both of the following:

(1) some or all of the research appearing on the list and found by the reviewer(s) to involve no more than minimal risk,

(2) minor changes in previously approved research during the period (of one year or less) for which approval is authorized.

Under an expedited review procedure, the review may be carried out by the IRB chairperson or by one or more experienced reviewers designated by the chairperson from among members of the IRB. In reviewing the research, the reviewers may exercise all of the authorities of the IRB except that the reviewers may not disapprove the research. A research activity may be disapproved only after review in accordance with the non-expedited procedure set forth in §46.108(b).

(c) Each IRB which uses an expedited review procedure shall adopt a method for keeping all members advised of research proposals which have been approved under the procedure.

(d) The Department or Agency head may restrict, suspend, terminate, or choose not to authorize an institution's or IRB's use of the expedited review procedure.

§46.111 Criteria for IRB approval of research.

(a) In order to approve research covered by this policy the IRB shall determine that all of the following requirements are satisfied:

(1) Risks to subjects are minimized: (i) by using procedures which are consistent with sound research design and which do not unnecessarily expose subjects to risk, and (ii) whenever appropriate, by using procedures already being performed on the subjects for diagnostic or treatment purposes.

(2) Risks to subjects are reasonable in relation to anticipated benefits, if any, to subjects, and the importance of the knowledge that may reasonably be expected to result. In evaluating risks and benefits, the IRB should consider only those risks and benefits that may result from the research (as distinguished from risks and benefits of therapies subjects would receive even if not participating in the research). The IRB should not consider possible long-range effects of applying knowledge gained in the research (for example, the possible effects of the research on public policy) as among those research risks that fall within the purview of its responsibility.

(3) Selection of subjects is equitable. In making this assessment the IRB should take into account the purposes of the research and the setting in which the research will be conducted and should be particularly cognizant of the special problems of research involving vulnerable populations, such as children, prisoners, pregnant women, mentally disable persons, or economically or educationally disadvantaged persons.

(4) Informed consent will be sought from each prospective subject or the subject's legally authorized representative, in accordance with, and to the extent required by §46.116.

(5) Informed consent will be appropriately documented, in accordance with, and to the extent required by §46.117.

(6) When appropriate, the research plan makes adequate provision for monitoring the data collected to ensure the safety of subjects.

(7) When appropriate, there are adequate provisions to protect the privacy of subjects and to maintain the confidentiality of data.

(b) When some or all of the subjects are likely to be vulnerable to coercion or undue influence, such as children, prisoners, pregnant women, mentally disabled persons, or economically or educationally disadvantaged persons, additional safeguards have been included in the study to protect the rights and welfare of these subjects.

§46.112 Review by institution.

Research covered by this policy that has been approved by an IRB may be subject to further appropriate review and approval or disapproval by officials of the institution. However, those officials may not approve the research if it has not been approved by an IRB.

§46.113 Suspension or termination of IRB approval of research.

An IRB shall have authority to suspend or terminate approval of research that is not being conducted in accordance with the IRB's requirements or that has been associated with unexpected serious harm to subjects. Any suspension or termination or approval shall include a statement of the reasons for the IRB's action and shall be reported promptly to the investigator, appropriate institutional officials, and the Department or Agency head.

(Approved by the Office of Management and Budget under Control Number 9999–0020.)

§46.114 Cooperative research.

Cooperative research projects are those projects covered by this policy which involve more than one institution. In the conduct of cooperative research projects, each institution is responsible for safeguarding the rights and welfare of human subjects and for complying with this policy. With the approval of the Department or Agency head, an institution participating in a cooperative project may enter into a joint review arrangement, rely upon the review of another qualified IRB, or make similar arrangements for avoiding duplication of effort.

§46.115 IRB records.

(a) An institution, or when appropriate an IRB, shall prepare and maintain adequate documentation of IRB activities, including the following:

   (1) Copies of all research proposals reviewed, scientific evaluations, if any, that accompany the proposals, approved sample consent documents, progress reports submitted by investigators, and reports of injuries to subjects.

   (2) Minutes of IRB meetings which shall be in sufficient detail to show attendance at the meetings; actions taken by the IRB; the vote on these actions including the number of members voting for, against, and abstaining; the basis for requiring changes in or disapproving research; and a written summary of the discussion of controverted issues and their resolution.

   (3) Records of continuing review activities.

   (4) Copies of all correspondence between the IRB and the investigators.

   (5) A list of IRB members in the same detail as described in §46.103(b)(3).

   (6) Written procedures for the IRB in the same detail as described in §46.103(b)(4) and §46.103(b)(5).

   (7) Statements of significant new findings provided to subjects, as required by §46.116(b)(5).

(b) The records required by this policy shall be retained for at least 3 years, and records relating to research which is conducted shall be retained for at least 3 years after completion of the research. All records shall be accessible for inspection and copying by authorized representatives of the Department or Agency at reasonable times and in a reasonable manner.

(Approved by the Office of Management and Budget under Control Number 9999–0020.)

§46.116 General requirements for informed consent.

Except as provided elsewhere in this policy, no investigator may involve a human being as a subject in research covered by this policy unless the investigator has obtained the legally effective informed consent of the subject or the subject's legally authorized representative. An investigator shall seek such consent only under circumstances that provide the prospective subject or the representative sufficient opportunity to consider whether or not to participate and that minimize the possibility of coercion or undue influence. The information that is given to the subject or the representative shall be in language understandable to the subject or the representative. No informed consent, whether oral or written, may include any exculpatory language through which the subject or the representative is made to waive or appear to waive any of the subject's legal rights, or releases or appears to release the investigator, the sponsor, the institution or its agents from liability for negligence.

(a) Basic elements of informed consent. Except as provided in paragraph (c) or (d) of this section, in seeking informed consent the following information shall be provided to each subject:

   (1) a statement that the study involves research, an explanation of the purposes of the research and the expected duration of the subject's participation, a description of the procedures to be followed, and identification of any procedures which are experimental;

   (2) a description of any reasonably foreseeable risks or discomforts to the subject;

   (3) a description of any benefits to the subject or to others which may reasonably be expected from the research;

   (4) a disclosure of appropriate alternative procedures or courses of treatment, if any, that might be advantageous to the subject;

   (5) a statement describing the extent, if any, to which confidentiality of records identifying the subject will be maintained;

   (6) for research involving more than minimal risk, an explanation as to whether any compensation and an explanation as to whether any medical treatments are available if injury occurs and, if so, what they consist of, or where further information may be obtained;

   (7) an explanation of whom to contact for answers to pertinent questions about the research and research subjects' rights, and whom to contact in

the event of a research-related injury to the subject; and

(8) a statement that participation is voluntary, refusal to participate will involve no penalty or loss of benefits to which the subject is otherwise entitled, and the subject may discontinue participation at any time without penalty or loss of benefits to which the subject is otherwise entitled.

(b) additional elements of informed consent. When appropriate, one or more of the following elements of information shall also be provided to each subject:

(1) a statement that the particular treatment or procedure may involve risks to the subject (or to the embryo or fetus, if the subject is or may become pregnant) which are currently unforeseeable;

(2) anticipated circumstances under which the subject's participation may be terminated by the investigator without regard to the subject's consent;

(3) any additional costs to the subject that may result from participation in the research;

(4) the consequences of a subject's decision to withdraw from the research and procedures for orderly termination of participation by the subject;

(5) A statement that significant new findings developed during the course of the research which may relate to the subject's willingness to continue participation will be provided to the subject; and

(6) the approximate number of subjects involved in the study.

(c) An IRB may approve a consent procedure which does not include, or which alters, some or all of the elements of informed consent set forth above, or waive the requirement to obtain informed consent provided the IRB finds and documents that:

(1) the research or demonstration project is to be conducted by or subject to the approval of state or local government officials and is designed to study, evaluate, or otherwise examine: (i) public benefit or service programs; (ii) procedures for obtaining benefits or services under those programs; (iii) possible changes in or alternatives to those programs or procedures; or (iv) possible changes in methods or levels of payment for benefits or services under those programs; and

(2) the research could not practicably be carried out without the waiver or alteration.

(d) An IRB may approve a consent procedure which does not include, or which alters, some or all of the

elements of informed consent set forth in this section, or waive the requirements to obtain informed consent provided the IRB finds and documents that:

(1) the research involves no more than minimal risk to the subjects;

(2) the waiver or alteration will not adversely affect the rights and welfare of the subjects;

(3) the research could not practicably be carried out without the waiver or alteration; and,

(4) whenever appropriate, the subjects will be provided with additional pertinent information after participation.

(e) The informed consent requirements in this policy are not intended to preempt any applicable Federal, State, or local laws which require additional information to be disclosed in order for informed consent to be legally effective.

(f) Nothing in this policy is intended to limit the authority of a physician to provide emergency medical care, to the extent the physician is permitted to do so under applicable Federal, State, or local law.

(Approved by the Office of Management and Budget under Control Number 9999–0020.)

§46.117 Documentation of informed consent.

(a) Except as provided in paragraph (c) of this section, informed consent shall be documented by the use of a written consent form approved by the IRB and signed by the subject or the subject's legally authorized representative. A copy shall be given to the person signing the form.

(b) Except as provided in paragraph (c) of this section, the consent form may be either of the following:

(1) A written consent document that embodies the elements of informed consent required by §46.116. This form may be read to the subject or the subject's legally authorized representative, but in any event, the investigator shall give either the subject or the representative adequate opportunity to read it before it is signed; or

(2) A short form written consent document stating that the elements of informed consent required by §46.116 have been presented orally to the subject or the subject's legally authorized representative. When this method is used, there shall be a witness to the oral presentation. Also, the IRB shall approve a written summary of what is to be said to the subject or the representative.

Only the short form itself is to be signed by the subject or the representative. However, the witness shall sign both the short form and a copy of the summary, and the person actually obtaining consent shall sign a copy of the summary. A copy of the summary shall be given to the subject or the representative, in addition to a copy of the short form.

(c) An IRB may waive the requirement for the investigator to obtain a signed consent form for some or all subjects if it finds either:

(1) That the only record linking the subject and the research would be the consent document and the principal risk would be potential harm resulting from a breach of confidentiality. Each subject will be asked whether the subject wants documentation linking the subject with the research, and the subject's wishes will govern; or

(2) That the research presents no more than minimal risk of harm to subjects and involves no procedures for which written consent is normally required outside of the research context.

In cases in which the documentation requirement is waived, the IRB may require the investigator to provide subjects with a written statement regarding the research.

(Approved by the Office of Management and Budget under Control Number 9999–0020.)

§46.118 Applications and proposals lacking definite plans for involvement of human subjects.

Certain types of applications for grants, cooperative agreements, or contracts are submitted to departments or agencies with the knowledge that subjects may be involved within the period of support, but definite plans would not normally be set forth in the application or proposal. These include activities such as institutional type grants when selection of specific projects is the institution's responsibility; research training grants in which the activities involving subjects remain to be selected; and projects in which human subjects' involvement will depend upon completion of instruments, prior animal studies, or purification of compounds. These applications need not be reviewed by an IRB before an award may be made. However, except for research exempted or waived under §46.101 (b) or (i), no human subjects may be involved in any project supported by these awards until the project has been reviewed and approved by the IRB, as provided in this policy, and certification submitted, by the institution, to the Department or Agency.

§46.119 Research undertaken without the intention of involving human subjects.

In the event research is undertaken without the intention of involving human subjects, but it is later proposed to involve human subjects in the research, the research shall first be reviewed and approved by an IRB, as provided in this policy, a certification submitted, by the institution, to the Department or Agency, and final approval given to the proposed change by the Department or Agency.

§46.120 Evaluation and disposition of applications and proposals for research to be conducted or supported by a Federal Department or Agency.

(a) The Department or Agency head will evaluate all applications and proposals involving human subjects submitted to the Department or Agency through such officers and employees of the Department or Agency and such experts and consultants as the Department or Agency head determines to be appropriate. This evaluation will take into consideration the risks to the subjects, the adequacy of protection against these risks, the potential benefits of the research to the subjects and others, and the importance of the knowledge gained or to be gained.

(b) On the basis of this evaluation, the Department or Agency head may approve or disapprove the application or proposal, or enter into negotiations to develop an approvable one.

§46.121 [Reserved]

§46.122 Use of Federal funds.

Federal funds administered by a Department or Agency may not be expended for research involving human subjects unless the requirements of this policy have been satisfied.

§46.123 Early termination of research support: Evaluation of applications and proposals.

(a) The Department or Agency head may require that Department or Agency support for any project be terminated or suspended in the manner prescribed in applicable program requirements, when the Department or Agency head finds an institution has materially failed to comply with the terms of this policy.

(b) In making decisions about supporting or approving applications or proposals covered by this policy the Department or Agency head may take into account, in addition to all other eligibility requirements and program criteria, factors such as whether the applicant has been subject to a termination or suspension under paragraph (a) of this section and whether the applicant or the person or persons who would direct or has/have directed the scientific and technical aspects of an activity has/have, in the judgment of the Department or Agency head, materially failed to discharge responsibility for the protection of the rights and welfare of human subjects (whether or not the research was subject to Federal regulation).

§46.124 Conditions.

With respect to any research project or any class of research projects the Department or Agency head may impose additional conditions prior to or at the time of approval when in the judgment of the Department or Agency head additional conditions are necessary for the protection of human subjects.

§46.201 To what do these regulations apply?

(a) Except as provided in paragraph (b) of this section, this subpart applies to all research involving pregnant women, human fetuses, neonates of uncertain viability, or nonviable neonates conducted or supported by the Department of Health and Human Services (DHHS). This includes all research conducted in DHHS facilities by any person and all research conducted in any facility by DHHS employees.

(b) The exemptions at Sec. 46.101(b)(1) through (6) are applicable to this subpart.

(c) The provisions of Sec. 46.101(c) through (i) are applicable to this subpart. Reference to State or local laws in this subpart and in Sec. 46.101(f) is intended to include the laws of federally recognized American Indian and Alaska Native Tribal Governments.

(d) The requirements of this subpart are in addition to those imposed under the other subparts of this part.

§46.202 Definitions.

The definitions in Sec. 46.102 shall be applicable to this subpart as well. In addition, as used in this subpart:

(a) Dead fetus means a fetus that exhibits neither heartbeat, spontaneous respiratory activity, spontaneous movement of voluntary muscles, nor pulsation of the umbilical cord.

(b) Delivery means complete separation of the fetus from the woman by expulsion or extraction or any other means.

(c) Fetus means the product of conception from implantation until delivery.

(d) Neonate means a newborn.

(e) Nonviable neonate means a neonate after delivery that, although living, is not viable.

(f) Pregnancy encompasses the period of time from implantation until delivery. A woman shall be assumed to be pregnant if she exhibits any of the pertinent presumptive signs of pregnancy, such as missed menses, until the results of a pregnancy test are negative or until delivery.

(g) Secretary means the Secretary of Health and Human Services and any other officer or employee of the Department of Health and Human Services to whom authority has been delegated.

(h) Viable, as it pertains to the neonate, means being able, after delivery, to survive (given the benefit of available medical therapy) to the point of independently maintaining heartbeat and respiration. The Secretary may from time to time, taking into account medical advances, publish in the Federal Register guidelines to assist in determining whether a neonate is viable for purposes of this subpart. If a neonate is viable then it may be included in research only to the extent permitted and in accordance with the requirements of subparts A and D of this part.

§46.203 Duties of IRBs in connection with research involving pregnant women, fetuses, and neonates.

In addition to other responsibilities assigned to IRBs under this part, each IRB shall review research covered by this subpart and approve only research which satisfies the conditions of all applicable sections of this subpart and the other subparts of this part.

§46.204 Research involving pregnant women or fetuses.

Pregnant women or fetuses may be involved in research if all of the following conditions are met:

(a) Where scientifically appropriate, preclinical studies, including studies on pregnant animals, and clinical studies, including studies on nonpregnant women, have been conducted and provide data for assessing potential risks to pregnant women and fetuses;

(b) The risk to the fetus is caused solely by interventions or procedures that hold out the prospect of direct benefit for the woman or the fetus; or, if there is no such prospect of benefit, the risk to the fetus is not greater than minimal and the purpose of the research is the development of important biomedical knowledge which cannot be obtained by any other means;

(c) Any risk is the least possible for achieving the objectives of the research;

(d) If the research holds out the prospect of direct benefit to the pregnant woman, the prospect of a direct benefit both to the pregnant woman and the fetus, or no prospect of benefit for the woman nor the fetus when risk to the fetus is not greater than minimal and the purpose of the research is the development of important biomedical knowledge that cannot be obtained by any other means, her consent is obtained in accord with the informed consent provisions of subpart A of this part;

(e) If the research holds out the prospect of direct benefit solely to the fetus then the consent of the pregnant woman and the father is obtained in accord with the informed consent provisions of subpart A of this part, except that the father's consent need not be obtained if he is unable to consent because of unavailability, incompetence, or temporary incapacity or the pregnancy resulted from rape or incest.

(f) Each individual providing consent under paragraph (d) or (e) of this section is fully informed regarding the reasonably foreseeable impact of the research on the fetus or neonate;

(g) For children as defined in Sec. 46.402(a) who are pregnant, assent and permission are obtained in accord with the provisions of subpart D of this part;

(h) No inducements, monetary or otherwise, will be offered to terminate a pregnancy;

(i) Individuals engaged in the research will have no part in any decisions as to the timing, method, or procedures used to terminate a pregnancy; and

(j) Individuals engaged in the research will have no part in determining the viability of a neonate

§46.205 Research involving neonates.

(a) Neonates of uncertain viability and nonviable neonates may be involved in research if all of the following conditions are met:

(1) Where scientifically appropriate, preclinical and clinical studies have been conducted and provide data for assessing potential risks to neonates.

(2) Each individual providing consent under paragraph (b)(2) or (c)(5) of this section is fully informed regarding the reasonably foreseeable impact of the research on the neonate.

(3) Individuals engaged in the research will have no part in determining the viability of a neonate.

(4) The requirements of paragraph (b) or (c) of this section have been met as applicable.

(b) Neonates of uncertain viability. Until it has been ascertained whether or not a neonate is viable, a neonate may not be involved in research covered by this subpart unless the following additional conditions have been met:

(1) The IRB determines that:

(i) The research holds out the prospect of enhancing the probability of survival of the neonate to the point of viability, and any risk is the least possible for achieving that objective, or

(ii) The purpose of the research is the development of important biomedical knowledge which cannot be obtained by other means and there will be no added risk to the neonate resulting from the research; and

(2) The legally effective informed consent of either parent of the neonate or, if neither parent is able to consent because of unavailability, incompetence, or temporary incapacity, the legally effective informed consent of either parent's legally authorized representative is obtained in accord with subpart A of this part, except that the consent of the father or his legally authorized representative need not be obtained if the pregnancy resulted from rape or incest.

(c) Nonviable neonates. After delivery nonviable neonate may not be involved in research covered by this subpart unless all of the following additional conditions are met:

(1) Vital functions of the neonate will not be artificially maintained;

(2) The research will not terminate the heartbeat or respiration of the neonate;

(3) There will be no added risk to the neonate resulting from the research;

(4) The purpose of the research is the development of important biomedical knowledge that cannot be obtained by other means; and

(5) The legally effective informed consent of both parents of the neonate is obtained in accord with subpart A of this part, except that the waiver and alteration provisions of Sec. 46.116(c) and (d) do not apply. However, if either parent is unable to consent because of unavailability, incompetence, or temporary incapacity, the informed consent of one parent of a nonviable neonate will suffice to meet the requirements of this paragraph (c)(5), except that the consent of the father need not be obtained if the pregnancy resulted from rape or incest. The consent of a legally authorized representative of either or both of the parents of a nonviable neonate will not suffice to meet the requirements of this paragraph (c)(5).

(d) Viable neonates. A neonate, after delivery, that has been determined to be viable may be included in research only to the extent permitted by and in accord with the requirements of subparts A and D of this part.

§46.206 Research involving, after delivery, the placenta, the dead fetus or fetal material.

(a) Research involving, after delivery, the placenta; the dead fetus; macerated fetal material; or cells, tissue, or organs excised from a dead fetus, shall be conducted only in accord with any applicable Federal, State, or local laws and regulations regarding such activities.

(b) If information associated with material described in paragraph (a) of this section is recorded for research purposes in a manner that living individuals can be identified, directly or through identifiers linked to those individuals, those individuals are research subjects and all pertinent subparts of this part are applicable.

§46.207 Research not otherwise approvable which presents an opportunity to understand, prevent, or alleviate a serious problem affecting the health or welfare of pregnant women, fetuses, or neonates.

The Secretary will conduct or fund research that the IRB does not believe meets the requirements of Sec. 46.204 or Sec. 46.205 only if:

(a) The IRB finds that the research presents a reasonable opportunity to further the understanding, prevention, or alleviation of a serious problem affecting the health or welfare of pregnant women, fetuses or neonates; and

(b) The Secretary, after consultation with a panel of experts in pertinent disciplines (for example: science, medicine, ethics, law) and following opportunity for public review and comment, including a public meeting announced in the Federal Register, has determined either:

(1) That the research in fact satisfies the conditions of Sec. 46.204, as applicable; or

(2) The following:

(i) The research presents a reasonable opportunity to further the understanding, prevention, or alleviation of a serious problem affecting the health or welfare of pregnant women, fetuses or neonates;

(ii) The research will be conducted in accord with sound ethical principles; and

(iii) Informed consent will be obtained in accord with the informed consent provisions of

subpart A and other applicable subparts of this part.

Subpart C: Additional DHHS Protections Pertaining to Biomedical and Behavioral Research Involving Prisoners as Subjects
Source: 43 FR 53655, Nov. 16, 1978.

§46.301 Applicability.

(a) The regulations in this subpart are applicable to all biomedical and behavioral research conducted or supported by the Department of Health and Human Services involving prisoners as subjects.

(b) Nothing in this subpart shall be construed as indicating that compliance with the procedures set forth herein will authorize research involving prisoners as subjects, to the extent such research is limited or barred by applicable State or local law.

(c) The requirements of this subpart are in addition to those imposed under the other subparts of this part.

§46.302 Purpose.

Inasmuch as prisoners may be under constraints because of their incarceration which could affect their ability to make a truly voluntary and uncoerced decision whether or not to participate as subjects in research, it is the purpose of this subpart to provide additional safeguards for the protection of prisoners involved in activities to which this subpart is applicable.

§46.303 Definitions.

As used in this subpart:

(a) "Secretary" means the Secretary of Health and Human Services and any other officer or employee of the Department of Health and Human Services to whom authority has been delegated.

(b) "DHHS" means the Department of Health and Human Services.

(c) "Prisoner" means any individual involuntarily confined or detained in a penal institution. The term is intended to encompass individuals sentenced to such an institution under a criminal or civil statute, individuals detained in other facilities by virtue of statutes or commitment procedures which provide alternatives to criminal prosecution or incarceration in a penal institution, and individuals detained pending arraignment, trial, or sentencing.

(d) "Minimal risk" is the probability and magnitude of physical or psychological harm that is normally encountered in the daily lives, or in the routine medical, dental, or psychological examination of healthy persons.

§46.304 Composition of Institutional Review Boards where prisoners are involved.

In addition to satisfying the requirements in §46.107 of this part, an Institutional Review Board, carrying out responsibilities under this part with respect to research covered by this subpart, shall also meet the following specific requirements:

(a) A majority of the Board (exclusive of prisoner members) shall have no association with the prison(s) involved, apart from their membership on the Board.

(b) At least one member of the Board shall be a prisoner, or a prisoner representative with appropriate background and experience to serve in that capacity, except that where a particular research project is reviewed by more than one Board only one Board need satisfy this requirement.

§46.305 Additional duties of the Institutional Review Boards where prisoners are involved.

(a) In addition to all other responsibilities prescribed for Institutional Review Boards under this part, the Board shall review research covered by this subpart and approve such research only if it finds that:

(1) the research under review represents one of the categories of research permissible under §46.306(a)(2);

(2) any possible advantages accruing to the prisoner through his or her participation in the research, when compared to the general living conditions, medical care, quality of food, amenities and opportunity for earnings in the prison, are not of such a magnitude that his or her ability to weigh the risks of the research against the value of such advantages in the limited choice environment of the prison is impaired;

(3) the risks involved in the research are commensurate with risks that would be accepted by nonprisoner volunteers;

(4) procedures for the selection of subjects within the prison are fair to all prisoners and immune from arbitrary intervention by prison authorities or prisoners. Unless the principal investigator provides to the Board justification in writing for following some other procedures, control subjects must be selected randomly from the group of available prisoners who meet the characteristics needed for that particular research project;

(5) the information is presented in language which is understandable to the subject population;

(6) adequate assurance exists that parole boards will not take into account a prisoner's participation in the research in making decisions regarding parole, and each prisoner is clearly informed in advance that participation in the research will have no effect on his or her parole; and

(7) where the Board finds there may be a need for follow-up examination or care of participants after the end of their participation, adequate provision has been made for such examination or care, taking into account the varying lengths of individual prisoners' sentences, and for informing participants of this fact.

(b) The Board shall carry out such other duties as may be assigned by the Secretary.

(c) The institution shall certify to the Secretary, in such form and manner as the Secretary may require, that the duties of the Board under this section have been fulfilled.

§46.306 Permitted research involving prisoners.

(a) Biomedical or behavioral research conducted or supported by DHHS may involve prisoners as subjects only if:

(1) the institution responsible for the conduct of the research has certified to the Secretary that the Institutional Review Board has approved the research under §46.305 of this subpart; and

(2) in the judgment of the Secretary the proposed research involves solely the following:

(A) study of the possible causes, effects, and processes of incarceration, and of criminal behavior, provided that the study presents no more than minimal risk and no more than inconvenience to the subjects;

(B) study of prisons as institutional structures or of prisoners asincarcerated persons, provided that the study presents no more than minimal risk and no more than inconvenience to the subjects;

(C) research on conditions particularly affecting prisoners as a class (for example, vaccine trials and other research on hepatitis which is much more prevalent in prisons than elsewhere; and research on social and psychological problems such as alcoholism, drug addiction, and sexual assaults) provided that the study may proceed only after the Secretary has consulted with appropriate experts including experts in penology, medicine, and ethics, and published notice, in the Federal Register, of his intent to approve such research; or

(D) research on practices, both innovative and accepted, which have the intent and reasonable probability of improving the health or well-being of the subject. In cases in which those studies require the assignment of prisoners in a manner consistent with protocols approved by the IRB to control groups which may not benefit from the research, the study may proceed only after the Secretary has consulted with appropriate experts, including experts in penology, medicine, and ethics, and published notice, in the Federal Register, of the intent to approve such research.

(b) Except as provided in paragraph (a) of this section, biomedical or behavioral research conducted or supported by DHHS shall not involve prisoners as subjects.

Subpart D: Additional DHHS Protections for Children Involved as Subjects in Research

Source: 48 FR 9818, March 8, 1983; 56 FR 28032, June 18, 1991.

§46.401 To what do these regulations apply?

(a) This subpart applies to all research involving children as subjects, conducted or supported by the Department of Health and Human Services.

(1) This includes research conducted by Department employees, except that each head of an Operating Division of the Department may adopt such nonsubstantive, procedural modifications as may be appropriate from an administrative standpoint.

(2) It also includes research conducted or supported by the Department of Health and Human Services outside the United States, but in appropriate circumstances, the Secretary may, under paragraph (i) of §46.101 of Subpart A, waive the applicability of some or all of the requirements of these regulations for research of this type.

(b) Exemptions at §46.101(b)(1) and (b)(3) through (b)(6) are applicable to this subpart. The exemption at §46.101(b)(2) regarding educational tests is also applicable to this subpart. However, the exemption at §46.101(b)(2) for research involving survey or interview procedures or observations of public behavior does not apply to research covered by this subpart, except for research involving observation of public behavior when the investigator(s) do not participate in the activities being observed.

(c) The exceptions, additions, and provisions for waiver as they appear in paragraphs (c) through (i) of §46.101 of Subpart A are applicable to this subpart.

§46.402 Definitions.

The definitions in §46.102 of Subpart A shall be applicable to this subpart as well. In addition, as used in this subpart:

(a) "Children" are persons who have not attained the legal age for consent to treatments or procedures involved in the research, under the applicable law of the jurisdiction in which the research will be conducted.

(b) "Assent" means a child's affirmative agreement to participate in research. Mere failure to object should not, absent affirmative agreement, be construed as assent.

(c) "Permission" means the agreement of parent(s) or guardian to the participation of their child or ward in research.

(d) "Parent" means a child's biological or adoptive parent.

(e) "Guardian" means an individual who is authorized under applicable State or local law to consent on behalf of a child to general medical care.

§46.403 IRB duties.

In addition to other responsibilities assigned to IRBs under this part, each IRB shall review research covered by this subpart and approve only research which satisfies the conditions of all applicable sections of this subpart.

§46.404 Research not involving greater than minimal risk.

DHHS will conduct or fund research in which the IRB finds that no greater than minimal risk to children is presented, only if the IRB finds that adequate provisions are made for soliciting the assent of the children and the permission of their parents or guardians, as set forth in §46.408.

§46.405 Research involving greater than minimal risk but presenting the prospect of direct benefit to the individual subjects.

DHHS will conduct or fund research in which the IRB finds that more than minimal risk to children is presented by an intervention or procedure that holds out the prospect of direct benefit for the individual subject, or by a monitoring procedure that is likely to contribute to the subject's well-being, only if the IRB finds that:

(a) the risk is justified by the anticipated benefit to the subjects;

(b) the relation of the anticipated benefit to the risk is at least as favorable to the subjects as that presented by available alternative approaches; and

(c) adequate provisions are made for soliciting the assent of the children and permission of their parents or guardians, as set forth in §46.408.

§46.406 Research involving greater than minimal risk and no prospect of direct benefit to individual subjects, but likely to yield generalizable knowledge about the subject's disorder or condition.

DHHS will conduct or fund research in which the IRB finds that more than minimal risk to children is presented by an intervention or procedure that does not hold out the prospect of direct benefit for the individual subject, or by a monitoring procedure which is not likely to contribute to the well-being of the subject, only if the IRB finds that:

(a) the risk represents a minor increase over minimal risk;

(b) the intervention or procedure presents experiences to subjects that are reasonably commensurate with those inherent in their actual or expected medical, dental, psychological, social, or educational situations;

(c) the intervention or procedure is likely to yield generalizable knowledge about the subjects' disorder or condition which is of vital importance for the understanding or amelioration of the subjects' disorder or condition; and

(d) adequate provisions are made for soliciting assent of the children and permission of their parents or guardians, as set forth in §46.408.

§46.407 Research not otherwise approvable which presents an opportunity to understand, prevent, or alleviate a serious problem affecting the health or welfare of children.

DHHS will conduct or fund research that the IRB does not believe meets the requirements of §46.404, §46.405, or §46.406 only if:

(a) the IRB finds that the research presents a reasonable opportunity to further the understanding, prevention, or alleviation of a serious problem affecting the health or welfare of children; and

(b) the Secretary, after consultation with a panel of experts in pertinent disciplines (for example: science, medicine, education, ethics, law) and following

opportunity for public review and comment, has determined either:

(1) that the research in fact satisfies the conditions of §46.404, §46.405, or §46.406, as applicable, or
     (2) the following:
       (i) the research presents a reasonable opportunity to further the understanding, prevention, or alleviation of a serious problem affecting the health or welfare of children;

       (ii) the research will be conducted in accordance with sound ethical principles;

       (iii) adequate provisions are made for soliciting the assent of children and the permission of their parents or guardians, as set forth in §46.408.

§46.408 Requirements for permission by parents or guardians and for assent by children.

(a) In addition to the determinations required under other applicable sections of this subpart, the IRB shall determine that adequate provisions are made for soliciting the assent of the children, when in the judgment of the IRB the children are capable of providing assent. In determining whether children are capable of assenting, the IRB shall take into account the ages, maturity, and psychological state of the children involved. This judgment may be made for all children to be involved in research under a particular protocol, or for each child, as the IRB deems appropriate. If the IRB determines that the capability of some or all of the children is so limited that they cannot reasonably be consulted or that the intervention or procedure involved in the research holds out a prospect of direct benefit that is important to the health or well-being of the children and is available only in the context of the research, the assent of the children is not a necessary condition for proceeding with the research. Even where the IRB determines that the subjects are capable of assenting, the IRB may still waive the assent requirement under circumstances in which consent may be waived in accord with §46.116 of Subpart A.

(b) In addition to the determinations required under other applicable sections of this subpart, the IRB shall determine, in accordance with and to the extent that consent is required by §46.116 of Subpart A, that adequate provisions are made for soliciting the permission of each child's parents or guardian. Where parental permission is to be obtained, the IRB may find that the permission of one parent is sufficient for research to be conducted under §46.404 or §46.405. Where research is covered by §46.406 and §46.407 and permission is to be obtained from parents, both parents must give their permission unless one parent is deceased, unknown, incompetent, or not reasonably available, or when only one parent has legal responsibility for the care and custody of the child.

(c) In addition to the provisions for waiver contained in §46.116 of Subpart A, if the IRB determines that a research protocol is designed for conditions or for a subject population for which parental or guardian permission is not a reasonable requirement to protect the subjects (for example, neglected or abused children), it may waive the consent requirements in Subpart A of this part and paragraph (b) of this section, provided an appropriate mechanism for protecting the children who will participate as subjects in the research is substituted, and provided further that the waiver is not inconsistent with Federal, State, or local law. The choice of an appropriate mechanism would depend upon the nature and purpose of the activities described in the protocol, the risk and anticipated benefit to the research subjects, and their age, maturity, status, and condition.

(d) Permission by parents or guardians shall be documented in accordance with and to the extent required by §46.117 of Subpart A.

(e) When the IRB determines that assent is required, it shall also determine whether and how assent must be documented.

§46.409 Wards.

(a) Children who are wards of the State or any other agency, institution, or entity can be included in research approved under §46.406 or §46.407 only if such research is:

(1) related to their status as wards; or

(2) conducted in schools, camps, hospitals, institutions, or similar settings in which the majority of children involved as subjects are not wards.

(b) If the research is approved under paragraph (a) of this section, the IRB shall require appointment of an advocate for each child who is a ward, in addition to any other individual acting on behalf of the child as guardian or in loco parentis. One individual may serve as advocate for more than one child. The advocate shall be an individual who has the background and experience to act in, and agrees to act in, the best interests of the child for the duration of the child's participation in the research and who is not associated in any way (except in the role as advocate or member of the IRB) with the research, the investigator(s), or the guardian organization.

SUMMARY REPORT OF THE INTERNATIONAL SUMMIT CONFERENCE ON BIOETHICS TOWARDS AN INTERNATIONAL ETHIC FOR RESEARCH INVOLVING HUMAN SUBJECTS

1987

• • •

Twenty-six delegates, nominated by the heads of state of the Economic Summit nations, by the European Economic Community, and by the World Health Organization, met at the fourth Bioethics Summit Conference in Ottawa, Canada, on April 5–10, 1987. The Summary Report addresses the major areas discussed at the conference and presents both the background and the major recommendations of the delegates for improving the protection of research subjects throughout the world. The recommendations are shown in boldface within the text.

I. Introduction

Rapid progress in bioscience has created an urgent need for continuing development of national standards of ethics in research with human subjects. The growing interdependence of nations throughout the world has stimulated a need for internationally agreed upon standards and practices based on a careful continuing dialogue and reflection on values. The delegates at the fourth International Summit Conference on Bioethics worked towards these goals. They focused not only on the principles, but more specifically on the practice and procedures guaranteeing their implementation.

The fourth in a series of annual bioethics summit meetings initiated by Prime Minister Nakasone in 1984, this meeting reflected deeply on an area important to the entire practice of bioscience and medical research. It is hoped that the discussions and recommendations will benefit national practices, and contribute to improved international standards.

We, the delegates to this meeting, invite the Prime Minister of Canada, the Right Honourable Brian Mulroney, to present this report to the next Economic Summit Conference, to be held in Italy in June, 1987.

2. Underlying Principles and Practices: Development and Implementation of National Ethics Standards

The underlying principles for the ethics of research with human subjects are defined in national and international codes. These include respect for individuals, contribution to the well-being of peoples, and the equitable distribution of potential risks and benefits throughout society. Even though only very general international guidelines have been accepted, as yet, uniform practices are not widely accepted due to national and cultural differences.

Though need for societal review of research proposals is generally accepted, there are great differences in how countries and even institutions within some countries carry out this review. Only some of these variations can be ascribed to the cultural differences which are an essential background to societal standards.

As national standards are established, consideration must be given to evolving international guidelines for research involving human subjects. These will permit research jointly undertaken between nations and amongst groups of nations using common protocols, stimulate sharing of research results amongst nations and avoid unnecessary duplication and multiplication of research efforts.

The question of how common standards can best be developed and implemented considering the present diversity in practice and the complexity of the biomedical research enterprise occupied much of the discussion.

For that reason, the delegates recommend that, **in order to safeguard the rights and well-being of patients and research subjects, research ethics committees should be established in all countries. All research projects involving human subjects must be submitted for approval to a research ethics committee.**

It is further recommended that **these committees should be comprised of medical experts, and of experts outside the medical profession (e.g. theologians, moral philosophers, lawyers and lay members who represent the general public). Lawyers acting professionally for an institution, and others having a financial interest or potentially conflicting interest in the institution or the research in question should not serve on the ethics committee adjudicating that research. Furthermore, the committees should be of a size which is sufficient to allow for the inclusion of the three groups (medical experts, outside experts and lay members) and small enough to make efficient work possible.**

Delegates also considered the means of operation, freedoms and accountabilities of the research ethics committees. The decisions which they must take often reflect fine-tuning of competing values, and the scientific, technical or cultural environments within which they work may vary. Therefore, some differences of views between research ethics committees should be expected. Delegates were of the view

that, while there may well be a need for nations to monitor the functioning of local research ethics committees, the highest standards can best be assured if they are given responsibility and authority for the review of research ethics in their institutions; as well, their effect will be enhanced if seen by researchers and society as working with the research process in a collegial sense rather than in an adversarial mode.

3. Sharing the Risks

Three groups in society can be identified as carrying risks and benefits. The researchers or clinicians who carry out the trials and other research carry the primary burdens of ethical responsibility for protection of the research subjects. In the context of drug testing, the risks and costs of developing a new drug or device remain with the manufacturer. Nevertheless, the human beings on whom the research is performed carry the most direct risks of research, but can gain the benefits of the higher standards. Society or mankind as a whole is the ultimate beneficiary from research towards improved health standards, and for that reason, the delegates recommend **that human research subjects be fully informed concerning the availability or the lack of availability of mechanisms of care and compensation to subjects who are injured as a result of their participation in research.** The delegates encourage member nations to establish and implement appropriate mechanisms for care and compensation in areas where they do not presently exist.

4. Public Participation

The delegates agreed that the imposition of societal standards on the sensitive areas raised by medical research demand the involvement of the general public. Public involvement is required not only in the development of consensus but also in consideration of individual research proposals to ensure full and open discussion which might otherwise be uncritical or too narrowly based. The multi-disciplinary character of research ethics committees provides for both public accountability and credibility.

5. Research with Those with Restricted Ability to Give Consent

The overriding purpose of ethics review is the protection of the research subjects. An essential component of this protection, enunciated in all international codes of ethics is that each research subject must consent freely, and with full information, to participate in the research. However, those who are legally incompetent cannot, by definition, give their consent. Delegates focused their discussion of this issue on research with children, while recognizing that similar concerns arise with adults who are mentally handicapped and with other vulnerable populations.

All delegates accepted the need for therapeutic research with children. Such research would be of potentially direct benefit to the well-being of the individual subjects.

Non-therapeutic research with children poses special problems. While such research is necessary if treatment of childhood diseases is to advance, there was agreement that such research could only be considered under the following conditions: the specific project must be approved by a research ethics committee all needed knowledge must have been obtained through research with adults or animals, there must be no valid alternative to the use of children in the research; a valid proxy consent (by family, guardians, ombudsman, those with power of attorney or others) must have been obtained for each research subject; and, to the extent possible, the child should have given assent. Thus, it was the view of most delegates that needed non-therapeutic research on children, if within the limitations just mentioned and if involving minimal or no risk to such children, should not be precluded.

6. Research with Embryos

The integrity and uniqueness of human life in its earliest embryonic stages of formation must be accorded great respect. Generally, current forms of control of research procedures and manipulation of human embryos are not legislative in nature. In fact, in the almost total absence of legislation, research on the embryo is presently, for the most part, governed by the self-regulatory efforts of scientific and professional bodies, the centres themselves, and the review by ethics committees, local and national. Voluntary licensing control exists, for example in England, but there was consensus on the need to regulate the current anarchic proliferation and operation of in vitro fertilization centres in some countries as an interim measure while acquiring the experience necessary for effective legislation. Thus the delegates recommended **the need to keep in balance the professional liberty for clinical treatment and for scientific inquiry in the interest of progress in medical knowledge and skill while upholding regard for the human interest in the embryo. To this end, the delegates recommend the supervision and control of centres offering in vitro fertilization, of related treatments for infertility and of those conducting embryo research. Procedure should be regulated according to appropriate guidelines administered by a competent authority.**

All delegates recognized the preciousness of the human embryo. Nevertheless, different positions were taken with respect to the possibility of permitting research on the human embryo.

Several questions were raised with respect to the applicability of legal concepts of "ownership" (more properly discussed in terms of legitimate interest in) and control of human embryos during storage or after the death of the donors. Questions were also raised concerning penal sanction as opposed to professional regulation.

Considering the experimental nature of in vitro fertilization, its low success rate and the unknown long term effect of these procedures, which though "therapeutic" in nature for the infertile have implications for the manipulation and control of human life, **any work with embryos even as a treatment for infertility should be regarded as developmental procedures that are experimental in nature and therefore should be closely monitored.**

7. Pilot Studies and the Introduction of Novel Therapies

Delegates debated the special problem of ethics review of pilot studies or preliminary studies of medical innovations. Such studies were viewed as a phase between the initial observations on one or a few patients and the start of a full fledged protocol-based program.

Delegates recognized that it is often not easy to be sure whether an intervention by a physician should be regarded as a treatment undertaken only in the patient's best interest, or whether it is guided also by an intent to gain scientific knowledge.

The decision on when a research intent is present in therapy is a determination to be made by the physician. It was the opinion of the delegates that, if the health professional has any doubt whether the intervention is in fact research, the issue would best be brought to the attention of the ethics committee.

In reviewing the novel therapy of research, delegates recommended that **they should be subject to the same ethical judgements that apply to all research protocols. Special consideration should be given to limiting the number of subjects entered into pilot studies and to monitoring closely and frequently.**

In ethics review of pilot studies as in that of other proposed research, the delegates agreed that provision should be made for a mechanism to re-examine a research project rejected by a research ethics committee if the investigator should request it. Such a mechanism should be of a sort which would not invite the overriding of local decisions by a higher or distant authority. It should maintain the collaborative nature of the relationship between the researcher and the ethics committee, rather than encourage an adversarial relationship. It was also agreed that there should be a greater exchange of information between research ethics committees.

8. Industrial Research

Industries are a major source of medical innovation. Also much of their research is mandated by national standards for licensing drugs or devices. This research involves both animals and human beings and is often carried out in a number of countries. For that reason, the interactions between industries, governments and sometimes universities are of great concern.

Differences in the way ethics standards are interpreted and implemented can have direct economic effects. Lack of consistency can adversely affect national and commercial interests as well as the safety of research subjects. Delegates recommended that, at the very least, **a nation should not allow or support, in other countries, research which does not conform to ethics review standards at least equivalent to those in force within the nation.** Nations and industries should develop international accords which strive for common attitudes and the exchangeability of standards and for mutual trust. Nations and industries should also identify emerging technologies to foster early discussion of the ethical concerns. Such interaction might help the equitable distribution of effort in research and development.

Delegates also discussed the ethical concerns raised by the growing pace of commercialization of biomedical products. The increasingly close links between university-based and industry-based research mean that academic physicians or institutions may have financial interests in the outcome of the research; any such potential conflicts of interest should be declared in the research ethics review process. Moreover, it was the opinion of some delegates that we should develop and implement values which integrate ethics and economic interests.

Delegates also discussed the effects of confidentiality, and of compensation of research subjects. The confidentiality of commercially sensitive material may not be consistent with the requirements for ethics review. In addition, payment can induce subjects, especially those of more limited means, to participate in research, and may lead to financial competition for research subjects. With respect to both industrial and other research, concern was expressed over whether patients will be compensated for adverse effects which may on rare occasions arise from research.

Much industrial research and other biomedical research depends on research with animals. Delegates recommended that **in all research we must continue to insist that animal research precede research on humans, while recognizing the obligation to reduce the number of animals required to a minimum wherever possible and to encourage alternative methods for assessing safety and efficacy.**

Much of the regulatory testing of new drugs still requires the use of animals. In this regard, delegates recommended that **governmental agencies continuously modernize their own regulatory requirements to ensure that they do not demand test results of safety and toxicology which are no longer relevant or which can be replaced by satisfactory alternatives requiring fewer animals.**

9. The Selection of Research Topics and Directed Research

Researchers consider many scientific, social and other factors when choosing research topics; choices are also made in the context of national policies and systems of support as well as national policies and practices in respect to ethics. In some instances, this results in an apparent imbalance between the research topics being chosen and major global needs for research in fields such as fertility regulation and tropical diseases.

International research programs can provide a successful mechanism to promote and carry out research in those areas which are neglected, sensitive and/or economically unattractive to national researchers. These programs can make extensive use of the international scientific community and can apply high standards of scientific and ethical review to carry out research in the areas of high global priority which are difficult to address on a national basis. Those nations with the means to support research have an obligation to devote some of those resources to the research needs of nations without such means.

The group recommended that **research should focus upon the development of knowledge in broad fields of science with the aim of achieving a fundamental understanding of biological processes, even those which might not appear to have direct application over the short or longer term.** It is seen as a scientific infrastructure of further advance. It was also recommended that **the results of research should be applied as rapidly and as effectively as possible.**

Large scale support for narrowly focussed research on specific diseases without the necessary foundation of scientific knowledge was seen as rarely, if ever, successful. Also the failure to implement the results of research for the benefit of mankind has, in itself, serious ethical implications.

10. Towards Improved Ethics Standards: Biomedical Research in an Interdependent World

The last decade has witnessed profound growth in improved communication and common endeavor among nations. As well, movement has begun towards international agreement on research with human subjects.

Delegates are certain that meaningful international agreement is not only possible but necessary, and urge the Heads of States to work toward ensuring that practice accords with principles in all aspects of research involving human subjects.

The delegates accept that society should make the human subject an active and educated participant in a process in which he or she contributes from a sense of basic human altruism and a desire to serve the common good, rather than as a "subject of research" as has sometimes been the case in the past.

The further refinement and expansion of national standards of research ethics with human subjects across political and cultural boundaries demand continuing investigation into the ethical problems of biomedical research. Furthermore while agreeing on the necessity for this ethical review process, the delegates recommended that **these committees themselves, their operations and their functions be studied.**

According to the delegates, research ethics should always be integrated into clinical decision making. The delegates recommended that *education in medical ethics for physicians, investigators and medical students be intensified and that the media and public be informed.*

Delegates also recommended that special attention be given to the ethical issues involved in epidemiological studies which can be as intrusive of human dignity and privacy as medical intervention. In particular, the regulation of confidentiality, which may both restrict the exchange and gathering of information and may at the same time fail adequately to protect the subject of such epidemiological studies, requires examination.

In regard to dissemination of principles, statements by way of declaration are laudable and necessary. However, if such statements are to have proper binding power, they must be known and an effort made to ensure compliance with

them. To assist in this endeavor and in view of the importance of continuing dialogue, delegates recommended the **establishment of appropriate fora devoted to the issues arising in research with human subjects.**

Conclusions

This conference affirmed the growing importance of international agreement and cooperation on both the elaboration of principle and on the implementation of ethics review processes in medical research involving human subjects. To this end, the establishment of multi-disciplinary research ethics review bodies for the examination of research protocols was considered essential, as was further study and communication among nations.

Implementation of effective ethics review processes demands the enhanced education in medical ethics both of those involved in research and of the greater public.

The development of national and international standards for research with human subjects and their implementation must continue to aim at the protection of more vulnerable subjects.

The promulgation of ethics standards for research across nations and cultures should focus on areas of concern, as well as on international needs that are not being met.

RECOMMENDATION NO. R (90) 3 OF THE COMMITTEE OF MINISTERS TO MEMBER STATES CONCERNING MEDICAL RESEARCH ON HUMAN BEINGS

Council of Europe

1990

• • •

In their recommendation concerning medical research on human beings, adopted February 6, 1990, the Committee of Ministers of the Council of Europe recommended that the governments of member states adopt legislation or take any other measures to ensure the implementation of the principles articulated as well as ensuring that the provisions adopted be brought to the knowledge of all persons concerned. When the recommendation was adopted, the representative of the Federal Republic of Germany reserved the right of his government to comply with it or not. Although delegates from other countries were not so explicit, other European countries are entitled to the same reservation.

The Committee of Ministers, under the terms of Article 15.b of the Statute of the Council of Europe,

. . .

Being aware of the fact that the advancement of medical science and practice is dependent on knowledge and discovery which necessitate, as a last resort, experimentation on human beings;

Being convinced that medical research should never be carried out contrary to human dignity;

Considering the paramount concern to be the protection of the person undergoing medical research;

Considering that particular protection should be given to certain groups of persons;

Considering that every person has a right to accept or to refuse to undergo medical research and that no one should be forced to undergo it;

Considering that medical research on human beings should take into account ethical principles, and should also be subject to legal provisions;

Realising that in member states existing legal provisions are either divergent or insufficient in this field;

Noting the wish and the need to harmonise legislation,

Recommends the governments of member states:

a. to adopt legislation in conformity with the principles appended to this recommendation, or to take any other measures in order to ensure their implementation;

b. to ensure that the provisions so adopted are brought to the knowledge of all persons concerned.

Principles Concerning Medical Research on Human Beings

Scope and Definition

For the purpose of application of these principles, medical research means any trial and experimentation carried out on human beings, the purpose of which or one of the purposes of which is to increase medical knowledge.

Principle 1

Any medical research must be carried out within the framework of a scientific plan and in accordance with the following principles.

Principle 2

1. In medical research the interests and well-being of the person undergoing medical research must always prevail over the interests of science and society.

2. The risks incurred by a person undergoing medical research must be kept to a minimum. The risks should not be disproportionate to the benefits to that person or the importance of the aims pursued by the research.

Principle 3

1. No medical research may be carried out without the informed, free, express and specific consent of the person undergoing it. Such consent may be freely withdrawn at any phase of the research and the person undergoing the research should be informed, before being included in it, of his right to withdraw his consent.

2. The person who is to undergo medical research should be given information on the purpose of the research and the methodology of the experimentation. He should also be informed of the foreseeable risks and inconveniences to him of the proposed research. This information should be sufficiently clear and suitably adapted to enable consent to be given or refused in full knowledge of the relevant facts.

3. The provisions of this principle should apply also to a legal representative and to a legally incapacitated person having the capacity of understanding, in the situations described in Principles 4 and 5.

Principle 4

A legally incapacitated person may only undergo medical research where authorized by Principle 5 and if his legal representative, or an authority or an individual authorised or designated under his national law, consents. If the legally incapacitated person is capable of understanding, his consent is also required and no research may be undertaken if he does not give his consent.

Principle 5

1. A legally incapacitated person may not undergo medical research unless it is expected to produce a direct and significant benefit to his health.

2. However, by way of exception, national law may authorise research involving a legally incapacitated person which is not of direct benefit to his health when that person offers no objection, provided that the research is to the benefit of persons in the same

category and that the same scientific results cannot be obtained by research on persons who do not belong to this category.

Principle 6

Pregnant or nursing women may not undergo medical research where their health and/or that of the child would not benefit directly unless this research is aimed at benefiting other women and children who are in the same position and the same scientific results cannot be obtained by research on women who are not pregnant or nursing.

Principle 7

Persons deprived of liberty may not undergo medical research unless it is expected to produce a direct and significant benefit to their health.

Principle 8

In an emergency situation, notwithstanding Principle 3, where a patient is unable to give a prior consent, medical research can be carried out only when the following conditions are fulfilled:

—the research must have been planned to be carried out in the emergency in question;

—the systematic research plan must have been approved by an ethics committee;

—the research must be intended for the direct health benefit of the patient.

Principle 9

Any information of a personal nature obtained during medical research should be treated as confidential.

Principle 10

Medical research may not be carried out unless satisfactory evidence as to its safety for the person undergoing research is furnished.

Principle 11

Medical research that is not in accordance with scientific criteria in its design and cannot answer the questions posed is unacceptable even if the way it is to be carried out poses no risk to the person undergoing research.

Principle 12

1. Medical research must be carried out under the responsibility of a doctor or a person who exercises full clinical responsibility and who possesses appropriate knowledge and qualifications to meet any clinical contingency.

2. The responsible doctor or other person referred to in the preceding paragraph should enjoy full professional independence and should have the power to stop the research at any time.

Principle 13

1. Potential subjects of medical research should not be offered any inducement which compromises free consent. Persons undergoing medical research should not gain any financial benefit. However, expenses and any financial loss may be refunded and in appropriate cases a modest allowance may be given for any inconvenience inherent in the medical research.

2. If the person undergoing research is legally incapacitated, his legal representatives should not receive any form of remuneration whatever, except for the refund of their expenses.

Principle 14

1. Persons undergoing medical research and/or their dependents should be compensated for injury and loss caused by the medical research.

2. Where there is no existing system providing compensation for the persons concerned, states should ensure that sufficient guarantees for such compensation are provided.

3. Terms and conditions which exclude or limit, in advance, compensation to the victim should be considered to be null and void.

Principle 15

All proposed medical research plans should be the subject of an ethical examination by an independent and multidisciplinary committee.

Principle 16

Any medical research which is:

—unplanned, or

—contrary to any of the preceding principles, or

—in any other way contrary to ethics or law, or

—not in accordance with scientific methods in its design and cannot answer the questions posed should be prohibited or, if it has already begun, stopped or revised, even if it poses no risk to the person(s) undergoing the research.

INTERNATIONAL ETHICAL GUIDELINES FOR BIOMEDICAL RESEARCH INVOLVING HUMAN SUBJECTS

Council for International Organizations of Medical Sciences (CIOMS) in collaboration with the World Health Organization

1993, 2002

• • •

The 1993 guidelines were updated beginning in 1998. The document's acknowledgements states that "the 2002 text, which supersedes that of 1993, consists of a statement of general ethical principles, a preamble and 21 guidelines, with an introduction and a brief account of earlier declarations and guidelines. Like the 1982 and 1993 Guidelines, the present publication is designed to be of use, particularly to low-resource countries, in defining national policies on the ethics of biomedical research, applying ethical standards in local circumstances, and establishing or redefining adequate mechanisms for ethical review of research involving human subjects."

<http://www.cioms.ch/frame_guidelines_nov_2002.htm>

• • •

Introduction

This is the third in the series of international ethical guidelines for biomedical research involving human subjects issued by the Council for International Organizations of Medical Sciences since 1982. Its scope and preparation reflect well the transformation that has occurred in the field of research ethics in the almost quarter century since CIOMS first undertook to make this contribution to medical sciences and the ethics of research. The CIOMS Guidelines, with their stated concern for the application of the Declaration of Helsinki in developing countries, necessarily reflect the conditions and the needs of biomedical research in those countries, and the implications for multinational or transnational research in which they may be partners.

An issue, mainly for those countries and perhaps less pertinent now than in the past, has been the extent to which ethical principles are considered universal or as culturally relative—the universalist versus the pluralist view. The challenge to international research ethics is to apply universal ethical principles to biomedical research in a multicultural world with a multiplicity of health-care systems and considerable variation in standards of health care. The Guidelines take the position that research involving human subjects must not violate any universally applicable ethical standards, but acknowledge that, in superficial aspects, the application of the ethical principles, e.g., in relation to individual autonomy and informed consent, needs to take account of cultural values, while respecting absolutely the ethical standards.

Related to this issue is that of the human rights of research subjects, as well as of health professionals as researchers in a variety of sociocultural contexts, and the contribution that international human rights instruments can make in the application of the general principles of ethics to research involving human subjects. The issue concerns largely, though not exclusively, two principles: respect for autonomy and protection of dependent or vulnerable persons and populations. In the preparation of the Guidelines the potential contribution in these respects of human rights instruments and norms was discussed, and the Guideline drafters have represented the views of commentators on safeguarding the corresponding rights of subjects.

Certain areas of research are not represented by specific guidelines. One such is human genetics. It is, however, considered in Guideline 18 Commentary under *Issues of confidentiality in genetics research*. The ethics of genetics research was the subject of a commissioned paper and commentary.

Another unrepresented area is research with products of conception (embryo and fetal research, and fetal tissue research). An attempt to craft a guideline on the topic proved unfeasible. At issue was the moral status of embryos and fetuses and the degree to which risks to the life or well-being of these entities are ethically permissible.

In relation to the use of comparators in controls, commentators have raised the question of standard of care to be provided to a control group. They emphasize that standard of care refers to more than the comparator drug or other intervention, and that research subjects in the poorer countries do not usually enjoy the same standard of all-round care enjoyed by subjects in richer countries. This issue is not addressed specifically in the Guidelines.

In one respect the Guidelines depart from the terminology of the Declaration of Helsinki. 'Best current intervention' is the term most commonly used to describe the active comparator that is ethically preferred in controlled clinical trials. For many indications, however, there is more than one established 'current' intervention and expert clinicians do not agree on which is superior. In other circumstances in which there are several established 'current' interventions, some expert clinicians recognize one as superior to the rest; some commonly prescribe another because the superior intervention may be locally unavailable, for example, or prohibitively expensive or unsuited to the capability of particular patients to adhere to a complex and rigorous regimen. 'Established effective intervention' is the term used in Guideline 11 to refer to all such interventions, including the best and the various alternatives to the best. In some cases an ethical review committee may determine that it is ethically acceptable to use an established effective intervention as a comparator, even in cases where such an intervention is not considered the best current intervention.

The mere formulation of ethical guidelines for biomedical research involving human subjects will hardly resolve all the moral doubts that can arise in association with much research, but the Guidelines can at least draw the attention of sponsors, investigators and ethical review committees to the need to consider carefully the ethical implications of research protocols and the conduct of research, and thus conduce to high scientific and ethical standards of biomedical research.

International Instruments and Guidelines

The first international instrument on the ethics of medical research, the Nuremberg Code, was promulgated in 1947 as a consequence of the trial of physicians (the Doctors' Trial) who had conducted atrocious experiments on unconsenting prisoners and detainees during the second world war. The Code, designed to protect the integrity of the research subject, set out conditions for the ethical conduct of research involving human subjects, emphasizing their voluntary consent to research.

The Universal Declaration of Human Rights was adopted by the General Assembly of the United Nations in 1948. To give the Declaration legal as well as moral force, the General Assembly adopted in 1966 the International Covenant on Civil and Political Rights. Article 7 of the Covenant states "*No one shall be subjected to torture or to cruel, inhuman or degrading treatment or punishment. In particular, no one shall be subjected without his free consent to medical or scientific experimentation*". It is through this statement that society expresses the fundamental human value that is held to govern all research involving human subjects—the protection of the rights and welfare of all human subjects of scientific experimentation.

The Declaration of Helsinki, issued by the World Medical Association in 1964, is the fundamental document in the field of ethics in biomedical research and has influenced the formulation of international, regional and national legislation and codes of conduct. The Declaration, amended several times, most recently in 2000 (Appendix 2), is a comprehensive international statement of the ethics of research involving human subjects. It sets out ethical guidelines for physicians engaged in both clinical and nonclinical biomedical research.

Since the publication of the CIOMS 1993 Guidelines, several international organizations have issued ethical guidance on clinical trials. This has included, from the World Health Organization, in 1995, *Guidelines for Good Clinical Practice for Trials on Pharmaceutical Products*; and from the International Conference on Harmonisation of Technical Requirements for Registration of Pharmaceuticals for Human Use (ICH), in 1996, *Guideline on Good Clinical Practice*, designed to ensure that data generated from clinical trials are mutually acceptable to regulatory authorities in the European Union, Japan and the United States of America. The Joint United Nations Programme on HIV/AIDS published in 2000 the UNAIDS Guidance Document *Ethical Considerations in HIV Preventive Vaccine Research*.

In 2001 the Council of Ministers of the European Union adopted a Directive on clinical trials, which will be binding in law in the countries of the Union from 2004. The Council of Europe, with more than 40 member States, is developing a Protocol on Biomedical Research, which will be an additional protocol to the Council's 1997 Convention on Human Rights and Biomedicine.

Not specifically concerned with biomedical research involving human subjects but clearly pertinent, as noted above, are international human rights instruments. These are mainly the Universal Declaration of Human Rights, which, particularly in its science provisions, was highly influenced by the Nuremberg Code; the International Covenant on Civil and Political Rights; and the International Covenant on Economic, Social and Cultural Rights. Since the Nuremberg experience, human rights law has expanded to include the protection of women (Convention on the Elimination of All Forms of Discrimination Against Women) and children (Convention on the Rights of the Child). These and other such international instruments endorse in terms of human rights the general ethical principles that underlie the CIOMS International Ethical Guidelines.

General Ethical Principles

All research involving human subjects should be conducted in accordance with three basic ethical principles, namely respect for persons, beneficence and justice. It is generally agreed that these principles, which in the abstract have equal moral force, guide the conscientious preparation of proposals for scientific studies. In varying circumstances they may be expressed differently and given different moral weight, and their application may lead to different decisions or courses of action. The present guidelines are directed at the application of these principles to research involving human subjects.

Respect for persons incorporates at least two fundamental ethical considerations, namely:

a) respect for autonomy, which requires that those who are capable of deliberation about their personal choices should be treated with respect for their capacity for self-determination; and

b) protection of persons with impaired or diminished autonomy, which requires that those who are dependent or vulnerable be afforded security against harm or abuse.

Beneficence refers to the ethical obligation to maximize benefits and to minimize harms. This principle gives rise to norms requiring that the risks of research be reasonable in the light of the expected benefits, that the research design be sound, and that the investigators be competent both to conduct the research and to safeguard the welfare of the research subjects. Beneficence further proscribes the deliberate infliction of harm on persons; this aspect of beneficence is sometimes expressed as a separate principle, **nonmaleficence** (do no harm).

Justice refers to the ethical obligation to treat each person in accordance with what is morally right and proper, to give each person what is due to him or her. In the ethics of research involving human subjects the principle refers primarily to **distributive justice,** which requires the equitable distribution of both the burdens and the benefits of participation in research. Differences in distribution of burdens and benefits are justifiable only if they are based on morally relevant distinctions between persons; one such distinction is vulnerability. "Vulnerability" refers to a substantial incapacity to protect one's own interests owing to such impediments as lack of capability to give informed consent, lack of alternative means of obtaining medical care or other expensive necessities, or being a junior or subordinate member of a hierarchical group. Accordingly, special provision must be made for the protection of the rights and welfare of vulnerable persons.

Sponsors of research or investigators cannot, in general, be held accountable for unjust conditions where the research is conducted, but they must refrain from practices that are likely to worsen unjust conditions or contribute to new inequities. Neither should they take advantage of the relative inability of low-resource countries or vulnerable populations to protect their own interests, by conducting research inexpensively and avoiding complex regulatory systems of industrialized countries in order to develop products for the lucrative markets of those countries.

In general, the research project should leave low-resource countries or communities better off than previously or, at least, no worse off. It should be responsive to their health needs and priorities in that any product developed is made reasonably available to them, and as far as possible leave the population in a better position to obtain effective health care and protect its own health.

Justice requires also that the research be responsive to the health conditions or needs of vulnerable subjects. The subjects selected should be the least vulnerable necessary to accomplish the purposes of the research. Risk to vulnerable subjects is most easily justified when it arises from interventions or procedures that hold out for them the prospect of direct health-related benefit. Risk that does not hold out such prospect must be justified by the anticipated benefit to the population of which the individual research subject is representative.

Preamble

The term "research" refers to a class of activity designed to develop or contribute to generalizable knowledge. Generalizable knowledge consists of theories, principles or relationships, or the accumulation of information on which they are based, that can be corroborated by accepted scientific methods of observation and inference. In the present context "research" includes both medical and behavioural studies pertaining to human health. Usually "research" is modified by the adjective "biomedical" to indicate its relation to health.

Progress in medical care and disease prevention depends upon an understanding of physiological and pathological processes or epidemiological findings, and requires at some time research involving human subjects. The collection, analysis and interpretation of information obtained from research involving human beings contribute significantly to the improvement of human health.

Research involving human subjects includes:

—studies of a physiological, biochemical or pathological process, or of the response to a specific intervention—whether physical, chemical or psychological—in healthy subjects or patients;

—controlled trials of diagnostic, preventive or therapeutic measures in larger groups of persons, designed to demonstrate a specific generalizable response to these measures against a background of individual biological variation;

—studies designed to determine the consequences for individuals and communities of specific preventive or therapeutic measures; and

—studies concerning human health-related behaviour in a variety of circumstances and environments.

Research involving human subjects may employ either observation or physical, chemical or psychological intervention; it may also either generate records or make use of existing records containing biomedical or other information about individuals who may or may not be identifiable from the records or information. The use of such records and the protection of the confidentiality of data obtained from those records are discussed in *International Guidelines for Ethical Review of Epidemiological Studies (CIOMS, 1991)*.

The research may be concerned with the social environment, manipulating environmental factors in a way that could affect incidentally-exposed individuals. It is defined in broad terms in order to embrace field studies of pathogenic organisms and toxic chemicals under investigation for health-related purposes.

Biomedical research with human subjects is to be distinguished from the practice of medicine, public health and other forms of health care, which is designed to contribute directly to the health of individuals or communities. Prospective subjects may find it confusing when research and practice are to be conducted simultaneously, as when research is designed to obtain new information about the efficacy of a drug or other therapeutic, diagnostic or preventive modality.

As stated in Paragraph 32 of the Declaration of Helsinki, "In the treatment of a patient, where proven prophylactic, diagnostic and therapeutic methods do not exist or have been ineffective, the physician, with informed consent from the patient, must be free to use unproven or new prophylactic, diagnostic and therapeutic measures, if in the physician's judgement it offers hope of saving life, re-establishing health or alleviating suffering. Where possible, these measures should be made the object of research, designed to evaluate their safety and efficacy. In all cases, new information should be recorded and, where appropriate, published. The other relevant guidelines of this Declaration should be followed."

Professionals whose roles combine investigation and treatment have a special obligation to protect the rights and welfare of the patient-subjects. An investigator who agrees to act as physician-investigator undertakes some or all of the legal and ethical responsibilities of the subject's primary-care physician. In such a case, if the subject withdraws from the research owing to complications related to the research or in the exercise of the right to withdraw without loss of benefit, the physician has an obligation to continue to provide medical care, or to see that the subject receives the necessary care in the health-care system, or to offer assistance in finding another physician.

Research with human subjects should be carried out only by, or strictly supervised by, suitably qualified and experienced investigators and in accordance with a protocol that clearly states: the aim of the research; the reasons for proposing that it involve human subjects; the nature and degree of any known risks to the subjects; the sources from which it is proposed to recruit subjects; and the means proposed for ensuring that subjects' consent will be adequately informed and voluntary. The protocol should be scientifically and ethically appraised by one or more suitably constituted review bodies, independent of the investigators.

New vaccines and medicinal drugs, before being approved for general use, must be tested on human subjects in clinical trials; such trials constitute a substantial part of all research involving human subjects.

The Guidelines

GUIDELINE 1: *Ethical justification and scientific validity of biomedical research involving human beings*

The ethical justification of biomedical research involving human subjects is the prospect of discovering new ways of benefiting people's health. Such research can be ethically justifiable only if it is carried out in ways that respect and protect, and are fair to, the subjects of that research and are morally acceptable within the communities in which the research is carried out. Moreover, because scientifically invalid research is unethical in that it exposes research subjects to risks without possible benefit, investigators and sponsors must ensure that proposed studies involving human subjects conform to generally accepted scientific principles and are based on adequate knowledge of the pertinent scientific literature.

COMMENTARY ON GUIDELINE 1

Among the essential features of ethically justified research involving human subjects, including research with identifiable human tissue or data, are that the research offers a means of developing information not otherwise obtainable, that the design of the research is scientifically sound, and that the investigators and other research personnel are competent. The methods to be used should be appropriate to the objectives of the research and the field of study. Investigators and sponsors must also ensure that all who participate in the conduct of the research are qualified by virtue of their education and experience to perform competently in their roles. These considerations should be adequately reflected in the research protocol submitted for review and clearance to scientific and ethical review committees (Appendix I).

Scientific review is discussed further in the Commentaries to Guidelines 2 and 3: *Ethical review committees and Ethical review of externally sponsored research.* Other ethical aspects of research are discussed in the remaining guidelines and their commentaries. The protocol designed for submission for review and clearance to scientific and ethical review committees should include, when relevant, the items specified in Appendix I, and should be carefully followed in conducting the research.

GUIDELINE 2: *Ethical review committees*

All proposals to conduct research involving human subjects must be submitted for review of their scientific merit and ethical acceptability to one or more scientific review and ethical review committees. The review committees must be independent of the research team, and any direct financial or other material benefit they may derive from the research should not be contingent on the outcome of their review. The investigator must obtain their approval or clearance before undertaking the research. The ethical review committee should conduct further reviews as necessary in the course of the research, including monitoring of the progress of the study.

COMMENTARY ON GUIDELINE 2

Ethical review committees may function at the institutional, local, regional, or national level, and in some cases at the international level. The regulatory or other governmental authorities concerned should promote uniform standards across committees within a country, and, under all systems, sponsors of research and institutions in which the investigators are employed should allocate sufficient resources to the review process. Ethical review committees may receive money for the activity of reviewing protocols, but under no circumstances may payment be offered or accepted for a review committee's approval or clearance of a protocol.

Scientific review. According to the Declaration of Helsinki (Paragraph 11), medical research involving humans must conform to generally accepted scientific principles, and be based on a thorough knowledge of the scientific literature, other relevant sources of information, and adequate laboratory and, where indicated, animal experimentation. Scientific review must consider, inter alia, the study design, including the provisions for avoiding or minimizing risk and for monitoring safety. Committees competent to review and approve scientific aspects of research proposals must be multidisciplinary.

Ethical review. The ethical review committee is responsible for safeguarding the rights, safety, and well-being of the research subjects. Scientific review and ethical review

cannot be separated: scientifically unsound research involving humans as subjects is ipso facto unethical in that it may expose them to risk or inconvenience to no purpose; even if there is no risk of injury, wasting of subjects' and researchers' time in unproductive activities represents loss of a valuable resource. Normally, therefore, an ethical review committee considers both the scientific and the ethical aspects of proposed research. It must either carry out a proper scientific review or verify that a competent expert body has determined that the research is scientifically sound. Also, it considers provisions for monitoring of data and safety.

If the ethical review committee finds a research proposal scientifically sound, or verifies that a competent expert body has found it so, it should then consider whether any known or possible risks to the subjects are justified by the expected benefits, direct or indirect, and whether the proposed research methods will minimize harm and maximize benefit. (See Guideline 8: *Benefits and risks of study participation.*) If the proposal is sound and the balance of risks to anticipated benefits is reasonable, the committee should then determine whether the procedures proposed for obtaining informed consent are satisfactory and those proposed for the selection of subjects are equitable.

Ethical review of emergency compassionate use of an investigational therapy. In some countries, drug regulatory authorities **require that the so-called compassionate or humanitarian use of an investigational treatment be reviewed by an ethical review committee as though it were research. Exceptionally, a physician may undertake the compassionate use of an investigational therapy before obtaining the approval or clearance of an ethical review committee, provided three criteria are met: a patient needs emergency treatment, there is some evidence of possible effectiveness of the investigational treatment, and there is no other treatment available that is known to be equally effective or superior. Informed consent should be obtained according to the legal requirements and cultural standards of the community in which the intervention is carried out. Within one week the physician must report to the ethical review committee the details of the case and the action taken, and an independent health-care professional must confirm in writing to the ethical review committee the treating physician's judgment that the use of the investigational intervention was justified according to the three specified criteria.** (See also Guideline 13 Commentary section: *Other vulnerable groups.*)

National (centralized) or local review. Ethical review committees may be created under the aegis of national or local health administrations, national (or centralized) medical research councils or other nationally representative bodies. In a highly centralized administration a national, or centralized, review committee may be constituted for both the scientific and the ethical review of research protocols. In countries where medical research is not centrally administered, ethical review is more effectively and conveniently undertaken at a local or regional level. The authority of a local ethical review committee may be confined to a single institution or may extend to all institutions in which biomedical research is carried out within a defined geographical area. The basic responsibilities of ethical review committees are:

- to determine that all proposed interventions, particularly the administration of drugs and vaccines or the use of medical devices or procedures under development, are acceptably safe to be undertaken in humans or to verify that another competent expert body has done so;
- to determine that the proposed research is scientifically sound or to verify that another competent expert body has done so;
- to ensure that all other ethical concerns arising from a protocol are satisfactorily resolved both in principle and in practice;
- to consider the qualifications of the investigators, including education in the principles of research practice, and the conditions of the research site with a view to ensuring the safe conduct of the trial; and
- to keep records of decisions and to take measures to follow up on the conduct of ongoing research projects.

Committee membership. National or local ethical review committees should be so composed as to be able to provide complete and adequate review of the research proposals submitted to them. It is generally presumed that their membership should include physicians, scientists and other professionals such as nurses, lawyers, ethicists and clergy, as well as lay persons qualified to represent the cultural and moral values of the community and to ensure that the rights of the research subjects will be respected. They should include both men and women. When uneducated or illiterate persons form the focus of a study they should also be considered for membership or invited to be represented and have their views expressed.

A number of members should be replaced periodically with the aim of blending the advantages of experience with those of fresh perspectives.

A national or local ethical review committee responsible for reviewing and approving proposals for externally sponsored research should have among its members or consultants persons who are thoroughly familiar with the customs and traditions of the population or community concerned and sensitive to issues of human dignity.

Committees that often review research proposals directed at specific diseases or impairments, such as HIV/AIDS or paraplegia, should invite or hear the views of individuals or bodies representing patients with such diseases or impairments. Similarly, for research involving such subjects as children, students, elderly persons or employees, committees should invite or hear the views of their representatives or advocates.

To maintain the review committee's independence from the investigators and sponsors and to avoid conflict of interest, any member with a special or particular, direct or indirect, interest in a proposal should not take part in its assessment if that interest could subvert the member's objective judgment. Members of ethical review committees should be held to the same standard of disclosure as scientific and medical research staff with regard to financial or other interests that could be construed as conflicts of interest. A practical way of avoiding such conflict of interest is for the committee to insist on a declaration of possible conflict of interest by any of its members. A member who makes such a declaration should then withdraw, if to do so is clearly the appropriate action to take, either at the member's own discretion or at the request of the other members. Before withdrawing, the member should be permitted to offer comments on the protocol or to respond to questions of other members.

Multi-centre research. Some research projects are designed to be conducted in a number of centres in different communities or countries. Generally, to ensure that the results will be valid, the study must be conducted in an identical way at each centre. Such studies include clinical trials, research designed for the evaluation of health service programmes, and various kinds of epidemiological research. For such studies, local ethical or scientific review committees are not normally authorized to change doses of drugs, to change inclusion or exclusion criteria, or to make other similar modifications. They should be fully empowered to prevent a study that they believe to be unethical. Moreover, changes that local review committees believe are necessary to protect the research subjects should be documented and reported to the research institution or sponsor responsible for the whole research programme for consideration and due action, to ensure that all other subjects can be protected and that the research will be valid across sites.

To ensure the validity of multi-centre research, any change in the protocol should be made at every collaborating centre or institution, or, failing this, explicit inter-centre comparability procedures must be introduced; changes made at some but not all will defeat the purpose of multi-centre research. For some multi-centre studies, scientific and ethical review may be facilitated by agreement among centres to accept the conclusions of a single review committee; its members could include a representative of the ethical review committee at each of the centres at which the research is to be conducted, as well as individuals competent to conduct scientific review. In other circumstances, a centralized review may be complemented by local review relating to the local participating investigators and institutions. The central committee could review the study from a scientific and ethical standpoint, and the local committees could verify the practicability of the study in their communities, including the infrastructures, the state of training, and ethical considerations of local significance.

In a large multi-centre trial, individual investigators will not have authority to act independently, with regard to data analysis or to preparation and publication of manuscripts, for instance. Such a trial usually has a set of committees which operate under the direction of a steering committee and are responsible for such functions and decisions. The function of the ethical review committee in such cases is to review the relevant plans with the aim of avoiding abuses.

Sanctions. Ethical review committees generally have no authority to impose sanctions on researchers who violate ethical standards in the conduct of research involving humans. They may, however, withdraw ethical approval of a research project if judged necessary. They should be required to monitor the implementation of an approved protocol and its progression, and to report to institutional or governmental authorities any serious or continuing non-compliance with ethical standards as they are reflected in protocols that they have approved or in the conduct of the studies. Failure to submit a protocol to the committee should be considered a clear and serious violation of ethical standards.

Sanctions imposed by governmental, institutional, professional or other authorities possessing disciplinary power should be employed as a last resort. Preferred methods of control include cultivation of an atmosphere of mutual trust, and education and support to promote in researchers and in sponsors the capacity for ethical conduct of research.

Should sanctions become necessary, they should be directed at the non-compliant researchers or sponsors. They may include fines or suspension of eligibility to receive research funding, to use investigational interventions, or to practise medicine. Unless there are persuasive reasons to do otherwise, editors should refuse to publish the results of research conducted unethically, and retract any articles that are subsequently found to contain falsified or fabricated data or to have been based on unethical research. Drug regulatory authorities should consider refusal to accept unethically obtained data submitted in support of an application for authorization to market a product. Such sanctions, however, may deprive of benefit not only the errant researcher or sponsor but also that segment of society intended to benefit from the research; such possible consequences merit careful consideration.

Potential conflicts of interest related to project support. Increasingly, biomedical studies receive funding from commercial firms. Such sponsors have good reasons to support research methods that are ethically and scientifically acceptable, but cases have arisen in which the conditions of funding could have introduced bias. It may happen that investigators have little or no input into trial design, limited access to the raw data, or limited participation in data interpretation, or that the results of a clinical trial may not be published if they are unfavourable to the sponsor's product. This risk of bias may also be associated with other sources of support, such as government or foundations. As the persons directly responsible for their work, investigators should not enter into agreements that interfere unduly with their access to the data or their ability to analyse the data independently, to prepare manuscripts, or to publish them. Investigators must also disclose potential or apparent conflicts of interest on their part to the ethical review committee or to other institutional committees designed to evaluate and manage such conflicts. Ethical review committees should therefore ensure that these conditions are met. See also *Multi-centre research,* above.

GUIDELINE 3: *Ethical review of externally sponsored research*

An external sponsoring organization and individual investigators should submit the research protocol for ethical and scientific review in the country of the sponsoring organization, and the ethical standards applied should be no less stringent than they would be for research carried out in that country. The health authorities of the host country, as well as a national or local ethical review committee, should ensure that the proposed research is responsive to the health needs and priorities of the host country and meets the requisite ethical standards.

COMMENTARY ON GUIDELINE 3

Definition. The term *externally sponsored research* refers to research undertaken in a host country but sponsored, financed, and sometimes wholly or partly carried out by an external international or national organization or pharmaceutical company with the collaboration or agreement of the appropriate authorities, institutions and personnel of the host country.

Ethical and scientific review. Committees in both the country of the sponsor and the host country have responsibility for conducting both scientific and ethical review, as well as the authority to withhold approval of research proposals that fail to meet their scientific or ethical standards. As far as possible, there must be assurance that the review is independent and that there is no conflict of interest that might affect the judgement of members of the review committees in relation to any aspect of the research. When the external sponsor is an international organization, its review of the research protocol must be in accordance with its own independent ethical-review procedures and standards.

Committees in the external sponsoring country or international organization have a special responsibility to determine whether the scientific methods are sound and suitable to the aims of the research; whether the drugs, vaccines, devices or procedures to be studied meet adequate standards of safety; whether there is sound justification for conducting the research in the host country rather than in the country of the external sponsor or in another country; and whether the proposed research is in compliance with the ethical standards of the external sponsoring country or international organization.

Committees in the host country have a special responsibility to determine whether the objectives of the research are responsive to the health needs and priorities of that country. The ability to judge the ethical acceptability of various aspects of a research proposal requires a thorough understanding of a community's customs and traditions. The ethical review committee in the host country, therefore, must have as either members or consultants persons with such understanding; it will then be in a favourable position to determine the acceptability of the proposed means of obtaining informed consent and otherwise respecting the rights of prospective subjects as well as of the means proposed to protect the welfare of the research subjects. Such persons should be able, for example, to indicate suitable members of the community to serve as intermediaries between investigators and subjects, and to advise on whether material benefits or inducements may be regarded as appropriate in the light of a community's gift-exchange and other customs and traditions.

When a sponsor or investigator in one country proposes to carry out research in another, the ethical review committees in the two countries may, by agreement, undertake to review different aspects of the research protocol. In short, in respect of host countries either with developed capacity for independent ethical review or in which external sponsors and investigators are contributing substantially to such capacity, ethical review in the external, sponsoring country may be limited to ensuring compliance with broadly stated ethical standards. The ethical review committee in the host country can be expected to have greater competence for reviewing the detailed plans for compliance, in view of its better understanding of the cultural and moral values of the population in which it is proposed to conduct the research; it is also likely to be in a better position to monitor compliance in the course of a study. However, in respect of research in host countries with inadequate capacity for independent ethical review, full review by the ethical review committee in the external sponsoring country or international agency is necessary.

GUIDELINE 4: *Individual informed consent*

For all biomedical research involving humans the investigator must obtain the voluntary informed consent of the prospective subject or, in the case of an individual who is not capable of giving informed consent, the permission of a legally authorized representative in accordance with applicable law. Waiver of informed consent is to be regarded as uncommon and exceptional, and must in all cases be approved by an ethical review committee.

COMMENTARY ON GUIDELINE 4

General considerations. Informed consent is a decision to participate in research, taken by a competent individual who has received the necessary information; who has adequately understood the information; and who, after considering the information, has arrived at a decision without having been subjected to coercion, undue influence or inducement, or intimidation.

Informed consent is based on the principle that competent individuals are entitled to choose freely whether to participate in research. Informed consent protects the individual's freedom of choice and respects the individual's autonomy. As an additional safeguard, it must always be complemented by independent ethical review of research proposals. This safeguard of independent review is particularly important as many individuals are limited in their capacity to give adequate informed consent; they include young children, adults with severe mental or behavioural disorders, and persons who are unfamiliar with medical concepts and technology (See Guidelines 13, 14, 15).

Process. Obtaining informed consent is a process that is begun when initial contact is made with a prospective subject and continues throughout the course of the study. By informing the prospective subjects, by repetition and explanation, by answering their questions as they arise, and by ensuring that each individual understands each procedure, investigators elicit their informed consent and in so doing manifest respect for their dignity and autonomy. Each individual must be given as much time as is needed to reach a decision, including time for consultation with family members or others. Adequate time and resources should be set aside for informed-consent procedures.

Language. Informing the individual subject must not be simply a ritual recitation of the contents of a written document. Rather, the investigator must convey the information, whether orally or in writing, in language that suits the individual's level of understanding. The investigator must bear in mind that the prospective subject's ability to understand the information necessary to give informed consent depends on that individual's maturity, intelligence, education and belief system. It depends also on the investigator's ability and willingness to communicate with patience and sensitivity.

Comprehension. The investigator must then ensure that the prospective subject has adequately understood the information. The investigator should give each one full opportunity to ask questions and should answer them honestly, promptly and completely. In some instances the investigator may administer an oral or a written test or otherwise determine whether the information has been adequately understood.

Documentation of consent. Consent may be indicated in a number of ways. The subject may imply consent by voluntary actions, express consent orally, or sign a consent form. As a general rule, the subject should sign a consent form, or, in the case of incompetence, a legal guardian or other duly authorized representative should do so. The ethical review committee may approve waiver of the requirement of a signed consent form if the research carries no more than minimal risk—that is, risk that is no more likely and not greater than that attached to routine medical or psychological examination—and if the procedures to be used are only those for which signed consent forms are not customarily required outside the research context. Such waivers may also be approved when existence of a signed consent form would be an unjustified threat to the subject's confidentiality. In some cases, particularly when the information is complicated, it is advisable to give subjects information sheets to retain; these may resemble consent forms in all respects except that subjects are not required to sign them. Their wording should be cleared by the ethical review committee. When consent has been obtained orally, investigators are responsible for providing documentation or proof of consent.

Waiver of the consent requirement. Investigators should never initiate research involving human subjects without obtaining each subject's informed consent, unless they have received explicit approval to do so from an ethical review committee. However, when the research design involves no more than minimal risk and a requirement of individual informed consent would make the conduct of the research impracticable (for example, where the research involves only excerpting data from subjects' records), the ethical review committee may waive some or all of the elements of informed consent.

Renewing consent. When material changes occur in the conditions or the procedures of a study, and also periodically in long-term studies, the investigator should once again seek informed consent from the subjects. For example, new information may have come to light, either from the study or from other sources, about the risks or benefits of products being tested or about alternatives to them. Subjects should be given such information promptly. In many clinical trials, results are not disclosed to subjects and investigators until the study is concluded. This is ethically acceptable if an ethical review committee has approved their non-disclosure.

Cultural considerations. In some cultures an investigator may enter a community to conduct research or approach prospective subjects for their individual consent only after obtaining permission from a community leader, a council of elders, or another designated authority. Such customs must be respected. In no case, however, may the permission of a community leader or other authority substitute for individual informed consent. In some populations the use of a number of local languages may complicate the communication of information to potential subjects and the ability of an investigator to ensure that they truly understand it. Many people in all cultures are unfamiliar with, or do not readily understand, scientific concepts such as those of placebo or randomization. Sponsors and investigators should develop culturally appropriate ways to communicate information that is necessary for adherence to the standard required in the informed consent process. Also, they should describe and justify in the research protocol the procedure they plan to use in communicating information to subjects. For collaborative research in developing countries the research project should, if necessary, include the provision of resources to ensure that informed consent can indeed be obtained legitimately within different linguistic and cultural settings.

Consent to use for research purposes biological materials (including genetic material) from subjects in clinical trials. Consent forms for the research protocol should include a separate section for clinical-trial subjects who are requested to provide their consent for the use of their biological specimens for research. Separate consent may be appropriate in some cases (e.g., if investigators are requesting permission to conduct basic research which is not a necessary part of the clinical trial), but not in others (e.g., the clinical trial requires the use of subjects' biological materials).

Use of medical records and biological specimens. Medical records and biological specimens taken in the course of clinical care may be used for research without the consent of the patients/subjects only if an ethical review committee has determined that the research poses minimal risk, that the rights or interests of the patients will not be violated, that their privacy and confidentiality or anonymity are assured, and that the research is designed to answer an important question and would be impracticable if the requirement for informed consent were to be imposed. Patients have a right to know that their records or specimens may be used for research. Refusal or reluctance of individuals to agree to participate would not be evidence of impracticability sufficient to warrant waiving informed consent. Records and specimens of individuals who have specifically rejected such uses in the past may be used only in the case of public health emergencies. (See Guideline 18 Commentary, *Confidentiality between physician and patient*)

Secondary use of research records or biological specimens. Investigators may want to use records or biological specimens that another investigator has used or collected for use, in another institution in the same or another country. This raises the issue of whether the records or specimens contain personal identifiers, or can be linked to such identifiers, and by whom. (See also Guideline 18: *Safeguarding confidentiality*) If informed consent or permission was required to authorize the original collection or use of such records or specimens for research purposes, secondary uses are generally constrained by the conditions specified in the original consent. Consequently, it is essential that the original consent process anticipate, to the extent that this is feasible, any foreseeable plans for future use of the records or specimens for research. Thus, in the original process of seeking informed consent a member of the research team should discuss with, and, when indicated, request the permission of, prospective subjects as to: i) whether there will or could be any secondary use and, if so, whether such secondary use will be limited with regard to the type of study that may be performed on such materials; ii) the conditions under which investigators will be required to contact the research subjects for additional authorization for secondary use; iii) the investigators' plans, if any, to destroy or to strip of personal identifiers the records or specimens; and iv) the rights of subjects to request destruction or anonymization of biological specimens or of records or parts of records that

they might consider particularly sensitive, such as photographs, videotapes or audiotapes.

(See also Guidelines 5: *Obtaining informed consent: Essential information for prospective research subjects;* 6: *Obtaining informed consent: Obligations of sponsors and investigators;* and 7: *Inducement to participate.*)

GUIDELINE 5: *Obtaining informed consent: Essential information for prospective research subjects*

Before requesting an individual's consent to participate in research, the investigator must provide the following information, in language or another form of communication that the individual can understand:

1. that the individual is invited to participate in research, the reasons for considering the individual suitable for the research, and that participation is voluntary;

2. that the individual is free to refuse to participate and will be free to withdraw from the research at any time without penalty or loss of benefits to which he or she would otherwise be entitled;

3. the purpose of the research, the procedures to be carried out by the investigator and the subject, and an explanation of how the research differs from routine medical care;

4. for controlled trials, an explanation of features of the research design (e.g., randomization, double-blinding), and that the subject will not be told of the assigned treatment until the study has been completed and the blind has been broken;

5. the expected duration of the individual's participation (including number and duration of visits to the research centre and the total time involved) and the possibility of early termination of the trial or of the individual's participation in it;

6. whether money or other forms of material goods will be provided in return for the individual's participation and, if so, the kind and amount;

7. that, after the completion of the study, subjects will be informed of the findings of the research in general, and individual subjects will be informed of any finding that relates to their particular health status;

8. that subjects have the right of access to their data on demand, even if these data lack immediate clinical utility (unless the ethical review committee has approved temporary or permanent non-disclosure of data, in which case the subject should be informed of, and given, the reasons for such non-disclosure);

9. any foreseeable risks, pain or discomfort, or inconvenience to the individual (or others) associated with participation in the research, including

risks to the health or well-being of a subject's spouse or partner;

10. the direct benefits, if any, expected to result to subjects from participating in the research

11. the expected benefits of the research to the community or to society at large, or contributions to scientific knowledge;

12. whether, when and how any products or interventions proven by the research to be safe and effective will be made available to subjects after they have completed their participation in the research, and whether they will be expected to pay for them;

13. any currently available alternative interventions or courses of treatment;

14. the provisions that will be made to ensure respect for the privacy of subjects and for the confidentiality of records in which subjects are identified;

15. the limits, legal or other, to the investigators' ability to safeguard confidentiality, and the possible consequences of breaches of confidentiality;

16. policy with regard to the use of results of genetic tests and familial genetic information, and the precautions in place to prevent disclosure of the results of a subject's genetic tests;

17. to immediate family relatives or to others (e.g., insurance companies or employers) without the consent of the subject;

18. the sponsors of the research, the institutional affiliation of the investigators, and the nature and sources of funding for the research;

19. the possible research uses, direct or secondary, of the subject's medical records and of biological specimens taken in the course of clinical care (See also Guidelines 4 and 18 Commentaries);

20. whether it is planned that biological specimens collected in the research will be destroyed at its conclusion, and, if not, details about their storage (where, how, for how long, and final disposition) and possible future use, and that subjects have the right to decide about such future use, to refuse storage, and to have the material destroyed (See Guideline 4 Commentary);

21. whether commercial products may be developed from biological specimens, and whether the participant will receive monetary or other benefits from the development of such products;

22. whether the investigator is serving only as an investigator or as both investigator and the subject's physician;

23. the extent of the investigator's responsibility to provide medical services to the participant;

24. that treatment will be provided free of charge for specified types of research-related injury or for

complications associated with the research, the nature and duration of such care, the name of the organization or individual that will provide the treatment, and whether there is any uncertainty regarding funding of such treatment;

25. in what way, and by what organization, the subject or the subject's family or dependants will be compensated for disability or death resulting from such injury (or, when indicated, that there are no plans to provide such compensation);

26. whether or not, in the country in which the prospective subject is invited to participate in research, the right to compensation is legally guaranteed;

27. that an ethical review committee has approved or cleared the research protocol.

GUIDELINE 6: *Obtaining informed consent: Obligations of sponsors and investigators*

Sponsors and investigators have a duty to:

- refrain from unjustified deception, undue influence, or intimidation;

- seek consent only after ascertaining that the prospective subject has adequate understanding of the relevant facts and of the consequences of participation and has had sufficient opportunity to consider whether to participate;

- as a general rule, obtain from each prospective subject a signed form as evidence of informed consent—investigators should justify any exceptions to this general rule and obtain the approval of the ethical review committee (See Guideline 4 Commentary, *Documentation of consent*);

- renew the informed consent of each subject if there are significant changes in the conditions or procedures of the research or if new information becomes available that could affect the willingness of subjects to continue to participate; and,

- renew the informed consent of each subject in long-term studies at pre-determined intervals, even if there are no changes in the design or objectives of the research.

COMMENTARY ON GUIDELINE 6

The investigator is responsible for ensuring the adequacy of informed consent from each subject. The person obtaining informed consent should be knowledgeable about the research and capable of answering questions from prospective subjects. Investigators in charge of the study must make themselves available to answer questions at the request of subjects. Any restrictions on the subject's opportunity to ask questions and receive answers before or during the research undermines the validity of the informed consent.

In some types of research, potential subjects should receive counselling about risks of acquiring a disease unless they take precautions. This is especially true of HIV/AIDS vaccine research (UNAIDS Guidance Document *Ethical Considerations in HIV Preventive Vaccine Research, Guidance Point 14*).

Withholding information and deception. Sometimes, to ensure the validity of research, investigators withhold certain information in the consent process. In biomedical research, this typically takes the form of withholding information about the purpose of specific procedures. For example, subjects in clinical trials are often not told the purpose of tests performed to monitor their compliance with the protocol, since if they knew their compliance was being monitored they might modify their behaviour and hence invalidate results. In most such cases, the prospective subjects are asked to consent to remain uninformed of the purpose of some procedures until the research is completed; after the conclusion of the study they are given the omitted information. In other cases, because a request for permission to withhold some information would jeopardize the validity of the research, subjects are not told that some information has been withheld until the research has been completed. Any such procedure must receive the explicit approval of the ethical review committee.

Active deception of subjects is considerably more controversial than simply withholding certain information. Lying to subjects is a tactic not commonly employed in biomedical research. Social and behavioural scientists, however, sometimes deliberately misinform subjects to study their attitudes and behaviour. For example, scientists have pretended to be patients to study the behaviour of healthcare professionals and patients in their natural settings.

Some people maintain that active deception is never permissible. Others would permit it in certain circumstances. Deception is not permissible, however, in cases in which the deception itself would disguise the possibility of the subject being exposed to more than minimal risk. When deception is deemed indispensable to the methods of a study the investigators must demonstrate to an ethical review committee that no other research method would suffice; that significant advances could result from the research; and that nothing has been withheld that, if divulged, would cause a reasonable person to refuse to participate. The ethical review committee should determine the consequences for the subject of being deceived, and whether and how deceived subjects should be informed of the deception upon completion of the research. Such informing, commonly called

"debriefing", ordinarily entails explaining the reasons for the deception. A subject who disapproves of having been deceived should be offered an opportunity to refuse to allow the investigator to use information thus obtained. Investigators and ethical review committees should be aware that deceiving research subjects may wrong them as well as harm them; subjects may resent not having been informed when they learn that they have participated in a study under false pretences. In some studies there may be justification for deceiving persons other than the subjects by either withholding or disguising elements of information. Such tactics are often proposed, for example, for studies of the abuse of spouses or children. An ethical review committee must review and approve all proposals to deceive persons other than the subjects. Subjects are entitled to prompt and honest answers to their questions; the ethical review committee must determine for each study whether others who are to be deceived are similarly entitled.

Intimidation and undue influence. Intimidation in any form invalidates informed consent. Prospective subjects who are patients often depend for medical care upon the physician/investigator, who consequently has a certain credibility in their eyes, and whose influence over them may be considerable, particularly if the study protocol has a therapeutic component. They may fear, for example, that refusal to participate would damage the therapeutic relationship or result in the withholding of health services. The physician/investigator must assure them that their decision on whether to participate will not affect the therapeutic relationship or other benefits to which they are entitled. In this situation the ethical review committee should consider whether a neutral third party should seek informed consent.

The prospective subject must not be exposed to undue influence. The borderline between justifiable persuasion and undue influence is imprecise, however. The researcher should give no unjustifiable assurances about the benefits, risks or inconveniences of the research, for example, or induce a close relative or a community leader to influence a prospective subject's decision. (See also Guideline 4: *Individual informed consent.*)

Risks. Investigators should be completely objective in discussing the details of the experimental intervention, the pain and discomfort that it may entail, and known risks and possible hazards. In complex research projects it may be neither feasible nor desirable to inform prospective participants fully about every possible risk. They must, however, be informed of all risks that a 'reasonable person' would consider material to making a decision about whether to participate, including risks to a spouse or partner associated with trials of, for example, psychotropic or genital-tract medicaments. (See also Guideline 8 Commentary, *Risks to groups of persons.*)

Exception to the requirement for informed consent in studies of emergency situations in which the researcher anticipates that many subjects will be unable to consent. Research protocols are sometimes designed to address conditions occurring suddenly and rendering the patients/subjects incapable of giving informed consent. Examples are head trauma, cardiopulmonary arrest and stroke. The investigation cannot be done with patients who can give informed consent in time and there may not be time to locate a person having the authority to give permission. In such circumstances it is often necessary to proceed with the research interventions very soon after the onset of the condition in order to evaluate an investigational treatment or develop the desired knowledge. As this class of emergency exception can be anticipated, the researcher must secure the review and approval of an ethical review committee before initiating the study. If possible, an attempt should be made to identify a population that is likely to develop the condition to be studied. This can be done readily, for example, if the condition is one that recurs periodically in individuals; examples include grand mal seizures and alcohol binges. In such cases, prospective subjects should be contacted while fully capable of informed consent, and invited to consent to their involvement as research subjects during future periods of incapacitation. If they are patients of an independent physician who is also the physician-researcher, the physician should likewise seek their consent while they are fully capable of informed consent. In all cases in which approved research has begun without prior consent of patients/subjects incapable of giving informed consent because of suddenly occurring conditions, they should be given all relevant information as soon as they are in a state to receive it, and their consent to continued participation should be obtained as soon as is reasonably possible.

Before proceeding without prior informed consent, the investigator must make reasonable efforts to locate an individual who has the authority to give permission on behalf of an incapacitated patient. If such a person can be located and refuses to give permission, the patient may not be enrolled as a subject. The risks of all interventions and procedures will be justified as required by Guideline 9 (*Special limitations on risks when research involves individuals who are not capable of giving consent*). The researcher and the ethical review committee should agree to a maximum time of involvement of an individual without obtaining either the individual's informed consent or authorization according to the applicable legal system if the person is not able to give consent. If by that time the researcher has not obtained either consent or permission—owing either to a failure to contact a representative or to a refusal of either the patient or the person or body authorized to give permission—the participation of the patient as a subject must be discontinued. The patient or the person or body providing authorization should be offered an opportunity to forbid the use of data derived from participation of the patient as a subject without consent or permission.

Where appropriate, plans to conduct emergency research without prior consent of the subjects should be publicized within the community in which it will be carried out. In the design and conduct of the research, the ethical review committee, the investigators and the sponsors should be responsive to the concerns of the community. If there is cause for concern about the acceptability of the research in the community, there should be a formal consultation with representatives designated by the community. The research should not be carried out if it does not have substantial support in the community concerned. (See Guideline 8 Commentary, *Risks to groups of persons.*)

Exception to the requirement of informed consent for inclusion in clinical trials of persons rendered incapable of informed consent by an acute condition. Certain patients with an acute condition that renders them incapable of giving informed consent may be eligible for inclusion in a clinical trial in which the majority of prospective subjects will be capable of informed consent. Such a trial would relate to a new treatment for an acute condition such as sepsis, stroke or myocardial infarction. The investigational treatment would hold out the prospect of direct benefit and would be justified accordingly, though the investigation might involve certain procedures or interventions that were not of direct benefit but carried no more than minimal risk; an example would be the process of randomization or the collection of additional blood for research purposes. For such cases the initial protocol submitted for approval to the ethical review committee should anticipate that some patients may be incapable of consent, and should propose for such patients a form of proxy consent, such as permission of the responsible relative. When the ethical review committee has approved or cleared such a protocol, an investigator may seek the permission of the responsible relative and enroll such a patient.

GUIDELINE 7: *Inducement to participate*

Subjects may be reimbursed for lost earnings, travel costs and other expenses incurred in taking part in a study; they may also receive free medical services. Subjects, particularly those who receive no direct benefit from research, may also be paid or otherwise compensated for inconvenience and time spent. The payments should not be so large, however, or the medical services so extensive as to induce prospective subjects to consent to participate in the research against their better judgment ("undue inducement"). All payments, reimbursements and medical services provided to research subjects must have been approved by an ethical review committee.

COMMENTARY ON GUIDELINE 7

Acceptable recompense. Research subjects may be reimbursed for their transport and other expenses, including lost earnings, associated with their participation in research. Those who receive no direct benefit from the research may also receive a small sum of money for inconvenience due to their participation in the research. All subjects may receive medical services unrelated to the research and have procedures and tests performed free of charge.

Unacceptable recompense. Payments in money or in kind to research subjects should not be so large as to persuade them to take undue risks or volunteer against their better judgment. Payments or rewards that undermine a person's capacity to exercise free choice invalidate consent. It may be difficult to distinguish between suitable recompense and undue influence to participate in research. An unemployed person or a student may view promised recompense differently from an employed person. Someone without access to medical care may or may not be unduly influenced to participate in research simply to receive such care. A prospective subject may be induced to participate in order to obtain a better diagnosis or access to a drug not otherwise available; local ethical review committees may find such inducements acceptable. Monetary and in-kind recompense must, therefore, be evaluated in the light of the traditions of the particular culture and population in which they are offered, to determine whether they constitute undue influence. The ethical review committee will ordinarily be the best judge of what constitutes reasonable material recompense in particular circumstances. When research interventions or procedures that do not hold out the prospect of direct benefit present more than minimal risk, all parties involved in the research—sponsors, investigators and ethical review committees—in both funding and host countries should be careful to avoid undue material inducement.

Incompetent persons. Incompetent persons may be vulnerable to exploitation for financial gain by guardians. A guardian asked to give permission on behalf of an incompetent person should be offered no recompense other than a refund of travel and related expenses.

Withdrawal from a study. A subject who withdraws from research for reasons related to the study, such as

unacceptable side-effects of a study drug, or who is withdrawn on health grounds, should be paid or recompensed as if full participation had taken place. A subject who withdraws for any other reason should be paid in proportion to the amount of participation. An investigator who must remove a subject from the study for willful noncompliance is entitled to withhold part or all of the payment.

GUIDELINE 8: *Benefits and risks of study participation*

For all biomedical research involving human subjects, the investigator must ensure that potential benefits and risks are reasonably balanced and risks are minimized.

- Interventions or procedures that hold out the prospect of direct diagnostic, therapeutic or preventive benefit for the individual subject must be justified by the expectation that they will be at least as advantageous to the individual subject, in the light of foreseeable risks and benefits, as any available alternative. Risks of such 'beneficial' interventions or procedures must be justified in relation to expected benefits to the individual subject.
- Risks of interventions that do not hold out the prospect of direct diagnostic, therapeutic or preventive benefit for the individual must be justified in relation to the expected benefits to society (generalizable knowledge). The risks presented by such interventions must be reasonable in relation to the importance of the knowledge to be gained.

COMMENTARY ON GUIDELINE 8

The Declaration of Helsinki in several paragraphs deals with the well-being of research subjects and the avoidance of risk. Thus, considerations related to the well-being of the human subject should take precedence over the interests of science and society (Paragraph 5); clinical testing must be preceded by adequate laboratory or animal experimentation to demonstrate a reasonable probability of success without undue risk (Paragraph 11); every project should be preceded by careful assessment of predictable risks and burdens in comparison with foreseeable benefits to the subject or to others (Paragraph 16); physician-researchers must be confident that the risks involved have been adequately assessed and can be satisfactorily managed (Paragraph 17); and the risks and burdens to the subject must be minimized, and reasonable in relation to the importance of the objective or the knowledge to be gained (Paragraph 18).

Biomedical research often employs a variety of interventions of which some hold out the prospect of direct therapeutic benefit (beneficial interventions) and others are administered solely to answer the research question (non-beneficial interventions). Beneficial interventions are justified as they are in medical practice by the expectation that they will be at least as advantageous to the individuals concerned, in the light of both risks and benefits, as any available alternative. Non-beneficial interventions are assessed differently; they may be justified only by appeal to the knowledge to be gained. In assessing the risks and benefits that a protocol presents to a population, it is appropriate to consider the harm that could result from forgoing the research.

Paragraphs 5 and 18 of the Declaration of Helsinki do not preclude well-informed volunteers, capable of fully appreciating risks and benefits of an investigation, from participating in research for altruistic reasons or for modest remuneration.

Minimizing risk associated with participation in a randomized controlled trial. In randomized controlled trials subjects risk being allocated to receive the treatment that proves inferior. They are allocated by chance to one of two or more intervention arms and followed to a predetermined end-point. (Interventions are understood to include new or established therapies, diagnostic tests and preventive measures.) An intervention is evaluated by comparing it with another intervention (a control), which is ordinarily the best current method, selected from the safe and effective treatments available globally, unless some other control intervention such as placebo can be justified ethically (See Guideline 11).

To minimize risk when the intervention to be tested in a randomized controlled trial is designed to prevent or postpone a lethal or disabling outcome, the investigator must not, for purposes of conducting the trial, withhold therapy that is known to be superior to the intervention being tested, unless the withholding can be justified by the standards set forth in Guideline 11. Also, the investigator must provide in the research protocol for the monitoring of research data by an independent board (Data and Safety Monitoring Board); one function of such a board is to protect the research subjects from previously unknown adverse reactions or unnecessarily prolonged exposure to an inferior therapy. Normally at the outset of a randomized controlled trial, criteria are established for its premature termination (stopping rules or guidelines).

Risks to groups of persons. Research in certain fields, such as epidemiology, genetics or sociology, may present risks to the interests of communities, societies, or racially or ethnically defined groups. Information might be published that could stigmatize a group or expose its members to discrimination. Such information, for example,

could indicate, rightly or wrongly, that the group has a higher than average prevalence of alcoholism, mental illness or sexually transmitted disease, or is particularly susceptible to certain genetic disorders. Plans to conduct such research should be sensitive to such considerations, to the need to maintain confidentiality during and after the study, and to the need to publish the resulting data in a manner that is respectful of the interests of all concerned, or in certain circumstances not to publish them. The ethical review committee should ensure that the interests of all concerned are given due consideration; often it will be advisable to have individual consent supplemented by community consultation.

[The ethical basis for the justification of risk is elaborated further in Guideline 9]

GUIDELINE 9: *Special limitations on risk when research involves individuals who are not capable of giving informed consent*

When there is ethical and scientific justification to conduct research with individuals incapable of giving informed consent, the risk from research interventions that do not hold out the prospect of direct benefit for the individual subject should be no more likely and not greater than the risk attached to routine medical or psychological examination of such persons. Slight or minor increases above such risk may be permitted when there is an overriding scientific or medical rationale for such increases and when an ethical review committee has approved them.

COMMENTARY ON GUIDELINE 9

The low-risk standard: Certain individuals or groups may have limited capacity to give informed consent either because, as in the case of prisoners, their autonomy is limited, or because they have limited cognitive capacity. For research involving persons who are unable to consent, or whose capacity to make an informed choice may not fully meet the standard of informed consent, ethical review committees must distinguish between intervention risks that do not exceed those associated with routine medical or psychological examination of such persons and risks in excess of those.

When the risks of such interventions do not exceed those associated with routine medical or psychological examination of such persons, there is no requirement for special substantive or procedural protective measures apart from those generally required for all research involving members of the particular class of persons. When the risks are in excess of those, the ethical review committee must find: 1) that the research is designed to be responsive to the disease affecting the prospective subjects or to conditions to which they are particularly susceptible; 2) that the risks of the research interventions are only slightly greater than those associated with routine medical or psychological examination of such persons for the condition or set of clinical circumstances under investigation; 3) that the objective of the research is sufficiently important to justify exposure of the subjects to the increased risk; and 4) that the interventions are reasonably commensurate with the clinical interventions that the subjects have experienced or may be expected to experience in relation to the condition under investigation.

If such research subjects, including children, become capable of giving independent informed consent during the research, their consent to continued participation should be obtained.

There is no internationally agreed, precise definition of a "slight or minor increase" above the risks associated with routine medical or psychological examination of such persons. Its meaning is inferred from what various ethical review committees have reported as having met the standard. Examples include additional lumbar punctures or bone-marrow aspirations in children with conditions for which such examinations are regularly indicated in clinical practice. The requirement that the objective of the research be relevant to the disease or condition affecting the prospective subjects rules out the use of such interventions in healthy children.

The requirement that the research interventions be reasonably commensurate with clinical interventions that subjects may have experienced or are likely to experience for the condition under investigation is intended to enable them to draw on personal experience as they decide whether to accept or reject additional procedures for research purposes. Their choices will, therefore, be more informed even though they may not fully meet the standard of informed consent.

(See also Guidelines 4: *Individual informed consent;* 13: *Research involving vulnerable persons;* 14: *Research involving children;* and 15: *Research involving individuals who by reason of mental or behavioural disorders are not capable of giving adequately informed consent.*)

GUIDELINE 10: *Research in populations and communities with limited resources*

Before undertaking research in a population or community with limited resources, the sponsor and the investigator must make every effort to ensure that:

- the research is responsive to the health needs and the priorities of the population or community in which it is to be carried out; and

- any intervention or product developed, or knowledge generated, will be made reasonably available for the benefit of that population or community.

COMMENTARY ON GUIDELINE 10

This guideline is concerned with countries or communities in which resources are limited to the extent that they are, or may be, vulnerable to exploitation by sponsors and investigators from the relatively wealthy countries and communities.

Responsiveness of research to health needs and priorities. The ethical requirement that research be responsive to the health needs of the population or community in which it is carried out calls for decisions on what is needed to fulfil the requirement. It is not sufficient simply to determine that a disease is prevalent in the population and that new or further research is needed: the ethical requirement of "responsiveness" can be fulfilled only if successful interventions or other kinds of health benefit are made available to the population. This is applicable especially to research conducted in countries where governments lack the resources to make such products or benefits widely available. Even when a product to be tested in a particular country is much cheaper than the standard treatment in some other countries, the government or individuals in that country may still be unable to afford it. If the knowledge gained from the research in such a country is used primarily for the benefit of populations that can afford the tested product, the research may rightly be characterized as exploitative and, therefore, unethical.

When an investigational intervention has important potential for health care in the host country, the negotiation that the sponsor should undertake to determine the practical implications of "responsiveness", as well as "reasonable availability", should include representatives of stakeholders in the host country; these include the national government, the health ministry, local health authorities, and concerned scientific and ethics groups, as well as representatives of the communities from which subjects are drawn and non-governmental organizations such as health advocacy groups. The negotiation should cover the health-care infrastructure required for safe and rational use of the intervention, the likelihood of authorization for distribution, and decisions regarding payments, royalties, subsidies, technology and intellectual property, as well as distribution costs, when this economic information is not proprietary. In some cases, satisfactory discussion of the availability and distribution of successful products will necessarily engage international organizations, donor governments and bilateral agencies, international nongovernmental organizations, and the private sector. The development of a health-care infrastructure should be facilitated at the onset so that it can be of use during and beyond the conduct of the research.

Additionally, if an investigational drug has been shown to be beneficial, the sponsor should continue to provide it to the subjects after the conclusion of the study, and pending its approval by a drug regulatory authority. The sponsor is unlikely to be in a position to make a beneficial investigational intervention generally available to the community or population until some time after the conclusion of the study, as it may be in short supply and in any case cannot be made generally available before a drug regulatory authority has approved it.

For minor research studies and when the outcome is scientific knowledge rather than a commercial product, such complex planning or negotiation is rarely, if ever, needed. There must be assurance, however, that the scientific knowledge developed will be used for the benefit of the population.

Reasonable availability. The issue of "reasonable availability" is complex and will need to be determined on a case-by-case basis. Relevant considerations include the length of time for which the intervention or product developed, or other agreed benefit, will be made available to research subjects, or to the community or population concerned; the severity of a subject's medical condition; the effect of withdrawing the study drug (e.g., death of a subject); the cost to the subject or health service; and the question of undue inducement if an intervention is provided free of charge.

In general, if there is good reason to believe that a product developed or knowledge generated by research is unlikely to be reasonably available to, or applied to the benefit of, the population of a proposed host country or community after the conclusion of the research, it is unethical to conduct the research in that country or community. This should not be construed as precluding studies designed to evaluate novel therapeutic concepts. As a rare exception, for example, research may be designed to obtain preliminary evidence that a drug or a class of drugs has a beneficial effect in the treatment of a disease that occurs only in regions with extremely limited resources, and it could not be carried out reasonably well in more developed communities. Such research may be justified ethically even if there is no plan in place to make a product available to the population of the host country or community at the conclusion of the preliminary phase of its development. If the concept is found to be valid, subsequent phases of the research could result in a product that could be made reasonably available at its conclusion.

(See also Guidelines 3: *Ethical review of externally sponsored research;* 12, *Equitable distribution of burdens and benefits;* 20: *Strengthening capacity for ethical and scientific*

review and biomedical research; and 21: *Ethical obligation of external sponsors to provide health-care services.*)

GUIDELINE II: *Choice of control in clinical trials*

As a general rule, research subjects in the control group of a trial of a diagnostic, therapeutic, or preventive intervention should receive an established effective intervention. In some circumstances it may be ethically acceptable to use an alternative comparator, such as placebo or "no treatment".

Placebo may be used:

- when there is no established effective intervention;
- when withholding an established effective intervention would expose subjects to, at most, temporary discomfort or delay in relief of symptoms;
- when use of an established effective intervention as comparator would not yield scientifically reliable results and use of placebo would not add any risk of serious or irreversible harm to the subjects.

COMMENTARY ON GUIDELINE II

General considerations for controlled clinical trials. The design of trials of investigational diagnostic, therapeutic or preventive interventions raises interrelated scientific and ethical issues for sponsors, investigators and ethical review committees. To obtain reliable results, investigators must compare the effects of an investigational intervention on subjects assigned to the investigational arm (or arms) of a trial with the effects that a control intervention produces in subjects drawn from the same population and assigned to its control arm. Randomization is the preferred method for assigning subjects to the various arms of the clinical trial unless another method, such as historical or literature controls, can be justified scientifically and ethically. Assignment to treatment arms by randomization, in addition to its usual scientific superiority, offers the advantage of tending to render equivalent to all subjects the foreseeable benefits and risks of participation in a trial.

A clinical trial cannot be justified ethically unless it is capable of producing scientifically reliable results. When the objective is to establish the effectiveness and safety of an investigational intervention, the use of a placebo control is often much more likely than that of an active control to produce a scientifically reliable result. In many cases the ability of a trial to distinguish effective from ineffective interventions (its assay sensitivity) cannot be assured unless the control is a placebo. If, however, an effect of using a placebo would be to deprive subjects in the control arm of an established effective intervention, and thereby to expose them to serious harm, particularly if it is irreversible, it would obviously be unethical to use a placebo.

Placebo control in the absence of a current effective alternative. The use of placebo in the control arm of a clinical trial is ethically acceptable when, as stated in the Declaration of Helsinki (Paragraph 29), "no proven prophylactic, diagnostic or therapeutic method exists." Usually, in this case, a placebo is scientifically preferable to no intervention. In certain circumstances, however, an alternative design may be both scientifically and ethically acceptable, and preferable; an example would be a clinical trial of a surgical intervention, because, for many surgical interventions, either it is not possible or it is ethically unacceptable to devise a suitable placebo; for another example, in certain vaccine trials an investigator might choose to provide for those in the 'control' arm a vaccine that is unrelated to the investigational vaccine.

Placebo-controlled trials that entail only minor risks. A placebo-controlled design may be ethically acceptable, and preferable on scientific grounds, when the condition for which patients/subjects are randomly assigned to placebo or active treatment is only a small deviation in physiological measurements, such as slightly raised blood pressure or a modest increase in serum cholesterol; and if delaying or omitting available treatment may cause only temporary discomfort (e.g., common headache) and no serious adverse consequences. The ethical review committee must be fully satisfied that the risks of withholding an established effective intervention are truly minor and short-lived.

Placebo control when active control would not yield reliable results. A related but distinct rationale for using a placebo control rather than an established effective intervention is that the documented experience with the established effective intervention is not sufficient to provide a scientifically reliable comparison with the intervention being investigated; it is then difficult, or even impossible, without using a placebo, to design a scientifically reliable study. This is not always, however, an ethically acceptable basis for depriving control subjects of an established effective intervention in clinical trials; only when doing so would not add any risk of serious harm, particularly irreversible harm, to the subjects would it be ethically acceptable to do so. In some cases, the condition at which the intervention is aimed (for example, cancer or HIV/AIDS) will be too serious to deprive control subjects of an established effective intervention.

This latter rationale (when active control would not yield reliable results) differs from the former (trials that entail only minor risks) in emphasis. In trials that entail only minor risks the investigative interventions are aimed at relatively trivial conditions, such as the common cold or hair loss; forgoing an established effective intervention for the duration of a trial deprives control subjects of only minor benefits. It is for this reason that it is not unethical to use a placebo-control design. Even if it were possible to design a so-called "non-inferiority", or "equivalency", trial using an active control, it would still not be unethical in these circumstances to use a placebo-control design. In any event, the researcher must satisfy the ethical review committee that the safety and human rights of the subjects will be fully protected, that prospective subjects will be fully informed about alternative treatments, and that the purpose and design of the study are scientifically sound. The ethical acceptability of such placebo-controlled studies increases as the period of placebo use is decreased, and when the study design permits change to active treatment ("escape treatment") if intolerable symptoms occur.

Exceptional use of a comparator other than an established effective intervention. An exception to the general rule is applicable in some studies designed to develop a therapeutic, preventive or diagnostic intervention for use in a country or community in which an established effective intervention is not available and unlikely in the foreseeable future to become available, usually for economic or logistic reasons. The purpose of such a study is to make available to the population of the country or community an effective alternative to an established effective intervention that is locally unavailable. Accordingly, the proposed investigational intervention must be responsive to the health needs of the population from which the research subjects are recruited and there must be assurance that, if it proves to be safe and effective, it will be made reasonably available to that population. Also, the scientific and ethical review committees must be satisfied that the established effective intervention cannot be used as comparator because its use would not yield scientifically reliable results that would be relevant to the health needs of the study population. In these circumstances an ethical review committee can approve a clinical trial in which the comparator is other than an established effective intervention, such as placebo or no treatment or a local remedy.

However, some people strongly object to the exceptional use of a comparator other than an established effective intervention because it could result in exploitation of poor and disadvantaged populations. The objection rests on three arguments:

- Placebo control could expose research subjects to risk of serious or irreversible harm when the use of an established effective intervention as comparator could avoid the risk.
- Not all scientific experts agree about conditions under which an established effective intervention used as a comparator would not yield scientifically reliable results.

• An economic reason for the unavailability of an established effective intervention cannot justify a placebo-controlled study in a country of limited resources when it would be unethical to conduct a study with the same design in a population with general access to the effective intervention outside the study.

Placebo control when an established effective intervention is not available in the host country. The question addressed here is: when should an exception be allowed to the general rule that subjects in the control arm of a clinical trial should receive an established effective intervention?

The usual reason for proposing the exception is that, for economic or logistic reasons, an established effective intervention is not in general use or available in the country in which the study will be conducted, whereas the investigational intervention could be made available, given the finances and infrastructure of the country.

Another reason that may be advanced for proposing a placebo-controlled trial is that using an established effective intervention as the control would not produce scientifically reliable data relevant to the country in which the trial is to be conducted. Existing data about the effectiveness and safety of the established effective intervention may have been accumulated under circumstances unlike those of the population in which it is proposed to conduct the trial; this, it may be argued, could make their use in the trial unreliable. One reason could be that the disease or condition manifests itself differently in different populations, or other uncontrolled factors could invalidate the use of existing data for comparative purposes.

The use of placebo control in these circumstances is ethically controversial, for the following reasons:

• Sponsors of research might use poor countries or communities as testing grounds for research that would be difficult or impossible in countries where there is general access to an established effective intervention, and the investigational intervention, if proven safe and effective, is likely to be marketed in countries in which an established effective intervention is already available and it is not likely to be marketed in the host country.

• The research subjects, both active-arm and control-arm, are patients who may have a serious, possibly life-threatening, illness. They do not normally have access to an established effective intervention currently available to similar patients in many other countries. According to the requirements of a scientifically reliable trial, investigators, who may be their attending physicians, would be expected to enroll some of those patients/subjects in the placebo-control arm. This would appear to be a violation of the physician's fiduciary duty of undivided loyalty to the patient, particularly in cases in which known effective therapy could be made available to the patients.

An argument for exceptional use of placebo control may be that a health authority in a country where an established effective intervention is not generally available or affordable, and unlikely to become available or affordable in the foreseeable future, seeks to develop an affordable intervention specifically for a health problem affecting its population. There may then be less reason for concern that a placebo design is exploitative, and therefore unethical, as the health authority has responsibility for the population's health, and there are valid health grounds for testing an apparently beneficial intervention. In such circumstances an ethical review committee may determine that the proposed trial is ethically acceptable, provided that the rights and safety of subjects are safeguarded.

Ethical review committees will need to engage in careful analysis of the circumstances to determine whether the use of placebo rather than an established effective intervention is ethically acceptable. They will need to be satisfied that an established effective intervention is truly unlikely to become available and implementable in that country. This may be difficult to determine, however, as it is clear that, with sufficient persistence and ingenuity, ways may be found of accessing previously unattainable medicinal products, and thus avoiding the ethical issue raised by the use of placebo control.

When the rationale of proposing a placebo-controlled trial is that the use of an established effective intervention as the control would not yield scientifically reliable data relevant to the proposed host country, the ethical review committee in that country has the option of seeking expert opinion as to whether use of an established effective intervention in the control arm would invalidate the results of the research.

An "equivalency trial" as an alternative to a placebo-controlled trial. An alternative to a placebo-control design in these circumstances would be an "equivalency trial", which would compare an investigational intervention with an established effective intervention and produce scientifically reliable data. An equivalency trial in a country in which no established effective intervention is available is not designed to determine whether the investigational intervention is superior to an established effective intervention currently used somewhere in the world; its purpose is, rather, to determine whether the investigational intervention is, in effectiveness and safety, equivalent to, or almost equivalent to, the established effective intervention. It would be hazardous to conclude, however, that an intervention demonstrated to be equivalent, or almost equivalent, to an established effective intervention is better than nothing or superior to whatever intervention is available in the country; there may be substantial differences between the results of superficially identical clinical trials carried out in different countries. If there are such differences, it would be scientifically acceptable and ethically preferable to conduct such 'equivalency' trials in countries in which an established effective intervention is already available.

If there are substantial grounds for the ethical review committee to conclude that an established effective intervention will not become available and implementable, the committee should obtain assurances from the parties concerned that plans have been agreed for making the investigational intervention reasonably available in the host country or community once its effectiveness and safety have been established. Moreover, when the study has external sponsorship, approval should usually be dependent on the sponsors and the health authorities of the host country having engaged in a process of negotiation and planning, including justifying the study in regard to local healthcare needs.

Means of minimizing harm to placebo-control subjects. Even when placebo controls are justified on one of the bases set forth in the guideline, there are means of minimizing the possibly harmful effect of being in the control arm.

First, a placebo-control group need not be untreated. An add-on design may be employed when the investigational therapy and a standard treatment have different mechanisms of action. The treatment to be tested and placebo are each added to a standard treatment. Such studies have a particular place when a standard treatment is known to decrease mortality or irreversible morbidity but a trial with standard treatment as the active control cannot be carried out or would be difficult to interpret [*International Conference on Harmonisation (ICH) Guideline: Choice of Control Group and Related Issues in Clinical Trials, 2000*]. In testing for improved treatment of life-threatening diseases such as cancer, HIV/AIDS, or heart failure, add-on designs are a particularly useful means of finding improvements in interventions that are not fully effective or may cause intolerable side-effects. They have a place also in respect of treatment for epilepsy, rheumatism and osteoporosis, for example, because withholding of established effective therapy could result in progressive disability, unacceptable discomfort or both.

Second, as indicated in Guideline 8 Commentary, when the intervention to be tested in a randomized controlled trial is designed to prevent or postpone a lethal or disabling outcome, the investigator minimizes harmful effects of placebo-control studies by providing in the research protocol for the monitoring of research data by an independent Data and Safety Monitoring Board (DSMB). One function of such a board is to protect the research subjects from previously unknown adverse reactions; another is to avoid unnecessarily prolonged exposure to an inferior therapy. The board fulfils the latter function by means of interim analyses of the data pertaining to efficacy to ensure that the trial does not continue beyond the point at which an investigational therapy is demonstrated to be effective. Normally, at the outset of a randomized controlled trial, criteria are established for its premature termination (stopping rules or guidelines).

In some cases the DSMB is called upon to perform "conditional power calculations", designed to determine the probability that a particular clinical trial could ever show that the investigational therapy is effective. If that probability is very small, the DSMB is expected to recommend termination of the clinical trial, because it would be unethical to continue it beyond that point.

In most cases of research involving human subjects, it is unnecessary to appoint a DSMB. To ensure that research is carefully monitored for the early detection of adverse events, the sponsor or the principal investigator appoints an individual to be responsible for advising on the need to consider changing the system of monitoring for adverse events or the process of informed consent, or even to consider terminating the study.

GUIDELINE 12: *Equitable distribution of burdens and benefits in the selection of groups of subjects in research*

Groups or communities to be invited to be subjects of research should be selected in such a way that the burdens and benefits of the research will be equitably distributed. The exclusion of groups or communities that might benefit from study participation must be justified.

COMMENTARY ON GUIDELINE 12

General considerations: Equity requires that no group or class of persons should bear more than its fair share of the burdens of participation in research. Similarly, no group should be deprived of its fair share of the benefits of research, short-term or long-term; such benefits include the direct benefits of participation as well as the benefits of the new knowledge that the research is designed to yield. When burdens or benefits of research are to be apportioned unequally among individuals or groups of persons, the criteria for unequal distribution should be morally justifiable and not arbitrary. In other words, unequal allocation must not be inequitable. Subjects should be drawn from the qualifying population in the general geographic area of the trial without regard to race, ethnicity, economic status or gender unless there is a sound scientific reason to do otherwise.

In the past, groups of persons were excluded from participation in research for what were then considered good reasons. As a consequence of such exclusions, information about the diagnosis, prevention and treatment of diseases in such groups of persons is limited. This has resulted in a serious class injustice. If information about the management of diseases is considered a benefit that is distributed within a society, it is unjust to deprive groups of persons of that benefit. Such documents as the Declaration of Helsinki and the UNAIDS Guidance Document *Ethical Considerations in HIV Preventive Vaccine Research,* and the policies of many national governments and professional societies, recognize the need to redress these injustices by encouraging the participation of previously excluded groups in basic and applied biomedical research.

Members of vulnerable groups also have the same entitlement to access to the benefits of investigational interventions that show promise of therapeutic benefit as persons not considered vulnerable, particularly when no superior or equivalent approaches to therapy are available.

There has been a perception, sometimes correct and sometimes incorrect, that certain groups of persons have been overused as research subjects. In some cases such overuse has been based on the administrative availability of the populations. Research hospitals are often located in places where members of the lowest socioeconomic classes reside, and this has resulted in an apparent overuse of such persons. Other groups that may have been overused because they were conveniently available to researchers include students in investigators' classes, residents of long-term care facilities and subordinate members of hierarchical institutions. Impoverished groups have been overused because of their willingness to serve as subjects in exchange for relatively small stipends. Prisoners have been considered ideal subjects for Phase I drug studies because of their highly regimented lives and, in many cases, their conditions of economic deprivation.

Overuse of certain groups, such as the poor or the administratively available, is unjust for several reasons. It is unjust to selectively recruit impoverished people to serve as research subjects simply because they can be more easily induced to participate in exchange for small payments. In most cases, these people would be called upon to bear the burdens of research so that others who are better off could enjoy the benefits. However, although the burdens of research should not fall disproportionately on socio-economically disadvantaged groups, neither should such groups be categorically excluded from research protocols. It would not be unjust to selectively recruit poor people to serve as subjects in research designed to address problems that are prevalent in their group—malnutrition, for example. Similar considerations apply to institutionalized groups or those whose availability to the investigators is for other reasons administratively convenient.

Not only may certain groups within a society be inappropriately overused as research subjects, but also entire communities or societies may be overused. This has been particularly likely to occur in countries or communities with insufficiently well-developed systems for the protection of the rights and welfare of human research subjects. Such overuse is especially questionable when the populations or communities concerned bear the burdens of participation in research but are extremely unlikely ever to enjoy the benefits of new knowledge and products developed as a result of the research. (See Guideline 10: *Research in populations and communities with limited resources.*)

GUIDELINE 13: *Research involving vulnerable persons*

Special justification is required for inviting vulnerable individuals to serve as research subjects and, if they are selected, the means of protecting their rights and welfare must be strictly applied.

COMMENTARY ON GUIDELINE 13

Vulnerable persons are those who are relatively (or absolutely) incapable of protecting their own interests. More formally, they may have insufficient power, intelligence, education, resources, strength, or other needed attributes to protect their own interests.

General considerations. The central problem presented by plans to involve vulnerable persons as research subjects is that such plans may entail an inequitable distribution of the burdens and benefits of research participation. Classes of individuals conventionally considered vulnerable are those with limited capacity or freedom to consent or to decline to consent. They are the subject of specific guidelines in this document (Guidelines 14,15) and include children, and persons who because of mental or behavioural disorders are incapable of giving informed consent. Ethical justification of their involvement usually requires that investigators satisfy ethical review committees that:

- the research could not be carried out equally well with less vulnerable subjects;

- the research is intended to obtain knowledge that will lead to improved diagnosis, prevention or treatment of diseases or other health problems characteristic of, or unique to, the vulnerable class-either the actual subjects or other similarly situated members of the vulnerable class;
- research subjects and other members of the vulnerable class from which subjects are recruited will ordinarily be assured reasonable access to any diagnostic, preventive or therapeutic products that will become available as a consequence of the research;
- the risks attached to interventions or procedures that do not hold out the prospect of direct health-related benefit will not exceed those associated with routine medical or psychological examination of such persons unless an ethical review committee authorizes a slight increase over this level of risk (Guideline 9); and,
- when the prospective subjects are either incompetent or otherwise substantially unable to give informed consent, their agreement will be supplemented by the permission of their legal guardians or other appropriate representatives.

Other vulnerable groups. The quality of the consent of prospective subjects who are junior or subordinate members of a hierarchical group requires careful consideration, as their agreement to volunteer may be unduly influenced, whether justified or not, by the expectation of preferential treatment if they agree or by fear of disapproval or retaliation if they refuse. Examples of such groups are medical and nursing students, subordinate hospital and laboratory personnel, employees of pharmaceutical companies, and members of the armed forces or police. Because they work in close proximity to investigators, they tend to be called upon more often than others to serve as research subjects, and this could result in inequitable distribution of the burdens and benefits of research.

Elderly persons are commonly regarded as vulnerable. With advancing age, people are increasingly likely to acquire attributes that define them as vulnerable. They may, for example, be institutionalized or develop varying degrees of dementia. If and when they acquire such vulnerability-defining attributes, and not before, it is appropriate to consider them vulnerable and to treat them accordingly.

Other groups or classes may also be considered vulnerable. They include residents of nursing homes, people receiving welfare benefits or social assistance and other poor people and the unemployed, patients in emergency rooms, some ethnic and racial minority groups, homeless persons, nomads, refugees or displaced persons, prisoners, patients

with incurable disease, individuals who are politically powerless, and members of communities unfamiliar with modern medical concepts. To the extent that these and other classes of people have attributes resembling those of classes identified as vulnerable, the need for special protection of their rights and welfare should be reviewed and applied, where relevant.

Persons who have serious, potentially disabling or life-threatening diseases are highly vulnerable. Physicians sometimes treat such patients with drugs or other therapies not yet licensed for general availability because studies designed to establish their safety and efficacy have not been completed. This is compatible with the Declaration of Helsinki, which states in Paragraph 32: " *In the treatment of a patient, where proven…therapeutic methods do not exist or have been ineffective, the physician, with informed consent from the patient, must be free to use unproven or new…therapeutic measures, if in the physician's judgement it offers hope of saving life, re-establishing health or alleviating suffering*". Such treatment, commonly called 'compassionate use', is not properly regarded as research, but it can contribute to ongoing research into the safety and efficacy of the interventions used.

Although, on the whole, investigators must study less vulnerable groups before involving more vulnerable groups, some exceptions are justified. In general, children are not suitable for Phase I drug trials or for Phase I or II vaccine trials, but such trials may be permissible after studies in adults have shown some therapeutic or preventive effect. For example, a Phase II vaccine trial seeking evidence of immunogenicity in infants may be justified when a vaccine has shown evidence of preventing or slowing progression of an infectious disease in adults, or Phase I research with children may be appropriate because the disease to be treated does not occur in adults or is manifested differently in children (Appendix 3: *The phases of clinical trials of vaccines and drugs*).

GUIDELINE 14: *Research involving children*

Before undertaking research involving children, the investigator must ensure that:

- the research might not equally well be carried out with adults;
- the purpose of the research is to obtain knowledge relevant to the health needs of children;
- a parent or legal representative of each child has given permission;
- the agreement (assent) of each child has been obtained to the extent of the child's capabilities; and,

• a child's refusal to participate or continue in the research will be respected.

COMMENTARY ON GUIDELINE 14

Justification of the involvement of children in biomedical research. The participation of children is indispensable for research into diseases of childhood and conditions to which children are particularly susceptible (cf. vaccine trials), as well as for clinical trials of drugs that are designed for children as well as adults. In the past, many new products were not tested for children though they were directed towards diseases also occurring in childhood; thus children either did not benefit from these new drugs or were exposed to them though little was known about their specific effects or safety in children. Now it is widely agreed that, as a general rule, the sponsor of any new therapeutic, diagnostic or preventive product that is likely to be indicated for use in children is obliged to evaluate its safety and efficacy for children before it is released for general distribution.

Assent of the child. The willing cooperation of the child should be sought, after the child has been informed to the extent that the child's maturity and intelligence permit. The age at which a child becomes legally competent to give consent differs substantially from one jurisdiction to another; in some countries the "age of consent" established in their different provinces, states or other political subdivisions varies considerably. Often children who have not yet reached the legally established age of consent can understand the implications of informed consent and go through the necessary procedures; they can therefore knowingly agree to serve as research subjects. Such knowing agreement, sometimes referred to as assent, is insufficient to permit participation in research unless it is supplemented by the permission of a parent, a legal guardian or other duly authorized representative.

Some children who are too immature to be able to give knowing agreement, or assent, may be able to register a 'deliberate objection', an expression of disapproval or refusal of a proposed procedure. The deliberate objection of an older child, for example, is to be distinguished from the behaviour of an infant, who is likely to cry or withdraw in response to almost any stimulus. Older children, who are more capable of giving assent, should be selected before younger children or infants, unless there are valid scientific reasons related to age for involving younger children first.

A deliberate objection by a child to taking part in research should always be respected even if the parents have given permission, unless the child needs treatment that is not available outside the context of research, the investigational intervention shows promise of therapeutic benefit, and there is no acceptable alternative therapy. In such a case, particularly if the child is very young or immature, a parent or guardian may override the child's objections. If the child is older and more nearly capable of independent informed consent, the investigator should seek the specific approval or clearance of the scientific and ethical review committees for initiating or continuing with the investigational treatment. If child subjects become capable of independent informed consent during the research, their informed consent to continued participation should be sought and their decision respected.

A child with a likely fatal illness may object or refuse assent to continuation of a burdensome or distressing intervention. In such circumstances parents may press an investigator to persist with an investigational intervention against the child's wishes. The investigator may agree to do so if the intervention shows promise of preserving or prolonging life and there is no acceptable alternative treatment. In such cases, the investigator should seek the specific approval or clearance of the ethical review committee before agreeing to override the wishes of the child.

Permission of a parent or guardian. The investigator must obtain the permission of a parent or guardian in accordance with local laws or established procedures. It may be assumed that children over the age of 12 or 13 years are usually capable of understanding what is necessary to give adequately informed consent, but their consent (assent) should normally be complemented by the permission of a parent or guardian, even when local law does not require such permission. Even when the law requires parental permission, however, the assent of the child must be obtained.

In some jurisdictions, some individuals who are below the general age of consent are regarded as "emancipated" or "mature" minors and are authorized to consent without the agreement or even the awareness of their parents or guardians. They may be married or pregnant or be already parents or living independently. Some studies involve investigation of adolescents' beliefs and behaviour regarding sexuality or use of recreational drugs; other research addresses domestic violence or child abuse. For studies on these topics, ethical review committees may waive parental permission if, for example, parental knowledge of the subject matter may place the adolescents at some risk of questioning or even intimidation by their parents.

Because of the issues inherent in obtaining assent from children in institutions, such children should only exceptionally be subjects of research. In the case of institutionalized children without parents, or whose parents are not legally authorized to grant permission, the ethical review committee may require sponsors or investigators to provide it with the opinion of an independent, concerned, expert advocate for institutionalized children as to the propriety of undertaking the research with such children.

Observation of research by a parent or guardian. A parent or guardian who gives permission for a child to participate in research should be given the opportunity, to a reasonable extent, to observe the research as it proceeds, so as to be able to withdraw the child if the parent or guardian decides it is in the child's best interests to do so.

Psychological and medical support. Research involving children should be conducted in settings in which the child and the parent can obtain adequate medical and psychological support. As an additional protection for children, an investigator may, when possible, obtain the advice of a child's family physician, paediatrician or other health-care provider on matters concerning the child's participation in the research.

(See also Guideline 8: *Benefits and risks of study participation;* Guideline 9: *Special limitations on risks when subjects are not capable of giving consent;* and Guideline 13: *Research involving vulnerable persons.*)

GUIDELINE 15: *Research involving individuals who by reason of mental or behavioural disorders are not capable of giving adequately informed consent*

Before undertaking research involving individuals who by reason of mental or behavioural disorders are not capable of giving adequately informed consent, the investigator must ensure that:

- such persons will not be subjects of research that might equally well be carried out on persons whose capacity to give adequately informed consent is not impaired;
- the purpose of the research is to obtain knowledge relevant to the particular health needs of persons with mental or behavioural disorders;
- the consent of each subject has been obtained to the extent of that person's capabilities, and a prospective subject's refusal to participate in research is always respected, unless, in exceptional circumstances, there is no reasonable medical alternative and local law permits overriding the objection; and,
- in cases where prospective subjects lack capacity to consent, permission is obtained from a responsible family member or a legally authorized representative in accordance with applicable law.

COMMENTARY ON GUIDELINE 15

General considerations. Most individuals with mental or behavioural disorders are capable of giving informed consent; this Guideline is concerned only with those who are not capable or who because their condition deteriorates become temporarily incapable. They should never be subjects of research that might equally well be carried out on persons in full possession of their mental faculties, but they are clearly the only subjects suitable for a large part of research into the origins and treatment of certain severe mental or behavioural disorders.

Consent of the individual. The investigator must obtain the approval of an ethical review committee to include in research persons who by reason of mental or behavioural disorders are not capable of giving informed consent. The willing cooperation of such persons should be sought to the extent that their mental state permits, and any objection on their part to taking part in any study that has no components designed to benefit them directly should always be respected. The objection of such an individual to an investigational intervention intended to be of therapeutic benefit should be respected unless there is no reasonable medical alternative and local law permits overriding the objection. The agreement of an immediate family member or other person with a close personal relationship with the individual should be sought, but it should be recognized that these proxies may have their own interests that may call their permission into question. Some relatives may not be primarily concerned with protecting the rights and welfare of the patients. Moreover, a close family member or friend may wish to take advantage of a research study in the hope that it will succeed in "curing" the condition. Some jurisdictions do not permit third-party permission for subjects lacking capacity to consent. Legal authorization may be necessary to involve in research an individual who has been committed to an institution by a court order.

Serious illness in persons who because of mental or behavioural disorders are unable to give adequately informed consent. Persons who because of mental or behavioural disorders are unable to give adequately informed consent and who have, or are at risk of, serious illnesses such as HIV infection, cancer or hepatitis should not be deprived of the possible benefits of investigational drugs, vaccines or devices that show promise of therapeutic or preventive benefit, particularly when no superior or equivalent therapy or prevention is available. Their entitlement to access to such therapy or prevention is justified ethically on the same grounds as is such entitlement for other vulnerable groups.

Persons who are unable to give adequately informed consent by reason of mental or behavioural disorders are, in general, not suitable for participation in formal clinical trials except those trials that are designed to be responsive to their particular health needs and can be carried out only with them.

(See also Guidelines 8: *Benefits and risks of study participation;* 9: *Special limitations on risks when subjects are not capable of giving consent;* and 13: *Research involving vulnerable persons.*)

GUIDELINE 16: *Women as research subjects*

Investigators, sponsors or ethical review committees should not exclude women of reproductive age from biomedical research. The potential for becoming pregnant during a study should not, in itself, be used as a reason for precluding or limiting participation. However, a thorough discussion of risks to the pregnant woman and to her fetus is a prerequisite for the woman's ability to make a rational decision to enroll in a clinical study. In this discussion, if participation in the research might be hazardous to a fetus or a woman if she becomes pregnant, the sponsors/investigators should guarantee the prospective subject a pregnancy test and access to effective contraceptive methods before the research commences. Where such access is not possible, for legal or religious reasons, investigators should not recruit for such possibly hazardous research women who might become pregnant.

COMMENTARY ON GUIDELINE 16

Women in most societies have been discriminated against with regard to their involvement in research. Women who are biologically capable of becoming pregnant have been customarily excluded from formal clinical trials of drugs, vaccines and medical devices owing to concern about undetermined risks to the fetus. Consequently, relatively little is known about the safety and efficacy of most drugs, vaccines or devices for such women, and this lack of knowledge can be dangerous.

A general policy of excluding from such clinical trials women biologically capable of becoming pregnant is unjust in that it deprives women as a class of persons of the benefits of the new knowledge derived from the trials. Further, it is an affront to their right of self-determination. Nevertheless, although women of childbearing age should be given the opportunity to participate in research, they should be helped to understand that the research could include risks to the fetus if they become pregnant during the research.

Although this general presumption favours the inclusion of women in research, it must be acknowledged that in some parts of the world women are vulnerable to neglect or harm in research because of their social conditioning to submit to authority, to ask no questions, and to tolerate pain and suffering. When women in such situations are potential subjects in research, investigators need to exercise special care in the informed consent process to ensure that they have adequate time and a proper environment in which to take decisions on the basis of clearly given information.

Individual consent of women: In research involving women of reproductive age, whether pregnant or non-pregnant, only the informed consent of the woman herself is required for her participation. In no case should the permission of a spouse or partner replace the requirement of individual informed consent. If women wish to consult with their husbands or partners or seek voluntarily to obtain their permission before deciding to enroll in research, that is not only ethically permissible but in some contexts highly desirable. A strict requirement of authorization of spouse or partner, however, violates the substantive principle of respect for persons.

A thorough discussion of risks to the pregnant woman and to her fetus is a prerequisite for the woman's ability to make a rational decision to enroll in a clinical study. For women who are not pregnant at the outset of a study but who might become pregnant while they are still subjects, the consent discussion should include information about the alternative of voluntarily withdrawing from the study and, where legally permissible, terminating the pregnancy. Also, if the pregnancy is not terminated, they should be guaranteed a medical follow-up.

GUIDELINE 17: *Pregnant women as research participants.*

Pregnant women should be presumed to be eligible for participation in biomedical research. Investigators and ethical review committees should ensure that prospective subjects who are pregnant are adequately informed about the risks and benefits to themselves, their pregnancies, the fetus and their subsequent offspring, and to their fertility.

Research in this population should be performed only if it is relevant to the particular health needs of a pregnant woman or her fetus, or to the health needs of pregnant women in general, and, when appropriate, if it is supported by reliable evidence from animal experiments, particularly as to risks of teratogenicity and mutagenicity.

COMMENTARY ON GUIDELINE 17

The justification of research involving pregnant women is complicated by the fact that it may present risks and potential benefits to two beings—the woman and the fetus—as well as to the person the fetus is destined to become. Though the decision about acceptability of risk should be made by the mother as part of the informed consent process, it is desirable in research directed at the health of the fetus to obtain the father's opinion also, when possible. Even when evidence concerning risks is unknown or ambiguous, the decision about acceptability of risk to the fetus should be made by the woman as part of the informed consent process.

Especially in communities or societies in which cultural beliefs accord more importance to the fetus than to the woman's life or health, women may feel constrained to participate, or not to participate, in research. Special safeguards should be established to prevent undue inducement to pregnant women to participate in research in which interventions hold out the prospect of direct benefit to the fetus. Where fetal abnormality is not recognized as an indication for abortion, pregnant women should not be recruited for research in which there is a realistic basis for concern that fetal abnormality may occur as a consequence of participation as a subject in research.

Investigators should include in protocols on research on pregnant women a plan for monitoring the outcome of the pregnancy with regard to both the health of the woman and the short-term and long-term health of the child.

GUIDELINE 18: *Safeguarding confidentiality*

The investigator must establish secure safeguards of the confidentiality of subjects' research data. Subjects should be told the limits, legal or other, to the investigators' ability to safeguard confidentiality and the possible consequences of breaches of confidentiality.

COMMENTARY ON GUIDELINE 18

Confidentiality between investigator and subject. Research relating to individuals and groups may involve the collection and storage of information that, if disclosed to third parties, could cause harm or distress. Investigators should arrange to protect the confidentiality of such information by, for example, omitting information that might lead to the identification of individual subjects, limiting access to the information, anonymizing data, or other means. During the process of obtaining informed consent the investigator should inform the prospective subjects about the precautions that will be taken to protect confidentiality.

Prospective subjects should be informed of limits to the ability of investigators to ensure strict confidentiality and of the foreseeable adverse social consequences of breaches of confidentiality. Some jurisdictions require the reporting to appropriate agencies of, for instance, certain communicable diseases or evidence of child abuse or neglect. Drug regulatory authorities have the right to inspect clinical-trial records, and a sponsor's clinical-compliance audit staff may require and obtain access to confidential data. These and similar limits to the ability to maintain confidentiality should be anticipated and disclosed to prospective subjects.

Participation in HIV/AIDS drug and vaccine trials may impose upon the research subjects significant associated risks of social discrimination or harm; such risks merit consideration equal to that given to adverse medical consequences of the drugs and vaccines. Efforts must be made to reduce their likelihood and severity. For example, subjects in vaccine trials must be enabled to demonstrate that their HIV seropositivity is due to their having been vaccinated rather than to natural infection. This may be accomplished by providing them with documents attesting to their participation in vaccine trials, or by maintaining a confidential register of trial subjects, from which information can be made available to outside agencies at a subject's request.

Confidentiality between physician and patient. Patients have the right to expect that their physicians and other health-care professionals will hold all information about them in strict confidence and disclose it only to those who need, or have a legal right to, the information, such as other attending physicians, nurses, or other health-care workers who perform tasks related to the diagnosis and treatment of patients. A treating physician should not disclose any identifying information about patients to an investigator unless each patient has given consent to such disclosure and unless an ethical review committee has approved such disclosure.

Physicians and other health care professionals record the details of their observations and interventions in medical and other records. Epidemiological studies often make use of such records. For such studies it is usually impracticable to obtain the informed consent of each identifiable patient; an ethical review committee may waive the requirement for informed consent when this is consistent with the requirements of applicable law and provided that there are secure safeguards of confidentiality. (See also Guideline 4 Commentary: *Waiver of the consent requirement.*) In institutions in which records may be used for research purposes without the informed consent of patients, it is advisable to notify patients generally of such practices; notification is usually by means of a statement in patient-information brochures. For research limited to patients' medical records, access must be approved or cleared by an ethical review committee and must be supervised by a person who is fully aware of the confidentiality requirements.

Issues of confidentiality in genetic research. An investigator who proposes to perform genetic tests of known clinical or predictive value on biological samples that can be linked to an identifiable individual must obtain the informed consent of the individual or, when indicated, the permission of a legally authorized representative. Conversely, before performing a genetic test that is of known predictive value or gives reliable information about a known heritable condition, and individual consent or permission has not been obtained, investigators must see that biological samples are fully anonymized and unlinked; this ensures that no information about specific individuals can be derived from such research or passed back to them.

When biological samples are not fully anonymized and when it is anticipated that there may be valid clinical or research reasons for linking the results of genetic tests to research subjects, the investigator in seeking informed consent should assure prospective subjects that their identity will be protected by secure coding of their samples (encryption) and by restricted access to the database, and explain to them this process.

When it is clear that for medical or possibly research reasons the results of genetic tests will be reported to the subject or to the subject's physician, the subject should be informed that such disclosure will occur and that the samples to be tested will be clearly labelled.

Investigators should not disclose results of diagnostic genetic tests to relatives of subjects without the subjects' consent. In places where immediate family relatives would usually expect to be informed of such results, the research protocol, as approved or cleared by the ethical review committee, should indicate the precautions in place to prevent such disclosure of results without the subjects' consent; such plans should be clearly explained during the process of obtaining informed consent.

GUIDELINE 19: *Right of injured subjects to treatment and compensation*

Investigators should ensure that research subjects who suffer injury as a result of their participation are entitled to free medical treatment for such injury and to such financial or other assistance as would compensate them equitably for any resultant impairment, disability or handicap. In the case of death as a result of their participation, their dependants are entitled to compensation. Subjects must not be asked to waive the right to compensation.

COMMENTARY ON GUIDELINE 19

Guideline 19 is concerned with two distinct but closely related entitlements. The first is the uncontroversial entitlement to free medical treatment and compensation for accidental injury inflicted by procedures or interventions performed exclusively to accomplish the purposes of research (non-therapeutic procedures). The second is the entitlement of dependants to material compensation for

death or disability occurring as a direct result of study participation. Implementing a compensation system for research-related injuries or death is likely to be complex, however.

Equitable compensation and free medical treatment. Compensation is owed to research subjects who are disabled as a consequence of injury from procedures performed solely to accomplish the purposes of research. Compensation and free medical treatment are generally not owed to research subjects who suffer expected or foreseen adverse reactions to investigational therapeutic, diagnostic or preventive interventions when such reactions are not different in kind from those known to be associated with established interventions in standard medical practice. In the early stages of drug testing (Phase I and early Phase II), it is generally unreasonable to assume that an investigational drug holds out the prospect of direct benefit for the individual subject; accordingly, compensation is usually owed to individuals who become disabled as a result of serving as subjects in such studies.

The ethical review committee should determine in advance: i) the injuries for which subjects will receive free treatment and, in case of impairment, disability or handicap resulting from such injuries, be compensated; and ii) the injuries for which they will not be compensated. Prospective subjects should be informed of the committee's decisions, as part of the process of informed consent. As an ethical review committee cannot make such advance determination in respect of unexpected or unforeseen adverse reactions, such reactions must be presumed compensable and should be reported to the committee for prompt review as they occur.

Subjects must not be asked to waive their rights to compensation or required to show negligence or lack of a reasonable degree of skill on the part of the investigator in order to claim free medical treatment or compensation. The informed consent process or form should contain no words that would absolve an investigator from responsibility in the case of accidental injury, or that would imply that subjects would waive their right to seek compensation for impairment, disability or handicap. Prospective subjects should be informed that they will not need to take legal action to secure the free medical treatment or compensation for injury to which they may be entitled. They should also be told what medical service or organization or individual will provide the medical treatment and what organization will be responsible for providing compensation.

Obligation of the sponsor with regard to compensation. Before the research begins, the sponsor, whether a pharmaceutical company or other organization or institution, or a government (where government insurance is not precluded by law), should agree to provide compensation for any physical injury for which subjects are entitled to compensation, or come to an agreement with the investigator concerning the circumstances in which the investigator must rely on his or her own insurance coverage (for example, for negligence or failure of the investigator to follow the protocol, or where government insurance coverage is limited to negligence). In certain circumstances it may be advisable to follow both courses. Sponsors should seek adequate insurance against risks to cover compensation, independent of proof of fault.

GUIDELINE 20: *Strengthening capacity for ethical and scientific review and biomedical research*

Many countries lack the capacity to assess or ensure the scientific quality or ethical acceptability of biomedical research proposed or carried out in their jurisdictions. In externally sponsored collaborative research, sponsors and investigators have an ethical obligation to ensure that biomedical research projects for which they are responsible in such countries contribute effectively to national or local capacity to design and conduct biomedical research, and to provide scientific and ethical review and monitoring of such research.

Capacity-building may include, but is not limited to, the following activities:

- establishing and strengthening independent and competent ethical review processes/ committees
- strengthening research capacity
- developing technologies appropriate to health-care and biomedical research
- training of research and health-care staff
- educating the community from which research subjects will be drawn

COMMENTARY ON GUIDELINE 20

External sponsors and investigators have an ethical obligation to contribute to a host country's sustainable capacity for independent scientific and ethical review and biomedical research. Before undertaking research in a host country with little or no such capacity, external sponsors and investigators should include in the research protocol a plan that specifies the contribution they will make. The amount of capacity building reasonably expected should be proportional to the magnitude of the research project. A brief epidemiological study involving only review of medical records, for example, would entail relatively little, if any, such development, whereas a considerable contribution is to be expected of an external sponsor of, for instance, a large-scale vaccine field-trial expected to last two or three years.

The specific capacity-building objectives should be determined and achieved through dialogue and negotiation between external sponsors and host-country authorities. External sponsors would be expected to employ and, if necessary, train local individuals to function as investigators, research assistants or data managers, for example, and to provide, as necessary, reasonable amounts of financial, educational and other assistance for capacity-building. To avoid conflict of interest and safeguard the independence of review committees, financial assistance should not be provided directly to them; rather, funds should be made available to appropriate authorities in the host-country government or to the host research institution.

(See also Guideline 10: *Research in populations and communities with limited resources*)

GUIDELINE 21: *Ethical obligation of external sponsors to provide health-care services*

External sponsors are ethically obliged to ensure the availability of:

- health-care services that are essential to the safe conduct of the research;
- treatment for subjects who suffer injury as a consequence of research interventions; and,
- services that are a necessary part of the commitment of a sponsor to make a beneficial intervention or product developed as a result of the research reasonably available to the population or community concerned.

COMMENTARY ON GUIDELINE 21

Obligations of external sponsors to provide health-care services will vary with the circumstances of particular studies and the needs of host countries. The sponsors' obligations in particular studies should be clarified before the research is begun. The research protocol should specify what health-care services will be made available, during and after the research, to the subjects themselves, to the community from which the subjects are drawn, or to the host country, and for how long. The details of these arrangements should be agreed by the sponsor, officials of the host country, other interested parties, and, when appropriate, the community from which subjects are to be drawn. The agreed arrangements should be specified in the consent process and document.

Although sponsors are, in general, not obliged to provide health-care services beyond that which is necessary for the conduct of the research, it is morally praiseworthy to do so. Such services typically include treatment for diseases contracted in the course of the study. It might, for example, be agreed to treat cases of an infectious disease contracted during a trial of a vaccine designed to provide immunity to that disease, or to provide treatment of incidental conditions unrelated to the study.

The obligation to ensure that subjects who suffer injury as a consequence of research interventions obtain medical treatment free of charge, and that compensation be provided for death or disability occurring as a consequence of such injury, is the subject of Guideline 19, on the scope and limits of such obligations.

When prospective or actual subjects are found to have diseases unrelated to the research, or cannot be enrolled in a study because they do not meet the health criteria, investigators should, as appropriate, advise them to obtain, or refer them for, medical care. In general, also, in the course of a study, sponsors should disclose to the proper health authorities information of public health concern arising from the research.

The obligation of the sponsor to make reasonably available for the benefit of the population or community concerned any intervention or product developed, or knowledge generated, as a result of the research is considered in Guideline 10: *Research in populations and communities with limited resources.*

Appendix I

ITEMS TO BE INCLUDED IN A PROTOCOL (OR ASSOCIATED DOCUMENTS) FOR BIOMEDICAL RESEARCH INVOLVING HUMAN SUBJECTS.

(Include the items relevant to the study/project in question)

1. Title of the study;
2. A summary of the proposed research in lay/non-technical language;
3. A clear statement of the justification for the study, its significance in development and in meeting the needs of the country /population in which the research is carried out;
4. The investigators' views of the ethical issues and considerations raised by the study and, if appropriate, how it is proposed to deal with them;
5. Summary of all previous studies on the topic, including unpublished studies known to the investigators and sponsors, and information on previously published research on the topic, including the nature, extent and relevance of animal studies and other preclinical and clinical studies;
6. A statement that the principles set out in these Guidelines will be implemented;
7. An account of previous submissions of the protocol for ethical review and their outcome;
8. A brief description of the site(s) where the research is to be conducted, including information about the adequacy of facilities for the safe and appropriate conduct of the research, and relevant demographic and epidemiological information about the country or region concerned;
9. Name and address of the sponsor;
10. Names, addresses, institutional affiliations, qualifications and experience of the principal investigator and other investigators;
11. The objectives of the trial or study, its hypotheses or research questions, its assumptions, and its variables;
12. A detailed description of the design of the trial or study. In the case of controlled clinical trials the description should include, but not be limited to, whether assignment to treatment groups will be randomized (including the method of randomization), and whether the study will be blinded (single blind, double blind), or open;
13. The number of research subjects needed to achieve the study objective, and how this was statistically determined;
14. The criteria for inclusion or exclusion of potential subjects, and justification for the exclusion of any groups on the basis of age, sex, social or economic factors, or for other reasons;
15. The justification for involving as research subjects any persons with limited capacity to consent or members of vulnerable social groups, and a description of special measures to minimize risks and discomfort to such subjects;
16. The process of recruitment, e.g., advertisements, and the steps to be taken to protect privacy and confidentiality during recruitment;
17. Description and explanation of all interventions (the method of treatment administration, including route of administration, dose, dose interval and treatment period for investigational and comparator products used);
18. Plans and justification for withdrawing or withholding standard therapies in the course of the research, including any resulting risks to subjects;
19. Any other treatment that may be given or permitted, or contraindicated, during the study;
20. Clinical and laboratory tests and other tests that are to be carried out;
21. Samples of the standardized case-report forms to be used, the methods of recording therapeutic response (description and evaluation of methods and frequency of measurement), the follow-up procedures, and, if applicable, the measures proposed to

determine the extent of compliance of subjects with the treatment;

22. Rules or criteria according to which subjects may be removed from the study or clinical trial, or (in a multi-centre study) a centre may be discontinued, or the study may be terminated;

23. Methods of recording and reporting adverse events or reactions, and provisions for dealing with complications;

24. The known or foreseen risks of adverse reactions, including the risks attached to each proposed intervention and to any drug, vaccine or procedure to be tested;

25. For research carrying more than minimal risk of physical injury, details of plans, including insurance coverage, to provide treatment for such injury, including the funding of treatment, and to provide compensation for research-related disability or death;

26. Provision for continuing access of subjects to the investigational treatment after the study, indicating its modalities, the individual or organization responsible for paying for it, and for how long it will continue;

27. For research on pregnant women, a plan, if appropriate, for monitoring the outcome of the pregnancy with regard to both the health of the woman and the short-term and long-term health of the child;

28. The potential benefits of the research to subjects and to others;

29. The expected benefits of the research to the population, including new knowledge that the study might generate;

30. The means proposed to obtain individual informed consent and the procedure planned to communicate information to prospective subjects, including the name and position of the person responsible for obtaining consent;

31. When a prospective subject is not capable of informed consent, satisfactory assurance that permission will be obtained from a duly authorized person, or, in the case of a child who is sufficiently mature to understand the implications of informed consent but has not reached the legal age of consent, that knowing agreement, or assent, will be obtained, as well as the permission of a parent, or a legal guardian or other duly authorized representative;

32. An account of any economic or other inducements or incentives to prospective subjects to participate, such as offers of cash payments, gifts, or free services or facilities, and of any financial obligations assumed by the subjects, such as payment for medical services;

33. Plans and procedures, and the persons responsible, for communicating to subjects information arising from the study (on harm or benefit, for example), or from other research on the same topic, that could affect subjects' willingness to continue in the study;

34. Plans to inform subjects about the results of the study;

35. The provisions for protecting the confidentiality of personal data, and respecting the privacy of subjects, including the precautions that are in place to prevent disclosure of the results of a subject's genetic tests to immediate family relatives without the consent of the subject;

36. Information about how the code, if any, for the subjects' identity is established, where it will be kept and when, how and by whom it can be broken in the event of an emergency;

37. Any foreseen further uses of personal data or biological materials;

38. A description of the plans for statistical analysis of the study, including plans for interim analyses, if any, and criteria for prematurely terminating the study as a whole if necessary;

39. Plans for monitoring the continuing safety of drugs or other interventions administered for purposes of the study or trial and, if appropriate, the appointment for this purpose of an independent data-monitoring (data and safety monitoring) committee;

40. A list of the references cited in the protocol;

41. The source and amount of funding of the research: the organization that is sponsoring the research and a detailed account of the sponsor's financial commitments to the research institution, the investigators, the research subjects, and, when relevant, the community;

42. The arrangements for dealing with financial or other conflicts of interest that might affect the judgement of investigators or other research personnel: informing the institutional conflict-of-interest committee of such conflicts of interest; the communication by that committee of the pertinent details of the information to the ethical review committee; and the transmission by that committee to the research subjects of the parts of the information that it decides should be passed on to them;

43. The time schedule for completion of the study;

44. For research that is to be carried out in a developing country or community, the contribution that the sponsor will make to capacity-building for scientific and ethical review and for biomedical research in the host country, and an assurance that the capacity-building objectives are in keeping with the values and expectations of the subjects and their communities;

45. Particularly in the case of an industrial sponsor, a contract stipulating who possesses the right to publish the results of the study, and a mandatory obligation to prepare with, and submit to, the principal investigators the draft of the text reporting the results;

46. In the case of a negative outcome, an assurance that the results will be made available, as appropriate, through publication or by reporting to the drug registration authority;

47. Circumstances in which it might be considered inappropriate to publish findings, such as when the findings of an epidemiological, sociological or genetics study may present risks to the interests of a community or population or of a racially or ethnically defined group of people;

48. A statement that any proven evidence of falsification of data will be dealt with in accordance with the policy of the sponsor to take appropriate action against such unacceptable procedures.

Appendix 2

WORLD MEDICAL ASSOCIATION DECLARATION OF HELSINKI

<www.wma.net>

Appendix 3

THE PHASES OF CLINICAL TRIALS OF VACCINES AND DRUGS

Vaccine development

Phase I refers to the first introduction of a candidate vaccine into a human population for initial determination of its safety and biological effects, including immunogenicity. This phase may include studies of dose and route of administration, and usually involves fewer than 100 volunteers.

Phase II refers to the initial trials examining effectiveness in a limited number of volunteers (usually between 200 and 500); the focus of this phase is immunogenicity.

Phase III trials are intended for a more complete assessment of safety and effectiveness in the prevention of disease, involving a larger number of volunteers in a multicentre adequately controlled study.

Drug development

Phase I refers to the first introduction of a drug into humans. Normal volunteer subjects are usually studied to determine levels of drugs at which toxicity is observed. Such studies are followed by dose-ranging studies in patients for safety and, in some cases, early evidence of effectiveness.

Phase II investigation consists of controlled clinical trials designed to demonstrate effectiveness and relative safety. Normally, these are performed on a limited number of closely monitored patients.

Phase III trials are performed after a reasonable probability of effectiveness of a drug has been established and are intended to gather additional evidence of effectiveness for specific indications and more precise definition of drug-related adverse effects. This phase includes both controlled and uncontrolled studies.

Phase IV trials are conducted after the national drug registration authority has approved a drug for distribution or marketing. These trials may include research designed to explore a specific pharmacological effect, to establish the incidence of adverse reactions, or to determine the effects of long-term administration of a drug. Phase IV trials may also be designed to evaluate a drug in a population not studied adequately in the pre-marketing phases (such as children or the elderly) or to establish a new clinical indication for a drug. Such research is to be distinguished from marketing research, sales promotion studies, and routine post-marketing surveillance for adverse drug reactions in that these categories ordinarily need not be reviewed by ethical review committees (see Guideline 2).

SECTION V.

ETHICAL DIRECTIVES PERTAINING
TO THE WELFARE AND USE OF ANIMALS

• • •

I. **Veterinary Medicine**

Veterinarian's Oath, American Veterinary Medical
Association (AVMA) [1954, revised 1969, 1999]

Principles of Veterinary Medical Ethics, American
Veterinary Medical Association (AVMA) [revised
1993]

2. **Research Involving Animals**

International Guiding Principles for Biomedical
Research Involving Animals, Council for
International Organizations of Medical Sciences
(CIOMS), World Health Organization [1984]

Principles for the Utilization and Care of Vertebrate
Animals Used in Testing, Research, and
Education, U.S. Interagency Research Animal
Committee [1985]

Ethics of Animal Investigation, Canadian Council on
Animal Care [revised 1989]

Australian Code of Practice for the Care and Use of
Animals for Scientific Purposes, National Health
and Medical Research Council, Commonwealth
Scientific and Industrial Research Organization,
and Australian Agricultural Council [revised 1989,
1997]

World Medical Association Statement on Animal
Use in Biomedical Research, World Medical
Association [1989]

Guidelines for Ethical Conduct in the Care and Use
of Animals, American Psychological Association
[1985, revised 1992]

Principles and Guidelines for the Use of Animals in
Precollege Education, Institute of Laboratory
Animal Resources, National Research Council
[1989]

Concern for the humane treatment of animals was expressed in the nineteenth century in both the United Kingdom and the United States through societies organized for the prevention of cruelty to animals. The Cruelty to Animals Act, enacted by the British Parliament in 1876, was among the earliest and most comprehensive laws for the protection of animals. Antivivisection proposals were made to the New York State legislature in the nineteenth century, but it was not until 1966 that the United States government enacted the Animal Welfare Act (7 U.S.C. 2131 et seq.), which, with accompanying regulations administered by the U.S. Department of Agriculture (USDA), is the most comprehensive code for the promotion of animal welfare in the United States.

I. Veterinary Medicine

Documents focusing on the ethics of veterinary medicine are similar to those pertaining to human health care except that they are concerned both with the patient (animal) and the client (owner).

VETERINARIAN'S OATH

American Veterinary Medical Association (AVMA)

1954, REVISED 1969, 1999

• • •

Originally adopted by the AVMA House of Delegates in 1954, the Veterinarian's Oath was revised in 1969. Phrases regarding "the promotion of public health, and the advancement of medical knowledge" were added to the oath. Others were dropped, including a specific pledge to "temper pain with anesthesia where indicated" and one not to use professional knowledge "contrary to the laws of humanity." The 1969 version of the oath, printed below, is administered to the graduating classes at many veterinary colleges. The oath was amended by the Executive Board, November 1999.

<http://www.avma.org/membshp/about.asp>

Being admitted to the profession of veterinary medicine, I solemnly swear to use my scientific knowledge and skills for the benefit of society through the protection of animal health, the relief of animal suffering, the conservation of animal resources, the promotion of public health, and the advancement of medical knowledge.

I will practice my profession conscientiously, with dignity, and in keeping with the principles of veterinary medical ethics.

I accept as a lifelong obligation the continual improvement of my professional knowledge and competence.

PRINCIPLES OF VETERINARY MEDICAL ETHICS

American Veterinary Medical Association (AVMA)

REVISED 1993

• • •

Whereas animal research guidelines focus on the treatment of animals being used primarily for human purposes, veterinary medicine is concerned with balancing the interests and welfare of the patient (animal) and those of the client (owner). As a professionally generated ethics document, the AVMA's Principles of Veterinary Medical Ethics in many ways parallels the structure, content, and function of professional documents in human health care. The following are excerpts from the principles.

• • •

Attitude and Intent

The *Principles of Veterinary Medical Ethics* are purposely constructed in a general and broad manner, but veterinarians who accept the Golden Rule as a guide for general conduct and make a reasonable effort to abide by the *Principles of Veterinary Medical Ethics* in professional life will have little difficulty with ethics.

The honor and dignity of our profession rest in our obedience to a just and reasonable code of ethics set forth as a guide to the members. The object of this code, however, is more far-reaching, for exemplary professional conduct not only upholds honor and dignity, but also enlarges our sphere of usefulness, exalts our social standards, and promotes the science we cultivate. Briefly stated, our code of ethics is the foundation of our individual and collective efforts. It is the solemn duty of all members of the Association to deport themselves in accordance with the spirit of this code.

These *Principles of Veterinary Medical Ethics* are intended as aspirational goals. This code is not intended to cover the entire field of veterinary medical ethics. Professional life is too complex to classify one's duties and obligations to clients, colleagues, and fellow citizens into a set of rules.

General Concepts

The *Principles of Veterinary Medical Ethics* are intended to aid veterinarians individually and collectively in maintaining a high level of ethical conduct. They are standards by which an individual may determine the propriety of conduct in relationships with clients, colleagues, and the public. A high standard of professional behavior is expected of all members of the profession.

Veterinarians should be good citizens and participate in activities to advance community welfare. They should conduct themselves in a manner that will enhance the worthiness of their profession.

Professional associations of veterinarians should adopt the AVMA *Principles of Veterinary Medical Ethics* or a similar code, and each should establish an active committee on ethics.

State veterinary associations should include reports or discussions on professional ethics in the programs of their meetings.

Teaching of ethics and professional concepts should be intensified in the educational programs of the colleges of veterinary medicine.

The *Principles of Veterinary Medical Ethics* should be subjected to review with the object of clarification of any obscure parts and the amendment of any inadequate or inappropriate items. A determined effort should be made to encourage compliance with the *Principles* in their entirety.

Guidelines for Professional Behavior

1. In their relations with others, veterinarians should speak and act on the basis of honesty and fairness.

2. Veterinarians should consider first the welfare of the patient for the purpose of relieving suffering and disability while causing a minimum of pain or fright. Benefit to the patient should transcend personal advantage or monetary gain in decisions concerning therapy.

3. Veterinarians should not employ professional knowledge and attainments nor render services under terms and conditions which tend to interfere with the free exercise of judgment and skill or tend to cause a deterioration of the quality of veterinary service.

4. Veterinarians should seek for themselves and their profession the respect of their colleagues, their clients, and the public through courteous verbal interchange, considerate treatment, professional appearances, professionally acceptable procedures, and the utilization of current professional and scientific knowledge. Veterinarians should be concerned with the affairs and welfare of their communities, including the public health.

5. Veterinarians should respect the rights of clients, colleagues, and other health professionals. No member shall belittle or injure the professional standing of another member of the profession or unnecessarily condemn the character of that person's professional acts in such a manner as to be false or misleading.

6. Veterinarians may choose whom they will serve. Once they have undertaken care of a patient they must not neglect the patient. In an emergency, however, they should render service to the best of their ability.

7. Veterinarians should strive continually to improve veterinary knowledge and skill, making available to their colleagues the benefit of their professional attainments, and seeking, through consultation, assistance of others when it appears that the quality of veterinary service may be enhanced thereby.

8. Advertising or solicitation of clients by veterinarians should adhere to the Advertising Regulations, and should in no case be false, misleading, or deceptive.

9. The veterinary profession should safeguard the public and itself against veterinarians deficient in moral character or professional competence. Veterinarians should observe all laws, uphold the honor and dignity of the profession, and accept its self-imposed discipline.

10. The responsibilities of the veterinary profession extend not only to the patient but also to society. The health of the community as well as the patient deserves the veterinarian's interest and participation in nonprofessional activities and organizations.

• • •

Referrals, Consultations, and Relationships with Clients

Consultations and referrals should be offered or sought whenever it appears that the quality of veterinary service will be enhanced thereby.

Consultations should be conducted in a spirit of professional cooperation between the consultant and the attending veterinarian to assure the client's confidence in and respect for veterinary medicine.

When a fellow practitioner or a diagnostic laboratory, research, academic, or regulatory veterinarian is called into consultation by an attending veterinarian, findings and discussions with the client shall be handled in such a manner as to avoid criticism of the attending veterinarian by the consultant or the client, if that criticism is false or misleading.

When in the course of authorized official duty it is necessary for a veterinarian to render service in the field of another veterinarian, it will be considered unethical to offer free or compensated service or advice other than that which comes strictly within the scope of the official duty, unless the client and attending veterinarian agree.

Consultants must not revisit the patient or communicate in person with the client without the knowledge of the attending veterinarian.

Diagnostic laboratory, research, academic, or regulatory veterinarians in the role of consultants shall deport themselves in the same manner as fellow practitioners whether they are private, commercial, or public functionaries.

In dealing with referrals, veterinarians acting as consultants should not take charge of a case or problem without the consent of the client and notification of the referring veterinarian.

The first veterinarian to handle a case has an obligation to other veterinarians that the client may choose to consult about the same case. The first veterinarian should readily withdraw from the case, indicating the circumstances on the records, and should be willing to forward copies of the medical records to other veterinarians who request them.

A veterinarian may refuse to accept a client or a patient, but should not do so solely because the client has previously contacted another veterinarian.

If for any reason a client requests referral to another veterinarian or veterinary institution, the attending veterinarian should be willing to honor the request and facilitate the necessary arrangements.

The following suggestions are offered for consideration by veterinarians in dealing with clients with whom they are not acquainted or for whom they have not previously rendered service:

1) Conduct yourself in word and action as if the person had been referred to you by a colleague. Try to determine by careful questioning whether the client has consulted another veterinarian and if so, the veterinarian's name, diagnosis, and treatment. It may be advisable to contact the previous veterinarian to ascertain the original diagnosis and treatment before telling the client how you plan to handle the case.
2) Describe your diagnosis and intended treatment carefully so that the client will be generally satisfied with the professional contact.
3) Consider the advisability of notifying the previous veterinarian(s) of your diagnosis and therapy.
4) If your colleague's actions reflect professional incompetence or neglect or abuse of the patient, call it to your colleague's attention and, if appropriate, to the attention of officers or practice committees of the local or state veterinary associations or the proper regulatory agency. Remember that a client

who is abruptly changing veterinarians is often under severe stress and is likely to overstate or misstate the causes for differences with the other practitioner.

Confidentiality

The ethical ideals of the veterinary profession imply that a doctor of veterinary medicine and the veterinarian's staff will protect the personal privacy of clients, unless the veterinarian is required, by law, to reveal the confidences or unless it becomes necessary in order to protect the health and welfare of the individual, the animals, and/or others whose health and welfare may be endangered.

Emergency Service

Every practitioner has a moral and ethical responsibility to provide service when because of accidents or other emergencies involving animals it is necessary to save life or relieve suffering. Since veterinarians cannot always be available to provide this service, veterinarians should cooperate with colleagues to assure that emergency services are provided consistent with the needs of the locality.

Frauds

Members of the Association shall avoid the impropriety of employing misrepresentations to attract public attention.

When employed by the buyer to examine an animal for purchase, it is unethical to accept a fee from the seller. The acceptance of such a fee is prima facie evidence of fraud. On the other hand, it is deemed unethical to criticize unfairly an animal about to be sold. The veterinarian's duty in this connection is to be a just and honest referee.

When veterinarians know that surgery has been requested with intent to deceive a third party, they will have engaged in an unethical practice if they perform or participate in the operation.

Secret Remedies

It is unethical and unprofessional for veterinarians to promote, sell, prescribe, or use any product the ingredient formula of which has not been revealed to them.

Genetic Defects

Performance of surgical procedures in all species for the purpose of concealing genetic defects in animals to be shown, raced, bred, or sold as breeding animals is unethical. However, should the health or welfare of the individual patient require correction of such genetic defects, it is recommended that the patient be rendered incapable of reproduction.

Alliance with Unqualified Persons

No member shall willfully place professional knowledge, attainments, or services at the disposal of any lay body, organization, group, or individual by whatever name called, or however organized, for the purpose of encouraging unqualified groups and individuals to diagnose and prescribe for the ailments and diseases of animals.

. . .

Therapy, Determination of

Determination of therapy must not be relegated to secondary consideration with remuneration of the veterinarian being the primary interest. The veterinarian's obligation to uphold the dignity and honor of the profession precludes entering into an arrangement whereby, through commission or rebates, judgment on choice of treatment would be influenced by considerations other than needs of the patient, welfare of the client, or safety to the public.

. . .

Vaccination Clinics

Definition: The term vaccination clinics applies to either privately or publicly supported activities in which veterinarians are engaged in mass immunization of pet animals. Usually, animals are brought into points of assembly by their owners or caretakers in response to a notification that immunization services will be available. Characteristically, these clinics do not provide the opportunity for the participating veterinarians to (1) conduct a physical examination of the individual animals to be immunized, (2) obtain a history of past immunization or prior disease, or (3) advise individual owners on follow-up immunization and health care.

Scientific and Technical Considerations—Rabies vaccination for the purpose of protecting the public health may be achieved in a rabies vaccination clinic.

When the primary objective is to protect the animal patient's health, clinical examination of the patient including proper history taking, is an essential and necessary part of a professionally acceptable immunization procedure.

Such a clinical examination is expected to be provided without regard to where the vaccination procedure is performed.

. . .

Drugs, Practitioner's Responsibility in the Choice of

Practitioners of veterinary medicine, in common with practitioners in other branches of medicine, are fully responsible for their actions with respect to a patient from the time they accept the case until it is released from their care. In the choice of drugs, biologics, or other treatments, they are expected to use their professional judgment in the interests of the patient, based upon their knowledge of the condition, the probable effects of the treatment, and the available scientific evidence which may affect these decisions. If the preponderance of professional judgement is, or seems to be, contrary to theirs, the burden upon the practitioners to sustain their judgment becomes heavier. Nevertheless, the judgment is theirs and theirs alone.

. . .

Dispensing, Marketing, and Merchandising

Dispensing is the direct distribution of veterinary products to clients for their use on the supposition that the veterinarian has knowledge of the particular case or general conditions relating to the current health status of the animals involved and has established a veterinarian client patient relationship. A veterinarian client patient relationship is characterized by these attributes:

1) The veterinarian has assumed the responsibility for making medical judgments regarding the health of the animal(s) and the need for medical treatment, and the client (owner or other caretaker) has agreed to follow the instructions of the veterinarian; and when

2) There is sufficient knowledge of the animal(s) by the veterinarian to initiate at least a general or preliminary diagnosis of the medical condition of the animal(s). This means that the veterinarian has recently seen and is personally acquainted with the keeping and care of the animal(s) by virtue of an examination of the animal(s) and/or by medically appropriate and timely visits to the premises where the animal(s) are kept; and when

3) The practicing veterinarian is readily available for follow-up in case of adverse reactions or failure of the regimen of therapy.

In the veterinarian's office dispensing becomes the distributing of professional veterinary products by virtue of verbal information presented by the owner, as an adjunct to the knowledge gained previously by the practitioner. This is in contrast to a written prescription involving a pharmacist.

Marketing is interpreted to mean those efforts directed at stimulating and encouraging animal owners to make use of veterinary services and products for the purpose of improving animal health and welfare.

Merchandising is buying and selling of professional veterinary products without a veterinarian client patient relationship. Merchandising as defined here is unethical.

. . .

2. Research Involving Animals

Guidelines and regulations addressing the ethical treatment of animals, especially their use in scientific research, include those developed by groups involved in animal use and those generated by nonresearch groups.

INTERNATIONAL GUIDING PRINCIPLES FOR BIOMEDICAL RESEARCH INVOLVING ANIMALS

Council for International Organizations of Medical Sciences (CIOMS), World Health Organization

1984

. . .

The purpose of the guiding principles, approved in 1984, is to provide a conceptual and ethical framework for whatever regulations governing animal research a country chooses to adopt. The guiding principles reflect consultation with a large, representative sample of the international biomedical community as well as with representatives of animal welfare groups. They have gained general international acceptance and have served as a model for similar guidelines in specific countries, including the United States and Canada.

Basic Principles

I. The advancement of biological knowledge and the development of improved means for the protection of the health and wellbeing both of man and of animals require recourse to experimentation on intact live animals of a wide variety of species.

II. Methods such as mathematical models, computer simulation and in vitro biological systems should be used wherever appropriate.

III. Animal experiments should be undertaken only after due consideration of their relevance for human or animal health and the advancement of biological knowledge.

IV. The animals selected for an experiment should be of an appropriate species and quality, and the minimum number required, to obtain scientifically valid results.

V. Investigators and other personnel should never fail to treat animals as sentient, and should regard their proper care and use and the avoidance or minimization of discomfort, distress, or pain as ethical imperatives.

VI. Investigators should assume that procedures that would cause pain in human beings cause pain in other vertebrate species although more needs to be known about the perception of pain in animals.

VII. Procedures with animals that may cause more than momentary or minimal pain or distress should be performed with appropriate sedation, analgesia, or anaesthesia in accordance with accepted veterinary practice. Surgical or other painful procedures should not be performed on unanaesthetized animals paralysed by chemical agents.

VIII. Where waivers are required in relation to the provisions of article VII, the decisions should not rest solely with the investigators directly concerned but should be made, with due regard to the provisions of articles IV, V, and VI, by a suitably constituted review body. Such waivers should not be made solely for the purposes of teaching or demonstration.

IX. At the end of, or when appropriate during, an experiment, animals that would otherwise suffer severe or chronic pain, distress, discomfort, or disablement that cannot be relieved should be painlessly killed.

X. The best possible living conditions should be maintained for animals kept for biomedical purposes. Normally the care of animals should be under the supervision of veterinarians having experience in laboratory animal science. In any case, veterinary care should be available as required.

XI. It is the responsibility of the director of an institute or department using animals to ensure that investigators and personnel have appropriate qualifications or experience for conducting procedures on animals. Adequate opportunities shall be provided for in-service training, including the proper and humane concern for the animals under their care.

PRINCIPLES FOR THE UTILIZATION AND CARE OF VERTEBRATE ANIMALS USED IN TESTING, RESEARCH, AND EDUCATION

U.S. Interagency Research Animal Committee

1985

• • •

Developed in 1984 by the U.S. Interagency Research Animal Committee, which serves as a focal point for the discussion by federal agencies of issues involving the use of animals in research and testing, these principles are based on the CIOMS Guiding Principles. The U.S. principles are endorsed, implemented, and supplemented by the National Institutes of Health's Public Health Service Policy on Humane Care and Use of Laboratory Animals, which was revised in 1986, and the Guide for the Care and Use of Laboratory Animals, prepared by the Institute of Laboratory Animal Resources, National Academy of Sciences, in 1985. The Public Health Service (PHS) policy applies to all PHS researchers, grantees, and contractors who use warm-blooded vertebrates in research and testing. The policy requires compliance with the Animal Welfare Act (AWA) (7 U.S.C. 2131 et seq.) and the USDA regulations that implement it (9 CFR, Subchapter A—Animal Welfare).

The AWA was originally enacted in 1966 to impose civil and criminal penalties on persons who stole household pets and sold them to biomedical research facilities. It has been amended many times to provide additional protections for warm-blooded animals used in agriculture, the food and fiber industry, circuses, pet shops, and research. In 1985, the AWA was amended by P.L. 99–198 to require, among other provisions, the establishment of Animal Care and Use Committees to oversee animal housing and care and to review proposed research. Both the USDA regulations implementing the act and the PHS policy reference the Guide for the Care and Use of Laboratory Animals as the standard according to which programs for the care and use of laboratory animals will be judged.

The AWA and its accompanying regulations and the correlative Public Health Service Act and its accompanying PHS policy together with the guide constitute the fundamental documents that govern the care and use of animals used for research, testing, and teaching in the United States. Additionally, the Food and Drug Administration's Good Laboratory Practices regulations include similar provisions for the care and use of animals in testing sites used by the industry.

The development of knowledge necessary for the improvement of the health and well-being of humans as well as other animals requires in vivo experimentation with a wide variety of animal species. Whenever U.S. Government agencies develop requirements for testing, research, or training procedures involving the use of vertebrate animals, the following principles shall be considered; and whenever these agencies actually perform or sponsor such procedures, the responsible institutional official shall ensure that these principles are adhered to:

I. The transportation, care, and use of animals should be in accordance with the Animal Welfare Act (7 U.S.C. 2131 et seq.) and other applicable Federal laws, guidelines and policies.

II. Procedures involving animals should be designed and performed with due consideration of their relevance to human or animal health, the advancement of knowledge, or the good of society.

III. The animals selected for a procedure should be of an appropriate species and quality and the minimum number required to obtain valid results. Methods such as mathematical models, computer simulation, and in vitro biological systems should be considered.

IV. Proper use of animals, including the avoidance or minimization of discomfort, distress, and pain when consistent with sound scientific practices, is imperative. Unless the contrary is established, investigators should consider that procedures that cause pain or distress in human beings may cause pain or distress in other animals.

V. Procedures with animals that may cause more than momentary or slight pain or distress should be performed with appropriate sedation, analgesia, or anesthesia. Surgical or other painful procedures should not be performed on unanesthetized animals paralyzed by chemical agents.

VI. Animals that would otherwise suffer severe or chronic pain or distress that cannot be relieved should be painlessly killed at the end of the procedure or, if appropriate, during the procedure.

VII. The living conditions of animals should be appropriate for their species and contribute to their health and comfort. Normally, the housing, feeding, and care of all animals used for biomedical purposes must be directed by a veterinarian or other scientist trained and experienced in the proper care, handling, and use of the species being maintained or studied. In any case, veterinary care shall be provided as indicated.

VIII. Investigators and other personnel shall be appropriately qualified and experienced for conducting procedures on living animals. Adequate arrangements shall be made for their in-service training, including the proper and humane care and use of laboratory animals.

IX. Where exceptions are required in relation to the provision of these Principles, the decisions should not rest with the investigators directly concerned but should be made, with due regard to Principle II, by an appropriate review group such as an institutional animal research committee. Such exceptions should not be made solely for the purposes of teaching or demonstration.

ETHICS OF ANIMAL INVESTIGATION

Canadian Council on Animal Care

REVISED 1989

• • •

More detailed than the CIOMS and U.S. government principles, the Canadian Council on Animal Care's Ethics of Animal Investigation includes nine principles designed to be used in association with the CCAC's Guide to the Care and Use of Experimental Animals, a highly respected, two-volume document that provides detailed requirements for the humane use of animals in research, teaching, and testing.

The use of animals in research, teaching, and testing is acceptable only if it promises to contribute to understanding of fundamental biological principles, or to the development of knowledge that can reasonably be expected to benefit humans or animals.

Animals should be used only if the researcher's best efforts to find an alternative have failed. A continuing sharing of knowledge, review of the literature, and adherence to the Russell-Burch "3R" tenet of "Replacement, Reduction and Refinement" are also requisites. Those using animals should employ the most humane methods on the smallest number of appropriate animals required to obtain valid information.

The following principles incorporate suggestions from members of both the scientific and animal welfare communities, as well as the organizations represented on Council. They should be applied in conjunction with CCAC's "Guide to the Care and Use of Experimental Animals."

1. If animals must be used, they should be maintained in a manner that provides for their physical comfort and psychological well-being, according to CCAC's "Policy Statement on Social and Behavioural Requirements of Experimental Animals."

2. Animals must not be subjected to unnecessary pain or distress. The experimental design must offer them every practicable safeguard, whether in research, in teaching or in testing procedures; cost and convenience must not take precedence over the animal's physical and mental well-being.

3. Expert opinion must attest to the potential value of studies with animals. The following procedures,

which are restricted, require independent, external evaluation to justify their use:

i) burns, freezing injuries, fractures, and other types of trauma investigation in anesthetized animals, concomitant to which must be acceptable veterinary practices for the relief of pain, including adequate analgesia during the recovery period;

ii) staged encounters between predator and prey or between conspecifics where prolonged fighting and injury are probable.

4. If pain or distress are necessary concomitants to the study, these must be minimized both in intensity and duration. Investigators, animal care committees, grant review committees and referees must be especially cautious in evaluating the proposed use of the following procedures:

a) experiments involving withholding pre- and post-operative pain-relieving medication;

b) paralyzing and immobilizing experiments where there is no reduction in the sensation of pain;

c) electric shock as negative reinforcement;

d) extreme environmental conditions such as low or high temperatures, high humidity, modified atmospheres, etc., or sudden changes therein;

e) experiments studying stress and pain;

f) experiments requiring withholding of food and water for periods incompatible with the species specific psychological needs; such experiments should have no detrimental effect on the health of the animal;

g) injection of Freund's Complete Adjuvant (FCA). This must be carried out in accordance with "CCAC Guidelines on Immunization Procedures."

5. An animal observed to be experiencing severe, unrelievable pain or discomfort should immediately be humanely killed, using a method providing initial rapid unconsciousness.

6. While non-recovery procedures involving anesthetized animals, and studies involving no pain or distress are considered acceptable; the following experimental procedures inflict excessive pain and are thus unacceptable:

a) utilization of muscle relaxants or paralytics (curare and curare-like) alone, without anesthetics, during surgical procedures;

b) traumatizing procedures involving crushing, burning, striking or beating in unanesthetized animals.

7. Studies such as toxicological and biological testing, cancer research and infectious disease investigation may, in the past, have required continuation until

the death of the animal. However, in the face of distinct signs that such processes are causing irreversible pain or distress, alternative endpoints should be sought to satisfy both the requirements of the study and the needs of the animal.

8. Physical restraint should only be used after alternative procedures have been fully considered and found inadequate. Animals so restrained must receive exceptional care and attention, in compliance with species specific and general requirements as set forth in the "Guide."

9. Painful experiments or multiple invasive procedures on an individual animal, conducted solely for the instruction of students in the classroom, or for the demonstration of established scientific knowledge, cannot be justified. Audiovisual or other alternative techniques should be employed to convey such information.

AUSTRALIAN CODE OF PRACTICE FOR THE CARE AND USE OF ANIMALS FOR SCIENTIFIC PURPOSES

National Health and Medical Research Council, Commonwealth Scientific and Industrial Research Organization, and Australian Agricultural Council

REVISED 1989, 1997

• • •

The first Australian code was issued in 1969 and revised in 1979, 1982, 1985, and 1989. The current code encompasses all aspects of the care and use of animals for scientific purposes in medicine, biology, agriculture, veterinary and other animal sciences, industry, and teaching. Section 1 of the code, "General Principles for the Care and Use of Animals for Scientific Purposes," which is printed below, is similar to the CIOMS principles, but is unique in its inclusion of the principle that animals must not be taken from their natural habitats if others, bred in captivity, are available. In addition to general principles for the care and use of animals, the code specifies the responsibilities of researchers and institutions and the composition and function of Animal Experimentation Ethics Committees. It also provides guidelines for the acquisition and care of animals. It was most recently revised in 1997.

<http://www.health.gov.au/nhmrc/research/awc/pca.pdf>

For the guidance of Investigators, Institutions and Animal Experimentation Ethics Committees and all involved in the care and use of animals for scientific purposes.

1.1 Experiments on animals may be performed only when they are essential to obtain and establish significant information relevant to the understanding of humans or animals, to the maintenance and improvement of human or animal health and welfare, to the improvement of animal management or production, or to the achievement of educational objectives.

1.2 People who use animals for scientific purposes have an obligation to treat the animals with respect and to consider their welfare as an essential factor when planning and conducting experiments.

1.3 Investigators have direct and ultimate responsibility for all matters relating to the welfare of the animals they use in experiments.

1.4 Techniques which replace or complement animal experiments must be used wherever possible.

1.5 Experiments using animals may be performed only after a decision has been made that they are justified, weighing the scientific or educational value of the experiment against the potential effects on the welfare of the animals.

1.6 Animals chosen must be of an appropriate species with suitable biological characteristics, including behavioural characteristics, genetic constitution and nutritional, microbiological and general health status.

1.7 Animals must not be taken from their natural habitats if animals bred in captivity are available and suitable.

1.8 Experiments must be scientifically valid, and must use no more than the minimum number of animals needed.

1.9 Experiments must use the best available scientific techniques and must be carried out only by persons competent in the procedures they perform.

1.10 Experiments must not be repeated unnecessarily.

1.11 Experiments must be as brief as possible.

1.12 Experiments must be designed to avoid pain or distress to animals. If this is not possible, pain or distress must be minimised.

1.13 Pain and distress cannot be evaluated easily in animals and therefore investigators must assume that animals experience pain in a manner similar to humans. Decisions regarding the animals' welfare must be based on this assumption unless there is evidence to the contrary.

1.14 Experiments which may cause pain or distress of a kind and degree for which anaesthesia would normally be used in medical or veterinary practice must be carried out using anaesthesia appropriate to the species and the procedure. When it is not possible to use anaesthesia, such as in certain toxicological or animal production experiments or in animal models of disease, the end-point of the experiments must be as early as possible to avoid or minimise pain or distress to the animals.

1.15 Investigators must avoid using death as an experimental end-point whenever possible.

1.16 Analgesic and tranquilliser usage must be appropriate for the species and should at least parallel usage in medical or veterinary practice.

1.17 An animal which develops signs of pain or distress of a kind and degree not predicted in the proposal, must have the pain or distress alleviated promptly. If severe pain cannot be alleviated without delay, the animal must be killed humanely forthwith. Alleviation of such pain or distress must take precedence over finishing an experiment.

1.18 Neuromuscular blocking agents must not be used without appropriate general anaesthesia, except in animals where sensory awareness has been eliminated. If such agents are used, continuous or frequent intermittent monitoring of paralysed animals is essential to ensure that the depth of anaesthesia is adequate to prevent pain or distress.

1.19 Animals must be transported, housed, fed, watered, handled and used under conditions which are appropriate to the species and which ensure a high standard of care.

1.20 Institutions using animals for scientific purposes must establish Animal Experimentation Ethics Committees (AEECs) to ensure that all animal use conforms with the standards of this Code.

1.21 Investigators must submit written proposals for all animal experimentation to an AEEC which must take into account the expected value of the knowledge to be gained, the validity of the experiments, and all ethical and animal welfare aspects.

1.22 Experiments must not commence until written approval has been obtained from the AEEC.

1.23 The care and use of animals for all scientific purposes in Australia must be in accord with this Code of Practice, and with Commonwealth, State and Territory legislation.

WORLD MEDICAL ASSOCIATION STATEMENT ON ANIMAL USE IN BIOMEDICAL RESEARCH

World Medical Association

1989

• • •

Adopted by the Forty-first World Medical Assembly in Hong Kong, September 1989, the World Medical Association Statement on Animal

Use in Biomedical Research includes principles that affirm not only the need to respect the welfare of animals used for research but also the continued use of animals in biomedical research as essential, and it condemns the harassment of scientists by animal rights activists.

Preamble

Biomedical research is essential to the health and well-being of every person in our society. Advances in biomedical research have dramatically improved the quality and prolonged the duration of life throughout the world. However, the ability of the scientific community to continue its efforts to improve personal and public health is being threatened by a movement to eliminate the use of animals in biomedical research. This movement is spearheaded by groups of radical animal rights activists whose views are far outside mainstream public attitudes and whose tactics range from sophisticated lobbying, fund raising, propaganda and misinformation campaigns to violent attacks on biomedical research facilities and individual scientists.

The magnitude of violent animal rights activities is staggering. In the United States alone, since 1980, animal rights groups have staged more than 29 raids on U.S. research facilities, stealing over 2,000 animals, causing more than 7 million dollars in physical damages and ruining years of scientific research in the process. Animal activist groups have engaged in similar activities in Great Britain, Western Europe, Canada and Australia. Various groups in these countries have claimed responsibility for the bombing of cars, institutions, stores, and the private homes of researchers.

Animal rights violence has had a chilling effect on the scientific community internationally. Scientists, research organizations, and universities have been intimidated into altering or even terminating important research efforts that depend on the use of animals. Laboratories have been forced to divert thousands of research dollars for the purchase of sophisticated security equipment. Young people who might otherwise pursue a career in biomedical research are turning their sights to alternative professions.

Despite the efforts of many groups striving to protect biomedical research from animal activism, the response to the animal rights movement has been fragmented, underfunded, and primarily defensive. Many groups within the biomedical community are hesitant to take a public stand about animal activism because of fear of reprisal. As a result, the research establishment has been backed into a defensive posture. Its motivations are questioned, and the need for using animals in research is repeatedly challenged.

While research involving animals is necessary to enhance the medical care of all persons, we recognized also that humane treatment of research animals must be ensured.

Appropriate training for all research personnel should be prescribed and adequate veterinary care should be available. Experiments must comply with any rules or regulations promulgated to govern human handling, housing, care, treatment and transportation of animals.

International medical and scientific organizations must develop a stronger and more cohesive campaign to counter the growing threat to public health posed by animal activists. Leadership and coordination must be provided.

The World Medical Association therefore affirms the following principles:

1. Animal use in biomedical research is essential for continued medical progress.
2. The WMA Declaration of Helsinki requires that biomedical research involving human subjects should be based on animal experimentation, but also requires that the welfare of animals used for research be respected.
3. Humane treatment of animals used in biomedical research is essential.
4. All research facilities should be required to comply with all guiding principles for humane treatment of animals.
5. Medical Societies should resist any attempt to deny the appropriate use of animals in biomedical research because such denial would compromise patient care.
6. Although rights to free speech should not be compromised, the anarchistic element among animal right activists should be condemned.
7. The use of threats, intimidation, violence, and personal harassment of scientists and their families should be condemned internationally.
8. A maximum coordinated effort from international law enforcement agencies should be sought to protect researchers and research facilities from activities of a terrorist nature.

GUIDELINES FOR ETHICAL CONDUCT IN THE CARE AND USE OF ANIMALS

American Psychological Association

1985, REVISED 1992

• • •

Some professional associations, such as the American Psychological Association (APA), have developed their own guidelines governing research with animals, which reinforce and/or supplement all pertinent laws and other regulations. The APA produced one of the earliest and most complete sets of association guidelines pertaining to research on animals. Like other professional groups, the APA requires that individuals publishing research in APA journals attest to the fact that animal research was conducted in accordance with its guidelines.

I. Justification of the Research

A. Research should be undertaken with a clear scientific purpose. There should be a reasonable expectation that the research will a) increase knowledge of the processes underlying the evolution, development, maintenance, alteration, control, or biological significance of behavior; b) increase understanding of the species under study; or c) provide results that benefit the health or welfare of humans or other animals.

B. The scientific purpose of the research should be of sufficient potential significance to justify the use of animals. Psychologists should act on the assumption that procedures that would produce pain in humans will also do so in other animals.

C. The species chosen for study should be best suited to answer the question(s) posed. The psychologist should always consider the possibility of using other species, nonanimal alternatives, or procedures that minimize the number of animals in research, and should be familiar with the appropriate literature.

D. Research on animals may not be conducted until the protocol has been reviewed by the institutional animal care and use committee (IACUC) to ensure that the procedures are appropriate and humane.

E. The psychologist should monitor the research and the animals' welfare throughout the course of an investigation to ensure continued justification for the research.

II. Personnel

A. Psychologists should ensure that personnel involved in their research with animals be familiar with these guidelines.

B. Animal use procedures must conform with federal regulations regarding personnel, supervision, record keeping, and veterinary care.

C. Behavior is both the focus of study of many experiments as well as a primary source of information about an animal's health and well-being. It is therefore necessary that psychologists and their assistants be informed about the behavioral characteristics of their animal subjects, so as to be aware of normal, species-specific behaviors and unusual behaviors that could forewarn of health problems.

D. Psychologists should ensure that all individuals who use animals under their supervision receive explicit instruction in experimental methods and in the care, maintenance, and handling of the species being studied. Responsibilities and activities of all individuals dealing with animals should be consistent with their respective competencies, training, and experience in either the laboratory or the field setting.

III. Care and Housing of Animals

The concept of "psychological well-being" of animals is of current concern and debate and is included in Federal Regulations (United States Department of Agriculture [USDA], 1991). As a scientific and professional organization, APA recognizes the complexities of defining psychological well-being. Procedures appropriate for a particular species may well be inappropriate for others. Hence, APA does not presently stipulate specific guidelines regarding the maintenance of psychological well-being of research animals. Psychologists familiar with the species should be best qualified professionally to judge measures such as enrichment to maintain or improve psychological well-being of those species.

A. The facilities housing animals should meet or exceed current regulations and guidelines (USDA, 1990, 1991) and are required to be inspected twice a year (USDA, 1989).

B. All procedures carried out on animals are to be reviewed by a local IACUC to ensure that the procedures are appropriate and humane. The committee should have representation from within the institution and from the local community. In the event that it is not possible to constitute an appropriate local IACUC, psychologists are encouraged to seek advice from a corresponding committee of a cooperative institution.

C. Responsibilities for the conditions under which animals are kept, both within and outside of the context of active experimentation or teaching, rests with the psychologist under the supervision of the IACUC (where required by federal regulations) and with individuals appointed by the institution to oversee animal care. Animals are to be provided with humane care and healthful conditions during their stay in the facility. In addition to the federal requirements to provide for the psychological well-being of nonhuman primates used in research, psychologists are encouraged to consider enriching the environments of their laboratory animals and

should keep abreast of literature on well-being and enrichment for the species with which they work.

IV. Acquisition of Animals

A. Animals not bred in the psychologist's facility are to be acquired lawfully. The USDA and local ordinances should be consulted for information regarding regulations and approved suppliers.

B. Psychologists should make every effort to ensure that those responsible for transporting the animals to the facility provide adequate food, water, ventilation, space, and impose no unnecessary stress on the animals.

C. Animals taken from the wild should be trapped in a humane manner and in accordance with applicable federal, state, and local regulations.

D. Endangered species or taxa should be used only with full attention to required permits and ethical concerns. Information and permit applications can be obtained from the Fish and Wildlife Service, Office of Management Authority, U.S. Dept. of the Interior, 4401 N. Fairfax Dr., Rm. 432, Arlington, VA 22043, 703–358–2104. Similar caution should be used in work with threatened species or taxa.

V. Experimental Procedures

Humane consideration for the well-being of the animal should be incorporated into the design and conduct of all procedures involving animals, while keeping in mind the primary goal of experimental procedures—the acquisition of sound, replicable data. The conduct of all procedures is governed by Guideline I.

A. Behavioral studies that involve no aversive stimulation or overt sign of distress to the animal are acceptable. This includes observational and other noninvasive forms of data collection.

B. When alternative behavioral procedures are available, those that minimize discomfort to the animal should be used. When using aversive conditions, psychologists should adjust the parameters of stimulation to levels that appear minimal, though compatible with the aims of the research. Psychologists are encouraged to test painful stimuli on themselves, whenever reasonable. Whenever consistent with the goals of research, consideration should be given to providing the animals with control of the potentially aversive stimulation.

C. Procedures in which the animal is anesthetized and insensitive to pain throughout the procedure and is euthanized before regaining consciousness are generally acceptable.

D. Procedures involving more than momentary or slight aversive stimulation, which are not relieved by medication or other acceptable methods, should be undertaken only when the objectives of research cannot be achieved by other methods.

E. Experimental procedures that require prolonged aversive conditions or produce tissue damage or metabolic disturbances require greater justification and surveillance. This includes prolonged exposure to extreme environmental conditions, experimentally induced prey killing, or infliction of physical trauma or tissue damage. An animal observed to be in a state of severe distress or chronic pain that cannot be alleviated and is not essential to the purposes of the research should be euthanized immediately.

F. Procedures that use restraint must conform to federal regulations and guidelines.

G. Procedures involving the use of paralytic agents without reduction in pain sensation require particular prudence and humane concern. Use of muscle relaxants or paralytics alone during surgery, without general anesthesia, is unacceptable and shall not be used.

H. Surgical procedures, because of their invasive nature, require close supervision and attention to humane considerations by the psychologist. Aseptic (methods that minimize risks of infection) techniques must be used on laboratory animals whenever possible.

1. All surgical procedures and anesthetization should be conducted under the direct supervision of a person who is competent in the use of the procedures.

2. If the surgical procedure is likely to cause greater discomfort than that attending anesthetization, and unless there is specific justification for acting otherwise, animals should be maintained under anesthesia until the procedure is ended.

3. Sound postoperative monitoring and care, which may include the use of analgesics and antibiotics, should be provided to minimize discomfort and to prevent infection and other untoward consequences of the procedure.

4. Animals can not be subjected to successive surgical procedures unless these are required by the nature of the research, the nature of the surgery, or for the well-being of the animal. Multiple surgeries on the same animal must receive special approval from the IACUC.

I. When the use of an animal is no longer required by an experimental protocol or procedure, in order to minimize the number of animals used in research, alternatives to euthanasia should be considered. Such uses should be compatible with the goals of research and the welfare of the animal. Care should be taken that such an action does not expose the animal to multiple surgeries.

J. The return of wild-caught animals to the field can carry substantial risks, both to the formerly captive animals and to the ecosystem. Animals reared in the laboratory should not be released because, in most cases, they cannot survive or they may survive by disrupting the natural ecology.

K. When euthanasia appears to be the appropriate alternative, either as a requirement of the research or because it constitutes the most humane form of disposition of an animal at the conclusion of the research:

1. Euthanasia shall be accomplished in a humane manner, appropriate for the species, and in such a way as to ensure immediate death, and in accordance with procedures outlined in the latest version of the "American Veterinary Medical Association (AVMA) Panel on Euthanasia."

2. Disposal of euthanized animals should be accomplished in a manner that is in accordance with all relevant legislation, consistent with health, environmental, and aesthetic concerns, and approved by the IACUC. No animal shall be discarded until its death is verified.

VI. Field Research

Field research, because of its potential to damage sensitive ecosystems and ethologies, should be subject to IACUC approval. Field research, if strictly observational, may not require IACUC approval (USDA, 1989, pg. 36126).

A. Psychologists conducting field research should disturb their populations as little as possible—consistent with the goals of the research. Every effort should be made to minimize potential harmful effects of the study on the population and on other plant and animal species in the area.

B. Research conducted in populated areas should be done with respect for the property and privacy of the inhabitants of the area.

C. Particular justification is required for the study of endangered species. Such research on endangered species should not be conducted unless IACUC approval has been obtained and all requisite permits are obtained (see above, III D).

VII. Educational Use of Animals

APA has adopted separate guidelines for the educational use of animals in precollege education, including the use of animals in science fairs and demonstrations. For a copy of APA's "Ethical Guidelines for the Teaching of

Psychology in the Secondary Schools," write to: High School Teacher Affiliate Program, Education Directorate, APA, 750 First St., NE, Washington, DC 20002–4242.

A. Psychologists are encouraged to include instruction and discussion of the ethics and values of animal research in all courses that involve or discuss the use of animals.

B. Animals may be used for educational purposes only after review by a committee appropriate to the institution.

C. Some procedures that can be justified for research purposes may not be justified for educational purposes. Consideration should always be given to the possibility of using nonanimal alternatives.

D. Classroom demonstrations involving live animals can be valuable as instructional aids in addition to videotapes, films, or other alternatives. Careful consideration should be given to the question of whether this type of demonstration is warranted by the anticipated instructional gains.

PRINCIPLES AND GUIDELINES FOR THE USE OF ANIMALS IN PRECOLLEGE EDUCATION

Institute of Laboratory Animal Resources (ILAR) National Research Council

1989

• • •

The ILAR Principles and Guidelines provide guidance for improving the scientific integrity of precollege research and encouraging more humane study of animals in precollege education. They are designed to help schools implement changes in their use of animals in teaching programs to bring them more in line with current approaches to the use of animals in higher education and research.

The humane study of animals in precollege education can provide important learning experiences in science and ethics and should be encouraged. Maintaining classroom pets in preschool and grade school can teach respect for other species, as well as proper animal husbandry practices. Introduction of secondary school students to animal studies in closely supervised settings can reinforce those early lessons and teach the principles of humane care and use of animals in scientific inquiry. The National Research Council recommends compliance with the following principles whenever animals are used in precollege education or in science fair projects.

Principle 1

Observational and natural history studies that are not intrusive (that is, do not interfere with an animal's health or well-being or cause it discomfort) are encouraged for all classes of organisms. When an intrusive study of a living organism is deemed appropriate, consideration should be given first to using plants (including lower plants such as yeast and fungi) and invertebrates with no nervous systems or with primitive ones (including protozoa, planaria, and insects). Intrusive studies of invertebrates with advanced nervous systems (such as octopi) and vertebrates should be used only when lower invertebrates are not suitable and only under the conditions stated below in Principle 10.

Principle 2

Supervision shall be provided by individuals who are knowledgeable about and experienced with the health, husbandry, care, and handling of the animal species used and who understand applicable laws, regulations, and policies.

Principle 3

Appropriate care for animals must be provided daily, including weekends, holidays, and other times when school is not in session. This care must include

a. nutritious food and clean, fresh water;

b. clean housing with space and enrichment suitable for normal species behaviors; and

c. temperature and lighting appropriate for the species.

Principle 4

Animals should be healthy and free of disease that can be transmitted to humans or to other animals. Veterinary care must be provided as needed.

Principle 5

Students and teachers should report immediately to the school health authority all scratches, bites, and other injuries; allergies; or illnesses.

Principle 6

Prior to obtaining animals for educational purposes, it is imperative that the school develop a plan for their procurement and ultimate disposition. Animals must not be captured from or released into the wild without the approval of the responsible wildlife and public health officials. When euthanasia is necessary, it should be performed in accordance with the most recent recommendations of the American Veterinary Medical Association's Panel Report on Euthanasia (Journal of the American Veterinary Medical Association, 188[3]: 252–268, 1986, et seq.). It should be performed only by someone trained in the appropriate technique.

Principle 7

Students shall not conduct experimental procedures on animals that

a. are likely to cause pain or discomfort or interfere with an animal's health or well-being;

b. induce nutritional deficiencies or toxicities; or

c. expose animals to microorganisms, ionizing radiation, cancer-producing agents, or any other harmful drugs or chemicals capable of causing disease, injury, or birth defects in humans or animals.

In general, procedures that cause pain in humans are considered to cause pain in other vertebrates.

Principle 8

Experiments on avian embryos that might result in abnormal chicks or in chicks that might experience pain or discomfort shall be terminated 72 hours prior to the expected date of hatching. The eggs shall be destroyed to prevent inadvertent hatching.

Principle 9

Behavioral conditioning studies shall not involve aversive stimuli. In studies using positive reinforcement, animals should not be deprived of water; food deprivation intervals should be appropriate for the species but should not continue longer than 24 hours.

Principle 10

A plan for conducting an experiment with living animals must be prepared in writing and approved prior to initiating the experiment or to obtaining the animals. Proper experimental design of projects and concern for animal welfare are important learning experiences and contribute to respect for and appropriate care of animals. The plan shall be reviewed by a committee composed of individuals who have the knowledge to understand and evaluate it and who have the authority to approve or disapprove it. The written plan should include the following:

a. a statement of the specific hypotheses or principles to be tested, illustrated, or taught;

b. a summary of what is known about the subject under study, including references;

c. a justification for the use of the species selected and consideration of why a lower vertebrate or invertebrate cannot be used; and

d. a detailed description of the methods and procedures to be used, including experimental design; data analysis; and all aspects of animal procurement, care, housing, use, and disposal.

Exceptions

Exceptions to Principles 7–10 may be granted under special circumstances by a panel appointed by the school principal or his or her designee. This panel should consist of at least three individuals, including a science teacher, a teacher of a nonscience subject, and a scientist or veterinarian who has expertise in the subject matter involved. At least one panel member should not be affiliated with the school or science fair, and none should be a member of the student's family.

SECTION VI.

ETHICAL DIRECTIVES PERTAINING
TO THE ENVIRONMENT

• • •

World Charter for Nature, General Assembly of the United Nations [1982]

Rio Declaration on Environment and Development, United Nations Conference on Environment and Development [1992]

Conservation Policies of the Wildlife Society, The Wildlife Society [1988]

Code of Ethics for Members of the Society of American Foresters, Society of American Foresters [1976, amended 1986, 1992, 2000]

Code of Ethics and Standards of Practice for Environmental Professionals, National Association of Environmental Professionals [1979, revised 1994]

Code of Ethics, National Environmental Health Association [revised 1992]

Bioethics refers not only to the ethics of health care but also to the ethics of the life sciences, which include ecology and environmental sciences. Enhancing the health of plants, animals, and the entire biosphere has inherent moral value; it is also crucial for the protection and promotion of human health and well-being, which depend upon a healthy environment. Whether the environment is perceived to have intrinsic value, instrumental value, or both, society increasingly recognizes moral duties to preserve and nurture it and to foster a health-promoting relationship between humans and their environment. Many countries have laws and regulations designed to protect the environment and its resources through limitations on the emissions of industrial pollutants, hazardous waste disposal, recycling programs, and conservation policy.

The documents in this section fall into two categories: policy and professional conduct. They are issued both by professional groups and by a nonprofessional body, the United Nations. The editors have not attempted to include any of the myriad national and international laws and regulations pertaining to the environment, opting instead for more general policy statements.

WORLD CHARTER FOR NATURE

General Assembly of the United Nations

1982

• • •

A multinational task force began drafting the World Charter for Nature in 1975. Sponsored by thirty-four developing nations, it was adopted by the General Assembly of the United Nations on October 29, 1982, by a vote of 111 to 1, with the United States casting the sole dissenting vote.

The General Assembly,

Reaffirming the fundamental purposes of the United Nations, in particular the maintenance of international peace and security, the development of friendly relations among nations and the achievement of international co-operation in solving international problems of an economic, social, cultural, technical, intellectual or humanitarian character,

Aware that:

(a) Mankind is a part of nature and life depends on the uninterrupted functioning of natural systems which ensure the supply of energy and nutrients,

(b) Civilization is rooted in nature, which has shaped human culture and influenced all artistic and scientific achievement, and living in harmony with nature gives man the best opportunities for the development of his creativity, and for rest and recreation,

Convinced that:

(a) Every form of life is unique, warranting respect regardless of its worth to man, and, to accord other organisms such recognition, man must be guided by a moral code of action,

(b) Man can alter nature and exhaust natural resources by his action or its consequences and, therefore, must fully recognize the urgency of maintaining the stability and quality of nature and of conserving natural resources,

Persuaded that:

(a) Lasting benefits from nature depend upon the maintenance of essential ecological processes and life support systems, and upon the diversity of life forms, which are jeopardized through excessive exploitation and habitat destruction by man,

(b) The degradation of natural systems owing to excessive consumption and misuse of natural resources, as well as to failure to establish an appropriate economic order among peoples and among States, leads to the breakdown of the economic, social and political framework of civilization,

(c) Competition for scarce resources creates conflicts, whereas the conservation of nature and natural resources contributes to justice and the maintenance of peace and cannot be achieved until mankind learns to live in peace and to forsake war and armaments,

Reaffirming that man must acquire the knowledge to maintain and enhance his ability to use natural resources in a manner which ensures the preservation of the species and ecosystems for the benefit of present and future generations,

Firmly convinced of the need for appropriate measures, at the national and international, individual and collective, and private and public levels, to protect nature and promote international co-operation in this field,

Adopts, to these ends, the present World Charter for Nature, which proclaims the following principles of conservation by which all human conduct affecting nature is to be guided and judged.

I. General Principles

1. Nature shall be respected and its essential processes shall not be impaired.

2. The genetic viability on the earth shall not be compromised; the population levels of all life forms, wild and domesticated, must be at least sufficient for their survival, and to this end necessary habitats shall be safeguarded.

3. All areas of the earth, both land and sea, shall be subject to these principles of conservation; special protection shall be given to unique areas, to representative samples of all the different types of ecosystems and to the habitats of rare or endangered species.

4. Ecosystems and organisms, as well as the land, marine and atmospheric resources that are utilized by man, shall be managed to achieve and maintain optimum sustainable productivity, but not in such a way as to endanger the integrity of those other ecosystems or species with which they coexist.

5. Nature shall be secured against degradation caused by warfare or other hostile activities.

I. Functions

6. In the decision-making process it shall be recognized that man's needs can be met only by ensuring the proper functioning of natural systems and by respecting the principles set forth in the present Charter.

7. In the planning and implementation of social and economic development activities, due account shall be taken of the fact that the conservation of nature is an integral part of those activities.

8. In formulating long-term plans for economic development, population growth and the improvement of standards of living, due account shall be taken of the long-term capacity of natural systems to ensure the subsistence and settlement of the populations concerned, recognizing that this capacity may be enhanced through science and technology.

9. The allocation of areas of the earth to various uses shall be planned and due account shall be taken of the physical constraints, the biological productivity and diversity and the natural beauty of the areas concerned.

10. Natural resources shall not be wasted, but used with a restraint appropriate to the principles set forth in the present Charter, in accordance with the following rules:

    (a) Living resources shall not be utilized in excess of their natural capacity for regeneration;

    (b) The productivity of soils shall be maintained or enhanced through measures which safeguard their long-term fertility and the process of organic decomposition, and prevent erosion and all other forms of degradation;

    (c) Resources, including water, which are not consumed as they are used shall be reused or recycled;

    (d) Non-renewable resources which are consumed as they are used shall be exploited with restraint, taking into account their abundance, the rational possibilities of converting them for consumption, and the compatibility of their exploitation with the functioning of natural systems.

11. Activities which might have an impact on nature shall be controlled, and the best available technologies that minimize significant risks to nature or other adverse effects shall be used; in particular:

    (a) Activities which are likely to cause irreversible damage to nature shall be avoided;

    (b) Activities which are likely to pose a significant risk to nature shall be preceded by an exhaustive examination; their proponents shall demonstrate that expected benefits outweigh potential damage to nature, and where potential adverse effects are not fully understood, the activities should not proceed;

    (c) Activities which may disturb nature shall be preceded by assessment of their consequences, and environmental impact studies of development projects shall be conducted sufficiently in advance, and if they are to be undertaken, such activities shall be planned and carried out so as to minimize potential adverse effects;

    (d) Agriculture, grazing, forestry and fisheries practices shall be adapted to the natural characteristics and constraints of given areas;

    (e) Areas degraded by human activities shall be rehabilitated for purposes in accord with their natural potential and compatible with the well-being of affected populations.

12. Discharge of pollutants into natural systems shall be avoided and:

    (a) Where this is not feasible, such pollutants shall be treated at the source, using the best practicable means available;

    (b) Special precautions shall be taken to prevent discharge of radioactive or toxic wastes.

13. Measures intended to prevent, control or limit natural disasters, infestations and diseases shall be specifically directed to the causes of these scourges and shall avoid adverse side-effects on nature.

III. Implementation

14. The principles set forth in the present Charter shall be reflected in the law and practice of each State, as well as at the international level.

15. Knowledge of nature shall be broadly disseminated by all possible means, particularly by ecological education as an integral part of general education.

16. All planning shall include, among its essential elements, the formulation of strategies for the

conservation of nature, the establishment of inventories of ecosystems and assessments of the effects on nature of proposed policies and activities; all of these elements shall be disclosed to the public by appropriate means in time to permit effective consultation and participation.

17. Funds, programmes and administrative structures necessary to achieve the objective of the conservation of nature shall be provided.

18. Constant efforts shall be made to increase knowledge of nature by scientific research and to disseminate such knowledge unimpeded by restrictions of any kind.

19. The status of natural processes, ecosystems and species shall be closely monitored to enable early detection of degradation or threat, ensure timely intervention and facilitate the evaluation of conservation policies and methods.

20. Military activities damaging to nature shall be avoided.

21. States and, to the extent they are able, other public authorities, international organizations, individuals, groups and corporations shall:

    (a) Co-operate in the task of conserving nature through common activities and other relevant actions, including information exchange and consultations;

    (b) Establish standards for products and manufacturing processes that may have adverse effects on nature, as well as agreed methodologies for assessing these effects;

    (c) Implement the applicable international legal provisions for the conservation of nature and the protection of the environment;

    (d) Ensure that activities within their jurisdictions or control do not cause damage to the natural systems located within other States or in the areas beyond the limits of national jurisdiction;

    (e) Safeguard and conserve nature in areas beyond national jurisdiction.

22. Taking fully into account the sovereignty of States over their natural resources, each State shall give effect to the provisions of the present Charter through its competent organs and in co-operation with other States.

23. All persons, in accordance with their national legislation, shall have the opportunity to participate, individually or with others, in the formulation of decisions of direct concern to their environment, and shall have access to means of redress when their environment has suffered damage or degradation.

24. Each person has a duty to act in accordance with the provisions of the present Charter; acting

individually, in association with others or through participation in the political process, each person shall strive to ensure that the objectives and requirements of the present Charter are met.

RIO DECLARATION ON ENVIRONMENT AND DEVELOPMENT

United Nations Conference on Environment and Development

1992

• • •

The Rio Declaration on Environment and Development consists of twenty-seven principles for governing the economic and environmental behavior of individuals and states in the quest for global sustainability. The preamble to the declaration affirms the goal "of establishing a new and equitable global partnership" in the effort to develop international agreements that "respect the interests of all and protect the integrity of the global environmental and developmental system." It also recognizes "the integral and interdependent nature of the Earth, our home." The declaration was adopted by the United Nations Conference on Environment and Development at its meeting in Rio de Janeiro, June 3–14, 1992. The United States subscribes to the document. The text of the twenty-seven principles follows.

1. Human beings are at the centre of concerns for sustainable development. They are entitled to a healthy and productive life in harmony with nature.

2. States have, in accordance with the Charter of the United Nations and the principles of international law, the sovereign right to exploit their own resources pursuant to their own environmental and developmental policies, and the responsibility to ensure that activities within their jurisdiction or control do not cause damage to the environment of other States or of areas beyond the limits of national jurisdiction.

3. The right to development must be fulfilled so as to equitably meet developmental and environmental needs of present and future generations.

4. In order to achieve sustainable development, environmental protection shall constitute an integral part of the development process and cannot be considered in isolation from it.

5. All States and all people shall cooperate in the essential task of eradicating poverty as an indispensable requirement for sustainable development, in order to decrease the disparities in standards of

living and better meet the needs of the majority of the people of the world.

6. The special situation and needs of developing countries, particularly the least developed and those most environmentally vulnerable, shall be given special priority. International actions in the field of environment and development should also address the interests and needs of all countries.

7. States shall cooperate in a spirit of global partnership to conserve, protect and restore the health and integrity of the Earth's ecosystem. In view of the different contributions to global environmental degradation, States have common but differentiated responsibilities. The developed countries acknowledge the responsibility that they bear in the international pursuit of sustainable development in view of the pressures their societies place on the global environment and of the technologies and financial resources they command.

8. To achieve sustainable development and a higher quality of life for all people, States should reduce and eliminate unsustainable patterns of production and consumption and promote appropriate demographic policies.

9. States should cooperate to strengthen endogenous capacity-building for sustainable development by improving scientific understanding through exchanges of scientific and technological knowledge, and by enhancing the development, adaptation, diffusion and transfer of technologies, including new and innovative technologies.

10. Environmental issues are best handled with the participation of all concerned citizens, at the relevant level. At the national level, each individual shall have appropriate access to information concerning the environment that is held by public authorities, including information on hazardous materials and activities in their communities, and the opportunity to participate in decision-making processes. States shall facilitate and encourage public awareness and participation by making information widely available. Effective access to judicial and administrative proceedings, including redress and remedy, shall be provided.

11. States shall enact effective environmental legislation. Environmental standards, management objectives and priorities should reflect the environmental and developmental context to which they apply. Standards applied by some countries may be inappropriate and of unwarranted economic and social cost to other countries, in particular developing countries.

12. States should cooperate to promote a supportive and open international economic system that would lead to economic growth and sustainable development in all countries, to better address the problems of environmental degradation. Trade policy measures for environmental purposes should not constitute a means of arbitrary or unjustifiable discrimination or a disguised restriction on international trade. Unilateral actions to deal with environmental challenges outside the jurisdiction of the importing country should be avoided. Environmental measures addressing transboundary or global environmental problems should, as far as possible, be based on an international consensus.

13. States shall develop national law regarding liability and compensation for the victims of pollution and other environmental damage. States shall also cooperate in an expeditious and more determined manner to develop further international law regarding liability and compensation for adverse effects of environmental damage caused by activities within their jurisdiction or control to areas beyond their jurisdiction.

14. States should effectively cooperate to discourage or prevent the relocation and transfer to other States of any activities and substances that cause severe environmental degradation or are found to be harmful to human health.

15. In order to protect the environment, the precautionary approach shall be widely applied by States according to their capabilities. Where there are threats of serious or irreversible damage, lack of full scientific certainty shall not be used as a reason for postponing cost-effective measures to prevent environmental degradation.

16. National authorities should endeavour to promote the internalization of environmental costs and the use of economic instruments, taking into account the approach that the polluter should, in principle, bear the cost of pollution, with due regard to the public interest and without distorting international trade and investment.

17. Environmental impact assessment, as a national instrument, shall be undertaken for proposed activities that are likely to have a significant adverse impact on the environment and are subject to a decision of a competent national authority.

18. States shall immediately notify other States of any natural disasters or other emergencies that are likely to produce sudden harmful effects on the environment of those States. Every effort shall be made by the international community to help States so afflicted.

19. States shall provide prior and timely notification and relevant information to potentially affected States on

activities that may have a significant adverse transboundary environmental effect and shall consult with those States at an early stage and in good faith.

20. Women have a vital role in environmental management and development. Their full participation is therefore essential to achieve sustainable development.

21. The creativity, ideals, and courage of the youth of the world should be mobilized to forge a global partnership in order to achieve sustainable development and ensure a better future for all.

22. Indigenous people and their communities and other local communities have a vital role in environmental management and development because of their knowledge and traditional practices. States should recognize and duly support their identity, culture and interests and enable their effective participation in the achievement of sustainable development.

23. The environment and natural resources of people under oppression, domination and occupation shall be protected.

24. Warfare is inherently destructive of sustainable development. States shall therefore respect international law providing protection for the environment in times of armed conflict and cooperate in its further development, as necessary.

25. Peace, development and environmental protection are interdependent and indivisible.

26. States shall resolve all their environmental disputes peacefully and by appropriate means in accordance with the Charter of the United Nations.

27. States and people shall cooperate in good faith and in a spirit of partnership in the fulfillment of the principles embodied in this Declaration and in the further development of international law in the field of sustainable development.

CONSERVATION POLICIES OF THE WILDLIFE SOCIETY

The Wildlife Society

1988

• • •

In addition to national and international bodies, professional organizations, such as the Wildlife Society, also issue environmental policies. Founded in 1937, the Wildlife Society is dedicated to the wise

management and conservation of the world's wildlife resources. Excerpts from the society's Conservation Policies are printed below.

Human Populations

Burgeoning human populations continue to place an overwhelming and detrimental demand on many of the world's limited natural resources. Human degradation of terrestrial and aquatic communities is biologically unadvisable. Certain of these resources are irreplaceable, and others must be either preserved intact or managed carefully to ensure the integrity of the ecosystem and humanity. These resources will continue to decline or to sustain irreparable damage, despite scientific and technological advances, if the growth of the human population is not restrained.

The policy of The Wildlife Society, in regard to human populations is to:

1. Actively support an enlightened policy of population stabilization that will encourage the conservation of natural resources and enhance the quality of human existence.

2. Promote a better understanding of mankind's role in the world's ecosystems so as to minimize the contamination and harmful alteration of the global environment.

Environmental Quality

The demands that human societies make upon the earth and its biota inevitably result in environmental change. Many ecosystems have been exploited for immediate monetary profit rather than managed for sustained biotic yields. Careless or excessive exploitation often leads to unnecessary degradation of the environment. The common aim of mankind should be to perfect processes for deriving support from the environment without destroying its stability, diversity, productivity, or aesthetic values.

The policy of The Wildlife Society, in regard to environmental quality, is to:

1. Stimulate and support educational programs that emphasize mankind's dependence on functional ecosystems, and, consequently, the necessity for living in harmony with the environment.

2. Foster research designed to elucidate the complex biotic relationships of ecosystems.

3. Encourage the development and use of methods designed to reduce environmental degradation and to reclaim and reconstitute degraded ecosystems.

4. Contribute to the development of technologies, social systems, and individual behaviors that will

maintain the diversity and beauty of the environment.

The Management of Living Natural Resources

Human population growth jeopardizes mankind's existence. The continued well-being of mankind, and earth's other living natural resources, is dependent upon a healthy environment maintained through the skilled management of resources. As human populations increase, wild plant and animal habitats usually decrease. Many people presume that all wild habitats are untouched by humanity. Actually, few natural areas have escaped the influence of mankind. Often these influences have disrupted natural areas, thus requiring the need for scientific management of these areas and their associated living resources.

A "hands-off," non-manipulative policy for plant and animal resources eventually could result in reestablishing naturally-functioning plant and animal communities as wild areas, if mankind's ever-present impacts could be eliminated. In such areas the actions of nature would dominate and low-priority would be given to material human wants. Such areas have been and are being established where practicable.

Only limited amounts of land can be devoted to wild areas because of the demands of our growing human population. Land is required for housing, crops, mineral and timber production, manufacture and sale of goods, intensive recreation, and other necessary and desirable purposes. Plant and animal communities associated with these more intensive land uses, although often highly productive, are usually unnatural in that they lack the diversity and stability of unaltered communities. Applying sound land and water management practices to these altered lands can assist natural processes in providing habitat suitable for plants and animals which are forced to live in close association with human activities. Plant and animal populations also may be enhanced and optimized at levels within the land's ability to support them through proven professional resource management practices.

The Wildlife Society recognizes the serious implications of mankind's ever-increasing worldwide demands for living space, food, shelter and other products. It also recognizes a need for a policy of continued, intensified and improved management for earth's living resources.

The policy of The Wildlife Society, in regard to management of living natural resources, is to:

1. Support and strengthen scientific management as the rational instrument for maintaining, restoring, and enhancing plant and animal resources for the continued use and appreciation by humanity.

2. Encourage the development and dissemination of information to improve public understanding of the need for, and the positive benefits from, scientific management.

3. Encourage the retention or enhancement of habitat for native plants and animals on public and private lands.

4. Seek support for ethical restraints in the use of living natural resources.

5. Reaffirm our view that scientific management includes both the regulated harvest of the surplus of those species in plentiful supply, as well as the protection of those plant or animal species which are rare, threatened, or in danger of extinction.

Conservation Education

Worldwide growth of human populations is placing unprecedented demands and stresses on the world's finite natural resources. Satisfying human needs for energy, food, fibers, minerals, and wood products has the potential for further destruction of wildlife habitat and aesthetic resources. If these natural resources are to be given adequate consideration in the context of human needs, a sound program of conservation education is of paramount importance.

The educational process must contain four key elements if it is to be effective in enabling people to cope with resource problems. First, it must provide basic understanding of the properties and distribution of natural resources. Second, it must provide and encourage alternatives to current degrading resource uses and promote changes in life styles that can be accommodated by the existing resources base. Third, it must provide people with an understanding of the political, economic, and social processes by which changes in resource use can be effected. And last, it must lead to positive action in behalf of resource conservation.

The policy of The Wildlife Society, in regard to conservation education, is to:

1. Assist in the development and promotion of educational programs that will disseminate ecologically sound knowledge to advance wise management of wildlife and other natural resources.

2. Promote increased cooperation and communication among all agencies and groups concerned with conservation education and resource management.

3. Encourage members of the wildlife profession (a) to interpret and make readily available those results of wildlife research that citizens require for decision-making, and (b) to actively participate in the implementation of sound, publicly oriented programs in conservation education.

. . .

CODE OF ETHICS FOR MEMBERS OF THE SOCIETY OF AMERICAN FORESTERS

Society of American Foresters

1976, AMENDED 1986, 1992, 2000

. . .

In 1992 the Society of American Foresters adopted a new "land ethic canon" espousing "stewardship of" and "respect for the land." The 2000 version's preamble exhorts "foresters [to] seek to sustain and protect a variety of forest uses and attributes, such as aesthetic values, air and water quality, biodiversity, recreation, timber production, and wildlife habitat."

<http://www.safnet.org/who/codeofethics.cfm>

Preamble

Service to society is the cornerstone of any profession. The profession of forestry serves society by fostering stewardship of the world's forests. Because forests provide valuable resources and perform critical ecological functions, they are vital to the wellbeing of both society and the biosphere.

Members of the Society of American Foresters have a deep and enduring love for the land, and are inspired by the profession's historic traditions, such as Gifford Pinchot's utilitarianism and Aldo Leopold's ecological conscience. In their various roles as practitioners, teachers, researchers, advisers, and administrators, foresters seek to sustain and protect a variety of forest uses and attributes, such as aesthetic values, air and water quality, biodiversity, recreation, timber production, and wildlife habitat.

The purpose of this Code of Ethics is to protect and serve society by inspiring, guiding, and governing members in the conduct of their professional lives. Compliance with the code demonstrates members' respect for the land and their commitment to the long-term management of ecosystems, and ensures just and honorable professional and

human relationships, mutual confidence and respect, and competent service to society.

On joining the Society of American Foresters, members assume a special responsibility to the profession and to society by promising to uphold and abide by the following:

Principles and Pledges

1. Foresters have a responsibility to manage land for both current and future generations. We pledge to practice and advocate management that will maintain the long-term capacity of the land to provide the variety of materials, uses, and values desired by landowners and society.

2. Society must respect forest landowners' rights and correspondingly, landowners have a land stewardship responsibility to society. We pledge to practice and advocate forest management in accordance with landowner objectives and professional standards, and to advise landowners of the consequences of deviating from such standards.

3. Sound science is the foundation of the forestry profession. We pledge to strive for continuous improvement of our methods and our personal knowledge and skills; to perform only those services for which we are qualified; and in the biological, physical, and social sciences to use the most appropriate data, methods, and technology.

4. Public policy related to forests must be based on both scientific principles and societal values. We pledge to use our knowledge and skills to help formulate sound forest policies and laws; to challenge and correct untrue statements about forestry; and to foster dialogue among foresters, other professionals, landowners, and the public regarding forest policies.

5. Honest and open communication, coupled with respect for information given in confidence, is essential to good service. We pledge to always present, to the best of our ability, accurate and complete information; to indicate on whose behalf any public statements are made; to fully disclose and resolve any existing or potential conflicts of interest; and to keep proprietary information confidential unless the appropriate person authorizes its disclosure.

6. Professional and civic behavior must be based on honesty, fairness, good will, and respect for the law. We pledge to conduct ourselves in a civil and dignified manner; to respect the needs, contributions, and viewpoints of others; and to give due credit to others for their methods, ideas, or assistance.

CODE OF ETHICS AND STANDARDS OF PRACTICE FOR ENVIRONMENTAL PROFESSIONALS

National Association of Environmental Professionals

1979, REVISED 1994

• • •

The Code of the National Association of Environmental Professionals (NAEP) takes a broad view of environment, which includes physical, natural, and cultural systems. It is noteworthy that a New Jersey court ruled that the NAEP code of ethics be considered public policy in the state (Bowman v. Mobil Oil Corp., Civil Action No. 87–4093); as such, employees who abide by it cannot be fired for refusing to perform actions that directly contravene the code.

The objectives of Environmental Professionals are to conduct their personal and professional lives and activities in an ethical manner. Honesty, justice and courtesy form moral philosophy which, associated with a mutual interest among people, constitute the foundation of ethics. Environmental Professionals should recognize such a standard, not in passive observance, but as a set of dynamic principles guiding their conduct and way of life. It is their duty to practice their profession according to this Code of Ethics.

As the keystone of professional conduct is integrity, Environmental Professionals will discharge their duties with fidelity to the public, their employers, clients, and with fairness and impartiality to all. It is their duty to interest themselves in public welfare, and to be ready to apply their special knowledge for the benefit of mankind and their environment.

Creed

The objectives of an Environmental Professional are:

1. to recognize and attempt to reconcile societal and individual human needs with responsibility for physical, natural, and cultural systems.
2. to promote and develop policies, plans, activities and projects that achieve complementary and mutual support between natural and man-made, and present and future components of the physical, natural and cultural environment.

Ethics

As an Environmental Professional I will:

1. be personally responsible for the validity of all data collected, analyses performed, or plans developed by me or under my direction. I will be responsible and ethical in my professional activities.
2. encourage reason, planning, design, management and review of activities in a scientifically and technically objective manner. I will incorporate the best principles of the environmental sciences for the mitigation of environmental harm and enhancement of environmental quality.
3. not condone misrepresentation of work I have performed or that was performed under my direction.
4. examine all of my relationships or actions which could be legitimately interpreted as a conflict of interest by clients, officials, the public or peers. In any instance where I have a financial or personal interest in the activities with which they are directly or indirectly involved, I will make a full disclosure of that interest to my employer, client, or other affected parties.
5. not engage in conduct involving dishonesty, fraud, deceit, or misrepresentation or discrimination.
6. not accept fees wholly or partially contingent on the client's desired result where that desired result conflicts with my professional judgement.

Guidance for Practice as an Environmental Professional

As an Environmental Professional I will:

1. encourage environmental planning to begin in the earliest stages of project conceptualization.
2. recognize that total environmental management involves the consideration of all environmental factors including: technical, economic, ecological, and sociopolitical and their relationships.
3. incorporate the best principle of design and environmental planning when recommending measures to reduce environmental harm and enhance environmental quality.
4. conduct my analysis, planning, design and review my activities primarily in subject areas for which I am qualified, and shall encourage and recognize the participation of other professionals in subject areas where I am less experienced. I shall utilize and participate in interdisciplinary teams wherever practical to determine impacts, define and evaluate all reasonable alternatives to proposed actions, and assess short-term versus long-term productivity with and without the project or action.
5. seek common, adequate, and sound technical grounds for communication with and respect for the

contributions of other professionals in developing and reviewing policies, plans, activities, and projects.

6. determine that the policies, plans, activities, or projects in which I am involved are consistent with all governing laws, ordinances, guidelines, plans, and policies, to the best of my knowledge and ability.

7. encourage public participation at the earliest feasible time in an open and productive atmosphere.

8. conduct my professional activities in a manner that ensures consideration of technically and economically feasible alternatives.

Encourage Development of the Profession

As an Environmental Professional I will:

1. assist in maintaining the integrity and competence of my profession.

2. encourage education and research, and the development of useful technical information relating to the environmental field.

3. advertise and present my services in a manner that avoids the use of material and methods that may bring discredit to the profession.

CODE OF ETHICS

National Environmental Health Association

REVISED 1992

• • •

The National Environmental Health Association's Code of Ethics explicitly states that the environment is not restricted by political boundaries; *it must be viewed as a single entity. Health is recognized to be one of the fundamental rights of every human being, and those to whom the code applies have an obligation to work to provide a healthful environment for all. It is noteworthy that the code has a line for the member's signature, making it a personal pledge by the professional.*

As a member of the National Environmental Health Association, I acknowledge:

That I have an obligation to work to provide a healthful environment for all. I will uphold the standards of my profession, continually search for truths, and disseminate my findings. I will continually strive to keep myself fully informed on developments in the fields of public and environmental health and protection:

That I have an obligation to the public whose trust I hold and because of this, I will endeavor to the best of my ability to safeguard the public's health. I will be loyal to this trust in whatever governmental division, industry, or institution by which I am retained:

That the environment is not restricted by man-made political boundaries and therefore must be considered as a single entity;

That the enjoyment of the highest attainable standard of health is one of the fundamental rights of every human being without distinction of race, religion, cultural background, economic or social condition; and

That I will uphold the constitution and bylaws of the National Environmental Health Association and will at all times conduct myself in a manner worthy of my profession.

By my signature hereon, I acknowledge and affirm a realization of my personal responsibility to actively discharge these obligations.

CREDITS

• • •

SECTION I: DIRECTIVES ON HEALTH-RELATED RIGHTS AND PATIENT RESPONSIBILITIES

Constitution. World Health Organization. Reprinted by permission of the Organization.

Universal Declaration of Human Rights. *Yearbook of the United Nations 1948–49.* New York: Columbia University Press/United Nations, 1950, pp. 535–537. Reprinted by permission of the United Nations.

Rights of the Child. *Yearbook of the United Nations 1959.* New York: Columbia University Press/United Nations, 1960, pp. 198–199. Reprinted by permission of the United Nations.

Rights of Mentally Retarded Persons. *Yearbook of the United Nations 1971,* vol. 25. New York: United Nations, 1974, p. 368. Reprinted by permission of the United Nations.

A Patient's Bill of Rights. American Hospital Association. Reprinted by permission of the Association.

Declaration of Lisbon. World Medical Association. Reprinted by permission of the Association.

Declaration on Physician Independence. World Medical Association. Reprinted by permission of the Association.

Fundamental Elements. Council on Ethical and Judicial Affairs. *Code of Medical Ethics.* Chicago: American Medical Association, 1994. Reprinted by permission of the Association.

Patient Responsibilities. Council on Ethical and Judicial Affairs. *Code of Medical Ethics.* Chicago: American Medical Association, 2001. Reprinted by permission of the Association.

Patient Rights. *Accreditation Manual for Hospitals, 1994.* Oakbrook Terrace, IL: Joint Commission on Accreditation of Healthcare Organizations, 1994, sec. 4. Reprinted by permission of the Joint Commission.

SECTION II: ETHICAL DIRECTIVES FOR THE PRACTICE OF MEDICINE

Oath of Hippocrates. Ludwig Edelstein. "The Hippocratic Oath: Text, Translation and Interpretation." *Bulletin of the History of Medicine,* supplement 1 (1943): 1–64, p. 3. Reprinted by permission of the Johns Hopkins University Press.

Oath of Initiation. A. Menon and H. F. Haberman. "Oath of Initiation" (from the *Caraka Samhita*). Medical History 14 (1970): 295–296. Reprinted by permission of the BMJ Publishing Group, London.

Oath of Asaph. Translated by Dr. Suessman Munter for *Medical Ethics: A Compendium of Jewish Moral, Ethical and Religious Principles in Medical Practice,* ed. M. D. Tendler. 5th ed. New York: Committee on Religious Affairs, Federation of Jewish

Philanthropies, 1975, pp. 7–9. Reprinted by permission of the UJA-Federation of New York.

Advice to a Physician. Translated by Rahmatollah Eshraghi.

17 Rules of Enjuin. Translated by William O. Reinhardt, John Z. Bowers. *Western Medical Pioneers in Feudal Japan.* Baltimore: Johns Hopkins University Press, 1970, pp. 8–10. Reprinted by permission of the publisher.

Five Commandments and Ten Requirements. Translated by T'ao Lee. "Medical Ethics in Ancient China." *Bulletin of the History of Medicine* 13 (1943): 268–277. Reprinted by permission of the Johns Hopkins University Press.

A Physician's Ethical Duties. Translated and condensed by Rahmatollah Eshraghi.

Daily Prayer of a Physician. Translated by Harry Friedenwald. *Bulletin of the Johns Hopkins Hospital* 28 (1917): 260–261. Reprinted by permission of the Johns Hopkins University Press.

Code of Ethics (1847). *Code of Ethics.* New York: H. Ludwig & Co., 1848. American Medical Association. Reprinted by permission of the Association.

Venezuelan Code. "Codigo Venezolano de Moral Medica." In Luis Razetti, *Obras Completas: I. Deontologia Medica.* Caracas: Ministerio de Sanidad y Asistencia Social, 1963, pp. 111–135. The excerpt translated here is found on pp. 124–127.

Declaration of Geneva. World Medical Association. Reprinted by permission of the Association.

International Code. World Medical Association. Reprinted by permission of the Association.

Principles (1957). American Medical Association. Reprinted by permission of the Association.

Principles (1980). Council on Ethical and Judicial Affairs. *Code of Medical Ethics.* Chicago: American Medical Association, 1994. Reprinted by permission of the Association.

Principles (1993, 2001). Council on Ethical and Judicial Affairs. *Code of Medical Ethics.* Chicago: American Medical Association. Reprinted by permission of the Association.

Current Opinions. Council on Ethical and Judicial Affairs. Code of Medical Ethics. Chicago: American Medical Association. Reprinted by permission of the Association.

Moral and Technical Competence. American Academy of Ophthalmology. Reprinted by permission of the Academy.

Code of Ethics. American Osteopathic Association. Reprinted by permission of the Association.

Code of Ethics and Guide (1996). Canadian Medical Association. Reprinted by permission of the Association.

Code of Ethics and Guide. New Zealand Medical Association. Reprinted by permission of the Association.

Code of Ethics. Translated by Glenn A. Wilson. "Codigo de Etica del Colegio Medico de Chile." *Revista Medica de Chile* 112 (1984):516–522. Reprinted by permission of the Revista Medica de Chile.

Code of Medical Ethics. Translated by Hilde Bremmer Novaes. "Codigo de Etica Medica, Brasil." Conselho Federal de Medicina, Brasil. Reprinted by permission of the Council.

European Code. *World Medical Journal* 34, no. 5 (September/October 1987):66–69. Deutscher Aerzte-Verlag GmbH.

Code of Ethics for Doctors. Norske Laegeforening (Norwegian Medical Association). Reprinted by permission of the Association.

Final Report on Brain Death and Organ Transplantation. Japan Medical Association. Reprinted by permission of the Association.

Summary of the Report on Information. Japan Medical Association. Reprinted by permission of the Association.

Oath of Soviet Physicians. Translated by Zenonas Danilevicius. *Journal of the American Medical Association* 217 (1971): 834. Reprinted by permission of the American Medical Association.

Solemn Oath. Translated by Larisa Yurievna Podovalenko and Chris Speckhardt. *Kennedy Institute of Ethics Journal* 3, no. 4 (1993): 419. The Russian text of the oath was originally published in *Meditsinskaya Gazeta* (no. 44, 5 June 1992). Reprinted by permission of the Johns Hopkins University Press.

Regulations on Criteria for Medical Ethics. Translated by Shi Da-pu. *Kennedy Institute of Ethics Newsletter* 3, no. 4 (October 1989):3. Reprinted by permission of the Johns Hopkins University Press.

Ethical and Religious Directives. Copyright United States Conference of Catholic Bishops. Reprinted by permission of the Conference.

Health Ethics Guide (2000). Catholic Health Association of Canada. Reprinted by permission of the Association.

Oath of a Muslim Physician. Islamic Medical Association of North America. Reprinted by permission of the Islamic Medical Association.

Islamic Code. Islamic Organization for Medical Sciences (IOMS, Kuwait). Reprinted by permission of the Islamic Organization.

SECTION III: ETHICAL DIRECTIVES FOR OTHER HEALTH-CARE PROFESSIONS

Code for Nurses. International Council of Nurses. Copyright © 2000 by ICN—International Council of Nurses. Reprinted by permission of the Council.

Code for Nurses (2001). American Nurses' Association. Reprinted by permission of the Association.

Code of Ethics for Nursing. Canadian Nurses Association. Reprinted by permission of the Association.

Code of Ethics. American Chiropractic Association. Reprinted by permission of the Association.

Principles of Ethics. American Dental Association. Reprinted by permission of the Association.

Code of Ethics for the Profession of Dietetics. American Dietetic Association. Reprinted by permission of the Association.

Code of Ethics. American Association of Pastoral Counselors. Reprinted by permission of the Association.

Guidelines for the Chaplain's Role in Bioethics. College of Chaplains, Inc., American Protestant Health Association. Reprinted by permission of the Association.

Code of Ethics (1994). American Pharmacists Association. Reprinted by permission of the Association.

FIP Statement of Professional Standards: Code of Ethics for Pharmacists (1997). Fédération Internationale Pharmaceutique (FIP). Reprinted by permission of the Federation.

Code of Ethics and Guide. American Physical Therapy Association. Reprinted by permission of the Association.

Occupational Therapy Code. American Occupational Therapy Association. Reprinted by permission of the Association.

Code of Ethics. American Academy of Physician Assistants. Reprinted by permission of the Academy.

Ethical Principles of Psychologists. American Psychological Association. Reprinted by permission of the Association.

Code of Ethics. National Association of Social Workers. Reprinted by permission of the Association.

Code of Ethics. American College of Healthcare Executives. Reprinted by permission of the College.

Ethical Conduct. American Hospital Association. Reprinted by permission of the Association.

SECTION IV: ETHICAL DIRECTIVES FOR HUMAN RESEARCH

German Guidelines (1931). *International Digest of Health Legislation* 31, no. 2 (1980): 408–411.

Nuremberg Code. "Permissible Medical Experiments." *Trials of War Criminals Before the Nuremberg Military Tribunals Under Control Council Law No. 10: Nuremberg, October 1946–April 1949.* Washington, D.C.: U.S. Government Printing Office (n.d.), vol. 2, pp. 181–182.

Principles. *World Medical Journal* 2 (1955): 14–15.

Article Seven. *Yearbook of the United Nations 1958.* New York: Columbia University Press, p. 205. Reprinted by permission of the United Nations.

Declaration of Helsinki. World Medical Association. Reprinted by permission of the Association.

The Belmont Report. OPRR Reports. Washington, D.C.: U.S. Government Printing Office (1988) 201–778/80319.

DHHS Regulations. OPRR Reports. Washington, D.C.: U.S. Government Printing Office (1992) 0–307–551.

Summary Report. *Towards an International Ethic for Research with Human Beings: Proceedings of the International Summit Conference on Bioethics, April 5–10, 1987, Ottawa, Canada,* pp. 60–66. Ottawa, Ontario: Medical Research Council of Canada (1988). Reprinted by permission of the Council.

Recommendation No. R (90) 3. Council of Europe.

International Ethical Guidelines (2002). Council for International Organizations of Medical Sciences. Reprinted by permission of the Council.

SECTION V: ETHICAL DIRECTIVES PERTAINING TO THE WELFARE AND USE OF ANIMALS

Veterinarian's Oath. American Veterinary Medical Association. Reprinted by permission of the Association.

Principles of Veterinary Medicine. American Veterinary Medical Association. Reprinted by permission of the Association.

International Guiding Principles. Council for International Organizations of Medical Sciences. Reprinted by permission of the Council.

Principles for the Utilization and Care. NIH Guide Supplement for Grants and Contracts 14, no. 8 (June 25, 1985). Special Edition: Laboratory Animal Welfare, pp. 82–83. Washington, D.C.: U.S. Government Printing Office (1985) 527–967/30595.

Ethics of Animal Investigation. Canadian Council on Animal Care. Reprinted by permission of the Council.

Australian Code of Practice. National Health and Medical Research Council, Canberra, ACT. Reprinted by permission of the Council.

World Medical Association Statement. World Medical Association. Reprinted by permission of the Association.

Guidelines for Ethical Conduct. American Psychological Association. Reprinted by permission of the Association.

Principles and Guidelines. Institute of Laboratory Animal Resources, National Research Council. Reprinted by permission of the Council.

SECTION VI: ETHICAL DIRECTIVES PERTAINING TO THE ENVIRONMENT

World Charter. *Yearbook of the United Nations 1982,* vol. 36. New York: United Nations, pp. 1024–1026. Reprinted by permission of the United Nations.

Rio Declaration. *Yearbook of the United Nations 1992,* vol. 46. Dordrecht, The Netherlands: Martinus Nijhoff Publishers, pp. 670–672. Reprinted by permission of the United Nations.

Conservation Policies. The Wildlife Society. Reprinted by permission of the Society.

Code of Ethics for Members. Society of American Foresters. Reprinted by permission of the Society.

Code of Ethics and Standards of Practice. National Association of Environmental Professionals. Reprinted by permission of the Association.

Code of Ethics. National Environmental Health Association. Reprinted by permission of the Association.

APPENDIX II

ADDITIONAL RESOURCES IN BIOETHICS

In the intervening years since the revised edition of this Encyclopedia was published in 1995, the diversity and wealth of bioethics resources has once again increased enormously. The explosion of interest in this field continues to be demonstrated by the appearance of new periodicals devoted exclusively to bioethics along with increasing attention to bioethical issues by both general journals and specialty journals covering related disciplines, as well as the development of various organizational entities in bioethics.

The widespread availability of the Internet has had a great impact on the publication and accessibility of information. The preponderance of peer-reviewed bioethics literature continues to be published in print format, and is often now simultaneously offered via the Internet free or through subscriptions. These important sources of bioethics research are listed below, and the Web sites of most journals have been added to the list.

Another equally important development in the last decade is the institutionalization of bioethics concern by governments and professional groups around the world. In this update, the focus is restricted to national, international, regional and professional entities, most of which have Web sites. These groups supplement the peer-reviewed literature with what is called "gray literature." They are an important new entity involved in the exchange of ideas about contemporary ethical, legal, and public policy questions.

For the 1995 edition of this Encyclopedia, bioethics organizations, primarily those located in and fostered by academic institutions, that were developing library collections to support delineated courses of study, were highlighted. Many of those continue. Those academic programs that do not house special libraries of their own rely on bioethics collections in their respective universities, so those

libraries can be useful sites for bioethics research. Long lists of academic programs in bioethics can be found at many Web sites, including the Educational Opportunities page at <http://bioethics.georgetown.edu>.

This update provides a detailed look at the information services at the Kennedy Institute of Ethics at Georgetown University, as the first and most comprehensive library of its kind supporting bioethics research. Then, sources of periodical literature important to the field will be listed in two parts: A) Bioethics and Health Law Journals and B) General Philosophical, Scientific, and Medical Journals. Finally, the organization of bioethics endeavors in government and professional groups are shown, most with a Web address, arranged in the following categories: A) National Libraries of Bioethics, B) National Deliberative Bodies on Bioethics, C) Regional and International Bioethics Organizations, and D) Professional Groups.

I. Information Services of the Kennedy Institute of Ethics

Since the early 1970s the Kennedy Institute of Ethics has made a sustained effort to foster research and education in bioethics by collecting, analyzing, and disseminating bioethics information through various means. Its information services programs have grown significantly since the revised edition of this work was published in 1995, particularly with regard to free information services via the Internet.

Two long-standing information projects are: (1) the operation of a comprehensive bioethics library, the National Reference Center for Bioethics Literature (NRCBL), established in 1985 with support from the U.S. National Library of Medicine (NLM); and (2) the ongoing creation of bibliographic database records for the NLM, a project initiated in 1973. A third project joined these two in 1994 with support from what is now the U.S. National Human Genome Research Institute: the National Information Resource on Ethics and Human Genetics (NIREHG), which specifically tracks literature on the ethical, legal, and social implications of advances in genetics research and its applications. NIREHG hosts the Genetics and Ethics database at: http://bioethics.georgetown.edu/nirehg/index.html.

Originating from the Institute's ethics library, established in 1973 with funding from the Joseph P. Kennedy, Jr., Foundation, NRCBL now comprises more than 500 ongoing periodical subscriptions; 28,000 books; 200,000 cataloged, article-length documents; extensive archival materials pertaining to government organizations; 400 audiovisuals; and 500 course syllabi. Open to the public, it serves both on-site researchers and remote users through its reference desk service, through its toll-free number (1–888- BIO-ETHX, in the United States and Canada) and via email (bioethics@georgetown.edu). Services include the online database *ETHX on the Web,* reference service, custom database searches, a multifaceted publications program, document delivery, and a syllabus exchange clearinghouse for educators.

The Bioethics Information Retrieval Project, begun in 1975 and now operating under contract with the U.S. National Library of Medicine, contributes to making English-language literature accessible via two very large databases operated by the NLM: PubMed for journal articles and LOCATOR*plus* for books and chapters in books. The records in the predecessor BIOETHICSLINE® database (which was developed and augmented by the Project from 1975 through 2000), have been merged into one or the other of the aforementioned large databases. The closed BIOETHICSLINE database (1973–2000) continues to be distributed by Ovid and is archived at the NRCBL.

One of the early, major reasons for developing a bibliographic retrieval system for bioethics was to pull together the literature of a highly interdisciplinary field of study. In spite of the fact that specialty journals now exist, and that the major weeklies, such as *The Lancet* and *Science,* cover bioethical issues routinely, the literature is still widely dispersed.

Access to bioethics citations is available directly from the U.S. National Library of Medicine. Within PubMed, limiting searching to the "bioethics subset" serves to collect relevant materials, and in LOCATOR*plus* limiting searching to "ethics kie" similarly aggregates ethical works. Further instructions for searching these databases is at: http://bioethics.georgetown.edu/ir/bioline.htm.

An annual *Bibliography of Bioethics,* compiled from that portion of the literature selected for inclusion in NLM databases, has been published by the Kennedy Institute for almost three decades. Volume 29 for 2003 is estimated to include more than 5,000 citations. It will comprise two major sections: the first for journal articles, essays in books, and other similar materials; and the second for books.

NIREHG delivers many specialized services on its Web page, including updated Scope Notes on selected topics (eugenics, gene mapping, genetic counseling and screening, among others), and a bibliographic database of more than 19,000 entries called *Genetics and Ethics.*

II. Periodical Literature

Given the growth of interest in the field, it is not surprising that specialty journals have emerged that are devoted primarily to bioethical issues. A few have been published for decades, while others first appeared more recently. Some are affiliated with research organizations or professional societies. Publication information for several such periodicals is provided below in the section on Bioethics and Health Law Journals. This is not a comprehensive list, but it is representative of English-language sources. For information regarding foreign-language sources, readers may wish to contact the documentation centers mentioned below who are analyzing bioethics literature in other languages.

Since bioethical topics continue to receive a great deal of attention, the periodicals of contributing disciplines likewise continue to devote considerable space to pertinent issues. Medical, scientific, and philosophical journals that have consistently covered bioethics are also listed under General Philosophical, Scientific, and Medical Journals, below. Please note that U.S. offices are listed when available.

A. BIOETHICS AND HEALTH LAW JOURNALS

Accountability in Research, quarterly, published by: Gordon and Breach Publishing Group, c/o International Publishers Distributor, P.O. Box 32160, Newark, NJ 07102; <http://www.tandf.co.uk/journals/titles/08989621.html>; ISSN: 0898–9621.

American Journal of Bioethics (AJOB), quarterly, published by: MIT Press Journals, Five Cambridge Center, Cambridge, MA 02142; <http://mitpress.mit.edu>; ISSN: 1526–5161.

American Journal of Law and Medicine, quarterly, published by: American Society of Law, Medicine & Ethics, 765 Commonwealth Ave., 16th Floor, Boston, MA 02215; <http://www.aslme.org/>; ISSN: 0098–8588.

Bioethics (official journal of the International Association of Bioethics), five issues per year, published by: Blackwell Publishers Journals, Customer Services, P.O. Box 805, Oxford OX4 1FH, England; <http://www.bioethics-international.org/bioethics.html>; ISSN: 0269–9702.

Bioethics Forum, quarterly, published by: Midwest Bioethics Center, 1021–1025 Jefferson Street, Kansas City, MO 64105–1329; <http://www.midbio.org>;ISSN: 1065–7274.

Christian Bioethics, 3/year, published by: Swets & Zeitlinger, 440 Creamery Way, Suite A, Exton, PA 19341; <http://www.swets.nl/sps/journals/jhome.html>; ISSN: 1380–3603.

CQ: Cambridge Quarterly of Healthcare Ethics, quarterly, published by: Cambridge University Press, 110 Midland Ave., Port Chester, NY 10573- 4930; <http://journals.cambridge.org>; ISSN: 0963–1801.

Developing World Bioethics, semiannual, published by: Blackwell Publishers, 350 Main Street, Malden, MA 02148; <http://www.blackwellpublishers.co.uk>; ISSN: 1471–8731.

Ethics & Behavior, quarterly, published by: Lawrence Erlbaum Associates, Inc., Attn: Journals, 10 Industrial Avenue, Mahwah, NJ 07430–2262; <http://www.catchword.co.uk>; ISSN: 1050–8422.

Hastings Center Report, bimonthly, published by: The Hastings Center, 21 Malcolm Gordon Road, Garrison, NY 10524–5555; <http://www.thehastingscenter.org/;> ISSN: 0093–0334.

Health Care Analysis: An International Journal of Health Philosophy and Policy, quarterly, published by: John Wiley & Sons, Baffins Lane, Chichester, West Sussex, PO19 1UD England; <http://www.wiley.com/>; ISSN: 1065–3058.

Health Matrix: The Journal of Law-Medicine, biannual, Case Western Reserve University, School of Law, 11075 East Boulevard, Cleveland, OH 44106; <http://lawwww.cwru.edu/academic/healthMatrix/>; ISSN: 0748–383X.

HEC Forum (Healthcare Ethics Committee Forum), quarterly, published by: Kluwer Academic Publishers Group, P.O. Box 322,3300 AH Dordrecht, The Netherlands, or P.O. Box 358, Accord Station, Hingham, MA 02018–0358, <http://journals.kluweronline.com>; ISSN: 0956–2737.

International Journal of Bioethics/Journal International de Bioéthique, quarterly, published by: Editions Alexandre Lacassagne, 162, avenue Lacassagne, 69003 Lyon, France, <http://www.info-presse.fr/>; ISSN: 1287–7352.

IRB: Ethics & Human Research, bimonthly, published by: The Hastings Center, 21 Malcolm Gordon Rd., Garrison, NY 10524–5555, <http://www.thehastingscenter.org/;> ISSN: 0193–7758.

JONA's Healthcare Law, Ethics, and Regulation, quarterly, published by: Lippincott Williams & Wilkins, 16522 Hunters Green Parkway, Hagerstown, MD 21740–2116; <http://www.lww.com/>; ISSN: 1520–9229.

Journal of Clinical Ethics, quarterly, published by: Journal of Clinical Ethics, 12 South Market Street, Suite 300, Frederick, MD 21701; <http://www.clinicalethics.com/>; ISSN: 1046–7890.

Journal of Health Politics, Policy and Law, bimonthly, published by: Duke University Press, Journals Dept., P.O. Box 90660, Durham, NC 27708–0660, <http://www.jhppl.org/>; ISSN: 0361–6878.

The Journal of Law, Medicine & Ethics, quarterly, published by: American Society of Law, Medicine & Ethics, 765 Commonwealth Avenue, 16th Floor, Boston, MA 02215, <http://www.aslme.org/>; ISSN: 0277–8459.

Journal of Medical Ethics, includes *Medical Humanities* [ISSN: 1468–215X] in June and September as supplements; bimonthly, published by: St. Chloe House, The Avenue, Old Bussage, Glos GL6 8AT, United Kingdom; <http://jme.bmjjournals.com/>; ISSN: 0306–6800.

Journal of Medical Humanities, quarterly, published by: Kluwer, <http://www.kluweronline.com/>; ISSN: 1041–3545.

The Journal of Medicine and Philosophy, bimonthly, published by: Swets & Zeitlinger BV Publishers, P.O. Box 4508, Church Street Station, New York, NY 10261–4508, <http://www.swets.nl/swets/show>; ISSN: 0360–5310.

Kennedy Institute of Ethics Journal, quarterly, published by: Johns Hopkins University Press, 2715 North Charles Street, Baltimore, MD 21218–4319, <http://www.press.jhu.edu/press/index.htm>; ISSN: 1054–6863.

Medical Humanities, biannual (see *Journal of Medical Ethics* above), published by: BMJ Publishing Group, P.O. Box 590A, Kennebunkport, ME 04046; <http://mh.bmjjournals.com/>; ISSN: 1468–215X.

Medicine and Law, quarterly, published by: International Center for Health, Law and Ethics, University of Haifa,

Law Faculty, P.O. Box 6451, Haifa 31063, Israel; <http://research.haifa.ac.il/~medlaw/publications/hindex.htm>; ISSN: 0723–1393.

Medicine, Health Care and Philosophy, three issues per year, Kluwer Academic, 101 Philip Drive, Norwell, MA 02061; <http://journals.kluweronline.com;> ISSN: 1386–7423.

Milbank Quarterly, quarterly, published by: Blackwell Publishers, 238 Main Street, Cambridge, MA 02142; <http://www.blackwellpublishing.com/>; ISSN: 0887–378X.

National Catholic Bioethics Quarterly, quarterly, published by: The National Catholic Bioethics Center, 159 Washington Street, Boston, MA 02135; <http://www.ncbq.com/>; ISSN: 1532–5490.

New Zealand Bioethics Journal, three issues per year, Bioethics Centre, University of Otago, P.O. Box 913, Dunedin, New Zealand; <http://healthsci.otago.ac.nz/dsm/nzbj/NzBioethicsJournal.html>; ISSN: 1175–3455.

Nursing Ethics, bimonthly, published by: Arnold, c/o Turpin Distribution Services Ltd., Blackhorse Road, Letchworth, Hertfordshire SG6 1HN, England; <http://www.arnoldpublishers.com/journals/pages/nur_eth/aut.htm>; ISSN: 0969–7330.

Second Opinion, quarterly, published by: Park Ridge Center, 221 E. Ontario, Suite 800, Chicago, IL 60611–3215, ISSN: 0890–1570.

Theoretical Medicine and Bioethics, bimonthly, published by: Kluwer Academic Publishers, Drs A.M. Ultee, Van Godewijckstraat 30, P.O. Box 17, 3300 AA Dordrecht, The Netherlands, <http://www.kluweronline.com>; ISSN: 1386–7415.

Yale Journal of Health Policy, Law, and Ethics, biannual, published by: Yale Law School, P.O. Box 208215, New Haven, CT 06520–8215; <http://www.yale.edu/yjhple/>; ISSN: 1535–3532.

B. GENERAL PHILOSOPHICAL, SCIENTIFIC, AND MEDICAL JOURNALS

American Journal of Public Health, monthly, published by: American Public Health Association, 1015 15th St., NW, Washington, DC 20005; <http://www.ajph.org>; ISSN: 0090–0036.

Annals of Internal Medicine, twice per month, published by: Annals of Internal Medicine (on behalf of the American College of Physicians), P.O. Box 7777-R-0320,

Philadelphia, PA 19175; <http://www.annals.org>; ISSN: 0003–4819.

Archives of Internal Medicine, monthly, published by: American Medical Association, Subscription Department, P.O. Box 5201, Chicago, IL 60680–5201; <http://archinte.ama-assn.org/>; ISSN: 0003–9926.

BMJ (British Medical Journal), weekly, published by: British Medical Journal, P.O. Box 560B, Kennebunkport, ME 04046; <http://bmj.com>; ISSN: 0959–8146.

Ethics, quarterly, published by: University of Chicago Press, P.O. Box 37005, Chicago, IL 60637; <http://www.journals.uchicago.edu>; ISSN: 0014–1704.

JAMA: The Journal of the American Medical Association, weekly, published by: American Medical Association, Subscription Department, P.O. Box 5201, Chicago, IL 60680–5201, <http://jama.ama-assn.org>; ISSN: 0098–7484.

Journal of Applied Philosophy, three issues per year, published by: Blackwell Publishers, 108 Cowley Road, Oxford OX4 1JF United Kingdom; <http://www.blackwellpublishers.co.uk>; ISSN: 0264–3758.

The Lancet, weekly, published by: Williams & Wilkins, 428 East Preston Street, Baltimore, MD 21202; <http://www.thelancet.com/journal>; ISSN: 0099–5355.

Milbank Quarterly, quarterly, published by: Blackwell Publishers, 238 Main Street, Cambridge, MA 02142; <http://www.blackwellpublishing.com/>; ISSN: 0887–378X.

Nature, weekly, published by: Nature, P.O. Box 5055, Brentwood, TN 37024–9743; <http://www.nature.com/>; ISSN: 0028–0836.

New England Journal of Medicine, weekly, published by: New England Journal of Medicine, 1440 Main Street, Waltham, MA 02154–1649, <http://content.nejm.org>; ISSN: 0028–4793.

Philosophy & Public Affairs, quarterly, published by: Johns Hopkins University Press, 701 W. 40th Street, Baltimore, MD 21211–2190; <http://www.press.jhu.edu/press/index.htm>; ISSN: 0048–3915.

Science, weekly, published by: American Association for the Advancement of Science, P.O. Box 2032, Marion, OH 43305–0001; <http://www.sciencemag.com>; ISSN: 0036–8075.

Women's Health Issues, bimonthly, Elsevier Science Publishing Co., Regional Sales Office, P.O. Box 945, New York,

NY 10159–0945; <http://www.elsevier.com/>; ISSN: 1049–3867.

III. Governmental and Professional Bioethics Organizations

The ORGS database maintained by NRCBL now has more than one thousand entries. Only a selected subset can be listed here. Four categories have been selected because each represents in some way a group approach to the deliberation of bioethical problems. The first two groups are supported by their respective governments; the third benefits from international and regional support; and the final type of organization has the support of groups of professionals with common interests. The four categories are: A. National Libraries of Bioethics; B. National Deliberative Bodies on Bioethics; C. Regional and International Bioethics Organizations; and D. Professional Groups. Either a Web or postal address was required for candidate organizations to be included in this section. If the Web site offers an alternative English version, that is listed.

A. NATIONAL LIBRARIES OF BIOETHICS

With federal support, the following reference centers provide bioethics information to the public. Each contains resources unique to the language of its country.

FRANCE
Documentation center on ethics of life sciences and
  health (CDEI), (Centre de Documentation et
  d'Information en Éthique des Sciences de la Vie et de
  la Santé)
Institut National de la Santé et de la Recherche Médicale
  (INSERM)
71 rue Saint-Dominique
75007 Paris
<http://www.inserm.fr/servcom/servcom.nsf/
  (Web+Startup+P age)?ReadForm&english>

GERMANY
Deutsches Referenzzentrum für Ethik in den
  Biowissenschaften
Niebuhrstr. 53
D-53113 Bonn
<http://www.drze.de>

UNITED STATES
National Reference Center for Bioethics Literature
Joseph and Rose Kennedy Institute of Ethics
Georgetown University
Washington, DC 20057–1212
<http://bioethics.georgetown.edu>

B. NATIONAL DELIBERATIVE BODIES ON BIOETHICS

AUSTRALIA
Australian Health Ethics Committee
National Health and Medical Research Council; and
Health Ethics Section
Centre for Health Advice Policy & Ethics (CHAPE)
GPO Box 9848
Canberra ACT 2601
<http://www.health.gov.au/nhmrc>

AUSTRIA
Austrian Commission on Bioethics
Bundeskanzleramt
Hohenstaufengasse 3
1010 Vienna
<www.bka.gv.at/bka/bioethik/>

BELGIUM
Comité consultatif de Bioéthique de Belgique
C.A.E. Quartier Vésale—V416
Mme. Boxxon
19 bte 5 Bd. Pachéco
1010 Bruxelles
<http://www.health.fgov.be/bioeth/>

CANADA
National Council on Ethics in Human Research
  (NCEHR)
774 Echo Drive
Ottawa, Ontario K1S 5N8
<http://www.ncehr-cnerh.org>

DENMARK (Copenhagen)
Danish Council on Ethics
Ravnsborggade, 2–4
DK-2200 Copenhagen N
<http://www.etiskraad.dk>

FINLAND
National Advisory Board on Health Care Ethics
P.O. Box 33
(Kirkkokatu 14, Helsinki)
00023 Valtioneuvosto
<http://www.etene.org/>

National Advisory Board on Research Ethics
Mariankatu 5
FIN 00170 Helsinki
<http://pro.tsv.fi/tenk>

FRANCE
National Consultative Bioethics Committee
Le Comité Consultatif National d'Ethique pour les
    Sciences de la Vie et de la Santé
71, rue Saint-Dominique
75007 Paris
<http://www.ccne-ethique.org>

GERMANY
Der Nationale Ethikrat Berlin-Brandeburgische
    Akademie der Wissenchaft
Jägerstrasse 22/23
10117 Berlin
<http://www.ethikrat.org>

GREECE
Hellenic National Bioethics Commission
Evelpidon 47
113 62 Athens
<http://www.bioethics.gr>

INDIA
Indian Council of Medical Research
V. Ramalingaswami Bhawan
Ansari Nagar
New Delhi–110029
<http://icmr.nic.in/>

IRELAND
Irish Council for Bioethics
Comhairle Bitheitice na hÉireann
Academy House
19 Dawson Street
Dublin 2
<http://www.bioethics.ie>

ISRAEL
Israel Academy of Sciences and Humanities
Bioethics Advisory Committee
c/o Department of Science Teaching
The Weizmann Institute of Science
Rehovot 76100
<http://stwww.weizmann.ac.il/bioethics/index-e.html>

ITALY
Comitato Naztionale Italiano di Bioetica
Via Veneto, 56
00187 Roma
<http://www.governo.it/bioetica/eng/index.html>

LITHUANIA
Lithuanian Bioethics Committee
(Lietuvos bioetikos komitetas)
Vilniaus g. 33–230
LT-2001 Vilnius
<http://www.sam.lt/bioetika>

MALTA
The Bioethics Consultative Committee
c/o Department of Health
15, Merchants Street
Valletta
<http://www.synapse.net.mt/bioethics>

THE NETHERLANDS
Health Council
Standing Committee on Medical Ethics and Health Law
P.O. Box 16052
2500 BB The Hague
<http://www.gr.nl>

NEW ZEALAND
National Ethics Committee on Assisted Human
    Reproduction
Ministry of Health
133 Molesworth St
P.O. Box 5013, Wellington
<http://www.newhealth.govt.nz/>

Royal Commission on Genetic Modification
Ministry for the Environment
84 Boulcott Street
P.O. Box 10 362, Wellington
<http://www.gmcommission.govt.nz/>

NORWAY
The National Biotechnology Advisory Board
Prinsens gt. 18, Boks 522 Sentrum
0105 Oslo
<http://www.bion.no>

The National Committees for Research Ethics (Norway):
The National Committee for Medical Research
    Ethics, NEM
The National Committee for Research Ethics in Science
    and Technology, NENT
The National Committee for Research Ethics in the
    Social Sciences and the Humanities, NESH
Street address: Prinsensgate 18
Postal address: P.O. Box 522, Sentrum, N-0105 Oslo
<http://www.etikkom.no/Etikkom/Engelsk>

Department of Science and Technology
Philippine Council for Health Research and
    Development
3F DOST Main Bldg., DOST Compound
Gen. Santos Ave., Bicutan, Tagig, Metro Manila
<http://www.pchrd.dost.gov.ph/PCHRD/ethics/NEC.
    htm >

PORTUGAL
National Council on Ethics of Life Sciences
Conselho Nacional de Ética para as Ciências da Vida
Rue Prof. Gomes Teixeira
Edif PCM, 8
1399–022 Lisbon
<http://www.cnecv.gov.pt>

RUSSIA
National Committee on Bioethics
Volkhonka 14/1
119992 Moscow

SINGAPORE
Bioethics Advisory Committee
250 North Bridge Road
#15–01/02
Raffles City Tower
Singapore 179101
<http://www.bioethics-singapore.org/bac/index.jsp>

National Medical Ethics Committee (NMEC)
Ministry of Health
College of Medicine Building 16 College Road
Singapore 169854
<http://www.moh.gov.sg/nmec/nmec.html>

SOUTH AFRICA
Medical Research Council of South Africa, 2001
P.O. Box 19070
7505 Tygerberg
<http://www.mrc.ac.za/ethics/ethicshuman.htm>

SWEDEN
Swedish Gene Technology Board
<http://www.genteknik.se/>

Swedish National Council on Medical Ethics
Statens Medicinsk-etiska Rad
The Department of Justice
SE-103 33 Stockholm
<http://www.smer.gov.se/>

SWITZERLAND
Swiss National Advisory Commission on Biomedical
    Ethics
Nationale Ethikkommission im Bereich der
    Humanmedizin (NEK-CNE)
Bern
<http://www.nek-cne.ch/>

TURKEY
Bioethics Ad Hoc Committee for the Turkish National
    Commission for UNESCO
(Biyoetik _htisas Komitesi)
<http://www.unesco.org.tr>

UNITED KINGDOM
Advisory Committee on Genetic Testing
Department of Health
HGC Secretariat
Area 652C, Skipton House
80 London Road
London SE1 6LH
<http://www.doh.gov.uk/genetics/acgt/publications.htm >

Central Office for Research Ethics Committees
    (COREC)
Room 76, B Block
40 Eastbourne Terrace
London W2 3QR
<http://www.corec.org.uk>

Human Fertilisation and Embryology Authority
Paxton House
30 Artillery Lane
London E1 7LS
<http://www.hfea.gov.uk/>

Human Genetics Commission
Department of Health
Area 652C, Skipton House
80 London Road
London SE1 6LH
<http://www.hgc.gov.uk>

Nuffield Council on Bioethics
28 Bedford Square
London, WC1B 3EG
<http://www.nuffield.org/bioethics/>

Xenotransplantation Interim Regulatory Authority
    (UKXIRA)
UKXIRA Secretariat
Department of Health
Room 339, Wellington House
133–155 Waterloo Road
London SE1 8UG
<http://www.doh.gov.uk/ukxira/index.htm>

UNITED STATES
Department of Clinical Bioethics
National Institutes of Health
10 Center Drive Building 10, Room 1C118
Bethesda, MD 20892–1156
<http://www.bioethics.nih.gov/>

Department of Energy
Ethical, Legal, and Social Issues Program
Office of Science
U.S. Department of Energy
1000 Independence Avenue, SW
Washington, DC 20585
<http://www.ornl.gov/TechResources/Human_Genome/
  elsi/elsi.html >

National Human Genome Research Institute (NHGRI)
Ethical, Legal and Social Implications (ELSI) Program
National Institutes of Health
Building 31, Room B2B07
31 Center Drive, MSC 2033
Bethesda, MD 20892–2033
<http://www.genome.gov/page.cfm?pageID=10001618 >

The President's Council on Bioethics
1801 Pennsylvania Avenue, NW
Suite 600
Washington, DC 20006
<http://www.bioethics.gov>

C. REGIONAL AND INTERNATIONAL BIOETHICS ORGANIZATIONS

CENTRE FOR ASIAN AND INTERNATIONAL BIOETHICS
Faculty of Health Sciences
Ben Gurion University of the Negev
Beer-Sheva
Israel
<http://fohs.bgu.ac.il/toplevel/default.asp?DivType=
  CNT >

COUNCIL FOR INTERNATIONAL ORGANIZATIONS OF MEDICAL SCIENCES
World Health Organization
CH–1211 Geneva 27
Switzerland
<http://www.cioms.ch>

COUNCIL OF EUROPE
Bioethics Program, Legal Affairs
Council of Europe
F–67075 Strasbourg Cedex
France
<http://www.coe.int/T/E/Legal_affairs/Legal_co-
  operation/Bioethics/>

Steering Committee for Bioethics (CDBI, formerly
  CAHBI)
Council of Europe
Pièce 2004
67006 Strasbourg
France
<http://www.coe.int/T/E/Legal_Affairs/Legal_co-
  operation/Bioethics/CDBI/<

EUROPEAN ASSOCIATION OF CENTRES OF MEDICAL ETHICS (EACME)
c/o Mrs. A. Heijnen, Instituut voor Gezondheidsethiek
P.O. Box 616
6200 MD Maastricht
The Netherlands
<http://www.eacmeweb.com/en/>

EUROPEAN GROUP ON ETHICS IN SCIENCE AND NEW TECHNOLOGIES
c/o European Commission
B–1049 Brussels
Belgium
<http://europa.eu.int/comm/european_group_ethics/
  index_en.htm >

NORDIC COMMITTEE ON BIOETHICS
Rikhard Nymansväg 9 B
00370 Helsingfors
Finland
<http://www.ncbio.org/Html/eng_index.htm>

UNESCO
International Bioethics Committee
7, Place de Fontenoy
75700 Paris
France
(Includes a database of bioethics organizations.)
<http://www.unesco.org/ibc/>

D. PROFESSIONAL GROUPS

ALL INDIA ASSOCIATION OF BIOETHICS (AIBA)
c/o Dr.Jayapaul Azariah
No. 3, 8th Lane, 5th Cross Street, Indira Nagar,
Chennai 600 020
India
<http://www.biol.tsukuba.ac.jp/~macer/aiba.html#6>

AMERICAN SOCIETY FOR BIOETHICS AND HUMANITIES
4700 W. Lake
Glenview, IL 60025–1485
<http://www.asbh.org/>

ASIAN BIOETHICS ASSOCIATION
c/o Hyakudai Sakamoto, Ph.D., President
University Research Center, Nihon University
4–8-24 Kudan-Minami, Chiyoda-ku, Tokyo 102
Japan
<http://web.kssp.upd.edu.ph/philo/fora_BioethicsAsia.
  htm >

AUSTRALASIAN BIOETHICS ASSOCIATION
c/o School of Public Health and Community Medicine
University of NSW
NSW 2052
Australia
<http://www.australasian-bioethics.org.au/>

CANADIAN BIOETHICS SOCIETY
c/o Ms. Lydia Riddell
561 Rocky Ridge Bay NW
Calgary, Alberta T3G 4E7
Canada
<http://www.bioethics.ca/english/index.html>

FORUM FOR ETHICAL REVIEW COMMITTEES
  IN THE ASIAN AND WESTERN PACIFIC
  REGION (FERCAP)
c/o Dr. (Mrs.) N.A. Kshirsagar, Dean
Professor & Head, Dept. Clinical Pharmacology
'A' Bldg 4th Floor
TN Medical College & BYL Nair Ch. Hospital
Mumbai 400 008
India
<http://www.fercap.org/>

INTERNATIONAL ASSOCIATION OF BIOETHICS
Centre for Bioethics and Health Law
P.O. Box 80105
3508 TC Utrecht
The Netherlands
<http://bioethics-international.org>

INTERNATIONAL NETWORK ON FEMINIST
  APPROACHES TO BIOETHICS
(2003 sponsor of site)
<http://www.msu.edu/~hlnelson/fab/>

INTERNATIONAL SOCIETY OF BIOETHICS
Plaza del Humedal 3 (Edif. Gota de Leche)
33205 Gijón, Asturias
Spain
< http://www.sibi.org>

KOREAN BIOETHICS ASSOCIATION
c/o Dept of History of Medicine & Medical Humanities
Seoul National University College of Medicine
28 Yongon-dong, Chongno-gu, Seoul 110–799
Korea
<http://www.koreabioethics.net/>

PAN AMERICAN HEALTH ORGANIZATION
(World Health Organization [WHO])
Pan American Sanitary Bureau
Division of Health and Human Development
Program on Bioethics 525 Twenty-third Street, N.W.
Washington, DC 20037
<http://www.paho.org/>

Also:
Regional Program on Bioethics / Programa Regional de
  Bioetica
Avda. Providencia 1017. Piso 7 Providencia
Santiago de Chile, Chile

WORLD HEALTH ORGANIZATION
Ethics and Health
Avenue Appia 20
1211 Geneva 27, Switzerland
<http://www.who.int>

This resource is, to be sure, incomplete; any omissions are
the responsibility of the author. To recommend additions,
please email: goldstdo@georgetown.edu or fax: +202-
687–6770.

Prepared by:
Doris Mueller Goldstein, M.L.S., M.A.
Director, Library and Information Services
The Joseph and Rose Kennedy Institute of Ethics
Georgetown University
Washington, DC
March 2003

APPENDIX III

KEY LEGAL CASES IN BIOETHICS

Jacobson v. Massachusetts

197 U.S. 11 (1905)

• • •

The State of Massachusetts imposed a law mandating that all inhabitants either submit to a smallpox vaccination or pay a fine. Jacobson claimed that his liberty interest in caring for his own body and health was invaded when he was subjected to a fine for refusing to submit to the vaccination. The U.S. Supreme Court held that liberty rights were not absolute, but rather, could be limited to ensure equal enjoyment of rights by others. The Court cautioned, however, that their interpretation of the law did not give states the power to regulate in an arbitrary, oppressive, or unjust manner.

Schloendorff v. Society of the New York Hospital

105 N.E. 192 (N.Y. 1914)

• • •

Ms. Schloendorff, an inpatient at the Society of the New York Hospital, had a fibroid tumor removed. Following her operation Ms. Schloendorff developed gangrene in her arm, which necessitated the amputation of some of her fingers. Claming that she consented only to an examination and not to the actual surgery (the patient was under general anesthesia for both the exam and the surgery), Ms. Schloendorff sued the Hospital for her injuries. The highest court in the State of New York held that the Hospital was not liable. Despite this ruling, Justice Cardozo wrote that "[e]very

human being of adult years and sound mind has a right to determine what shall be done with his own body" (*Id.* at 129), marking the beginning of the development of the doctrine of informed consent.

Buck v. Bell

274 U.S. 200 (1927)

• • •

The State of Virginia enacted a law claiming that the welfare of society could legally be promoted by the careful sterilization of certain mentally defective individuals. Carrie Buck was described as "the daughter of a feeble-minded mother in the same institution, and the mother of an illegitimate feeble-minded child" (*Id.* at 205), and was targeted for sterilization by the state institution in which she lived. Since the sterilization was not deemed to be detrimental to Ms. Buck's general health, and since it was seen as a way to promote the general welfare of society by "prevent[ing] those who are manifestly unfit from continuing their kind" (*Id.* at 207), the U.S. Supreme Court upheld the forced sterilization. The Court explained, "[t]hree generations of imbeciles are enough" (*Id.*).

Skinner v. Oklahoma

316 U.S. 535 (1942)

• • •

Mr. Skinner was convicted of stealing chickens and subsequently convicted on two separate occasions of robbery with firearms. According to the terms of the Oklahoma Habitual Criminal Sterilization Act, Mr. Skinner could be sterilized for his acts as a repeated felon as long as the sterilization would not be detrimental to his general health. The U.S. Supreme Court held that state sterilization laws were subject to strict scrutiny to ensure that they did not violate the constitutional guarantee of equal protection. The Court based this holding on the notion that, "[m]arriage and procreation are fundamental to the very existence and survival of the race" (*Id.* at 541) and that the power to sterilize, if misused, "may have subtle, far reaching and devastating effects" (*Id.*). The Court ultimately found the Act unconstitutional because it called for the sterilization of only certain offenders and not others who committed equally reprehensible acts.

Prince v. Massachusetts

321 U.S. 158 (1944)

• • •

Betty Prince was accused of violating a statute prohibiting her from allowing her nine-year-old niece (over whom she had custody) to sell religious pamphlets from the street corner. Prince responded that her actions were protected by the First Amendment as well as by her rights as a parent. The U.S. Supreme Court upheld the statute, and explained that the "state has a wide range of power for limiting parental freedom and authority in things affecting the child's welfare; and that this includes, to some extent, matters of conscience and religious conviction" (*Id.* at 167). Courts restricting parental rights to make decisions about withholding medical care for minor children routinely cite this case.

Griswold v. Connecticut

381 U.S. 479 (1965)

• • •

Griswold, the Executive Director of the Planned Parenthood League of Connecticut, gave information and medical advice about contraception to married couples. Griswold and others were found guilty of violating Connecticut law forbidding the use of, or counseling about, contraceptives. Although not mentioned specifically in the United States Constitution, the U.S. Supreme Court extrapolated a zone of privacy from fundamental constitutional guarantees. The

Court held that the Connecticut law forbidding contraceptive use violated the privacy of the marital relationship and was therefore unconstitutional. In a subsequent opinion, the U.S. Supreme Court stated, "[i]f the right of privacy means anything, it is the right of the individual, married or single, to be free from unwarranted governmental intrusion into matters so fundamentally affecting a person as the decision whether to bear or beget a child" (*Eisenstadt v. Baird*, 405 U.S. 438, 453 (1972)) (declaring unconstitutional a Massachusetts statute prohibiting the distribution of contraceptives to single persons but allowing distribution to married persons).

Strunk v. Strunk

445 S.W.2D 145 (KY. 1967)

• • •

Tom Strunk was 28 years old and suffered from a fatal kidney disease. After exhaustive testing, it was determined that the only available kidney donor was Jerry Strunk, Tom's 27-year-old brother. Jerry Strunk was an incompetent, state-institutionalized individual with the approximate mental capacity of a six-year-old child. The Strunk parents petitioned the court for permission to proceed with the operation to transplant one of Jerry's kidneys to Tom. The highest court in Kentucky affirmed the lower court's authorization of the procedure. They based their decision on the conclusion that because of the close relationship between the brothers—noting in particular Jerry's family ties through Tom and the necessity of Tom's presence to Jerry's improvement—it would be in Jerry's best interest to have Tom alive.

Canterbury v. Spence

464 F.2D 762 (D.C. CIR. 1972)

• • •

Canterbury was a patient who suffered from back pain who sought surgical intervention after medical treatments failed to alleviate his pain. The physician did not inform Canterbury that there was a minor risk of paralysis associated with the surgery. Canterbury was recovering normally after the surgery when he suffered a fall that led to minor paralysis of his legs and urinary incontinence. Although Canterbury (via his mother) had given consent to the surgery, the consent it was not "informed." The physician protested that he had acted according to the custom of the profession (a professional standard of disclosure), but the Appellate Court held that the patient's right to make decisions about his or her own care affects the nature of what a physician must reveal—applying a "patient-oriented" standard of disclosure. They stated that the physician must provide the patient with "material" information to enable him/her to make an "intelligent choice." The standard of disclosure for informed consent continues to be debated today.

Roe v. Wade

410 U.S. 113 (1973)

• • •

The case arose from a challenge to a Texas statute declaring the attempt or actual procurement of an abortion, other than to save the life of the pregnant woman, a crime. The U.S. Supreme Court declared the statute unconstitutional, but made a series of findings that continue to affect reproductive law and policy. The Court, listing a variety of potential harms that might befall a woman with no choice of abortion, held that the right of privacy "is broad enough to encompass a woman's decision whether or not to terminate her pregnancy" (*Id.* at 153). Freedom to obtain an abortion is not absolute, since the Court noted that the state has an interest in protecting both potential human life and the health of the mother. Using the trimester framework as guideposts, the Court held that at different times in the pregnancy the interests of the State might become sufficiently compelling to sustain regulation of the interest of the pregnant woman in having an abortion. Finally, the Court explained that a fetus is not a "person" entitled to legal protection under the Fourteenth Amendment's Due Process and Equal Protection clauses.

The Supreme Court reexamined these issues in *Planned Parenthood of Southeastern Pennsylvania v. Casey*, 505 U.S. 833 (1992). The facts of the case revolved around specific provisions of a Pennsylvania abortion statute regulating consent, waiting periods, parental consent for minors, spousal notification, definitions of "medical emergency" and reporting requirements. The U.S. Supreme Court reaffirmed the holding in *Roe v. Wade* that a woman had a right to choose an abortion, but rejected *Roe's* trimester framework to favor a fetal viability notion for measuring state and individual interests. The Court stated that prior to fetal viability, the state could not impose an undue burden (described as a substantial obstacle) on the woman's right to choose to have an abortion. Specifically, the Court held that only Pennsylvania's spousal notification requirement imposed an undue burden and therefore invalidated only that provision.

O'Connor v. Donaldson

422 U.S. 563 (1975)

• • •

Kenneth Donaldson was committed as a mental patient to a Florida state hospital and kept confined there against his will for approximately 15 years; he subsequently sued the hospital claiming that his right to liberty had been violated. Donaldson was never accused of being a danger to society or incapable of taking care of himself. The U.S. Supreme Court held that finding a person to be mentally ill is not *per se* sufficient to justify the State's involuntarily confinement of that person. Further, the Court stated, "mere public intolerance or animosity cannot constitutionally justify the deprivation of a person's physical liberty" (*Id.* at 575).

Tarasoff v. Regents of the University of California

51 P.2D 334 (CAL. 1976)

• • •

A patient seeking psychotherapy confided to his therapist that he intended to kill Tatiana Tarasoff. The therapist did not warn the intended victim, nor did he notify persons likely to inform Ms. Tarasoff of her imminent peril. After Ms. Tarasoff was murdered, her parents sued the university, the psychotherapists involved in the case, and the campus police. The Supreme Court of California noted that "[w]hen a therapist determines, or pursuant to the standards of his profession should determine, that his patient presents a serious danger of violence to another, he incurs an obligation to use reasonable care to protect the intended victim against such danger. . .[which] may call for him to warn the intended victim or others likely to apprise the victim of the danger, to notify the police, or to take whatever other steps are reasonably necessary under the circumstances" (*Id.* at 340). The Court explained that at times of imminent and specific danger, the duty to warn outweighs the right of confidentiality.

In re Quinlan

355 A.2D 647 (N.J. 1976)

• • •

Karen Quinlan was characterized as existing in a persistent vegetative state, in which she retained some homeostatic function but would never regain cognitive function. Mr. Quinlan, Karen's father, sought the Court's permission to withdraw the life-sustaining mechanisms prolonging her eventual death. The Supreme Court of New Jersey held that the right of privacy was broad enough to encompass patients' decisions to decline medical care. The Court explained that the State's interest in preserving the sanctity of human life could ultimately be overcome by the rights of the individual. The Court cautioned that the right of choice was for Karen to exercise, but since she was incompetent, allowed the guardian and family to determine whether Karen would have wanted to remove support in these circumstances.

Superintendent of Belchertown State School v. Saikewicz

370 N.E.2D 417 (MASS. 1977)

• • •

Mr. Saikewicz was a mentally incompetent resident of a state facility who suffered from acute myeloblastic monocytic leukemia. Since he was unable to give informed consent for his treatment, the superintendent of the facility petitioned the court for appointment of a guardian to make decisions concerning Mr. Saikewicz's care. The appointed guardian noted that the illness was incurable, but could be managed with chemotherapy. The guardian explained that it would not be in Mr. Saikewicz's best interest to be treated, since the benefit of some uncertain extension of life would not outweigh the fear and pain caused by a treatment he had no ability to understand. The Supreme Court of Massachusetts recognized an individual's right to be free from unwanted medical intervention for an incurable illness. The Court ultimately applied the doctrine of substituted judgment, in which "the decision … [is] that which would be made by the incompetent person, if that person were competent, but taking into account the present and future incompetency of the individual as one of the factors which would necessarily enter into the decision-making process of the competent person" (*Id.* at 752–53). The Court concluded that the decision to withhold treatment was made with regard to Mr. Saikewicz's actual interests.

In re Conroy

486 A.2D 1209 (N.J. 1985)

• • •

The nephew and guardian of incompetent nursing home resident, Ms. Conroy, petitioned the Court to remove her nasogastric feeding tube. Ms. Conroy suffered from myriad conditions, and her physician felt that removal of the tube would hasten Ms. Conroy's eventual death. Ms. Conroy died, with the feeding tube intact, as the litigation was pending. The Supreme Court of New Jersey stated that if Ms. Conroy would have been competent to decline treatment, "[h]er interest in freedom from nonconsensual invasion of her bodily integrity would outweigh any state interest in preserving life or in safeguarding the integrity of the medical profession" (*Id.* at 1226). The Court noted that for incompetent patients, a subjective standard considering what the patient (if competent) would have wanted is the appropriate manner in which to make such decisions. The Court explained that when the formerly competent patient's wishes cannot be reliably determined, in rare circumstances it would be appropriate to withhold or withdraw life sustaining treatment if the benefits of removal outweigh the burdens.

In re Baby M

537 A.2D. 1227 (N.J. 1988)

• • •

Mr. Stern and Ms. Whitehead entered into a surrogacy contract in which Mr. Stern's sperm would be used to impregnate Ms. Whitehead. Upon delivering the child, Ms. Whitehead agreed to terminate any parental rights so that Ms. Stern (Mr. Stern's wife) could adopt the child. Mr. Whitehead (Ms. Whitehead's husband) agreed to rebut all presumptions of fatherhood. After delivering, Ms. Whitehead gave the baby to the Stern's temporarily, but then absconded with the child. The Supreme Court of New Jersey held that surrogacy contracts involving payment (such as this) were a violation of public policy. Further, the Court stated that Ms. Whitehead's parental rights would not be terminated as a result of the contract because surrogates had the right to change their minds and assert parental rights over the child in question. The Court noted that in this case the best interests of the child had to be considered, and awarded custody to Mr. Stern with visitation rights to Ms. Whitehead.

Cruzan v. Director, Missouri Department of Health

497 U.S. 261 (1990)

• • •

Nancy Cruzan entered a persistent vegetative state after sustaining injuries in an automobile accident and was supported by artificial nutrition and hydration. With the understanding that their daughter would never regain cognitive function, Nancy's parents petitioned the courts in Missouri to withdraw her artificial support. The Supreme Court of Missouri denied the Cruzan's request since they could not prove with clear and convincing evidence that Nancy would have wanted support withdrawn in such a circumstance. The U.S. Supreme Court reiterated the right of competent individuals to refuse medical treatment; however, the Court upheld Missouri's procedural requirement of meeting high evidentiary standards when incompetent's wishes are in question, based on the state's unqualified interest in preserving human life.

Davis v. Davis

842 S.W.2D 588 (TENN. 1992)

• • •

The case involved the disposition of seven cryogenically-preserved embryos subsequent to the divorce of Junior Lewis Davis and Mary Sue Davis. The embryos were stored at a fertility clinic, and were the combination of Mr. Davis' sperm and Mrs. Davis' ova. The only complication in the divorce proceeding was the disposition of the embryos: Mary Sue wanted to donate the embryos to a childless couple, Junior wanted to have the embryos destroyed. The Supreme Court of Tennessee concluded that embryos were neither "property" nor were they "persons," but instead occupied an interim category entitled to respect based on their potential for human life. The Court explained that if a prior contract concerning the embryo's disposition had been made, that it would have been valid in this situation. Absent a contract, the Court held that Tennessee's "interest in potential human life is insufficient to justify an infringement

on the gamete-providers' procreational autonomy" (*Id.* at 602). In a dispute between the procreational rights of two parties the Court stated that, in general, the party wishing to avoid procreation should prevail.

Johnson v. Calvert

851 P.2D 776 (CAL. 1993)

• • •

The Calverts entered into a surrogacy contract in which an embryo derived from their gametes was gestated by Ms. Johnson. Relations between the parties deteriorated, and Ms. Johnson demanded custody of the resulting child. The Supreme Court of California noted that under California law each child can only have one "natural" mother. Since there was no legislation specific to the issue, the Court ruled that the "natural" mother is the woman who "intended to procreate the child—that is, she who intended to bring about the birth of a child that she intended to raise as her own" (*Id.* at 500). Since the child would not have been born but for the Calverts' intention to have a child to raise as their own, Ms. Calvert was declared the "natural" mother.

Washington v. Glucksberg

521 U.S. 702 (1997)

• • •

The State of Washington prohibited assisted suicide, but specifically noted that withholding or withdrawing life-sustaining treatment was not suicide. Physicians, a non-profit organization, and terminally ill patients petitioned in federal court to have the statute declared an unconstitutional violation of their liberty interests protected by the Due Process clause of the Fourteenth Amendment. The U.S. Supreme Court held, "the 'right' to assistance in committing suicide is not a fundamental liberty interest protected by the Due Process Clause" (*Id.* at 727). The Court upheld the prohibition, because it was rationally related to Washington's interests in the preservation of human life, the public health problem of suicide prevention, protecting the integrity of the medical profession, protecting vulnerable populations, and avoiding a slippery slope toward euthanasia.

On the same day, the U.S. Supreme Court upheld New York's prohibition against assisted suicide in *Vacco v. Quill*, 521 U.S. 793 (1997). Physicians claimed that because New York permits refusal of life-sustaining treatment (which they saw as similar to physician-assisted suicide) the New York statute violated the Equal Protection clause of the Fourteenth Amendment. The U.S. Supreme Court maintained that there is a distinction between "letting a patient die and making that patient die" (*Id.* at 807); therefore it is consistent with the U.S. Constitution to treat the procedures differently.

COMPILED BY EMILY A. PETERSON

APPENDIX IV

ANNOTATED BIBLIOGRAPHY OF LITERATURE AND MEDICINE

This annotated bibliography focuses on literary works recognized for their portrayal of values issues in health care. It is not a bibliography of bioethics; the other essays in this encyclopedia provide bibliographies in those areas. Instead, this bibliography concentrates on stories, poems, plays, and essays that reveal conflicting values and differing perspectives in human interactions, especially under the pressure of illness and disability. Because literary works convey patients' stories as well as those of health care professionals and family members, they provide important resources for addressing issues in bioethics. This small selection makes no claim to being exhaustive; it is rather a sampling of significant works in literature and medicine. For a continuously growing online annotated bibliography of literature and medicine, see the Literature, Arts, and Medicine Database at <http://endeavor.med. nyu.edu/lit-med>.

General Essays, Memoirs, Stories of Cases

Broyard, Anatole. 1992. *Intoxicated by My Illness.* New York: Clarkson Potter 1992.

A literary critic and essayist thoughtfully observes his own experiences and feelings as he is dying. Several brilliant pieces comprise this work. Broyard writes about giving up his taste for irony. "Cancer cures you of irony. Perhaps my irony was all in my prostate." The work contains powerful and personal descriptions of his illness. He also portrays his personal physician and ponders what he would hope for in an ideal doctor. He closes with an abstract exploration of the meaning of death.

Coles, Robert. 1989. *The Call of Stories.* Boston: Houghton Mifflin Company.

This major work in literature and medicine contains clear arguments for the importance of stories in people's lives and in their health care. Coles sees patients as people who have stories and whose illnesses must be understood as parts of their life narratives. Learning from the great physician–writer William Carlos Williams, Coles understands that we need to respect each other's stories and learn from them.

Cousins, Norman. 1979. *Anatomy of an Illness.* New York: Norton.

This well-known autobiographical case history records how Cousins used humor and laughter to help cure his illness. Cousins checked himself out of the hospital and into a hotel room, where he ate better food, watched comedies, read jokes, and gave himself large doses of vitamin C. He attributes his returning health to the therapy of laughter, and to the capacity of the human mind and body to regenerate.

Davis, Cortney. 2001. *I Knew a Woman.* New York: Random House.

A nurse practitioner in an inner city Obstetrics & Gynecology clinic describes four of her women patients, from a fifteen-year-old homeless pregnant child to a mature woman struggling with cancer. Another of her patients is pregnant and drug addicted; a fourth suffers from pains that come from buried memories of sexual abuse. The stories of all four patients weave in and out of the narrator's own stories about herself, her own health and illness experiences, her own respectful appreciation of the female body.

Frank, Arthur. 1995. *The Wounded Storyteller.* Chicago: University of Chicago Press.

Frank argues that sick people are colonized by the health care profession, that takes over their bodies and their life stories. In order to heal, patients need to construct new narratives from the "narrative wreckage" of serious illness or injury. Frank describes three kinds of illness stories: (a) restitution narratives, where the patient returns to a previous state of health; (b) chaos narratives, where neither the patient (nor the health care professional) is in control; and (c) quest narratives, in which the patient understands his or her illness as a spiritual journey.

Gawande, Atul. 2002. *Complications: A Surgeon's Notes on an Imperfect Science.* New York: Henry Holt.

Written while Gawande was a resident in surgery, these essays explore many contemporary concerns about child abuse, informed consent, medical mistakes, chronic pain management—all grounded in stories about particular patients who are real people, not just reifications of disease and trauma. Gawande writes with wit and energy, gracing his penetrating insights with a tender humor.

Groopman, Jerome. 1997. *The Measure of our Days: New Beginnings at Life's End.* New York: Viking Press.

Groopman describes eight patients as they struggle with life-threatening illnesses and discover new understandings about themselves. More than medical cases, these narratives portray spiritual quests and new recognitions of what the patients have valued in their lives, sometimes bringing a dismayed awareness of mistakes and wrong turns, sometimes bringing peace and reconciliation. This articulate work also portrays a sensitive and caring physician.

Hilfiker, David. 1994. *Not All of Us Are Saints.* New York: Farrar, Straus & Giroux.

In the inner city of Washington, D.C., Dr. Hilfiker practices what he calls "poverty medicine." He devotes his time and skill to working with homeless men dying of AIDS. Most are African-American; many are addicted to drugs and alcohol as well as being sick with AIDS. Hilfiker encounters many uncomfortable differences between his white middle-class life and the poverty of the homeless dying men. His service to them goes beyond medical treatment.

Klass, Perri. 1987. *A Not Entirely Benign Procedure.* New York: G. P. Putnam.

This collection of autobiographical essays examines the experiences of a young woman in Harvard Medical School as she confronts the macho world of medicine. Originally published in *The New York Times* and other journals, these essays are often funny, always insightful, and sometimes troubling. Klass, who had a baby while she was at Harvard, records surprising discrepancies between what she was learning as a medical student and what she was experiencing as a

pregnant woman. She is especially aware of the power of language to label, dismiss, and silence people.

Kleinman, Arthur. 1988. *The Illness Narratives: Suffering, Healing and the Human Condition.* New York: Basic Books.

Kleinman explores the meanings of illness in a medical world that concentrates on the biological mechanisms of disease. The technical quest for control of symptoms overshadows and even prevents inquiry into multivocal meanings of the illness, to which powerful emotions and interests often are attached. Those meanings are bound up with the relationships of the patient with spouse, children, friends, caregivers, even the patient himself. Kleinman asserts that the multiple voices must be heard if the doctors are to deliver more effective and humane care.

Lorde, Audre. 1980. *The Cancer Journals.* Argyle, NY: Spinsters.

In this collection of journal entries, prose, and poetry, Audre Lorde ponders her breast cancer and mastectomy. As a lesbian and feminist, she is not interested in making her appearance attractive or even socially-acceptable to men, so she refuses reconstructive surgery or even wearing a prosthesis. She resists the culture that tries to hide the fact that a woman has had a mastectomy. She encourages women who have undergone that surgery to see themselves like Spartan warriors and to be proud of their scars. Her greatest comfort comes from supporting network of other women.

Lynch, Thomas. 1998. *The Undertaking: Life Studies from the Dismal Trade.* New York: Penguin.

This award-winning collection of essays describes Lynch's experiences and reflections on his career as an undertaker. Often finding humor and compassion in the funeral home environment, Lynch portrays the survivors as they try to deal with the death of friends and family. He recognizes the importance of rituals and community around the passage of death, and treats his subjects with a tenderness and wit that makes his writing thoroughly engaging.

Nuland, Sherwin. 1994. *How We Die: Reflections on Life's Final Chapter.* New York: Knopf .

Nuland believes that death is a normal biologic process, but Americans treat it as if it were an enemy to be fought off. Because so many deaths occur in hospitals, they are hidden from view and from public understanding, adding to fear of dying. Nuland writes that very few will "die with dignity." Physicians, patients, and families should allow nature to take its course instead of trying to do everything to keep someone alive. The "best" possible death reflects the hospice philosophy-it occurs in relative comfort, in the company of loved ones.

Remen, Rachel Naomi. 2000. *My Grandfather's Blessings.* New York: Riverhead Books.

Pediatrician and psychiatrist, Remen has a lifetime's experience working with cancer patients, others who are chronically or terminally ill and with those who are recovering from life-threatening illnesses. She discovers that many people, when forced deeply into their own vulnerability, transform their suffering into wisdom and appreciate their connections. They learn to serve and belong to one another, valuing authentic relationships.

Sacks, Oliver. 1984. *A Leg to Stand On.* New York: Harper Collins.

This is one of many books Sacks has written about his medical practice. In this work, Sacks recounts his own injury, hospitalization and long recovery, including a bout with depression. As a physician, he has a kind of double perspective (patient, doctor). As a patient, he feels alienated and alone, and he comes to realize how important caring relationships are between health care professionals and their patients. As a physician, he comes to understand the suffering of his patients.

Sontag, Susan. 1978. *Illness as Metaphor.* New York: Farrar, Straus & Giroux.

This classic argument says that using metaphorical thinking to describe illness is wrong because it is untruthful and misleading. Metaphors deny the direct approach, Sontag argues, and often lead to blaming the patient for contracting the disease. Cancer patients may be seen as life's losers with character flaws that cause the disease. Cancer invades and destroys, requiring an arsenal of weapons to fight it; military metaphors take over and the patient becomes the battleground.

Verghese, Abraham. 1994. *My Own Country: A Doctor's Story of a Town and Its People in the Age of AIDS.* Simon and Schuster.

Verghese is an Indian physician, born in Ethiopia and now practicing in America. In this collection, he describes caring for men and women with HIV/AIDS who have come home to their Tennessee families to die. He comes to understand rural people as they grapple with the realization that their sons are gay and are dying. He treats a woman infected by her husband (whose sister has also been infected by him) as they struggle to keep their condition private. He

tries to explain to his wife and his colleagues why he is caring for these AIDS patients.

Novels

Barker, Pat. 1991. *Regeneration.* London: Penguin.

During World War I, The English poets Sigfried Sassoon and Wilfred Owen met when both were patients in Craiglockhart War Hospital where they were under the care of Dr. W. Rivers. This powerful anti-war novel describes their resistance to the war, the "shell shocked" soldiers exposed to too many horrors, the efforts of Dr. Rivers to give them genuine healing through conversation about the origins of their ailments. Wilfred Owen wrote deeply moving poetry about the experiences of the common soldier [see entry in this bibliography]. He was killed a week before Armistice.

Bronte, Charlotte. 1983 (1847). *Jane Eyre.* New York: Bantum.

In this famous nineteenth century Gothic novel, Jane Eyre survives a typhus epidemic to be a governess for Rochester's illegitimate daughter. Jane sometimes hears weird laughter and odd noises. One night she finds Rochester unconscious in his bed that had been set on fire. Jane agrees to marry him, but at the wedding a man claims that Rochester is already married. His insane Creole wife is imprisoned on the third floor of the house. In her madness she finally burns down the house, blinding Rochester as he tries unsuccessfully to save her.

Camus, Albert. 1947. *The Plague.* Paris: Gallimard.

This great novel compares the bubonic plague and subsequent quarantine in Oran, Algeria, to other forms of occupation by war and colonization. Dr. Rieux, having just sent his wife to a sanitarium for her health, discovers dying rats as the city begins its nearly year-long struggle with plague. The novel explores many issues of isolation, of religious faith in times of great suffering, of the physician's commitment to providing health care at the continuing risk to his own life, of the public health efforts to defend against the invader.

Dickens, Charles. 1998 (1851). *The Old Curiosity Shop.* New York: Oxford.

Dickens's fourth novel mixes social realism and romance. Little Nell is forced to grow up quickly as she tries to manage her mentally ill grandfather's manipulative and destructive behavior. Characters often are physically distorted—a condition resulting from the industrial revolution. Through these characters, Dickens connects physical deformity and moral deformity. Little Nell is a golden haired beauty, as good as she is lovely. Quilp's misshapen body mirrors his depraved moral state, and Nell's physical wasting results from the moral disease of Victorian society.

Dostoevsky, Fyodor. 1960 (1864). *Notes from Underground.* New York: E. P. Dutton.

Exploiting the tensions between individual freedom and determinism, between atheism and belief in God, between faith in progress and human limitations, Dostoevsky portrays the contradictions that besiege modern humanity. As a religious philosopher, he sees man as fallen but free to choose; as a political historian he sees the West as fallen and in need of redemption; as a psychologist, he explores the problems of isolated and alienated people, driven by passions and capable of inspiration yet critical of utopian optimism. His protagonists can be vile and willfully disgusting, but they assert their freedom to be that way in the face of biological and social determinism.

Ellison, Ralph. 1972 (1952). *Invisible Man.* New York: Random House.

Combining brutal realism of a racist society with a surreal dreamy interior consciousness of his protagonist, Ellison portrays the invisibility of those who are seen only as stereotypes, never as real individuals. Trying to find his identity in this context, the unnamed protagonist naively expects to make it, but is continually expelled and rejected, confused and disillusioned. Mental hospital staff submit him to shock treatments and decide he is cured when he (they mistakenly believe) can no longer remember his name. He ends up living under a New York City manhole. The novel won the National Book Award in 1953.

Faulkner, William. 1987 (1930). *As I Lay Dying.* New York: Vintage.

This novel of grotesque humor follows a poor white family as it carries the mother's casket through hell and high water (literally) trying to keep the promise to bury her in her native town. This archetypal journey takes several days, so the decomposing body stinks. Trying to save the casket from being swept away in a flooded river, Cash, the eldest son, breaks a leg and so is forced to lie on top of the casket as the rickety wagon slowly lumbers along. Old Doc Peabody

eventually has to chip off the concrete the family poured on Cash's leg, so the leg can be set and cast. The profoundly dysfunctional family buries the mother and then picks up a new one on the way out of town.

Flaubert, Gustave. 1965 (1857). *Madame Bovary.* New York: W. W. Norton 1965.

In this great realist novel, the peasant Emma marries an elderly, bumbling doctor, Charles Bovary, who soon bores her. Neither of her inevitable love affairs work out, and since she cannot pay her debts or get anyone to help her, she commits suicide by swallowing arsenic. Flaubert tells this story in a detached, objective voice that makes no judgments but allows for a sense of inexorable determinism that will defeat anyone trying to escape the base and tedious everyday life.

Gaines, Ernest. 1993. *A Lesson Before Dying.* New York: Random House.

An inarticulate young black man, witness to his friends' murder of a white man, is convicted of murder himself and sentenced to death by an all white jury and judge. The narrator of this sensitive novel, a frustrated white school teacher, provides the condemned man with a way to express his feelings and thoughts about his confrontation with death. Both men grow as their relationship develops into empathy and caring, overcoming racial barriers, at least between the two of them.

Garcia Marquez, Gabriel. 1988. *Love in the Time of Cholera.* New York: Penguin.

Winner of the Nobel Prize for literature, Garcia Marquez is known for his "magic realism," in which brutally realistic events are interspersed with the fantastic and surrealistic, angels fall into pigsties, dead men live in their caskets for years, giant bodies wash up on the beach without showing any signs of decay. His stories reveal Latin American sociopolitical history while they express the symbolism and archetypes of folktale. In this novel, a complicated marriage between a woman and doctor lasts over fifty years, through cholera epidemics and political and personal turmoil. When the doctor dies, his wife reunites with an aged friend who has loved her since before she met the doctor.

Hurston, Zora Neal. 1990 (1937). *Their Eyes Were Watching God.* New York: Harper & Row.

Anthropologist Hurston creates a strong, determined African-American heroine who survives poverty and loveless marriages in which her husbands treated her like property. Finally free of them, she falls in love with a man who treats her as an equal partner; they work together on truck farms until he is bitten by a rabid dog. She cares for him, even though he becomes antagonistic, until he dies of rabies. She is at peace with herself at the end, having come to terms with life.

Huxley, Aldous. 1989 (1932). *Brave New World.* **New York: Harper.**

In this early version of genetic engineering, people are created in test tubes and chemically manipulated and conditioned to fill certain classes and roles. Henry Ford, the lord of mass production, has replaced God. Drugs keep the population happy, free sex replaces marriage and the family, everyone buys stuff whether they need it or not. The World Controller explains why keeping people contented is better than allowing them to think for themselves.

James, William. 1992 (1898). *The Turn of the Screw.* **New York: Oxford University Press.**

This ghost story can also be read as the hysterical writing of a mentally ill governess who "experiences" evil spirits haunting the two children she cares for. One spirit comes from a former governess who probably was pregnant and who died mysteriously (from suicide or from trying to abort the pregnancy?). The other spirit belongs to a valet who was killed in a fall. Suggestions of child abuse and other horrors come through the obsessions of the narrator.

Joyce, James. 1964 (1916). *Portrait of the Artist as a Young Man.* **New York: Viking Press.**

This famous pedagogical novel follows Stephen Dedalus from his infancy to young adulthood, from his father's storytelling to Aquinas' aesthetics. It also portrays the development of an artist growing up with an alcoholic father in an Ireland depressed both by English colonization and Catholic domination. The young man Stephen refuses to serve his home, his country or his church, determined to escape those nets by going into exile.

Kafka, Franz. 1972 (1915). *Metamorphosis,* **trans. Stanley Corngold.**

Mixing the ordinary and the surreal, Kafka takes everyday people and events and converts them to nightmare. Feeling trapped in a boring, mechanical job he had to support his family, Gregor Samsa wakes up one morning to find himself transformed into a giant cockroach. His sense of being metaphorically stepped on turns into fact. His family reacts with shock that evolves into shame and resentment; as his beetle self dries up and dies, they actively start supporting themselves. As his carcass gets dumped in the trash, they go off on a family vacation.

Lewis, Sinclair. 1925. *Arrowsmith.* **New York: Harcourt Brace.**

Martin Arrowsmith confronts the temptations and complexities typical of the medical professional: pure research vs. research for profit; public health vs. business interests; care for patients vs. laboratory research; individual standards vs. institutional demands; service to others vs. greed and power grabbing. Lewis satirizes many aspects of medicine, from the training in medical schools to the practice both in small towns and big cities. In the end, after being entangled in most of these conflicts, Arrowsmith decides to devote his life to research, where he can meet his standards of intellectual honesty.

Mann, Thomas. 1927 (1924). *The Magic Mountain.* **New York: Knopf.**

The protagonist, Hans, goes to visit a cousin in a tuberculosis sanitarium and remains there for seven years, struggling with his own critical illness and near death experiences while learning gradually through that suffering what is worth valuing. In addition to falling in love with a married woman who is also a patient in the TB sanitarium, Hans engages in challenging intellectual discussions with other patients about life and death, religion and politics. The beginning of the First World War brings an end to this retreat from the real world.

Maugham, Somerset. 1992 (1915). *Of Human Bondage.* **New York: Penguin.**

The orphaned Philip, who has a club foot, is sent away to boarding school where he struggles to grow up with children who are not crippled and who have parents to care for them. As he grows up, he tries awkwardly and often unsuccessfully to find fulfilling relationships with other people, especially women. After seeking possible careers in languages and art, Philip decides to take medical training to become a physician like his father.

Morrison, Toni. 1974. *Sula.* **New York: Alfred A. Knopf.**

This novel explores friendship between two African-American women—conventional nurturer (Nel) and a free spirit (Sula)—as they adjust to and rebel against their community and their families. Characters in this black rural town include the mentally-ill Shadrack, who creates National Suicide Day; drug-addicted Plum, whose mother burns him to death; Eva, Sula's grandmother, who lets a train run over her leg so she can collect insurance money and support her family. Sula and Nel, as young girls, accidentally cause Chicken Little's death, but they keep that dreadful secret to themselves.

Ondaatje, Michael. 1992. *The English Patient.* **New York: Random House.**

Near the end of World War II, four people retreat to an abandoned villa north of Florence: nurse Hana cares for the severely burned, dying English patient whose identity is unknown; Kip, a Sikh bomb-disposal expert, becomes Hana's lover; Caravaggio, a drug addicted friend of Hana's family, steals from her supply of morphine she uses to help the English patient. This award-winning novel explores the need for reaching across barriers of religion, race and nationality; both Caravaggio and the English patient have crossed boundaries as spies. The lyrical narrative moves in and out of the characters' memories as well as through chronological time.

Ozick, Cynthia. 1990. *The Shawl.* **New York: Random House.**

Holocaust survivor, Rosa, lives in a squalid one-room apartment in Miami, trying to endure day-to-day as she lives with her nightmare memories of the concentration camp. Rosa hid her baby daughter in a shawl, but her niece, Stella, took the shawl for herself. Rosa helplessly watched as a German camp guard threw her daughter against the electric barbed-wire fence. Now, decades later, Rosa talks to her dead child. An acquaintance she meets in a laundry tries to connect her to living in the present and caring about her own future.

Pasternak, Boris. 1958. *Doctor Zhivago.* **New York: Pantheon.**

This sprawling novel follows Dr. Zhivago as the Russian revolution spreads over the country. In his medical practice and in his poetry writing, the doctor is devoted to the imagination and intuition, so he earns the distrust of the Bolshevik dogmatists, and escapes with his family to a Ural mountain farm. His sensory appreciation of beauty attracts him to his lover, Lara, and to the mountains; his sense of justice makes him sympathetic with the peasants and those hurt by the war. His values are much larger and more humane than those driving the revolution.

Percy, Walker. 1980. *The Second Coming.* **New York: Farrar Straus & Giroux.**

A disillusioned retired lawyer, Will Barrett, struggles with his memories of his father's attempt to kill him and his father's suicide. Will finds everyone in his present world to be inauthentic and shallow; his depression is deepened by the materialistic values of his affluent society and by the false, superficial faith of the organized church. Meanwhile a mentally ill young woman, Allison, has escaped from a mental hospital and is living in a greenhouse when Will meets her. Allison loves the natural world and growing things. Her freshness and love of life heal Will; and she is healed by his love. The Second Coming refers to God's coming into their love.

Plath, Sylvia. 1981 (1963). *The Bell Jar.* **New York: Bantam.**

The novel draws on Plath's own experience with mental illness, with a suicide attempt and the following institutionalization in McLean psychiatric hospital. The protagonist, Esther, goes through shock therapy and develops a special relationship with her doctor. The Bell Jar refers metaphorically to being trapped inside a glass jar of depression. Esther gradually improves and is ready to leave McLean by the end of the novel. Plath herself, however, committed suicide the same year this book was published.

Shelley, Mary. 1992 (1918). *Frankenstein.* **London: Penguin.**

This classic novel examines what happens when a proud scientist steps over a line between the mortal and the divine and tries to create life himself. Dr. Frankenstein's creation is an ugly monster, yet one who wants to be loved and accepted. Finding only rejection, the creature turns malicious and murderous. He has no chance to learn civilized values or moral sensibility. Trying perhaps to take responsibility for his creation, Dr. Frankenstein pursues the monster at the cost of his own life.

Shem, Samuel [Stephen Bergman]. 1995 (1978). *House of God.* **New York: Dell.**

This irreverent and very popular novel satirizes the education and training of medical students and residents. The "House of God" refers to Beth Israel Hospital in Boston. The residents learn cynical definitions (GOMERS are elderly people who should Get Out of My Emergency Room) and laws (turf unpleasant patients to someone else's responsibility). Exhaustion and cynicism erode the ideal of the "caring" physician. Powerful physicians abuse those lower on the scale; patients get ignored. Still the comic perspective of the novel helps the medicine go down.

Solzhenitsyn, Alexander. 1968. *Cancer Ward*. New York: Dial.

The world of the dying is portrayed through the differing perspectives of thirteen patients brought together in the cancer ward where they suffer both their illnesses and the inflexible medical system. Most undergo radiation therapy though not many benefit from it. The ward becomes a metaphor for the totalitarian Soviet state afflicted by symbolic cancer that eats away at it vitality. The novel also explores the value of individual life in a culture that insists on the collective.

Tolstoy, Leo. 1935 (1886). *The Death of Ivan Ilyich*. London: Oxford University Press

This short novel is probably *the* most frequently taught work in the literature and medicine "canon." The work satirizes the tedium of everyday life, the chasing after trivial acquisitions, the hypocrisy of doctors and family, while their unexamined lives plod along. At the same time, Ilyich starts questioning his way of life when he confronts his own dying, and in that confrontation he resembles all humanity. The only honest person around him is the peasant servant, Gerasim, who helps Ilyich face the reality of death.

Drama

Albee, Edward. 1994. *Three Tall Women*. New York: Dutton.

Three women meet in a sick room. A frail, cranky old woman is in bed, her compassionate caregiver is middle-aged, and an impatient young woman comes to solve some financial problems. They discuss A's aging and the highlights of her life. At the end of the first act, the old woman has a stroke. In the second act, she is replaced by a dummy in the bed, and the three, all of whom turn out to be the same person at different times in her life, discuss with some humor and forgiveness how the young one evolved into the middle aged one and then into the elderly woman.

Beckett, Samuel. 1959. *Krapp's Last Tape*. London: Faber and Faber.

Nobel Laureate Beckett created several great tragicomedies, adapting music hall slapstick to tragedy in order to help his audiences laugh at our human condition. In this play, the clown-like Krapp is an old man, alone with his tape recorded commentaries made at earlier times in his life. As he listens to various earlier "selves" describing work or love or belief, he realizes he is not the same person he used to be. The dialogue between his past (on tape) and his present self helps him recognize that death is near, that he is through with former goals as he experiences a sense of loss and an uncertainty about his identity.

Chekhov, Anton. 1988 (1899). *Uncle Vanya*. London: Metheun.

Uncle Vanya is caretaker of an estate where his brother-in-law comes to live with his young wife, Yelena. The local doctor, Astrov, comes to treat the brother-in-law's gout and falls in love with Yelena. He is a good physician, but his love for Yelena is hopeless, and he consoles himself with alcohol. Like many of Chekhov's doctors, he has become disillusioned and alienated.

Coburn, D.L. 1977. *The Gin Game*. New York: French.

This prize winning tragicomedy takes place on the back porch of a charity nursing home where two patients, Fonsia and Weller, play gin rummy and talk about their lives. Both comment on the problems of trying to live in such a place, where the staff steal things, the food makes people sick, most patients are drugged and strapped in their wheelchairs. Both deny some truths about themselves that gradually emerge and the gin game gets more and more serious, Fonsia keeps winning without trying, and Weller gets furious.

Edson, Margaret. 1999. *Wit*. New York: Faber and Faber.

Winner of the Pulitzer Prize, this play opens with Vivian Bearing, a scholar of Donne's Holy Sonnets, being diagnosed with terminal ovarian cancer. She agrees to become a research subject, and tackles her full-dose chemotherapy with the same toughness and discipline she brought to her scholarship. Her doctors see her as research subject rather than a vulnerable patient; they have a very remote bedside manner. Vivian learns that she does want some compassion, some human sympathy, which Susie, her nurse, does give her. The play raises important issues about death and dying and about the complex mix of research and patient care.

Ibsen, Henrik. 1951 (1882). *An Enemy of the People*. New York: Viking Press.

When a scientist becomes a "whistle blower," warning of serious danger to public health in contaminated water supply, he discovers he is detested rather than thanked. Several vested interests make money on the system the way it is. They have the power to make him an outcast by turning the majority against him. The dynamic tension lies between an individual who knows he has the truth and the great majority that is wrong. In a democratic society, should the majority always rule?

Kopit, Arthur. 1978. *Wings.* New York: Hill and Wang.

This play opens inside the mind of a woman suffering a stroke, with confusions, disconnections, fragmented pieces of language and gibberish. At the same time, the caregivers are speaking normal language, though it sounds like nonsense to her. Later, in therapy, she hears a recording of herself and realizes she is speaking nonsense (though in her head she makes sense to herself). As she gradually improves through therapy, she connects again to her history, her identity.

Kushner, Tony. 1993 and 1994. *Angels in America. Part One: Millennium Approaches; Part Two: Perestroika.* New York: Theater Communication Group.

These plays both won Pulitzer Prizes. Grounded in American politics and its struggles with racism, anti-Semitism, homophobia, sexism, the play follows two men suffering with AIDS. One, a fictional version of the McCarthy lawyer Roy Cohn, denies he has the disease because he has power and influence (which, he says, gay men cannot have). The second sick man, Prior, has been selected by an Angel to be the next Prophet. Angel crashes through the ceiling at the end of Part One, and the audience has no choice but to accept this magical intrusion in a realistic play. Characters have to let go of their past and keep going even when they are suffering.

Marlowe, Christopher. 1959 (1588). *Doctor Faustus.* New York: Washington Square Press.

This classic play explores the timeless theme of a scholar wanting to know everything, to go beyond human boundaries, to have unlimited power because of that knowledge. So ambitious and prideful is Faustus that he is willing to sell his soul to the devil to gain that knowledge. Not only can he understand how the universe works; he can also call up Helen of Troy for his intellectual and sensual delight. The cost of this unlimited knowledge: Faustus is forever damned. A chorus warns at the end of the play that wise people will not try to "practice more than heavenly power permits."

McPherson, Scott. 1992. *Marvin's Room.* New York: Penguin: Plume.

Bessie, who has been caring for her invalid aunt and her father who is helpless after suffering a stroke, discovers she has leukemia. Bessie's sister, Lee, who has been out-of-touch for years, arrives with her two sons in the hopes that one of them might be a bone-marrow match for Bessie. Lee cannot stand the idea of devoting her life to caring for helpless aging relatives. She has plenty of trouble already trying to be a mother to her two sons, particularly Hank who has been committed to a mental hospital because he burned down the family home. While Bessie will die of leukemia, both Hank and Lee learn to care for each other and for the family.

Miller, Arthur. 1949. *Death of a Salesman.* New York: Viking Penguin.

Willy Loman, who used to have a somewhat successful career as a salesman, now finds himself depressed, without prospects, getting older and out-of-step with his contemporaries. He has lived on his dreams of making it, and has instilled the same kind of inflated assumptions in his son, Biff, who was once a high school football hero but is now a failure. Biff recognizes that his father has blown him full of hot air and that he's not a leader. Willy cannot take the deflation and commits suicide.

Molière, 1959 (c. 1666). *The Doctor in Spite of Himself.* New York: Viking.

This seventeenth century satire explains that even a woodcutter can set himself up as a physician and can practice medicine as effectively (or more so) than the trained professionals. The fake Latin jargon that the woodcutter spouts persuades the gullible patients that he knows what he is doing, and through a series of fortuitous events, he does manage to find out why the master's daughter has stopped talking. He then concludes that he likes this doctoring profession more than woodcutting and will probably make a career of it.

Nichols, Peter. 1967. *Joe Egg.* New York: Grove Press.

Joe Egg is a severely handicapped child, unable to talk or do anything for herself. Her parents, Bri and Sheila, make up personalities for her and invent little plays about all the reasons why their only child is a vegetable. The constant attention they must give Joe Egg means they cannot tend to each other's needs. Bri gets so desperate he actually tries to kill his child. In the end, the marriage cannot survive the relentless pressure of caregiving.

Pomerance, Bernard. 1979. *Elephant Man.* New York: Grove Press.

Severely deformed John Merrick is saved from being exhibited in a freak show by Dr. Treves, who admits him to his London hospital as a permanent patient. There Merrick becomes a favorite of the aristocracy, still on exhibit but to a different class. Based on the life of the real John Merrick, this play shows how the severely deformed can never be "normalized" even by those working hard to see past the deformity to the real person inside.

O' Neill, Eugene. 1956. *Long Day's Journey Into Night.* New Haven: Yale University Press.

This autobiographical play was written in 1941 but never produced until after O'Neill's death. The mother, Mary Tyrone, is a drug addict; the actor/father, James, is an alcoholic; the youngest brother, Edmund, is sick with tuberculosis; older brother, Jamie, who represents O'Neill, shows the marks of his own dissipation and cynicism. They struggle together with Mary's relapse into drugs, with the diagnosis of Edmund's TB, and James' refusal to spend money to send him to a private sanitarium.

Shaffer, Peter. 1975. *Equus.* New York: Avon Books.

A teenage boy has blinded several horses with a hoof pick. He comes under the care of the psychiatrist, Dysart, who gradually discovers that boy has mixed religion, sex, and horses into an orgiastic worship of his personal god, Equus. While Dysart knows he can help the boy, he envies the passion in the boy's worship and is reluctant to make him "normal," because that means taking away his worship. Without worship you shrink.

Shaw, George Bernard. 1946 (1908). *The Doctor's Dilemma.* New York: Penguin.

Four doctors gather in honor of their friend, Ridgeon, a research doctor who has his own theory of disease. A young Mrs. Dubechat asks Ridgeon to cure her husband of consumption. Ridgeon has only a limited amount of his special medicine, so he cannot treat all who come to him. Instead of curing the dishonest Mr. Dubechat, Ridgeon treats one of the doctors who also has consumption. Dubechat dies, which is convenient, since Ridgeon has fallen in love with Mrs. Dubechat. Shaw prefaced this play with an 88 page essay about medicine in England.

Shakespeare, William. 1948 (1606). *King Lear.* New York: Harcourt Brace Jovanovich.

The greatest of Shakespeare's tragedies, this play opens with the aged king giving up his kingdom, dividing it among his three daughters. Foolishly and willfully, he makes this a test of his daughters' love for him—whoever says she loves him the most will get the most land. Two older daughters lie but the youngest is honest. Lear reacts furiously, driving her out of the country. The demented old man finds himself unwanted and cast out by his older daughters. In the end the youngest daughter is murdered; Lear carries her in his arms in a heartbreaking final scene.

Sophocles. Oedipus at Colonus. 1982 (401 B.C.E.). New York: Viking Press.

The third play in the Theban trilogy (*Antigone* and *Oedipus the King* being the first two), the blind Oedipus, exiled from Thebes, goes to his birthplace near Athens. He is filthy, old, withered, his wild white hair flying in the wind. The prophesy many years before not only said Oedipus would kill his father and marry his mother; it also said he would die at Colonus and be a blessing to the Athenians who let him live among them. He manages to thwart Creon, who tries to trick him back to Thebes; he is reunited with his daughters/sisters; and dies/disappears at the prophesied secret spot.

Steinbeck, John. 1937. *Of Mice and Men.* New York: Viking Press.

Lennie, a large, very strong mentally retarded man, is buddies with George, who watches over Lennie as they move from one farm job to another during the depression. Both men long for a home—a little place where they could live off the fat of the land—but they have no money and have to move with the work. Lennie does not realize his own strength and often gets into trouble by misusing it. He accidentally kills a mouse and then a puppy and finally the wife of one of the farm bosses. To keep him from a life in prison, George shoots him in the head.

Vonnegut, Kurt. 1974. "Fortitude" in *Wampeters, Foma and Granfalloons.* New York: Dell.

Dr. Frankenstein has one patient: Sylvia Lovejoy. He has gradually replaced all her organs and limbs with mechanical devices that he runs from a large console. She is now just a head on top of a box, with lots of wires and tubes connecting her to the console. He also controls her moods, wakes her up, puts her to sleep. Sylvia raises questions about the quality of her life, and even tries to shoot herself, but her prosthetic arms have been constructed so as to prevent her from doing that. So she shoots Dr. Frankenstein instead. In the last scene both his head and hers are together, and they share all the artificial organs.

Williams, Tennessee. 1955. *Cat on a Hot Tin Roof.* **New York: New Directions.**

This tense drama opens with Big Daddy being brought back home from a hospital where he was diagnosed with terminal cancer. The doctor tells the family, but not Big Daddy. The two sons and their wives begin competing for his attention (and inheritance). Maggie tries to seduce her alcoholic husband Brick, who drowns his guilt about the death of his homosexual friend. Brick and Big Daddy drink and argue, each claiming the other isn't facing the truth ("a powerful odor of mendacity"). In the end Big Daddy makes Brick face his responsibility in his friend's death, Brick tells Big Daddy he's dying, and Maggie continues her seduction.

Short Stories

Borges, Jorge Luis. 1969. "The Immortals" in *The Aleph and Other Stories.* **New York: Dutton.**

The protagonist visits his gerontologist and learns that his doctor has a method of making people immortal. The doctor shows him a room where several heads are sitting on boxes with the rest of their bodies replaced by machinery. The narrator is terrified, changes his name, and moves away. This story stimulates interesting discussions about immortality research.

Canin, Ethan. 1988. "We Are Nighttime Travelers" in *The Emperor of the Air and Other Stories.* **Boston: Houghton Mifflin.**

An elderly, ill couple have been living with each other for a long time without any real physical or emotional contact. Frank, who spends most of his days at the aquarium reading poetry, knows he is near death. Francine finds scraps of romantic poems on the windowsills and fears an intruder. One night Frank, who has been leaving the romantic notes for his wife, takes Francine on a walk in the crystal snow and then kisses her in a rekindling of their love.

Doyle, Arthur Conan. 1893. *Round the Red Lamp.* **New York: Doubleday.**

This collection contains seventeen stories all dealing with physicians. Both Holmes and Dr. Watson use medical

methods of diagnosis to help them do their detective work. "The Doctors of Hoyland" is especially interesting in its dealing with sexism: a famous Dr. Smith, who moves into a town where Dr. Ripley has an established practice, turns out to be a woman. Dr. Ripley believes women cannot be doctors, that it is a biological and cultural impossibility. His belief changes when she treats his broken leg.

Forster, E.M. 1947. "Road to Colonus" in *Collected Tale of E.M. Forster.* **New York: Knopf .**

An aging Mr. Lucas and his unmarried daughter Ethel take a trip to Greece. At one place, he climbs into the hollow of a giant tree that has a spring bubbling out of it. In there he undergoes a kind of magical transformation and decides he will stay there the rest of his life. The family treats this behavior as demented, and forces him to go back to England. Later they learn that the old tree fell over the night they left, killing the people in the nearby inn. The story parallels Oedipus at Colonus, except that Mr. Lucas did not get to die in his sacred place.

Gaines, Ernest. 1963. "The Sky is Gray" in *Bloodline.* **New York: Doubleday.**

A child in rural Louisiana develops a toothache; he goes with his mother into Baton Rouge to find a dentist. The family is scrambling to survive, partly because the father is away in the army. The boy endures several racist experiences, from where he can sit on the bus to where he can eat in town, even to where he can get out of the freezing wind. His mother keeps urging him to be a man, well before most boys could consider such responsibility. The mother and son get some food and shelter from an unusual white couple who make arrangements for a different dentist to remove the boy's tooth.

Gilman, Charlotte Perkins. 1989 (1892). *The Yellow Wallpaper and Other Writings.* **New York: Bantam.**

This classic story in the literature and medicine canon is narrated by a young mother with a post-partum depression. Her patronizing physician–husband treats her like a child and forces her to take the Weir Mitchell "rest cure" and avoid all stimulation, even from books and writing. The narrator cannot stand the wallpaper in the room where she is kept, and gradually goes insane as she rips it off the wall. By the end she is crawling around the room through wallpaper scraps.

Hawthorne, Nathaniel. 1987. "Dr. Heidegger's Experiment" (1837); "The Birthmark" (1844); Rappaccini's Daughter" (1844) in *Selected Tales and Sketches.* New York: Penguin.

These three famous stories are cautionary tales, warning about scientist-researchers crossing ethical lines in their experiments on people. "The Birthmark," used by Leon Kass to open the deliberations of the President's Council on Bioethics, portrays a husband obsessed with removing a tiny birthmark on his wife's face. In his effort to make her perfect, to remove her flaw, he kills her. In Dr. Heidegger's experiment, he gives a "fountain of youth" elixir to four elderly friends who regress into their romantic youth, just for a few minutes. Then they age again, and feel worse for the contrasting experience.

Hemingway, Ernest. 1998. "Indian Camp" (1925); "Hills Like White Elephants" (1927); "God Rest You Merry, Gentlemen" (1925); "A Clean, Well-Lighted Place" (1926). *The Complete Short Stories of Ernest Hemingway.* New York: Charles Scribner.

"Indian Camp" is narrated by a boy who goes with his physician-father to an Indian camp where a woman is having trouble delivering her baby. The hubristic father performs a Caesarian with a jack-knife and fishing line without anesthesia; his pride get deflated when he realizes the woman's husband has slit his own throat in his anguish for her—all this in front of the doctor's young son. In "Hills Like White Elephants" a young couple argues over whether or not she should get an abortion. She wants the baby; he wants his freedom. "God Rest You Merry, Gentlemen" is a horrifying story of a teenager, terrified by his sexual awakening and believing sex was sinful, who requests a castration and tries to amputate his penis. The doctors are callous and incompetent. In "A Clean, Well-Lighted Place," depressed old men face the nothingness of darkness, the meaninglessness of life, the sense that there is no God ("our nada who art in nada, nada be thy name"). They want to stay up all night in a clean, well-lighted place so the nothingness is not so threatening.

Joyce, James. 1947 (1914). *Dubliners.* New York: Viking Press.

The first three of these stories are narrated by children, exposed to death, pederasty, and their own emotional turbulence. Young adults in the next few stories are trapped by the paralysis of Ireland, itself still dominated by England and the Catholic Church. In "Eveline," although the sailor promises her love and freedom, she is unable psychologically to break free from caring for her dominating father. In "Counterparts" an alcoholic father blunders at work, uses up his

money drinking, and comes home to beat his son. In the most famous of this collection, "The Dead," Gabriel moves from being full of himself to understanding that he really does not know his wife very well nor has he ever really been in love. He also realizes that his maiden aunts will die soon, and, like the snow falling all over Ireland, he is connected to all humanity, the living and the dead.

Lawrence, D. H. "Rocking Horse Winner"; "The Blind Man"; "The Prussian Officer" in *Selected Short Stories.* Cambridge, England: Cambridge University Press 1999.

Lawrence is best known for his penetrating psychological studies. In "Rocking Horse Winner," a boy is convinced that his mother would be happy if she had more money, so he frantically rides his rocking horse until he has a vision of the horse that will win the race. Then the gardener places the bet for him, and he wins every time; but his mother is never satisfied. The boy obsessively rocks himself to death. In "The Prussian Officer," a young peasant soldier engaged to be married becomes the unwilling victim of his officer's homosexual advances and kills him, with repercussions that lead to his own death.

Malamud, Bernard. 1997. "The Jewbird"; "Idiots First"; "In Retirement" in *Complete Stories.* New York: Robert Giroux.

Malamud treats difficult human problems with sensitivity and, sometimes, a little magic realism. In "Idiot's First," a desperate dying father tries to get his mentally retarded son on to a train. A devilish character, Ginzburg, appears in numerous locations trying to bring death before the father can get his son safely on his way. In "The Jewbird" an old, smelly talking crow arrives at a New York family's apartment and stays for a year, to the fury of the father and the benefit of the son. This fable-like story suggests problems aging relatives and their families have trying to live together. "In Retirement" describes a retired, widowed physician who develops a crush on a young woman in his apartment building and talks himself into believing they might have a relationship. She rejects him by throwing his torn up letter at him.

O'Connor, Flannery. 1971. *The Complete Stories.* New York: Farrar, Straus & Giroux.

Most of O'Connor's stories deal with "grotesques"—people who are physically and/or psychologically distorted—as they search for some kind of meaning in their lives. In "Good Country People," for instance, a large one-legged woman named Hulga thinks she is seducing an innocent Bible salesman, but he turns out to have pornographic cards and condoms in his hollow Bible, and he gleefully steals her glasses and her wooden leg. In "Revelation," Mrs. Turpin sits in a doctor's waiting room talking in a prejudiced, self-righteous way about "poor white trash, niggers," and others. A young woman with acne throws a book at her, tries to strangle her, and tells her to "go back to hell where you belong, you old warthog." When Mrs. Turpin demands of God what he means, she has a vision of poor white trash and blacks marching into heaven ahead of her.

Olsen, Tillie. 1961. "Tell Me a Riddle" in *Tell Me a Riddle*. New York: Dell.

An elderly woman develops cancer just at the time that she finally has raised all her children and has her house to herself. Her husband wants to move into a retirement village, but his wife just wants the peace and rhythm of home. They fight furiously. No one tells her she has cancer; instead they take her on one trip after another to see her children and grandchildren. She gets much sicker and is cared for in an apartment far from home by a grandchild who brings compassion and some real communication. The old couple holds hands in their sleep—a suggestion of reconciliation as she dies.

Ovid. 1955 (c. 15 b.c.e.). *Metamorphoses*. New York: Penguin.

Ovid's retelling of Greek and Roman myths combines such compelling narrative with beautiful writing that it has become a source for writers ever since. Beginning with the creation of the world and continuing to his own time, Ovid's stories tell of changes and transformations, often with great psychological suggestiveness. For instance, when the sculptor Pygmalion falls in love with his own statue, the goddess Venus changes it into a real woman. When Narcissus falls in love with his own reflection in the pool, he falls into it and drowns, transforming into the flower; and the poor nymph Echo, who loved Narcissus, fades away until nothing is left of her but her voice.

Poe, Edgar A. 1978. *Collected Works of Edgar Allen Poe*. Cambridge, MA: Harvard University Press.

Famous for his nightmare stories in gothic settings, Poe presents distorted characters in desperate situations. One of his most famous works, "The Tell Tale Heart," portrays a man so obsessed with the blind "evil" eye of his old neighbor that he kills him and buries him beneath the floorboards. When the police arrive to question him, the narrator hallucinates that he is hearing the old man's heart beating beneath the floor. Finally it gets so loud, he cannot stand it, and

confesses. In "Hop-Frog," the dwarf kept as a slave to entertain the king becomes so outraged at the king's brutal behavior that he concocts a way to burn him alive.

Selzer, Richard. 1998. *The Doctor Stories*. New York: Picador USA.

Selzer is one of the major physician–writers of the twentieth century. This collection brings together twenty-five of his stories, which have become part of the canon of literature and medicine. They include such classics as "Brute," "Imelda," "Mercy," and "Tube Feeding." Often the physician makes some kind of misjudgment or acts in a way he later regrets. In "Brute" an exhausted doctor, trying to control a drunk, unruly patient, sutures his earlobes to the bed so he has to hold still for stitches. Selzer's stories teach humility as well as respect for humanity.

Stevenson, Robert Louis. 1993 (1886). "The Strange Case of Dr. Jekyll and Mr. Hyde," in *Complete Stories*, Vol. 2. Edinburgh: Mainstream.

The classic story of the split personality or double presents Dr. Jekyll, who gives up medical practice for experimental research, and his alter-ego, Mr. Hyde, who is an evil man released from Dr. Jekyll when he has taken one of the research potions. Hyde kills a man, and Jekyll realizes that the only way he can prevent Hyde from killing others is to commit suicide, killing both personalities at the same time.

Walker, Alice. 1967. *In Love and Trouble*. Orlando, FL: Harcourt Brace Jovanovich.

This collection contains several powerful African-American tales, among them three stories often used in medical humanities: "To Hell with Dying," "Everyday Use," and "Strong Horse Tea." They present a view of health care that has nothing to do with hospitals or conventional medicine. Access to white people's doctors is not an option in "Strong Horse Tea." A wise old black woman knows the baby is dying, and sends the mother out to collect horse urine (not really for the baby, but to keep the mother occupied while the baby dies).

Williams, William Carlos. 1984. *The Doctor Stories*. New York: New Directions.

This is the most used collection of stories in the literature and medicine canon. Williams touches on many important themes: the addicted doctor in "Old Doc Rivers"; the physician who loses his temper and manhandles a terrified child in "The Use of Force"; the fatal misdiagnosis of a beloved child's infection in "Jean Beicke"; the simple reward of a sniff of snuff in "Ancient Gentility"; a close and respectful relationship with a mother in labor in "A Night in June"; a delight in helping an independent teenager clear up her acne in "The Girl with a Pimply Face." Williams' sensitivity to language and his great compassion for and interest in his fellow human beings enriches all his work.

Selected Books of Poetry

Selected individual poems of many major poets appear in the anthologies listed under Selected Anthologies of Literature and Medicine.

Abse, Dannie. 1977. *Collected Poems: 1948-1976.* London: Hutchinson.

Welsh physician–poet Dannie Abse's work often explores the world of medicine with the acute sensibility of one trained to observe in detail. Among his poems often used in medical humanities classes are "X-Ray," "Pathology of Colors," "Case History," "Carnal Knowledge."

Campo, Raphael. 1996. *What the Body Told.* Durham, NC: Duke University Press.

Physician-poet Campo devotes a section of this collection to poems about his clinical practice, often the horrors he faces: a twelve-year-old pregnant by her father; a three-year-old who has swallowed cocaine; a homeless man whose eyelids have frozen shut. Yet he meets these cases with compassion and a recognition of the common humanity he shares with them.

Coulehan, Jack. *The Knitted Glove,* 1991; *First Photographs of Heaven,*1994; *Medicine Stone: Poems,* 2002. Troy, ME: Nightshade Press.

Physician–poet Jack Coulehan writes sensitively and compassionately about his patients and their cultural contexts, whether he is treating Appalachian children for worms or seeking healing in a Native American dance. Coulehan also has several poems about Chekhov, the master physician-writer who set the standard for stories and drama.

Davis, Cortney. 1994. *The Body Flute.* East Hampton, MA: Adastra. 1997. *Details of Flesh.* Corvallis, OR: Calyx.

Nurse and writer Cortney Davis is talented both in poetry and prose. In these two collections of poems, she gives

vivid, sensual descriptions of nursing experiences, often identifying with her patients while enduring the mechanized hospital system. She has a special sensitivity to women and their illnesses.

Getsi, Lucia Cordell. 1992. *Intensive Care.* Minneapolis, MN: New Rivers Press.

As the poet's daughter, suffering from Guillain-Barre Syndrome, fights for her life, the mother suffers with her and surrounds her with love and support. These tough poems assert control over the chaos of illness. Getsi also notices the conditions of other patients. Many of the children with her daughter in the rehabilitation institute never see their mothers (who are dead, or abusive, or indifferent).

Gunn, Thom. 1992. *The Man with Night Sweats.* New York: Farrar Straus & Giroux.

These poems detail the many deaths from AIDS and the struggles of caregivers to try to be there through the dying process. Through the ravages of the plague, Gunn finds affirmation in love and compassion.

Hacker, Marilyn. 1994. *Winter Numbers.* New York: Norton.

A masterful sonnet sequence entitled "Cancer Winter" describes the author's experience with breast cancer, mastectomy, and return to health, but with concerns about disfigurement and its effect on her lover. She also compares her personal experience with universal tendencies: "My self-betraying body needs to grieve / at how hatreds metastasize."

Hall, Donald. 1998. *Without.* Boston: Houghton Mifflin.

The first half of this beautiful collection of poems traces the dying of Jane Kenyon, Hall's wife, from leukemia. At the center of the book, "Without" expresses his great loss at her death. The last half finds him struggling to deal with his grief, writing poem-letters to her with "news" about the family dog, Gus, and their friends' lives.

Lynch, Thomas. 1998. *Still Life in Milford.* New York: Norton.

Undertaker-poet Thomas Lynch has an Irishman's gift for storytelling and a tight control over his poetry. These poems range from laments to love poems. The are portraits of his home town, small enough that people know each other and suffer as a community when someone dies. As the funeral director in town, Lynch tends to the grieving survivors and keeps secrets the dead would probably not want revealed.

Olds, Sharon. 1992. *The Father.* New York: Alfred A. Knopf

These tough poems describe the poet sitting at her father's bedside as he is dying of cancer, dealing with disgusting smells, sounds and sights as his body disintegrates. But the poet's main struggle is with her own negative feelings about him: an alcoholic, divorced from her mother, not a warm or caring father.

Owen, Wilfred. 1986. *The Poems of Wilfred Owen,* ed. Jon Stallworthy. W. W. Norton.

The most important English poet of the First World War, Owen told the truth about the horror of war and its toll on the bodies and minds of young men. Many of his poems are classics, including "Arms and the Boy," "Dulce et Decorum Est," "Disabled," "Futility," "Mental Cases." Benjamin Britten selected Owen's poetry for his "War Requiem."

Shafer, Audrey. 2001. *Sleep Talker: Poems by a Doctor/ Mother.* Philadelphia, PA: Xlibris Corporation.

Physician and mother and poet, Audrey Shafer writes about how she balances and interweaves her medical career, her marriage and family, her writing. She explores the emotional experiences in all her contexts, sees her home life through the perspective of medicine and her medical career through the perspective of motherhood.

Stone, John. 1972. *The Smell of Matches.* Baton Rouge: Louisiana State University Press. 1980. *In All This Rain.* Baton Rouge: Louisiana State University Press. 1985. *Renaming the Streets.* Baton Rouge: Louisiana State University Press. 1998. *Where Water Begins: New Poems and Prose.* Baton Rouge: Louisiana State University Press.

Cardiologist and poet, John Stone set the standard for excellent poetry by doctor–poets. Many of his poems in these collections portray his experiences with patients, from his first heart surgery patient to a young teenager in labor. One of his most touching poems treat the difficult situation of having to tell family members a loved one has died. In his later work, he examines his own grieving process over the untimely death of his wife, including his sleep disorder.

Selected Anthologies of Literature and Medicine

Belli, Angela, and Coulehan, Jack, eds. 1998. *Blood and Bone: Poems by Physicians.* Iowa City: University of Iowa Press.

This anthology collects one hundred poems of contemporary physician–writers about their work in medicine. Many of today's most notable authors are included: John Stone, Jack Coulehan, Raphael Campo, Audrey Shafer, Marc Straus. The editors introduce the collection by discussing the connections between medicine and poetry: both require the ability to see and pay attention; the medical encounter is "the poetic act of…standing in the presence of suffering."

Chekhov, Anton. 2003. *Chekhov's Doctors,* ed. Jack Coulehan. Kent, OH: Kent State University Press.

Chekhov was a physician who made most of his living by writing. Of his hundreds of short stories, many focus on physicians. This collection gathers several excellent works, among them: "A Doctor's Visit," where a young doctor learns to empathize with his patient; "The Grasshopper," in which a doctor's devotion to science and his practice makes him a dull husband for his romantic wife who finds a lover; "Enemies," in which a doctor's own son has just died but he is called out on a medical emergency that turns out to be a hoax.

Davis, Cortney, and Schaefer, Judy, eds. 1995. *Between the Heartbeats: Poetry and Prose by Nurses.* Iowa City: University of Iowa Press.

This is the first major anthology devoted to the works of nurses who are also writers. The registered nurses in this anthology write honestly and thoughtfully about their experiences caring for patients. The collection helps to show that nurses' perspectives and understandings about health care are different from the physicians' and that those differences ought to be heard. Most, but not all, the nurses are women.

Donley, Carol, and Buckley, Sheryl, eds. 1996. *The Tyranny of the Normal: An Anthology.* Kent, OH: Kent State University Press.

This anthology collects stories and poems about physical disability. It opens with several critical essays that provide some theoretical approaches. The title comes from an essay by the literary critic, Leslie Fiedler, who finds people either rejecting disfigured "others" or trying to normalize them. "The Quasimodo Complex" is defined as a disfigured person's sense of his "otherness" through the reactions of people to him. The fictional sections of this collection focus on dwarfism, eating disorders, and physical disabilities caused by birth defects and accidents.

Donley, Carol, and Kohn, Martin, eds. 2002. *Recognitions: Doctors and Their Stories.* Kent, OH: Kent State University Press.

This anthology collects new works by physician–writers who have come to realize the struggle—sometimes tragic, sometimes triumphant, sometimes seemingly trivial—that is part of the calling to heal. Most of the essays and stories portray rewarding or educational experiences in the physician's life and work. The last piece in the collection is a parable by Richard Selzer. In it a dying patient lays hands on the physician in order to ease the doctor's suffering.

Haddad, Amy and Brown, K. H., eds. 1999. *The Arduous Touch: Women's Voices in Health Care.* West Lafayette, IN: Purdue University Press.

Contributors to this anthology are nurses, physicians, therapists, emergency room technologists, and many other women whose careers are in health care. Their essays, short stories, and poems are grouped into three categories: Power and Powerlessness, Vulnerability and Voice, Connection and Disconnection. Many also focus on issues in health care training when the women encounter experiences for the first time.

Kohn, Martin, Donley, Carol and Wear, Delese, eds. 1992. *Literature and Aging: An Anthology.* Kent, OH: Kent State University Press.

The editors have collected from well-known writers many poems, plays, and stories about aging, and have arranged them into four groups: aging and identity, aging and love, aging and the family, and aging and the community. The short plays include works by Edward Albee, Kurt Vonnegut, Harold Pinter, and Lady Gregory. Many major short story writers are included, such as Ernest Hemingway, Saul Bellow, Flannery O'Connor, Eudora Welty. Poets include Robert Frost, W.B. Yeats, Alice Walker, Anne Sexton.

Mukand, Jon, ed. 1994. *Articulations: The Body and Illness in Poetry.* Iowa City, IA: University of Iowa Press. [New edition of the original collection entitled *Sutured Words.*]

This seminal collection of twentieth-century American poetry gathers hundreds of poems on health care subjects, ranging from hospital experiences, death and dying experiences, views of physicians and nurses, views of families of ill patients, women's experiences, views of those with disabilities or mental illnesses, and social issues that impact health care. The anthology includes major writers, such as Anne Sexton, Sharon Olds, James Dickey, Langston Hughes, Lucille Clifton, Denise Levertov.

Reynolds, Richard, and Stone, John, eds. 2001. *On Doctoring: Stories, Poems and Essays,* 3rd edition. New York: Simon and Schuster.

This well-respected anthology is given to medical school students all across the country. It contains many of the "classic" stories and poems of the literature and medicine canon: poems from John Donne and John Keats to Raphael Campo and Jane Kenyon, stories from Anton Chekhov and William Carlos Williams to David Hilfiker and Ethan Canin. Each author is given a brief introduction.

Secundy, Marian Gray, ed. 1992. *Trials, Tribulations, and Celebrations: African-American Perspectives of Health, Aging and Loss.* Yarmouth, ME: Intercultural Press.

This anthology collects African-American poems, stories, and essays that describe the health care problems and experiences of black people, whose voices often are unheard or silenced. Included is Zora Neale Hurston's account of being forced into a utility closet in a white doctor's office so she would not be seen by white patients. The collection contains works by such well-known writers as Maya Angelou, Toni Cade Bambara, Gwendolyn Brooks, Langston Hughes, and Alice Walker.

Walker, Sue B., and Roffman, Rosaly D., eds. 1992. *Life on the Line: Selections on Words and Healing.* Mobile, AL: Negative Capability Press.

This huge collection of poems, stories, and essays is divided into sections that deal with Abuse, Death and Dying, Illness, Relationship, Memory, Ritual and Remedies, and an especially interesting group called "White Flags from the Silent Camp," a title taken from a Rita Dove poem.

BIBLIOGRAPHY

See the Literature, Arts, and Medicine Database at <http://endeavor. med.nyu.edu/lit-med/>.

FILM/VIDEO

DOCUMENTARIES

Best Boy. 1979. Ifex Films.

Mentally retarded man learns to make adjustments and move from his elderly parents' care to a sheltered home.

Complaints of a Dutiful Daughter. 1994. Women Make Movies.

Funny and compassionate story of Deborah Hoffman's mother suffering from Alzheimer's and eventually moving into a nursing home.

Dax's Case. 1985. Concern for Dying.

Severely burned man, who is blind and has lost most of his hands, asks to be allowed to die but his request is not granted. A classic conflict between patient autonomy and physician beneficence.

Death on Request. 1994. Fanlight Productions.

Euthanasia in the Netherlands. Man dying of ALS asks for euthanasia; his doctor comes to his home and complies with his wish.

On Our Own Terms. 2000. Public Affairs Television, Inc.

"Moyers on Dying in America"; four 90-minute parts. Efforts of patients and families to control pain and make end-of-life experiences better for all involved.

Strangers in Good Company. 1990. Touchstone.

Six elderly women have to find ways to survive when their bus breaks down in the wilderness. They learn from each other and help each other doing everything from catching frogs to making fish nets out of panty hose.

When Billy Broke His Head. 1994. Independent Television Service.

Brain damaged Billy tries hard to support himself, but like many others with disabilities, he finds himself discriminated against by the government and by institutions of culture. Good portraits of several politically active disabled people.

DRAMAS

Awakenings. 1990. Columbia Pictures.

Based on a story by Oliver Sacks, this film portrays a doctor using L-Dopa to awaken catatonic patients who were victims of encephalitis lethargica. Unfortunately his successes could not be permanent.

A Beautiful Mind. 2001. Universal Pictures.

A biography of Nobel Prize winning genius mathematician and his battle with schizophrenia, medication seeming both to control his illness and dilute his brilliance.

Born on the Fourth of July. 1989. MCA Universal.

The second of the Oliver Stone's Vietnam trilogy, this film follows an idealistic young soldier who comes home a paraplegic and depressed over his accidental killing of a fellow soldier.

Coming Home. 1978. MGM United Artists.

Marine sergeant comes back from Vietnam a paraplegic and tried to find ways to reconstruct his life. Inside the VA hospital he meets an old high school friend whose husband is serving overseas.

The Doctor. 1991. Touchstone Pictures.

Aggressive and remote surgeon becomes a patient himself, learning the hard way how a patient deserves some compassion and understanding.

The English Patient. 1996. Miramax.

A good film of the award-winning novel (see annotation under Ondaatje, Michael—Novels).

The Gin Game. 1984. Nederlander.

Jessica Tandy and Hume Cronyn play two combative residents of a nursing home (see annotation under Coburn, D.L.—Dramas).

Girl, Interrupted. 1999. Columbia Pictures.

An autobiographical story about a suicidal teenage girl admitted to McLean Hospital for the mentally ill in Boston. Also graphic portraits of other patients with eating disorders, depressions, and psychoses.

Lorenzo's Oil. 1992. MCA Home Video.

Parents take over the care of their child afflicted with a rare illness, dismissing conventional medical treatments and creating one of their own. The strains of caring for a critically ill child take their toll on the marriage.

Marvin's Room. 1996. Buena Vista Pictures.

(See annotations under McPherson, Scott—Dramas).

'Night, Mother. 1987. MCA Home Video.

A debate between a suicidal woman tired of her battle with chronic illness and her mother who tries unsuccessfully to persuade her to live.

One Flew Over the Cuckoo's Nest. 1997 (1975). 1997 Pioneer Entertainment.

A satirical film protesting coercive psychiatric treatment, shock therapy, and lobotomy, this film portrays sick and well patients, the later in the mental ward as an escape from the law or responsibilities.

Ordinary People. 1998 (1980). Paramount Home Video.

Family trying to deal with drowning death of one son, while his brother feels guilty about not being able to save him.

Rain Man. 1998 (1988). MGM Home Video.

A man expecting a big inheritance finds it is left to a brother he did not know existed. He discovers his brother is an autistic savant. The two travel together in a journey that undoes many of the prejudices and self-centeredness of the healthy one.

Regeneration (Behind the Lines). 1998. Artisan Entertainment.

A fine film of Pat Barker's historical fiction (see Barker, Pat—Novels).

What's Eating Gilbert Grape? 1993. Paramount Pictures.

A six hundred pound mother relies on her teenage son to take care of the family, including his brother who is mentally handicapped.

Whose Life Is It, Anyway? 1981. United Artists.

A sculptor becomes a quadriplegic because of an automobile accident. No longer able to use his hands creatively or to do anything for himself, he fights to be released from the hospital and taken off kidney dialysis so he can die.

Wit. 2001. HBO Home Video.

(See annotation under Edson, Margaret—Drama).

CAROL DONLEY

APPENDIX V

ACKNOWLEDGMENTS

Aging and the Aged: VI: Anti-Aging Interventions: Ethical and Social Issues

Support for the research reported in this entry comes from a research grant (1R01AGHG20916–01) from the National Institute on Aging and the National Human Genome Research Institute.

Biomedical Engineering

The author thanks Gerald M. Saidel of Case Western Reserve University's Biomedical Engineering Department for his contributions and comments on this article.

Death: I. Cultural Perspectives

Sections of this essay are based on Koenig and Davies (2003), by permission of the Institute of Medicine.

Deep Brain Stimulation

The author is indebted to my predecessor John C. Oakley who wrote "Electrical Stimulation of the Brain" for the 2nd edition of the *Encyclopedia of Bioethics.*

Embryo and Fetus: III. Embryonic Stem Cell Research

Work on this paper is roughly divided in two with John Harris taking responsibility for the section on ethical issues and Derek Morgan and Mary Ford for the one on legal and regulatory issues. Note that this paper draws on a number of previously published works, particularly Harris's "The Use of Human Embryonic Stem Cells in Research and Therapy" (a chapter in *A Companion to Genethics: Philosophy and the Genetic Revolution,* edited by Justine Burley and John Harris [Oxford: Basil Blackwell, 2002]) and Harris's "Stem Cells, Sex, and Procreation," an article to be published in *Cambridge Quarterly of Ethics.* Work on this paper was supported by a project grant from the European Commission for EUROSTEM under its "Quality of Life and Management of Living Resources" Programme, 2002.

Emotions

The author would like to thank Elisa Hurley for all her help in updating this article.

Fertility Control: II. Social and Ethical Issues

The author gratefully acknowledges contributions to an earlier edition of the *Encyclopedia* by Carole Joffe and Charles E. Curran.

Genetics and Human Behavior: I. Scientific and Research Issues

The author gratefully acknowledges the assistance of the National Science Foundation and NIH ELSI via a grant to AAAS-Hastings Center for support for his work in behavioral genetics.

Medical Ethics, History of Europe: Contemporary: IV. United Kingdom

With gratefully acknowledged advice from Richard Ashcroft and Kenneth Boyd.

Psychopharmacology

This work was supported, in part, by the National Institute of Mental Health grants MH49671, MH 43693, MH59101 and by the Department of Veterans Affairs.

Reproductive Technologies: III.
Fertility Drugs

Table entitled "Summary of Drugs Used to Stimulate Ovulation" used with permission of the New York State Task Force on Life and the Law. Published originally in the report, *Assisted Reproductive Technologies, Analysis and Recommendations for Public Policy* (1998).

Smoking

Research assistance by Rana Khalil.

INDEX

Page references to entire articles are in **boldface***. References to figures and tables are denoted by italics.*

American Physical Therapy
Association, 306
American Psychiatric Association (APA)
code of ethics, 1499
gender identity disorder (GID), 944,
946–947
Guidelines on Confidentiality, 496
homeless mentally ill, 1325
homosexuality, 1158–1159, 1163,
2436
sexual ethics, 2182, 2432
Task Force on Psychosurgery, 630
*See also Diagnostic and Statistical
Manual of Mental Disorders* (Ameri-
can Psychiatric Association)
American Psychoanalytic Association,
2182
American Psychological Association
deceptive studies, 2330
departmental subject pools, 2473
American Public Health Association,
2110, 2111, 2208
American Society for Bioethics and the
Humanities (ASBH)
*Core Competencies for Health Care
Ethics Consultation,* 843–846
creation of, 1535, 1536
American Society for Human Genetics,
1025
American Society for Reproductive Medi-
cine (ASRM), 964, 2272
American Society of Clinical
Oncology, 599
American Society of Gene Therapy, 1208
American Society of Human Genetics
Social Issues, 1023
American Society of Internal Medicine,
2023
American Society of Laboratory Animal
Practitioners, 2549
American Society of Nephrology (ASN),
651, 652
American Society of Reproductive Medi-
cine, 2283–2285, 2288–2289
Americans with Disabilities Act (ADA)
impaired professionals, 1235
long-term care, 1442
mental disabilities, 1777
overview, 668–672
rehabilitation, 2258, 2259
workplace accomodation, 408
*American Trucking Association v.
Whitman,* 787
American Veterinary Medicine Associa-
tion (AVMA), 2545, 2548, 2549
Americas, **1517–1552**
See also Latin America; Specific
countries
Amida, 1703
Am I My Parents' Keeper (Daniels), 1359
Amish Americans, 536

Amnesty International, 625
Amniocentesis, 855, 997, 1684
Amstad Report (Switzerland), 1629
Amsterdam College of Physicians, 1587
Amundsen, Darrel, 2552
AMWA (American Medical Women's
Association), 1748, 2588
Amygdalotomy, 2195, 2200
A.N. v. S.M., Sr., 2007
Anabaptists, 36
Analects, 509, 568
Anatman, 335–336
Anatomical study
animal experimentation, 166
Hinduism, 1147
history, 2498–2499
Anaximander, 572, 1213
Ancestors
African cultures, 2054
Confucianism and Daoism, 566,
568–569
Hinduism, 1144
India, 2079
pre-republican China, 1688
Ancient studies school of medicine, 1704
Ancient world
aging, views on, 109–110
contraception, 909
health and disease, concepts of,
1058–1059
medical ethics history, 1555–1582
medical prayers and oaths, 1488–1491
medicine as a profession, 1744
mental health, 1757–1758
Near East, 1659–1663
professional-patient relationship,
2133–2134
race, 2243
women healthcare professionals,
2584–2585
women's status, 2594
See also Egypt, ancient; Greece, ancient; Hebrews, ancient;
Mesopotamia; Persia; Rome, ancient
Anderson, Elizabeth Garrett, 2588
Anderson, Elizabeth S., 2293
Anderson, W. French, 1204, 1206
Andreae, Johann Valentin, 1061
Androcentrism
animal welfare, 192
environmental ethics, 765
feminism, 884
health and disease, concepts of, 1078
women's history, 2593
Anencephalic infants, 612, 1242, 1253
Anesthesia in animal research, 168
Anetzberger, Georgia, 53
Angels in America (Kushner), 1439
Anglican Church, 1916
Animal confinement, 2547
Animal husbandry, 449–455

Animal Intelligence (Romanes), 255
Animal Legal Defense Fund v. Espy, 182
*Animal Legal Defense Fund v.
Madigan,* 182
*Animal Legal Defense Fund v. Secretary of
Agriculture,* 182
Animal Liberation Front (ALF), 169
Animal Liberation (Singer), 169,
189, 190
Animal Machines (Harrison), 213
Animal magnetism, 152
Animal research, **166–183**
abolitionists, 174
aging process, 92, 94–97
antivivisection movement, 168–169,
1593, 1598
court cases, 182
defenses of, 172–174
Descartes, René, 1212
electrical stimulation of the brain, 630
embryo research, 713
exclusion of rats, mice and birds in
animal welfare regulations, 181
Germany, Austria and Switzerland,
1636–1637
history, 166–170, 254
human nature concepts, implications
of, 1218–1219
human research, as preliminary to,
2327
Jainism, 1340
laboratory animal veterinarians, 2546,
2548–2549
laws and policy, 178–182
Medical education, 1506
military testing, 171–172
objections to, 174–175
performance based standards, 181
philosophical issues, 170–178
protocol review, 181–182
psychosurgery, 2197–2198
reformers, 174–175
speciesism, 175–176
toxicity testing, 171
utilitarianism, 190–191, 194
Animal Research Act (Austria), 1636
*Animals' Rights Considered in Relation to
Social Progress* (Salt), 169
Animal Welfare Act, 178–182, 2546
Animal welfare and rights, **183–215**
animal rights movement, 167–168,
190–192, 194, 198
Arab world, 1675
biocentrism, 759–762
confinement, harm of, 213
contractarianism, 187–188, 526–527
death, human views of, 577–578
deep ecology, 192–193
despotism, 186
direct duty views, 189–193
disease, 1079

• • • B

Department of Ethics and Legal Affairs, 1541

Canadian Nurses Association (CNA), 1541

Cancer
artificial nutrition and hydration, 231
caregivers, 636
children, 345–347
diagnosis and treatment, **341–349**
ecogenetics, 967
familial ademomatous polyposis (FAP), 1027
fertility drugs, 2274
genetic counseling, 953–954
informal resources, 347–348
laetrile, 155, 161
models of care, 343–345
oncologists, 341–342, 347
oral contraceptives, 893
penile, 422
physician/patient relationship, 341–342, 343–345
radiation exposure, 777
remission *vs.* cure, 342
toxins, 777–778
warfare metaphor, 1835–1836
withholding food and water, 232

Cangiamilla, Francesco Emmanuel, 2137

Cannon, Ida, 2459

Cannon, Walter B., 741

Canon law
euthanasia, 1424
monastic medicine, 1570–1571

Canon of Medicine (Avicenna), 1666

Canterbury v. Spence, 1275, 1276, 1299–1300, 1307

Cantiollon, Richard, 2041

Capacity
autonomy, 246–247
competence, as distinct from, 1308
standards of, 490

Capital crimes, 625

Capital punishment. *See* Death penalty

Capitation payments, 1120, 1182, 1755

Caplan, Arthur L.
disease and health, concepts of, 308–309
embryos, moral status of, 311
medical research, obligation to participate in, 2344, 2373
required-request organ donation procedures, 1957–1958

Caplan, Bruce, 2257

Capron, Alexander Morgan, 1282

Captivity, animals in, 209–210

Caraka Samhitā
active killing, 1500
Ayurvedic medicine, 1681
death, 563
ethics of practice, 1146–1147
physicians' oath, 1489, 1682–1683

truth telling, 1501

Carbohydrate intolerance and oral contraception, 894

Carbon dioxide emissions, 427, 428, 788–789

Card, Claudia, 888

Cardiac assist devices. *See* Artificial hearts and cardiac assist devices

Cardiac research, 276

Cardiac transplantation, 608

Cardinal virtues, 815, 2554

Cardiopulmonary criteria for death determination, 616–617, 621

Cardiopulmonary resuscitation (CPR)
futility, 1720
nursing home care, 1451
practicing procedures on the newly deceased, 2016
presumed consent, 1417
public policy, 2235
See also Do not resuscitate (DNR) orders

Cardozo, Benjamin, 1281, 1307

Cards of Identity (Dennis), 990

CARE, 1226

Care, **349–374**
care of *vs.* care for, 362–363
children's welfare, 386–387
community responsibility for healthcare, 1102–1103
contemporary ethics, 367–372
defining, 365
Erikson, Erik, 355–356
feminism, 886–887, 889
Goethe's portrayal, 352
healthcare and the ethic of care, 361–366
history of notion, 349–359
infants, moral status of, 1249
Judaism, 1350
May, Rollo, 355
nursing, 370–371, 1901–1902, 1908, 1910–1911
privacy and confidentiality, 497
professional-patient relationship, 2155
social-compact model, 829–830
theories of, 300

Care ACT (Germany), 1632

Care and Protection of Beth, In re, 1262

Caregivers
abuse, 54–55
Alzheimer's disease, 636
burden of caregiving, 1455
cancer, 636
compassionate love, 483–488
compensation, 1447
exploitation, 887
home care, 1454–1456
women, 881–882, 886–887

Care of souls tradition, 350–352, 353

"The Care of the Patient" (Peabody), 363

Carey v. Population Services International, 915

Caring: A Feminine Approach to Ethics and Moral Education (Noddings), 799

Carnap, Rudolf, 2397

Caro, Joseph, 582–583

The Carolina (Holy Roman Empire statute), 1240

Carper, Barbara, 365–366, 1911

Carpozof, Benedict, 1240

Carrel, Alexis, 1944

Carrier screening, 1009–1010

Carr-Saunders, Alexander, 2043

Carse, Alisa L., 296

Carson, Rachel, 769, 966, 1044

Carter-Pokras, Olivia, 287

Cartwright, Samuel, 1847

Case control design, 2330

Case management, home care, 1456

Case method in ethical analysis, 378–379, 436–437

Case narrative, 1876–1878

Case reports, 2330

Cases, Materials, and Problems in Bioethics and Law (Shapiro and Spece), 1374

Case series, 2330

Casey v. Lewis, 2110

Cassel, Christine, 105

Cassell, Eric, 1052–1053

Cassiodorus, 1569–1570

Caste system, 240, 867, 1143–1144, 1682–1683

Casti Connubii (Pius XI), 849, 2064, 2066

Castle, William E., 848

Castrated males, 859–860

Casualty insurance, 1124–1125

The Casuist (periodical), 378

Casuistry, **374–380**
bioethics education, 295
care of souls tradition, 351
clinical ethics, 436
clinical ethics consultation, 441
in communitarian consensus building, 482
conflicting moral principles, 283
defined, 374, 377, 378
ethical theory, 379–380
moral judgment, 2383
normative theory, 812, 822

Catastrophic Diseases: Who Decides What? (Katz and Capron), 1282

Catechism, 1176

Categorical imperative, 1916

Catholicism. *See* Roman Catholicism

Catholic University of Uruguay, Department of Bioethics, 1549

Causal inference, 2400

Causalism in medicine, 1062

Causation
disease, 310–311, 792, 1600

free will, 934
  homosexuality, 1157–1159
  mental illness, 1792–1793
Cavazano-Calvo, Marina, 1204
Ceauşeçlu, Nicolae, 2097
Celestial Master Daoism, 540
Cell fusion, cloning by, *450*
Cell nuclear replacement (CNR),
  726–727
Cell senescence/telomere theory of ag-
  ing, 96
Cell transplants, 1896
Celsus, 1559, 1561
Center for Bioethics, Tuskegee Univer-
  sity, 1535
Center for Bioethics, University of
  Turku, 1640
Center for Bioethics of the Clinical
  Research Institute of Montreal, 1542
Center for Biologics Evaluation and
  Research, 1206
Center for Biomedical Ethics Develop-
  ment (Indonesia), 1717
Center for Human Bioethics,
  Melbourne, 302
Center for Human Caring, University of
  Colorado, 1910
Center for Laboratory Animal Wel-
  fare, 171
Center for Medical Ethics, ASCOFAME,
  1549
Center for Medical Ethics, University of
  Oslo, 302, 1640, 1649
Center for Midwifery and Nursing Eth-
  ics, 301
Centers for Disease Control and
  Prevention
    bioterrorism, 2229
    HIV reporting, 123–124
    infectious diseases and immigrants,
      1230
    primary prevention in genetics, 1010
    tissue transplantation regulation, 2513
    xenotransplantation, 1957
Central and Eastern European Associa-
  tion of Bioethics, 1649
Central Conference of American Rabbis
  (CCAR), 1174
Central Ethics Committee (Turkey),
  1671
Central European biothics history,
  1644–1650
Central Intelligence Agency, 428
Centralized healthcare systems,
  1117–1118, 1121
Centre for Applied Philosophy and Pub-
  lic Ethics, 1554
Centre for Philosophy and Health Care
  of Swansea, Wales, 1649
Centre for Social Ethics and Policy,
  University of Wales, 1619

Centre Lémanique d' Ethique (Switzer-
  land), 1628
Centre of Medical Law and Ethics,
  King's College, 1619
*Centuries of Childhood: A Social History of
  Family Life* (Ariès), 381
CERCLA (Comprehensive Environmental
  Response, Compensation, and Liability
  Act), 785, 786, 1044, 1047
Cerebral death. *See* Brain death
Cerlera, 1982
Certificates of confidentiality, 2116
Certification. *See* Licensure and
  certification
Cervical cap, 898
Cervical mucus method of contracep-
  tion, 898
Cesarean section, 1468–1469, 1471,
  1475
Chadwick, Edwin
  health reform, 2207
  industrialism, health effects of, 2139
  social medicine, 2453, 2454
Chakras, 1685
Challenges to theories of human nature,
  1210–1211
Chamberlen, Peter, III, 2586
Chamie, Joseph, 2055
Chance and free will, 934
Chan Chingchung, 1704
Chang Dao-ling, 540
Changelings, 1239
Change of sexual orientation, 1160,
  1166–1167
"Changing Ecological Values in the 21st
  Century" (meeting), 1885
Chang Kao, 1691
Le Chapelier law (France), 1591
Chaplaincy, healthcare. *See* Pastoral care
  and healthcare chaplaincy
Character
  physicians', 1586–1588
  virtue and, **2550–2556**
Charismatic religions
  Christians, 332, 333
  healing power, 1053
  leaders, 236
Charity
  hospitals, 1831
  Islam, 1333
  medieval physicians, 1577–1578
  organizational ethics, 1941,
    1943–1944
  philanthropy and, 362–363
  physicians', 1596
  professional-patient relationship, 2135,
    2136
Charlemagne, 1185
Charles Sturt University, 1554
Charles V, 1240
Charles VIII, 2585

Charlesworth, Max, 1554
Chastity, 413, 2079, 2080–2081
Châtauneuf, Louis-François Benoiston de,
  1590
Chauliac, Guy de, 1579–1580
Cheating, doping as, 2461–2462
Chekhov, Anton, 1651
Chemical abortion, 2–3, 16, 19, 25
Chemical and biological weapons, 1845,
  2558, 2569–2574
Chemical Waste Management, Inc., 1048
Chemical Weapons Convention, 2570
Chemnitz, Martin, 862
Chemotherapy, 557
Cheng-i Daoism, 541
Cheng Yen, 512
Ch'en Shih-kung, 1492, 1692
Cherkasky, Martin, 2457
Chesler, Phyllis, 2173, 2432
Chevron U.S.A. Inc. v. Echazabal, 671
Ch'ien fang (Sun), 1690
Chikunov, Aleksandr N., 514, 515–516
Child Abuse Amendments, 1258
Child abuse and neglect
  loss of parental authority, 388
  overview, 43–47
  reporting, 498–499, 1824
  substance abuse by pregnant women,
    1480–1481
Child Abuse Prevention and Treatment
  Act, 44
Childbirth, 1963
Child care, 2580
Children, **380–402**
  African religions, 85
  assent, 346, 389, 553, 1310,
    2013–2014
  brain death determination, 604
  cadaveric gamete donation,
    2303–2304
  cancer, 345–347
  child labor, 383
  child protective services, 45–46
  as commodities, 464–465
  custody issues, 1481–1482,
    2279–2280, 2292–2293
  decision making authority, 388–389
  diagnosis and prognosis
    disclosure, 551
  divorce, effect of, 876–877
  firearm safety, 1155
  gamete donation, 2286–2287
  genetic testing, 2018
  harm and sex selected children,
    2270–2271
  healthcare, 387–399
  healthcare coverage, 1128
  healthcare resource allocation,
    394–398
  history of childhood, 380–384
  homicide, 1154–1155

United Kingdom healthcare, 1614
Erde, Edmund, 1839
Erikson, Erik
    adult caring, 355–356
    aging, 113
    human virtue, 801
    psychodynamic therapy, 1783
Erlenmeyer-Kimling, Nikki, 974
Ersta Institute for Health Care Ethics,
    1640
Ervin, Fran, 2199
Escobar, Alfonso Llano, 1549
Escuela Latinoamericana de Bioética,
    1549
Esmein, Adhémar, 862
Esotericism, 1052
Esposito, Elaine, 606
Esquirol, Jean, 2478
Essay Concerning Human Understanding
    (Locke), 383, 2206
Essay on the Principle of Population
    (Malthus), 2041–2042
Essenes, 579
Essential care in resource allocation, 1101
Essentialism
    genetic, 994–995
    homosexuality, 1163–1164
    sexual behavior theory, 2412
Estelle v. Gamble, 57, 2108–2109, 2110
Eternal life, 584–585
Eternal Recurrence of the Same, 576
Eternal Treblinka (Patterson), 1152
Ether, 2500
*Ethical and Policy Issues in International
    Research* (National Bioethics Advisory
    Commission), 135, 2349, 2353–2354
"Ethical and Religious Directives for
    Catholic Health Facilities" (United
    States Catholic Conference), 1495,
    1499–1500, 1527, 1541
The Ethical Basis of Medical Practice
    (Sperry), 1527
Ethical research committees (ERCS), 392
Ethical vegetarianism, 197–198
"An Ethic for Same-Sex Relationships"
    (Farley), 1176
Ethics, **795–841**
    behavior genetics, 978–984
    concepts, 796
    epidemiology, 2217–2218
    evolution and, **1200–1204**
    Freud, Sigmund, 2179
    managed care, 1466–1467
    moral epistemology, 802–811
    narrative, 1434
    nursing, 1911
    pediatrics, **2017–2019**
    professional-patient relationship,
        2150–2157
    psychosurgery, **2193–2197**
    religion and morality, 834–840

reproductive technologies, 2298–2305
    sex selective reproductive technologies,
        2268–2271
    social and political theories, 824–833
    task of, 795–802
    in vitro fertilization, 2307–2310
    See also Bioethics; Clinical ethics;
        Medical ethics
Ethics advisory bodies, 713–714, 924,
    2308–2309
"Ethics and Clinical Research" (Beecher),
    2321, 2323
*Ethics and the Regulation of Clinical
    Research* (Levine), 468
Ethics Committee Research Group
    (ECRG), University of Pennsylvania,
    841, 842, 844
Ethics committees, **841–847**
    Australia, 1554
    Belgium, 1610–1611
    chaplains' role, 1976
    clinical consultation, 440
    clinical ethics, 434, 435, 436
    Germany, Austria and Switzerland,
        1630
    health services managers, 1140
    infant critical care decisions,
        1262–1263
    institutional ethics committees,
        444–446
    Ireland, 1625–1626
    Japan, 1711
    Netherlands, 1611
    Nordic countries, 1639
    nurses, exclusion of, 445
    organizational ethics, 1942–1943
    policy formation and review, 842–843
    professional-patient ethical conflicts,
        2157
    self-education, 842
    social workers, 2460
    See also Institutional review boards
        (IRBs); Research ethics committees
        (RECs)
Ethics consultation, 439–443, **841–847,**
    2157
"Ethics Guidelines for Human Genome/
    Gene Analysis Research" (Japan), 1711
Ethics-inquiry model of nursing ethics
    education, 300
Ethics Institute, University of Iceland,
    1640
Ethics Manual, American College of
    Physicians (ACP), 1265–1266,
    1268–1269
Ethics of Medical Practice (Song), 1694
*Die Ethik des Arztes als medicinischer
    Lehrgegenstand* (Ziemssen), 1593
Ethik in der Medizin (periodical), 1629
Ethikzentrum (Germany), 1628
Ethnocentrism, 215, 1535, 1726–1730

Ethnography
    bioethics and, 1535, 1726
    patterns of resort, 1072–1073
    See also Anthropology; Cultural issues
Ethnomedical practices, 155, 554
    See also Traditional medicine
Ethnopsychiatry, 1801–1809
Etiological view of disease, 1076
Etiquette, medical
    ancient Greece and Rome, 1557
    Middle Ages, 1570, 1576–1577
    nursing, 1899
    Percival on, 1596
    Renaissance and Enlightenment,
        1586–15887
    Royal College of Physicians, 1555
    code, 1492
Etymologies (Isidore of Seville), 863
Etzioni, Amitai, 1905
Eucharist, 330–331
Eudaimonia, 1211–1212
Eudaimonism, 798
Eudemos (Aristotle), 573
Eugenical News, 2223
Eugenic Protection Law (Japan), 1708,
    1712
Eugenics, **848–870**
    birth control, 901, 903
    Christianity, 861–863
    enhancement, 980
    ethical issues, 853–858
    euthanasia, 1421, 1425, 1427–1429
    genetic discrimination, 957–958
    Hinduism and Buddhism, 866–869
    history, 848–853, 978–979, 987–988
    human cloning, 458–459
    intelligence quotient theory, 1214
    Islam, 865–866
    Japan, 1707
    Judaism, 859–861
    medical ethics history, 1533
    Norplant, 916
    policy, 979–984
    political issues, 979
    prenatal testing, 1001, 1002
    public health law, 2223–2225
    religious law, **859–870**
    Russian medical ethics, 1656–1657
    Sparta, 381
    state-sponsored program, 994
    sterilization, 904, 918–919
Eugenics: A Journal of Race Betterment,
    2223
Eugenics Record Office, 848, 849,
    2223–2224
Europe
    Christian bioethics, 403
    feminism, 2596–2597
    health insurance, 1122–1123
    hospital history, 1185–1186,
        1187–1190

race/ethnicity, 217–218, 290, **992–996**
reductionism, 1385
Russian medical ethics, 1656–1657
schizophrenia, 1804
social determinants, 1218
specific causation, 1012
traits, 309–310
undesirable characteristics, 904
violence, 857–858, 976, 2251–2252
xenotransplantation, 2603
See also DNA identification; Eugenics
Genetic testing and screening, **996–1028,** *999*
Alzheimer's disease, 637
autonomy, 1018
central and eastern Europe, 1648
children, 2018
confidentiality, 499
disability, 988
discrimination, 409, 956, 1019
Eastern Orthodox Christianity, 696
eugenics, 852, 856
family ethics, 881
genetic discrimination, 409, **956–959,** 1017, 1019
genetic selection, 1003
Germany, Austria and Switzerland, 1635
informed consent, 1018
Judaism, 861
newborns, 1004–1007, 2018
pathological genotypes, determining, 1011–1012
pediatric genetic testing, 1025–1027, 2018
population screening, 1007–1015
predictive genetic testing, 1020–1027
privacy, 1019, 1023–1024, 2121–2122
public health issues, 1016–1020
relational responsibility, 1023
religious views, 738
screening/testing distinction, 1016–1017
sports performance potential, 2466–2467
workers, 1927–1928
Gene-trolling, 2117
Geneva Conventions, 1223, 2562
Geneva Medical School, 2587
Genital alteration. *See* Circumcision
Genital mutilation, female. *See* Circumcision, female
"Genius, and Inquiry into Its Laws and Consequences" (Galton), 2223
Genomic individuality, 711–712
Genotypic disease prevention, 1009, 1010–1014
Genre, literary, 1435
Gentleman doctors, 1589

Geographic issues
environmental health, 778–779, 780
hazardous wastes and toxic substances, 1045–1046
Georgetown approach to bioethics. *See* Principlism
George VI, 1615
Gerben v. Holsclaw, 669
Geriatric medicine, 106
German Drug Law Act, 1630
German Embryo Protection Act, 2309
German Federal Chamber of Physicians, 1630
German Society for Medical Law, 1631
Germany
abortion, 19, 1632–1633
animal research, 167, 1636
embryo research, 716, 1634–1635
ethics committees, 1630
genetic testing, 1635
modern era bioethics, 1627–1637
nineteenth century medical regulations, 1591
organ transplantation, 1635–1636
preimplantation embryo research, 924
psychiatry, 1807
racial classification, 2248
social insurance, 1132
in vitro fertilization, 1633
See also Nazi Germany
Germline, 707, 711
Germline therapy, 664, 856, 960–964, 1198
Germ theory, 1904
Gerontologist (periodical), 107
Gerry, Elbridge Thomas, 383
Gert, Bernard, 2102
Gesellschaften (Germany), 1629
Gestalt psychology, 260
Gestational ethics, 13
Gewirth, Alan
human dignity, 1195
Kantian theory, development of, 813
rational agency and morality, 806
Ghana, 1510
Al-Ghazālī, 42, 1673, 2057
Ghent University, 1610
Gibbs, Willard, 2143
Gifford, Fred, 310
"The Gift and the Market" (Campbell), 2516
The Gift (Mauss), 1954
Gift of Life Tax Credit Act, 1958
Gift paradigm of organ and tissue donation, 1953–1954, 2516
Gifts to healthcare professionals, 2023
Gill, Carol, 661
Gillick case (United Kingdom), 1617
Gilligan, Carol
care, 367, 370, 1911
law and bioethics, 1374

moral maturity scale, 886
power, competitive notion of, 1054
women's moral orientation, 272
Gillon, Raanan, 1268, 1619
Gilmore, Grant, 1374
Gin Lane (Hogarth), 1039
Ginsburg, Faye, 1384
Giovanella, Beppino, 243
Gisborne, Thomas, 1595
Glantz, Leonard H., 2013
Glantz, Stanton A., 2451
Glaser, Barney, 1068–1069
Glasgow University, 1619
Gleitman v. Cosgrove, 938
Global environmental justice, 430–432
Global warming. *See* Climate change
Glover, Jonathan, 272, 960, 1621
Glover Report to the European Commission, 2302
Glover v. Eastern Nebraska Community Office of Retardation, 2128
Glutathione S-transferase (GST), 967
Gluzman, Semyon, 2177
Gnosticism, 330, 2422
Goal-based views on euthanasia, 1413
God
African American religion, 84–85
cloning, 462–463
death, 581
Islam, 1335
Judaism, 1347
life as gift from, 1332
See also Image of God
Goddard, Henry, 904
Godwin, William, 1916–1917
Goering, Sara, 291
Goethe, Johann Wolfgang von, 352, 1241
Goffman, Erving, 1320, 2106
Goldberg, Kenneth, 107
Golden mean, doctrine of the, 1758
Golden Rule, 509
Golden Temple, 2447
Goldfarb v. Virginia State Bar, 80, 1749, 2170
Goldman, Alan H., 1165, 2437
Goldwater, Joseph, 2318
Gombrich, Ernst Hans, 1878
Gondishapur, 1665–1666
Gonsiorek, John C., 2432
Good
emotivism, 803–804
intuitionism, 803
naturalism, 805
Good, Mary Jo, 1726
Goodall, Jane, 2606
Good death
Christianity, 584, 585
Eastern Orthodox Christianity, 695
euthanasia, 1421
Judaism, 585

• • • H

Haber, Fritz, 2571
Habermas, Jürgen, 1607, 2504
Habitat and species extinction, 751
Habitual Criminal Sterilization Act, Oklahoma, 918
Hacking, Ian, 2526
Haddon, William, 1314, 2212
Hadiths
    abortion, 40–41
    circumcision, 425
    contraception, 2058
    religious authority, 238, 1331–1333
Hadrian, 1162
Haeckel, Ernst, 1427
Haggadah, 581
Hahnemann, Samuel Christian, 150, 161
Haider, S. M., 2052
Hair color and epigenetic effects, 448
Haiselden, J. J., 1427
Halakhah, 581, 1173–1174
Haldane, J. B. S., 848, 969
Hall, Marshall, 254
Halley, Edmund, 2206
Halsted, William S., 158
Halushka v. the University of Saskatchewan et al. (Canada), 1282, 1544
Haly Abbas, 1666
Hamer, Dean, 982, 1164, 2436
Hamilton, Jean, 276
Hamilton, William, 1202
Hamilton County v. Steele, 1305
Hanafis, 42, 1334
Hand, Augustus, 915
A Handbook for Confessors and Penitents (Azpilcueta), 376
Handicap, 656, 658
Handler, Joel, 2524
Hands on medical training, 1505–1506
Han dynasty, 509–510, 540
Hansen, Gerhard Armauer, 1593
Hansen, James, 427
Hansen, Michèle, 453
Happiness, 185
Harakas, Stanley, 2072
Haraway, Donna, 328, 885
Hardacre, Helen, 511
Hard determinism, 933
Hardenberg, Friedrich von, 1062
Harding, Sandra, 276, 885
Hardwig, John, 875, 878
Hare, R. M.
    mental illness diagnoses, 1796–1797
    universal prescriptivism, 804–805
    utilitarianism, 813
Hargobind, 2447
Hargrove, Eugene C., 758
Häring, Bernard, 1890
Härlin, Benedikt, 851
Harm, **1033–1038**

benefit and harm assymetry, 1034
children from reproductive technologies, 2300
compensation, 2154
definition, 937, 1033
divorce and children, 876–877
doping in sports, 2462–2465
future persons, 936–940
human cloning, 460
information disclosure, 1271, 1292
life as, 938–940
offenses, as distinct from, 1034
ordinary, 937–938
paternalism, 1987
pediatric genetic testing, 1026
placebo use in controlled trials, 2338
predicting, 1818–1819
public health, 2020, 2021
race-based genetic research, 995
reproductive autonomy, 2268
rights of conscience/harm to others, balancing, 518–519
sex selection, 2270–2271
sexual ethics, 2431–2432
smoking, 2449–2452
utopian eugenics, 980
want regard *vs.* ideal regard, 1036
Harman, Gilbert, 809
Harmful substances, legal control of, **1038–1043**
Harmlessness in Buddhism and Hinduism, 869
Harm reduction drug policy, 141, 1042
Harm to Self (Feinberg), 468
Harnack, Adolf, 1564
Harpham, Geoffrey Galt, 433
Harrell v. St. Mary's Hospital, 1305
Harris, John, 724, 725, 1137
Harris and Associates, 1276, 1277–1278
Harrison, Ruth, 213
Harrison Act, 1040
Harstock, Nancy, 885–886
Hart, H. L. A., 1377, 1889
Hartley, David, 254
Hartman, Nicolai, 2153
Harvard Educational Review, 1214
Harvard Law Review, 2122, 2126
Harvard Malpractice Study, 1460
Harvard Medical Practice Study, 1850
Harvard Medical School
    conflicts of interest policy, 474
    death determination criteria, 434, 602–603, 615–617, 1531
    exclusion of women, 2587
Harvard University, 1981
Harvey, William, 166, 321
Hasidic Jews, 861
Haskell, Thomas, 1744
Hastening death, actively, 2392–2395
Hastings Center

Behavioral Control Research Group, 630
Eastern European Program, 1649
establishment, 1536
founding, 1528
Guidelines on the Termination of Life-Sustaining Treatment and the Care of the Dying, 1152
Hastings Center Report
    feminism, 888
    Holocaust analogy, 1151, 1152
    law and bioethics, 1374
    race and bioethics, 291
Hathaway v. Worcester City Hospital, 919
Hatzopoulos, Haralambos, 2072
Hauerwas, Stanley
    abortion, 737
    family, 829
    genetic screening, 881
    physician-patient relationship, 1055
    suffering, physicians' obligation to relieve, 1967
    whole tradition communitarianism, 479
Havel, Vaclav, 833
Hawaii, 2445
Hawkins, Anne, 1085
Hawthorn, Geoffrey, 2527
Hayek, Friedrich A., 1354
Hayes, In re, 919
Hayflick, Leonard, 1137
Hayles, Katherine, 2518
Haynes, Brian, 2333
Hays, Isaac, 1519
Hays, Richard B., 1172–1173
Hazard Communication Standard, 1923
Hazardous Materials Transportation Act, 1044
Hazardous wastes, **1043–1050**
    See also Occupational safety and health
HCA, Inc. v. Miller, 1260, 1261
HCBS Waivers Program, 411
Headache, 895
Head trauma, 605
Healers and healing, **1050–1057**
    ancient cultures, 1058–1059
    Christian theology, 403–404
    Daoism, 543
    Eastern Orthodox Christianity, 692–693
    faith healing, 332
    Hebrews, ancient, 1661–1662
    Native Americans, 1883–1885
    Persia, ancient, 1665
    primitive peoples, 1058
    religious community, 1055–1056
Health
    ancient world, 1665, 1757
    Ayurvedic medicine, 1682
    climate change, impact of, 429

Janer, Félix, 1590
Jansenist theology, 377
Japan
    abortion, 23, 333, 338–339, 737, 1708
    ancient studies, 1704
    Buddhist views of death, 566–568
    Chinese-style medicine, 1702
    contaminated blood products, 1711–1712
    contemporary medical ethics, 1706–1712
    culture/religion interdependence, 838
    death determination, 623
    disease, 1679
    Dutch influence, 1705
    eugenics, 1707
    euthanasia, 1710
    German influence, 1706–1707
    human experimentation, 1707–1708
    life expectancy, 1709
    long-term care policy, 1131
    medical ethics history, 1701–1712
    mental health services, 1768
    mentally ill, treatment of the, 1710–1711
    mind-body unity, 1709–1710
    missionary physicians, 1703–1704
    modernization, 1706–1707
    national learning, 1704–1705
    Neo-Confucianism, 1704
    organ transplantation, 550, 1709–1710
    psychiatry, 1807
    public health, 1707
    racial classification, 2249
    relatedness, 1706, 1726–1727
    reproductive technologies, 1711
    Ritsuryo system, 1702–1704
    self-willed death, 567
    Seventeen Rules of Enjuin, 1497
    social death, 550
    socialization of children, 382
    unethical research, 2376
    in vitro fertilization, 1711
    vivisection, 1708
    Western medicine, 1705, 1706–1707
Japanese Association for Bioethics, 302, 1711
Japanese Association for Philosophical and Ethical Research in medicine, 1711
Japanese Association of Life Cooperatives Union, 1711
Japanese Criminal Code, 1708
Japanese Euthanasia Society, 1710
Japanese Mental Health Act, 1710
Japanese Nursing Association, 302
Japanese Society of Ethics, 1711
Japanese Society of Medical Law, 1711
Japan Medical Association (JMA)
    Bioethics Council, 1711

"Code of Medical Ethics," 1712
    physicians' ethics, 1708
Japan Society for Dying with Dignity, 1710
Jarvik, Lissy, 974
Jarvik, Robert, 226–227
Jarvis, Edward, 2207
Jaspers, Karl, 1063, 1791
Jastrow, Richard, 2517
Java Man, 1200
JCAH (Joint Commission on Accreditation of Hospitals), 1995
JCAHO (Joint Commission on Accreditation of Healthcare Organizations). *See* Joint Commission on Accreditation of Healthcare Organizations (JCAHO)
Jecker, Nancy, 369
Jefferson, Thomas, 1886, 2123
Jefferson Medical College of Philadelphia, 1649
Jefferson v. Griffin Spalding County Hospital Authority, 1482
Jeffries, Alex J., 677
Jehiel, Asher B., 582
Jehovah's Witnesses
    blood transfusions, 44–45, **1341–1346,** 2387–2388
    conscientious refusal, 515, 516
    parental loss of authority, 388
Jellinek, Elvin M., 145
Jenner, Edward, 2132, 2316
Jenness, et al. v. Forston, 671
Jennett, Bryan, 602
Jennings, Bruce, 522
Jennings, Herbert, 848, 1859
Jensen, Arthur, 981, 1214
Jensen, Peter S., 1785
Jeremiah, 1662
Jerome
    abortion, 1575
    Hippocratic Oath, 1490, 1564
    hospitals, 1185
    suicide, 1566
Jesuits, 376–377
Jesus
    care, 351
    as healer, 1060
    human dignity, 1197
    as physician, 1564–1565
    teachings, 375
Jevons, Stanley, 2326
Jewell, Wilson, 2207
Jew Ho v. Williamson, 2222
Jewish Chronic Disease Hospital, 1274, 1827, 2357
Jewish Medical Ethics (Jakobovits), 1527–1528
Jex-Blake, Sophia, 2588
J. Jeffrey, In re, 1481
JMA (Japan Medical Association). *See* Japan Medical Association (JMA)

Joas, Hans, 595
Johansson, Sten, 2049
John II, 1185
John Moore v. California Regents, 1386
John of Naples, 33
John Paul II, Pope
    contraception, 909
    homosexuality, 1176
    population policy, 2065–2069
    suffering, 1967
    xenotransplantation, 2607
Johns Hopkins Medical Center, 683, 2581, 2588
Johns Hopkins University, 158–159
Johnson, Ben, 2461–2462
Johnson, Deborah, 2508
Johnson, Gordon F., 2195
Johnson, Lawrence E., 762
Johnson, Lyndon B., 1722
Johnson, Mark, 1834
Johnson, Samuel, 168
Johnson Controls, Inc. v. UAW, 1923
Johnson Foundation, Robert Wood, 652
Johnson v. Calvert, 2280, 2292
Johnson v. Kokemoor, 1304
Johnson v. State, 1481, 1482
Johnson v. Thompson, 1400
Johnston, Ian, 1553
John XXI, Pope, 1571
John XXIII, Pope, 909, 2064
Joint Commission on Accreditation of Healthcare Organizations (JCAHO)
    clinical ethics consultation, 442
    dispute resolution mechanisms, 435, 439
    do not resuscitate (DNR) orders, 2235
    ethical issues mandate, 1181
    ethics committees educational efforts, 842
    ethics standards, 843
    nursing seat, 1906
    organizational ethics, 1095, 1941
    prisoner healthcare, 2110
Joint Commission on Accreditation of Hospitals (JCAH), 1995
Joint Commission on Mental Illness and Health, 1321, 1998
Joint United Nations Programme on HIV/AIDS (UNAIDS), 126, 2352
Joliet Prison, 2319
Jonas, Hans
    genetic technology, 458, 1856
    human body, 327
    research subjects and informed consent, 1283
    research subject selection, 2344, 2373
    student research subjects, 2473–2474
    technology and the environment, 2507–2508
Jones, Kathleen, 2175

Magico-religious medicine
  Japan, 1701–1703
  Southeast Asia, 1714–1715
Magyar, Imre, 1647
Mahābhārata, 240, 1684, 2078
Mahāparinibbāna Sutta, 565
Mahavagga, 1146
Mahāyāna Buddhism, 239, 334,
  336–339, 565
Mahidol University, Bioethics Study
  Group, 1717
Mahmud II, 1670
Mahoney, John, 717
Mahowald, Mary, 889
Maimon, Lois, 2146
Maimonides, Moses
  abortion, 29–30
  covenant with God, 1348
  duty to care for the sick, 1349
  human research, 2316
  prayer, 1488
  viability, 1351
Major depressive disorder (MDD), 400
Major life activity and the Americans
  with Disabilities Act, 670
Making Health Care Decisions (President's
  Commission for the Study of Ethical
  Problems in Medicine and Biomedi-
  cal and Behavioral Research), 1276,
  1285–1286, 2237, 2524–2525
Makrobiotik (Hufeland), 1061
Malan, David, 1783
Malaria, 792, 2319–2320
Male birth control pill, 893
Male circumcision, **420–424,** 425–426
Male contraception, 2097
Malette v. Shulman (Canada), 1543
Malherbe, Jean-François, 1607, 1610
Malikis, 42, 1334
The Malleus Maleficarum (Kraemer and
  Sprenger), 2586
Mallon, Mary, 2209
Malpractice, medical. *See* Medical
  malpractice
Malta, 1607
*Malthousianismos: To englema tes
  genoktonias* (Dionysiatou), 2071
Malthus, Thomas Robert, 1074,
  2041–2042, 2094
Mammals
  aging mechanisms, 97
  cloning, 449–454
Mamzer, 859–860
Man, Paul de, 1433
Managed care, **1463–1467**
  bioterrorism, 319
  commercialization, 2171
  consumer dissatisfaction, 1465–1466
  cost control, 1099, 1464–1465
  dentistry, 646
  development of, 1125

ethics, 1466–1467
hospitals, 1182
mental healthcare, 1767, 1787–1788
organizational ethics, 1941
See also Health maintenance organiza-
  tions (HMOs)
Managed risk agreements, 1444
Management, health services, **1138–1142**
Man-an-pō (Shozen), 1703
Manassein, Vjacheslav, 1651
Manchester Medical Ethical Association,
  1597
Mandatory arrest policies in domestic
  violence, 50–51
Mandatory compliance programs, 528
Mandatory HIV testing, 122, 123
Mandatory minimum sentences for drug
  offenses, 1042
Mandatory reporting, 498–499
Mandatory screening of newborns, 1004
Mandel, Emmanuel E., 1274
Manipulability approach to disease cau-
  sality, 310–311
Mann, John, 1783
MAOA genes, 857–858, 976
MAOIs (monoamine oxidase inhibitors),
  2187–2188
Mao Zedong, 1694–1696
Marcel, Gabriel, 323, 327
Marcus Aurelius, 574
Marcuse, Herbert, 2504
Marginalized groups
  epidemics, 790–794
  healthcare access, 1102
  See also Minorities; Stigmatization
Margolis, Joseph, 809, 1078
Marijuana, 1042–1043
Mark, Vernon, 2199
Marquis, Don, 10–11
Marriage
  African religions, 86
  ancient Greece and Rome, 2419
  Augustine, St., 2423
  circumcised females, 413–414
  cloning as threat to, 463–464
  consanguineous, 859, 862–863,
    865–866
  domestic abuse and patriarchal mar-
    riage, 49
  Eastern Orthodox Christianity,
    695–696
  gamete donation, 2285–2286
  Hinduism, 867–868, 1144
  Islam, 41–42, 2057
  Judaism, 2421
  legal notion, 877
  Protestantism, 2424
  same-sex marriage, 1166, 1176,
    2445–2446
  sexuality, 908
Marriage of Buzzanca, In re, 2292

Martin, Emily, 328
Martin v. Martin, 1398, 2389
Martyrdom, 2477, 2479
Marx, Carl Friedrich Heinrich,
  1425–1426, 1591
Marx, Karl
  human nature, 1216–1217
  marriage, 2426
  philosophical ethics, 801
  socialist justice, 1355
  technology and alienation, 2506
Marxism, 1644–1645
Masden v. Harrison, 1938
Mashaw, Jerry L., 2315
Maslow, Abraham, 260, 1761
Massachusetts General Hospital, 245,
  2459
Massachusetts Medical Society, 2588
Massachusetts State Board of Health,
  2208
Mastectomy, 2335–2336
Masters and Johnson, 2412
Master Settlement (tobacco settlement),
  2452
Mater et Magistra (John XXIII), 2065
Materialist view of human nature, 1213,
  1219
Maternal-fetal relationship, **1467–1485**
  analogy, 1840–1842
  conflict, 11–13, 686, 1473–1484
  ethical issues, 1472–1477
  legal issues, 1478–1484
  medical aspects, 1467–1472
  pregnant woman's duty to the fetus,
    1991
Maternalism and nursing, 371
Maternal mortality
  racial disparity, 287
  sub-Saharan Africa, 1510
  United States, 1467
Maternal Protection Law (Japan), 1712
Maternal serum alpha fetoprotein
  (MSAFP) screening, 998–1000
Maternal serum fetal cell recovery,
  997–998
Maternal thinking, 368
Mather, Cotton, 1517, 1519
Matlab experiment, 2084–2085
Matters of Life and Death (Dorff), 1174
Matthies v. Mastromonaco, 1304
Maturation, 380–381
Mature minor rules, 2005, 2014,
  2017–2018
Mauss, Marcel, 589, 1954
Maximin principle, 479
May, Roll, 355
May, William E., 1856
May, William F.
  acute illness, 1083
  contractarianism, 526
  profession, 2553

empirical methods, **746–748**
epidemiology, 2215–2220
human gene transfer research, 1204
law and bioethics, 1372
linguistic analysis in psychiatry, 1794
psychotherapy, 1783–1784
public health, 2215–2220
research, 746–747, **2326–2347**
student evaluation in bioethics education programs, 297
The Methods of Ethics (Sidgwick), 1858
Mexican Americans
    mental healthcare utilization rates, 1230
    research subjects, 1848
"Mexico City policy," 910
Meyer v. Nebraska, 2276
Michaels, Karin B., 2339
Michnik, Adam, 832–833
Microallocation of healthcare resources, 1107–1115
Middle Ages
    abortion, 1575–1576, 1581
    aging, 110
    anatomy, 2498–2499
    animal experimentation, 166
    body concept, 331
    Byzantine Christianity, 2135
    chastity belts, 413
    childhood, 381–382
    Christianity, 583–584
    epidemics, 790
    Europe, 2135–2136
    guilds, physicians' and surgeons', 1572–1574
    health and disease, 1060
    Hippocratic Oath, 1490
    homosexuality, 1162, 1164–1165
    hospitals, **1184–1186,** 2135
    infant abandonment, 1239
    infanticide, 1238–1240
    Judaism, 582
    licensure, 1571–1572
    medical ethics history, 1568–1582
    medicine as a profession, 1744–1745
    mental health, concepts of, 1758
    plague, 1579–1581
    professional-patient relationship, 2135–2136
    religious fasting, 331–332
    schooling, 382
    secular physicians, 1569–1570
    specialization, 2498–2499
    suicide, 2478
    women health professionals, 2585–2586
    women's status, 2595
Middle East
    female circumcision, 413
    medical ethics history, **1659–1679**

nursing ethics education, 302
religious conflict, 241
socialization of children, 382
See also Specific countries
Middle Path, 335
Midgley, Mary
    children, care of, 832
    moral duty, 1862
    moral principles, 767
    selfish genes, 1202
Midwest Ethics Committee Network of the Medical College of Wisconsin, 842
Midwifery, 149, 2586, 2588–2589
Mies, Maria, 2489
Mifepristone, 2–3, 16, 19, 25, 917–918
Migrant Health Program, 1230
Migration
    migrant programs, 2034
    population effects, 2042–2043
    population policy, **2087–2093**
    See also Immigrants and immigration; Refugees
Mikkelsen, Edward, 1068
Mild cognitive impairment (MCI), 634
Mild stage dementia, 635
Milgram, Stanley, 2330
Military
    animal research, 171–172
    chemical and biological weapons research, 2571–2573
    DNA identification, 679
    fertility encouragement for military might, 2097
    healthcare financing, 1118
    health insurance, 1127
    human research, 2319–2320
    medicine and war, 2560–2565
    mental health professionals, 674
    military personnel as research subjects, **1843–1846**
    nanotechnology, 1871, 1872
    national security research, 320, 505, 2572
    physicians, 2456, 2561–2565
    radiation studies, 2377
    toxins at military installations, 778
    triage, 2521–2522, 2563
    unethical research, 2377
    women physicians in World War I, 2590
    See also Warfare
Military metaphor of medicine, 1835–1837
Mill, James, 1213
Mill, John Stuart
    alcohol restrictions, 1041
    antipaternalism, 1986
    autonomy, 247, 468–469
    beneficence, 270
    consequentialist theories, 817
    death penalty, 628

family, 830
feminism, 1358
gender roles, 2426
good, 806
harm, 2020, 2268
homosexuality, morality of, 1165
human nature, 1213
individualism, 826
intervention limits, 1407
justice, 1357
libertarianism, 2153
liberty, 271
method of difference, 2328
morality, social enforcement of, 1377
paternalism, 1983–1984
power, 2020
public health laws, 2213
qualified supererogationism, 1917
quality of life owed to children, 939
research methodology, 2326, 2328
resource allocation, 394
self-regarding conduct, 2123, 2124
soft determinism, 933
utilitarianism, 189
veracity, 1265
Miller, Barbara, 2269
Miller, Bruce, 248
Miller, Franklin, 535
Miller v. Hospital Corporation of America, 1400
Milos Marilyn, 422
Mind-body dualism
    lack of in Daoism, 540
    mental illness, 1793
    philosophy, 322–324
    psychiatry, nineteenth century, 1760
    Western culture, 1072
Mind-body unity, 1709–1710
Mind cure, 152–153, 1760
Mind (periodical), 255
A Mind That Found Itself (Beers), 1998
Mind uploading, 2517
Mineness, 321, 322–325
Mine-related disabilities, 2567
Minilaparotomy, 899–900
Minimal independence, 1389, 1391
Minimally conscious state, 606–607
Minimal risk
    children, 392, 393
    definition, 1826, 2371
    incompetent research subjects, 2368–2370
Mining industry, 1046, 1922
Ministry of Health, Chinese, 1698
Minnesota Law Review, 2007
Minorities
    end-of-life care, 557
    environmental health, 778–779, 780
    family planning services, 907
    genetics, **992–996**

National Foundation for Medical Research (Belgium), 1610, 1611

National Guidelines for Biomedical Research Involving Human Subjects (Philippine Council for Health Research and Development), 1716

National Health Act (Japan), 1707

National Health and Medical Research Council (Australia), 1554, 1555

National health insurance
  Australia, 1553
  Canada, 1132, 1542–1543
  European countries, 2141
  southern Europe, 1605
  United Kingdom, 1132, 1190, 1191, 1614
  United States, 1094–1095, 1128, 1135, 1137, 1526, 2227

National Health Insurance Act (United Kingdom), 1190

National Health Service Act (United Kingdom), 1132, 1191, 1614

National Heart, Lung, and Blood Institute, 227, 1531

National Hospice and Palliative Care Organization, 1973

National Human Genome Research Institute, 2238–2239

National Inquiry into Medical Education (Australia), 1555

National Institute for Mental Health, 1767

National Institute for Occupational Safety and Health (NIOSH), 1922–1923

National Institute of Environmental Health Sciences, 968

National Institute on Aging (NIA), 106

National Institute on Drug Abuse (NIDA), 1042

National Institutes of Health (NIH)
  alternative therapies, 163
  animal research policy, 178–182
  appropriations, 2320
  Artificial Heart Assessment Panel, 226
  autoexperimentation, 245
  cardiac assist devices, 228
  Clinical Center, 2320–2321
  Consensus Development Conference, 1002
  decision making for end of life care, 487
  embryo research, 715
  epidemiology study bias, 2219
  "Group Consideration for Clinical Research Procedures Deviating from Accepted Medical Practice or Involving Unusual Hazard," 2312
  human gene transfer research (HGTR), 1205–1206
  human growth hormone study, 2371

human research guidelines, 2322
  life extension research, 1137
  National Center for Nursing Research, 1907
  National Institute on Aging (NIA), 106
  Office for Protection from Research Risks, 2324
  pain research budget, 1973
  "Points to Consider in the Design and Submission of Protocols for the Transfer of Recombinant DNA Molecules into One or More Human Subjects," 1206–1207
  Recombinant DNA Advisory Committee (RAC), 964
  research and patents, 2131
  research subject selection, 2345
  "The Science of the Placebo," 2030–2031
  training in research ethics, 2358

National Institutes of Health Revitalization Act, 289, 715, 2345, 2546

Nationalism, 579–580

National Kidney Foundation, National Donor Family Council, 2515

National Labor Relations Act, 1365–1366

National Labor Relations Board v. Jones & Laughlin Steel Corp., 1365

National League for Nursing (NLN), 1905–1906

National learning, school of, 1704–1705

National Medical Association, 1522

National Nanotechnology Initiative, 1871

National Organization for Women v. Scheidler, 27

National Organ Transplant Act, 1934, 1938–1939, 1958, 2512, 2513

National Policy Summit on Elder Abuse, 54

National Practitioner Data Bank, 1093, 1462

National Privacy Commission, 499

National Research Act, 630, 2313, 2357

National Research Council
  Committee on Models for Biomedical Research, 2327
  Committee on National Statistics, 2406
  learning standards, 2470
  slower population growth, 2036–2037

National Research Council of Thailand, 1716

National Research Ethics Committee (Finland), 1639

National Science Foundation, 534, 2518, 2520

National Security Agency (NSA), 2562

National security research, 320, 2572

National Statement on Ethical Conduct in Research Involving Humans (National Health and Medical Research Council), 1554

National Student Nurses' Association, 299

National Traffic and Motor Vehicle Safety Act, 1314

National Welfare Rights Organization (NWRO), 1995

National Women's Hospital in Auckland, 1554

Native Administration Act (South Africa), 1514

Native Americans
  adoption, 70
  death and dying, 555, 623
  healing, 1883–1885
  health and illness, 1883–1885
  healthcare financing, 1118
  health insurance, 1127
  religion, **1880–1886**
  spiritually-based *vs.* traditional medicine, 328
  suicide, 2479
  technology access, 536
  terminology, 1880–1881
  tribal names, 1881

Native Land Act (South Africa), 1514

Native wildlife and plants, 204

NATO (North Atlantic Treaty Organization), 1225

Natural contraceptive methods, 898–899

Natural Death Act (California), 1532

Natural Death Act (Virginia), 2127

Natural extinction, 751

Naturalism
  death, 577–578
  homosexuality, 1163
  human nature, 1213, 1219
  Native American ethics, 1881–1885
  overview, 805–806
  philosophy of science, 2400
  psychology, 254
  sexual behavior theory, 2412

Natural law, **1886–1894**
  Aquinas, Thomas, 1212
  autonomy, 1889–1892
  Catholicism, 1890–1891
  Christianity, 375–376
  history, 1376–1377
  human rights, 1222
  modern science, 1888–1889
  monotheistic religions, 836
  privacy right, 1891–1892
  religious authority, 240–241
  Stoicism, 574

Natural life cycle of humans, 114

Natural Sciences and Engineering Research Council of Canada (NSERC), 1545

experience of illness, 1081–1086
feedback and compassionate love, 486
healthcare teams, as members of, 2496–2497
information refusal, 1268–1269
metaphor, 342–343, 1085, 1438–1439
patterns of resort, 1072–1073
responsibilities, **1990–1994**
right to autonomy, 248–249
selection decisions, 1107
sick role, 1067–1069, 1079
solicitation of, 1692
virtues, 1992–1994
See also Advance directives; Competence, patient; Incompetent persons; Information disclosure and truthtelling; Informed consent; Patients' rights; Physician-patient relationship
"A Patient's Bill of Rights" (American Hospital Association)
adoption of, 1495–1496, 1532–1533, 1995
information disclosure, 1265
paternalism, 1501
treatment refusal, 1343
Patient Self-Determination Act
advanced consent, 2153
advance directives, 105, 651, 1136, 2235
clinical ethics, 435
contents, 1094
kidney dialysis, omission of, 651
long-term care, 1449–1450
Patients' rights, **1995–2004**
Australia, 1555
confidentiality, 496
history, 1995–1996
information disclosure, 1265–1269
Japan, 1709, 1711
law from the orientation of, 1373
medical ethics history, 1532–1533
mentally ill persons, 1321–1322, 1997–2003
privacy, 2127–2128
scientific publishing, 2405
southern European bioethics, 1605–1606
treatment refusal, 492–493, 2000–2001
See also Rights
Patients' Rights Declaration (Japan), 1709
Patients' Rights Legislation Movement (Japan), 1711
Patrinacos, Nicon, 2072
Patterns of resort in medical behavior, 1072–1073
Pauline Christianity, 580, 583, 1172
Paul of Tarsus, 375
Paulsen, Friedrich, 1594

Paul VI, Pope, 909, 2064–2067, 2425
Pavesich v. New England Life Insurance Co., 2126
Pavlov, Ivan
animal research, 2197
behaviorism, 256, 1216
eugenics, 1425
Pay equity, 1363
Peabody, Francis, 363–364
Pearl, Raymond, 848
The Pearl of Great Price, 1865–1866
Pearson, Karl, 849
Pedagogy of bioethics education, 295–296, 300, 304–306
Pedersen, Roger A., 722
Pediatric genetic testing and counseling, 953–954, 1025–1027, 2018
Pediatric intensive-care, 1245–1246, 1252–1257, **2012–2017**
Pediatric oncology, 345–347
Pediatrics
adolescents, **2004–2012**
consent, 2017
end-of-life care, 2014–2016, 2018–2019
ethical issues overview, **2017–2019**
informed consent, 2012–2014
international issues, 1246–1248
neuromuscular blocking agents, 2016
pain management, 2015
practicing procedures on the newly deceased, 2016
public health, **2020–2022**
technological advances, 1246
ventilator withdrawal, 2015–2016
Pedigree information, 950
Peel Committee (United Kingdom), 927, 928
Peele, Stanton, 147
Peer review, 2401–2402
See also Institutional review boards (IRBs); Research ethics committees (RECs)
Peking Union Medical College, 1693, 1695
Peking University, 510
Pellegrino, Edmund
beneficence, 271, 372
compassion, 1604
healing, 1050, 1051
patient refusal of information, 1268
virtues, 1735, 1992–1994, 2155
Pelling, Margaret, 1745
Pelvic inflammatory disease (PID), 893
Pemberton v. Tallahassee Memorial Regional Medical Center, 1305, 1482
Penance, 583–584
Penetrance in genetic diseases, 1021
Penfield, Wilder, 630
Peng, Li, 850
Penitential literature, 376

Pennsylvania Hospital, 1747
Pentecostal Christians, 327–328, 332
People for the Ethical Treatment of Animals (PETA), 169, 1152
Peoples' Commissariat for Health Care in the Russian Republic, 1652–1654
People v. Sanger, 915
People v. Stewart, 1480
People with AIDS Coalition, 125
Perception
pain, 1961–1962
values, 2540
Percival, Thomas
code of medical ethics, 1519
medical ethics field, importance to the, 1595–1597
professional ethics, 1492
terminal care, 1426
veracity, 1272, 1296
Percival's Medical Ethics (Leake), 1528
Percutaneous endoscopic gastrostomy (PEG), 230, 640
Peregrine, Michael, 1833
Perfected Ones, 540
Perfectionism, 184–187
Performance enhancement. *See* Enhancement
Performance standards in animal welfare regulation, 181
Peritoneal dialysis. *See* Kidney dialysis
Permanent coma, 605
Permanent unconsciousness, 605, 607
See also Persistent vegetative state (PVS)
Permission. *See* Assent, children's; Consent; Informed consent
Permission model of abortion policy, 20–22
Permissiveness, sexual, 2415–2417
Perrow, Charles, 1851
Persia, 1185, 1664–1666
Persian Gulf War, 1845, 2564, 2573
Persistent organic pollutants (POPs), 778
Persistent vegetative state (PVS)
artificial nutrition and hydration, 231, 232
overview, 605–606
pain, 1966
quality of life and the law, 1399–1400
terminology, 602
withholding food and water, 232
See also Quinlan, In re
Personal awareness training and end-of-life care, 601
Personal criteria for healthcare resources allocation, 1113
Personalism
care, 356–357
profession, 2166–2167
Personality, 587–588, 975

clinical ethics, 434
eugenics, 2224
informed consent, 1275
institutional review boards, 1940–1941
overview, 1848
racism, 2252
research bias, 276
subject misinformation, 2377
T.W., In re, 26
Twelve Step program, 146–147
Twice Dead (Lock), 550
Twinning, 710, 717, 923
Twins
behavior genetics, 972–973
cloning, 448
intelligence, 2244
organ transplantation, 1945
Two Sources of Morality and Religion (Bergson), 2507
Tyler, Edward, 548
Tyndall, John, 427
Typical disease cases, 1076
Tzu Chi Buddhist Compassion Foundation, 512

• • • U

Über das Zusammenseyn der Ärzte am Krankenbett (Stieglitz), 1591
Ubiquitous operator error, 1851
Uchida tubal ligation method, 899
UDDA (Uniform Determination of Death Act), 610–612, 620, 1531, 1532
Uganda, 1232, 2047
Ullambana Sūtra, 566
Ulrichs, Karl Heinrich, 1162
Ultrasound, 1144
Ulysses contract, 2609
Umi to dokuyaku (Endo), 1708
UNAIDS (Joint United Nations Programme on HIV/AIDS), 126, 2352
Uncertainty of treatment, 1267, 1300–1301
Uncommon Wisdom (Capra), 343
Underworld, 579
UNDP (United Nations Development Programme), 430, 1225
Unethical research, **2376–2379**
The Unexpected Legacy of Divorce (Wallerstein et al.), 876
UNFPA Funding Act, 911
UNICEF (United Nations International Children's Emergency Fund), 417, 418–419, 1225
Uniform anatomical Gift Act, 1531
Uniform Code of Military Justice, 2563
Uniform Determination of Death Act (UDDA), 610–612, 620, 1531, 1532

Uniform Requirements for the Submission of Manuscripts to Biomedical Journals (International Committee of Medical Journal Editors), 2401
Unilateral DNR orders, 684
Uninsured persons, 1126–1127, 1137, 1776
See also Access to healthcare
Union of American Hebrew Congregations (UAHC), 1174
Unions. *See* Labor unions
Unitarian Universalist Association, 2077
Unitary ethical theory, 436
United Church of Christ, 1177
United Kingdom
abortion, 21, 1616
adoption, 69
alcohol, 1039
animal welfare movement, 168
assisted suicide, 1615
behavior ethics research, 982, 983
bioethics, modern era, 1613–1621
bioethics education, 1619–1620
biological theories of human difference, 2245
brain death diagnosis criteria, 604
Committee on Homosexual Offenses and Prostitution, 1165–1166
death penalty, 627
Dickens and concept of childhood, 383
drug policy, 139
embryo research, 714, 716, 726
euthanasia, 1614–1615
factory acts, 2207
genetic discrimination, 958
healthcare justice, 1614
homosexuality, decriminalization of, 1165–1166
hospital history, 1188–1189, 1190–1191
human cloning, 726–730
human genetic engineering policy, 964
human research subjects, 1615–1616
infanticide, 1240–1241
informed consent, 1617
kidney dialysis provision, 1111
live aborted embryos and fetuses, research on, 928
medical ethics education in medical training, 293
mental health services, 1768
mental illness, 1797
National Health Service, 1132, 1190, 1191, 1614
nineteenth century medical ethics, 1595–1599
nursing ethics education, 301
palliative care, 1971
pet keeping, 205

pet legislation, 206
philosophical medical ethics, 1621
preimplantation embryo research, 924–925
privacy, 2126
professionalization of medicine, 1745
public health history, 2206–2207
refusal of life-sustaining treatment, 1615
religious influences on bioethics, 1620
reproductive technology, 1616–1617
selective nontreatment of infants, 1246, 1247
social justice, 1614
suicide, 1424
thalidomide, 1130
traditional medical ethics, 1621
war in Iraq, 2003–2004
workhouse infirmaries, 1189
United Kingdom Forum for Health Care Ethics and Law, 1620
United Kingdom Xenotransplantation Interim Regulatory Authority (IKXIRA), 2607
United Methodist Church, 2076
United Nations
African Charter on Human and Peoples' Rights, 1224
Commission on Environment and Development, 2491
Commission on Human Rights, 1223
Conference on Environment and Development, 430
Conference on Population, Mexico City, 2068
Convention on Biological Diversity, 748, 749
Convention on the Elimination of All Forms of Discrimination against Women, 1224
Convention on the Prohibition of the Development, Prevention and Stockpiling of Bacteriological and Toxin Weapons and on Their Destruction, 2571–2573
Convention on the Rights of the Child, 70, 399, 1244
Convention Relating to the Status of Refugees, 2088, 2089
Declaration of the Rights of the Child, 385, 388, 399
Declaration on the Elimination of Violence against Women, 48, 1224
Declaration on the Establishment of a New International Economic Order, 2092
Declaration on the Right to Development, 1224
Earth Summit in Rio de Janeiro, 748, 1885, 2605

Wolter, Allan B., 736
The Woman Rebel (periodical), 903, 915
Women
  abortion safety, 1–4
  academic medicine, **2577–2583,** 2589–2590
  African American, 49–50, 2580–2581
  African religions, 88
  athletes, 2467–2468
  bioethics field, contributions to the, 1535
  biomedical engineering, 314
  Buddhism, 339
  caregivers, 1455
  clinical trials, 2373–2374
  Confucianism, 511
  contraception, 2097–2098
  cross-cultural perspective, **2593–2600**
  Daoism, 543
  as different from men, 2593–2594
  egg donation, 2289
  epidemiology study bias, 2219
  eugenics, 848, 849
  family size, 2086
  gestational ethics, 13
  hazardous chemicals exposure, 1923
  health, 6, 2582
  health insurance coverage, 1126
  health professionals, 1522, 1573, 1585, 1670, **2577–2592**
  heart disease, 2409
  Hinduism and women's sexuality, 1144–1145
  historical perspective, **2593–2600**
  HIV/AIDS research, 275
  HIV infection, 131–132
  home care workers, 1456
  homicide, 1154
  immigrants, 1230
  Islam, 42, 1332
  lesbians, 1170, 2420, 2421
  medical students, 2591
  Middle Ages, 110
  oppression of, 418–419
  physicians, 1748
  psychiatry's patronizing attitude, 2173
  religion and autonomy of, 2054
  reproductive health, 889, 1923, 2096
   (*See also* Reproductive technologies)
  reproductive selection, 850
  research exclusion, 2410–2411
  research subjects, 2366–2367
  sati, 562–563, 2080
  sexism, **2408–2411**
  sex selection ban, 2270
  sexuality, 902–903, 2421
  social and political theory, 826–833
  socialization and caring as a gender role, 369
  stem cell research and women's rights, 722

  surrogate motherhood, 2293
  sustainable development, 2489
  traditional medicine practitioners, 1585
  underrepresentation in clinical trials, 2345
  as unpaid caregivers, 881–882, 886–887
  violence against, 47–52, 49–50
  volunteerism, 512
  western society, 2594–2596
  women's movements, 2598
  women's studies, 2593–2594
  See also Feminine ethics; Feminism; Gender; Pregnant women
Women and Madness (Chesler), 2432
Women-nature connections, 773–774
Women's Environmental and Development Organization (WEDO), 2489
Women's history, 2598–2599
Women's Medical Association, 2588
Women's Medical College of Pennsylvania, 2587
Women's Medical College of the New York Infirmary, 2587
Women's Medical Journal, 2588
Wonderwoman and Superman (Harris), 725
Wong, David, 809
Wons v. Public Health Trust, 2388
Wood, Carl, 1553
Wood, George, 1038
Wood, Nicholas S., 1255
Woodcock, George, 198
Woodruff, Wilford, 1865
Woodstock Theological Center, 1941
Woods v. White, 2110
Woodward, Beverly, 1312
Worcester, Alfred, 1426
Worcester State Hospital, 1977
Worden, J. William, 1029–1030
The Word of Wisdom, 1867
Work culture, 2581
Workers
  health insurance, 1122–1123
  immigrants, 2089
  just compensation, **1361–1363**
Workers' compensation, 1921–1922, 1924–1925
Workhouse infirmaries, 1189
Working group of Medical Ethics Committees (Germany), 1630
Working Group on Human Gene Therapy, 1205, 1206
Working women, 2597
Works (Philo), 1238
World Anti-Doping Agency, 1208, 2461
The World as Will and Idea (Schopenhauer), 576
World Bank

  fertility control programs, 2034
  migration and refugee programs, 2034
  World Development Report, 2036–2039
World Conference on Environment and Development in Rio de Janeiro, 748, 774, 2487–2489
World Congress on Law and Ethics, 302
World Conservation Strategy (IUCN, UNEP, WWF), 2488
World Development Report (World Bank), 2036–2039
World Federation of Neurology, Research Group on Huntington's Chorea, 1025
World Federation of Right to Die Societies, 1710
World Food Program (WFP), 1225
World Health Organization (WHO)
  abortion-related mortality statistics, 15–16
  AIDS research, 125–126
  alternative therapies, 163
  central and eastern Europe, help for, 1649
  disability definitions, 656–658
  domestic violence studies, 48
  female circumcision, denunciation of, 417, 418
  health definition, 57, 279–280, 1063, 1076
  Health-for-All initiative, 1130
  homosexuality, 1163
  human genetic engineering policy, 964
  incompetent mentally ill human research subjects, 1826
  International Council of Nurses (ICN) and, 1906
  intrauterine devices, 1675
  living organ donation, 1938
  multinational research guidelines, 2374–2375
  nursing education, 1905
  palliative care definition, 1970
  public health services in South Africa, 1514
  Quality of Life meeting, 487
  schizophrenia study, 1804
  standard of health, 1099
  WHO Collaborating Centers, 1905
  xenotransplantation, 2607
World Medical Association (WMA)
  benefits and burdens of research, 2346, 2348–2349
  Declaration of Geneva, 1223, 1491, 1499–1500
  International Code of Medical Ethics, 1493–1494, 1499–1500
  "Statement on Human Organ and Tissue Donation and Transplantation," 1938